Legal Aspects of Occupational Therapy

Legal Aspects of Occupational Therapy

Third Edition

Bridgit Dimond

MA, LLB, DSA, AHSM, Barrister-at-law,
Emeritus Professor of the University of Glamorgan

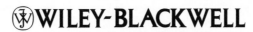

WILEY-BLACKWELL

A John Wiley & Sons, Ltd., Publication

This edition first published 2010
© 1997, 2004, 2010 by Bridgit Dimond

Blackwell Publishing was acquired by John Wiley & Sons in February 2007. Blackwell's publishing programme has been merged with Wiley's global Scientific, Technical, and Medical business to form Wiley-Blackwell.

First published 1997
Second edition 2004
Third edition 2009

Registered office
John Wiley & Sons Ltd, The Atrium, Southern Gate, Chichester, West Sussex, PO19 8SQ, United Kingdom

Editorial offices
9600 Garsington Road, Oxford, OX4 2DQ, United Kingdom
350 Main Street, Malden, MA 02148-5020, USA

For details of our global editorial offices, for customer services and for information about how to apply for permission to reuse the copyright material in this book please see our website at www.wiley.com/wiley-blackwell.

Library of Congress Cataloging-in-Publication Data
Dimond, Bridgit.
Legal aspects of occupational therapy / Bridgit Dimond. – 3rd ed.
p. cm.
Includes bibliographical references and index.
ISBN 978-1-4051-9654-3 (hardback : alk. paper) 1. Occupational therapy–Law and legislation–Great Britain.
2. Occupational therapists–Legal status, laws, etc.–Great Britain. I. Title.
[DNLM: 1. Occupational Therapy–legislation & jurisprudence–Great Britain.   WB 33 FA1 D582L 2010]
KD2968.T47D56 2010
344.4104′1–dc22
2010005812

A catalogue record for this book is available from the British Library.

Set in 10/12 pt Palatino by Toppan Best-set Premedia Limited
Printed and bound in Malaysia by Vivar Printing Sdn Bhd

1   2010

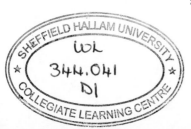

Contents

Foreword

Few will have failed to notice that we live and work in an increasingly litigious world. And while some might argue that legislation gives rise to burgeoning bureaucratic processes and a risk-adverse approach, others will recognise the role legislation plays in driving up the standards which govern our society.

Occupational therapy, alongside other health and social care professions, must be practised in a safe, ethical and transparent manner with due attention being paid to the rights of those receiving services. As undergraduates, occupational therapists will be offered an overview of key legislation relating to practice, and as students and later as qualified professionals they must be able to demonstrate an understanding of the legislative framework, as well as the application of the law, in relation to their particular working environment. From meeting a service user for the first time and agreeing a plan of intervention, through recording and implementing that plan, and dealing with the ensuing challenges and complexities, occupational therapists must be able to show that they work within the law.

Whether they be students, newly qualified practitioners, clinical experts, managers of services, educators or researchers, there will be aspects of the law that apply to their activities.

This book, with its guidance on all of the key legislation that currently applies to occupational therapists, is an essential guide to practice within a safe and lawful context. It will help therapists define the relevant legislation, clarify the associated duties incumbent upon them, assess risk and deliver their planned interventions in an appropriate and lawful manner. Once opened and consulted for the first time, I am confident that it will become an invaluable text for those within our profession, ensuring safe and lawful interventions and a true understanding of the legal context that applies to a broad spectrum of occupational therapy practice.

Julia Scott
Chief Executive, College of Occupational Therapists
May 2010

Preface to Third Edition

The aim of the third edition of this book is to provide an updated outline of the law relating to occupational therapy practice which is of direct relevance to occupational therapists (OTs). This third edition addresses the law relevant to occupational therapy against the complex background of major organisational and legal changes in health and social care. Further significant changes have occurred within the NHS and social services and in statute and case law over the past few years and this third edition attempts to cover these from the perspective of the OT. We at last have the legislation covering decision making on behalf of mentally incapacitated adults in the form of the Mental Capacity Act 2005, and the Mental Health Act 2007 makes significant changes to the Mental Health Act 1983, notably the introduction of supervised community treatment orders and independent mental health advocates.

As for the first and second editions, no previous legal knowledge is required and a similar format is followed for this edition. A new chapter covering pain management, palliative care and legal aspects relating to death has been added. It is hoped that this third edition will continue to prove to be a book for readers to dip into according to their needs and will provide the foundation for an ongoing development of legal knowledge.

Language is an important vehicle for demonstrating current philosophies and attitudes. I have preferred to use the term 'patient' or 'client' as appropriate to the context, rather than the term 'service user' which, to my mind, places those who receive health and social care on a par with railway commuters or gas and electricity consumers. Whilst the politically correct modern terminology does not recognise that certain individuals 'suffer' from specific conditions or are regarded as physically or mentally disabled, the law has not yet caught up with the modern language. Thus compensation is paid in negligence cases for 'pain and suffering'; the Chronic Sick and Disabled Persons Act 1970 is still the principal legislation on the duties of local authorities; the Disability Discrimination Act 1995 defines what is meant by a 'disabled person'; the Mental Health Act 1983 is concerned with the compulsory admission of those with mental disorder and with mentally disordered offenders; and the more recent Carers and Disabled Children Act 2000 still uses language which may not be acceptable to many occupational therapists.

I have therefore adopted the strategy that where legislation is being referred to, or cases cited, it is necessary to use the language used in that legislation. However, where the context permits, people are referred to as having disabilities or mental health issues, rather than being physically or mentally disabled.

Finally, modern usage suggests there are no 'elderly' people, instead there are 'older persons'. This may not be linguistically correct, since an 18-year-old is an older person in relation to a person below 16, but again where the context permits I have bowed to political correctness. The law has still not caught up with modern politically correct usage.

Preface to First Edition

Occupational therapists in the past have not sufficiently conveyed to the general public the complexity, extent and significance of their work in health and social care. Their contribution extends from the field of special care babies to the care of the elderly and bereaved and all intermediate stages of health, illness and social need, between birth and death. The legal issues which may arise are therefore vast and cover many areas of specialist law. It has been my task to provide the occupational therapist practitioner, student, manager and those in related professions and posts with an introduction to the laws which relate to the practice of occupational therapy. It is assumed that the reader will have no previous legal knowledge and a glossary has been provided to explain some of the technical legal language. It is essentially a book which is concerned with the practical aspects of the law as it applies to occupational therapy and examples of the specific legal concerns are derived to a considerable extent from the many questions raised with me by occupational therapists across the country. The anticipation is that this introduction to the law will enable the occupational therapist to develop the knowledge and awareness of the legal implications of her practice so that she can protect both her client and herself.

Terminology in relation to gender always causes concern and I have recognised the fact that the profession is mainly female and thus referred to the occupational therapist as 'she' or 'her'. This should be interpreted as including 'he' and 'him'. Persons cared for by occupational therapists are variously called 'patients, clients, residents, customers and consumers' and I have in the main used the term 'client', but where the context makes other terms more appropriate I have used these.

The statutory changes which took place in 1990 with the introduction of the internal market into healthcare and the developments within community care are still working their way through the role and profession of the occupational therapist. Further major changes are to come with a major reorganisation of the regulation of the professions supplementary to medicine. It is hoped that the knowledge obtained from this book on the law applying to occupational therapist will enable the reader to meet these challenges and continue to develop a comprehensive and high quality service to her clients.

Acknowledgements

I am once again considerably indebted to the College of Occupational Therapists for their whole-hearted support of this third edition and their unstinting assistance with materials and advice. I would like to thank the many occupational therapists working at the College and in specialist areas who have provided me with much help and information: Helen Carey, Julie Carr, Alyson Davies, Andrea Duffy, Maggie Ewer, Jo Griffin, Peter Hewitt, Katrina Hulme-Cross, Karen Jasinska, Anne Jenkins, Eric Johnson, Anne Joyce, Angela Kelsall, Ailsa Lawson, Sarah Lewis-Simms, Stephen Little, Sue Loughran, Sue Pengelly, Remy Reyes, Julie Roberts, Lorna Rutherford, Claire Smith, Genevieve Smyth, Beryl Steeden, Yasmin Yadi, Emily Van de Pol, Sara Vaughan and Clare Wiggins and many others.

Finally, I would like to record my indebtedness to my family and friends, who encouraged me in this work, in particular Bette, who read the typescript with her usual thoroughness and prepared the index and tables.

Abbreviations

ACAS	Advisory, Conciliation and Arbitration Service
ACOP	Approved Code of Practice
ACPC	Area Child Protection Committee
ADL	activities of daily living
AHP	Allied Health Professions
AOMH	Association of OTs in Mental Health
BAOT	British Association of Occupational Therapists
BCMA	British Complementary Medicine Association
CAFCASS	Child and Family Court Advisory and Support Service
CAM	complementary and alternative medicine
CDRP	Crime and Disorder Reduction Partnerships
CHAI	Commission of Healthcare Audit and Inspection
CHC	Community Health Council
CHI	Commission for Health Improvement
CNHC	Complementary and Natural Healthcare Council
CNST	Clinical Negligence Scheme for Trusts
COPE	Committee on Publication Ethics
COREC	Central Office for Research Ethics Committees
COSHH	Control of Substances Hazardous to Health
COT	College of Occupational Therapists
CPA	care programme approach; comprehensive performance assessment
CPD	continuing professional development
CPPH	Commission for Patient and Public Involvement in Health
CPR	Civil Procedure Rules
CPS	Crown Prosecution Service
CPSM	Council for Professions Supplementary to Medicine
CSCI	Commission for Social Care Inspection
CTO	community treatment order

DEE	Department for Education and Employment
DfES	Department for Education and Skill
DFG	disabled facility grant
DHA	district health authority
DISC	Disability and Information Centre
DNR	do not resuscitate
DH	Department of Health
DOLS	Deprivation of Liberty Safeguards
DRC	Disability Rights Commission
DSS	Department of Social Security
EC	European Community
EHR	electronic health record
EPIOC	electrically powered indoor/outdoor wheelchairs
EPR	electronic patient record
ESCR	electronic social care records
EWG	external working group
FHSA	family health services authorities
GDC	General Dental Council
GMC	General Medical Council
GSCC	General Social Care Council
HAI	hospital acquired infection
HASAW	Health and Safety at Work Act 1974
HEIs	Higher Education Institutes
HIS	hospital information system
HPC	Health Professions Council
HRDG	Health Records and Data Protection Review Group
HSC	Health and Safety Commission
HSE	Health and Safety Executive
IADL	instrumental activities of daily living
ICAS	Independent Complaints and Advice Services
ICES	Integrated Community Equipment Services
ICP	integrated care pathways
IM&T	information management and technology
IMCA	independent mental capacity advocates
ISA	Independent Safeguarding Authority
JP	Justice of the Peace
JVC	Joint Validation Committee
LA	local authority
LINKS	Local Involvement Networks
LOLER	Lifting Operations and Lifting Equipment Regulations
LREC	Local Research Ethics Committee
LSCB	Local Safeguarding Children Boards
LTPS	liabilities to third parties
MCA	Medicines Control Agency
MDA	Medical Devices Agency
MHAC	Mental Health Act Commission
MHRA	Medicines and Healthcare Products Regulatory Agency

MHRT	Mental Health Review Tribunal
MREC	Multi-Centre Research Ethics Committee
NAI	non-accidental injury
NAO	National Audit Office
NAPOT	National Association of Paediatric Occupational Therapists
NCSC	National Care Standards Commission
NHSLA	National Health Service Litigation Authority
NICE	National Council for Clinical Excellence
NMC	Nursing and Midwifery Council
NPSA	National Patient Safety Agency
NSF	National Service Frameworks
OOS	occupational overuse syndrome
OT	occupational therapist/occupational therapy
PACS	picture archiving and communication systems
PALS	Patient Advocacy and Liaison Service
PCMH	Plea and Case Management Hearing
PCT	Primary Care Trust
PES	property expenses scheme
PUWER	Provision and Use of Work Equipment Regulations
PVS	persistent vegetative state
QAA	Quality Assurance Agency for Higher Education
RADAR	Royal Association for Disability and Rehabilitation
RAE	research assessment exercise
RCP	Royal College of Psychiatrists
REC	Research Ethics Committee
RIDDOR 95	Reporting of Injuries, Diseases and Dangerous Occurrences (Regulations) 1995
RMO	responsible medical officer
RPST	Risk Pooling Schemes for Trusts
RSI	repetitive strain injury
SENDA	Special Educational Needs and Disability Act
SHA	strategic health authority
SOAD	second opinion appointed doctor
SRSC	Safety Representatives and Safety Committees (Regulations)
SRV	social role valorisation
SSD	social services department
SSI	Social Services Inspectorate
UKCCSG	United Kingdom Children's Cancer Study Group
UKOTRF	UK Occupational Therapy Research Foundation
VIAN	Voice for improvement action network
VTB	Vetting and Barring Scheme
WDC	Workforce Development Confederation
WFOT	World Federation of Occupational Therapists
WRULD	work-related upper limb disorder

1 Occupational Therapy

In attempting to identify the legal issues relevant to occupational therapy practice, I was immediately confronted by the problems in defining occupational therapy and identifying the scope and content of occupational therapy practice and what was properly to be regarded as within the extended scope of practice and what was outside both the scope and the extended scope of professional practice. To link the work of the occupational therapist (OT) in caring for the mentally disordered with anorexia or in looking at feeding regimes and working with dietitians, with the role in assessing and prescribing for wheelchairs, seemed impossible. Similarly, what has the work of the OT in special care baby units in common with that of her colleague in a forensic psychiatric unit? To provide a definition of occupational therapy which covers such diverse activities is a major challenge. This was taken up in a major review conducted by Louis Blom-Cooper in 1989 into the theory and practice of occupational therapy.

The report,[1] which was commissioned by the College of Occupational Therapists (COT), explored the changing demographic pattern and the growth in recognition of the need for a support service like occupational therapy to assist people to regain or develop their full potential.

Definition of occupational therapy

The first definition of an occupational therapist used by the Association of Occupational Therapists[2] was:

> Any person who is appointed as responsible for the treatment of patients by occupation and who is qualified by training and experience to administer the prescription of a Physician or Surgeon in the treatment of any patient by occupation.

Legal Aspects of Occupational Therapy, Third Edition By Bridgit Dimond
© 2010 Bridgit Dimond

Occupational therapy was defined by the Council for Professions Supplementary to Medicine (CPSM) booklet[3] as:

> the treatment of physical and psychiatric conditions using specific selected activities in order to help people who are temporarily or permanently disabled to recover independence and cope with everyday life. Therapists work in one of three main areas: with the physically disabled, with those with mental health problems, and with people who have learning disabilities.

This is much narrower than the definition which Blom-Cooper suggested in his Commission of Inquiry. The Commission's report adapted the definition of occupational therapy used by the COT and recommended its adoption:

> Occupational therapy is the assessment and treatment in conjunction and collaboration with other professional workers in the health and social services, of people of all ages with physical and mental health problems, through specifically selected and graded activities, in order to help them reach their maximum level of functioning and independence in all aspects of daily life, which include their personal independence, employment, social, recreational and leisure pursuits and their interpersonal relationships.

Stereotypes and core philosophy

The Blom-Cooper report discussed the outdated stereotypes of the profession associated with basket making and looked at changing the name to get away from the myths and out-of-date attitudes to the profession. It considered that the most suitable name would be 'ergotherapy', but recognised the limitations of this name because of its association with ergonomics and being too narrow. In the end the report abandoned the task of suggesting a name and made no recommendation on the title. The COT issued a statement on definition in May 1990[4] in line with that suggested in the Blom-Cooper report. It identified four facets of the therapeutic role:

- prevention
- habilitation and rehabilitation
- retraining and maintenance
- readjustment.

It also defined the other roles of the OT, i.e. the advisory and educational role and the management role.

In 2000 the COT suggested that an appropriate definition of the work of an occupational therapist would be:

> Occupational therapists treat people of all ages with mental and physical problems through meaningful occupation to improve everyday function and prevent disability.[5]

The heart of the OT's function has been widely debated. Thus Phillips and Renton[6] ask whether assessment of function should be the main aim of the OT's role. Jenkins and Brotherton[7] discuss an attempt to find a theoretical framework for occupational therapy. Some valuable insight into the philosophy behind occupational therapy as a profession was obtained from the third edition of Turner et al.'s classic work on occupational therapy.[8] The underlying thoughts and common links were identified as:

- individuals are each in a state which they wish to improve;
- the therapist uses activity as the medium for this improvement;
- individuals are aiming for the restoration or achievement of the skills required for daily life and have the capacity for change needed to achieve this;
- each person is an individual and inherently different from any other.

In order to achieve these objectives the OT must be skilled as a teacher, as a craftsman, as a purchaser and assessor of equipment and clients, as a therapist in understanding all mental and physical conditions, as a communicator, as a provider of healthcare, and so on. The law impacts upon them all. In their fifth edition the editors of this work note that there has been an enormous change in culture which

> has seen a growth in the need for occupational therapists to demonstrate that their interventions are based on sound clinical reasoning, with a specific brief to provide evidence for the efficacy of their practice. The introduction of clinical governance, evidence-based practice and quality audit has shaped the remit of therapists in health, social care and private practice.

The legal implications of this significant cultural change are enormous and can be seen throughout this text.

Annie Turner,[9] in her first chapter on the history and philosophy of occupational therapy, suggests that a philosophy on which to base the profession's practice, theory and research could consist of the following concepts:

- People are individuals and inherently different from one another.
- Occupation is fundamental to health and well-being.
- Where occupational performance has been interrupted a person can:
  - use occupation and/or activity to develop the adaptive skills required to acquire, maintain or restore occupational performance
  - modify their occupations and/or activities to facilitate occupational performance.

Since the Blom-Cooper report the attempt to define occupational therapy has been ongoing as the work of Jennifer Creek shows. In her MSc thesis[10] she discussed the complexity of identifying what OTs do and considered:

> Occupational Therapists' inability to explain to others what they do … in terms of the difficulty of expressing the breadth, complexity and subtlety of practice in language which is structured to communicate singularity and visibility and in contexts where men's styles of communication are privileged over women's.

She defined occupational therapy as a complex intervention.

> The difficulties of defining occupational therapy can be seen from the results of the COT commissioning Jennifer Creek in 2004[11] to develop standard terminology for OT which would include the definition of between 5 and 12 key terms plus the definition of occupational therapy itself. It was found that the Delphi approach (asking 42 expert OTs for their views in 10 rounds) whilst appropriate for producing a set of six definitions of key terms, failed to produce a single definition of occupational therapy. Instead of the number of possible definitions decreasing in each round it expanded as panel members struggled to find a way of capturing the complexity of occupational therapy within one or two sentences.[12]

When 37 definitions of occupational therapy were analysed, 107 elements were identified. These were organised into 7 categories: social position or status, aims or goals, domain of concern, client groups, tools/processes, services and principles of intervention. Jennifer Creek suggested that it may be that different definitions of occupational therapy, incorporating different categories of elements in each one, would be appropriate for use in different situations.

The conclusion was that:

> It is possible to conclude that no single definition of occupational therapy will be appropriate for all purposes. Using the materials, principles and processes described in this report, occupational therapists should be able to construct the definitions that they need to suit their own situations.

A COT/BAOT briefing note no 23 was published in 2006 on the definitions and core skills for OT. This used several definitions for use within the profession and for use with the public. Core skills were seen as collaboration with the client; assessment; enablement; problem solving; using activity as a therapeutic tool; group work and environmental adaptation. In 2008 the COT published a position statement on the value of occupational therapy and its contribution to adult social care users and their families.[13] This considers the value, the commitment of the OT and gives examples of best practice.

Ten roles of health professionals

In 2003 the DH set out the 10 key roles for allied health professionals. The following year the COT reviewed the ways these roles are being used by OTs and published a briefing note no 32 with BAOT. The 10 key roles were:

1. To develop extended clinical and practitioner roles which cross professional and organisational boundaries
2. To be a first point of contact for patient care including single assessment
3. To diagnose, request and assess diagnostic tests, and prescribe working with protocols where appropriate
4. To discharge and/or refer patients to other services, working with protocols where appropriate
5. To provide consultancy support to others promoting the AHP contribution to patient independence and functioning, training, developing, mentoring, teaching, informing and educating healthcare professionals, students, patients and carers
6. To manage and lead teams, projects, services and case loads, providing clinical leadership
7. To develop and apply the best available research evidence and evaluative thinking in all areas of practice
8. To play a central role in the promotion of health and well being
9. To take an active role in strategic planning and policy development for local organisations and services
10. To extend and improve collaboration with other professions and services including shared working practices and tools

Occupational therapy and the spiritual dimension

In the Casson Memorial Lecture 2001 Gwilym Wyn Roberts[14] considered the future development of higher level practice and stated that occupational therapy needed to consider a spiritual context of our work, our values and how we value ourselves.

The spiritual content and context of occupational therapy has been widely debated, including the influence of Eastern and Western philosophies.[15] Some have turned to Zen Buddhism as the foundation of occupational therapy practice. Kelly and McFarlane[16] emphasise the value of Chinese philosophy in providing the basis for a new, modified, holistic approach to occupational therapy. They also show the extent to which the principles are already being used, albeit indirectly, in occupational therapy management and treatment, for example the general systems theory and sensory integration theory. Lorraine Udell and Colin Chandler[17] discuss the role of the occupational therapist in addressing the spiritual needs of clients and note that in order to further discussion on this issue it is necessary to consider:

- the extent to which spirituality has an impact upon health and well-being
- the question of whether spirituality is a necessary component of holistic care
- the specific training and guidelines that would be needed.

This philosophy also has importance in relation to the terms in which the OT views her relationship with her client and the rights of the client. Non-interference and self-help are important features of a client-centred therapy.

This concern with the philosophy of the OT is taken further by Barnitt and Mayers.[18] They show that the starting point would appear to be an incompatibility in that humanists believe that individuals, not God, are responsible for their own existence while Christians look to God for rules and principles to guide behaviour.

Cunliffe[19] asks what rights patients have with a treatment containing philosophy, theory or spiritual belief. The answer must be that it is impossible to divest the therapy from any such content and, as Cunliffe emphasises, it is important that within occupational therapy the patients have a right to be informed of the philosophy, or spiritual belief, contained in the treatment. He adds descriptively that 'there is no difference between the surgeon's knife and a treatment belief that cuts theoretically, psychologically or spiritually in the wrong place'.

Inevitably OTs have become concerned with the relevance of occupational therapy to issues relating to the quality of life.[20]

Katrina Bannigan[21] urges every occupational therapist to communicate passionately what she or he does 'so that our vision shines through'.

Core knowledge and skills required by OTs

This ongoing debate as to the philosophy and function of occupational therapy will have a major impact in determining the relevant skills required.

The Blom-Cooper report identified the core knowledge and skills required by OTs under four headings, shown in Figure 1.1. (Reference should also be made to Chapter 5 on education and definition of core skills and competencies.)

Figure 1.1 Core knowledge and skill required by OTs as identified in the Blom-Cooper Report.

(1) Knowledge of the intelligence, physical strength, dexterity and personality attributes required to perform the tasks associated with a whole gamut of paid and unpaid occupations and valued leisure pursuits.

(2) The professional skill to assess potentialities and limitations of the physical and human environments to which patients have to adjust, and to judge how far these environments could be modified and at what cost to meet individual needs.

(3) Pedagogic skills required, first to teach people how to acquire or restore their maximum functional capacity, and second to supervise and encourage technically trained instructors and unqualified assistants in their tasks of implementing and monitoring therapeutic recommendations.

(4) The psychological knowledge and skills to deal with anxiety, depression and mood swings which are the frequent aftermath of serious threats to health or of continuing disability, and to motivate, or remotivate, those with temporary or persistent disabilities to achieve their maximum capacity.

Problems identified in the Blom-Cooper report

In discussing the attempt of the profession to establish its professional identity and autonomy, major problems were identified in the Blom-Cooper report:

- the dominant position of the medical profession in the provision of healthcare and the social work profession in the provision of social services
- the dependence of OTs on doctors and social workers for access to their clients
- the false and damaging stereotype that other staff and the public have of their function
- the pronounced female composition of the profession
- questions over occupational therapy's efficacy, a matter of increasing importance in the internal market.

There is unfortunately no clear evidence since the Blom-Cooper report was published, that all these weaknesses have been corrected. Whilst the internal market has been abolished, occupational therapists still need to show value added to the quality of life of their patients/clients and that they are a service which can provide significant benefits. Both the commissioners of OT care, consultants and clients must be convinced of the benefits which OTs can bring in the rehabilitation and social and healthcare of the vast majority of patients and clients.

Conclusions of the Blom-Cooper report

The report considered the role, function and organisation of the profession and reached the following conclusions:

- Occupational therapy is needed as an integral part of health and social service provision.
- Although there is room for devolution of some of the work at present performed by trained OTs to their helpers and clerical staff, there will be a continuing and expanding need for fully professional OTs.
- Further consideration should be given, in the long term if not in the immediate future, to the creation of a united profession of rehabilitation therapist, permitting post-qualification specialisation.
- In the decade following the report and increasingly into the twenty-first century occupational therapy should be largely relocated in the community care services.

Recommendations in the report addressed to the COT cover the topics shown in Figure 1.2.

Figure 1.2   Recommendations of the Blom-Cooper report.

- number and norms
- deployment
- recruitment
- preparation

- qualifying standards
- negotiating machinery
- professional enhancement

Developments since the Blom-Cooper report

The Blom-Cooper report was written at a time when the Government of the day had not indicated its intentions following the response to its White Paper, *Working for Patients: Caring for the 1990s* or following the Griffiths report, *Care in the Community: Agenda for Action*, 1988. It was therefore impossible in that uncertainty for the proposals of the inquiry to be precise. Since that time there have been fundamental changes in the organisation and management of health and social care; these are considered in detail in Chapters 17 and 18. These developments include: the implementation of the NHS and Community Care Act 1990, the Health Act 1999 and major changes in relation to the management of healthcare; the introduction and the abolition of the internal market; the establishment of NHS trusts; primary care trusts and care trusts and the introduction and the abolition of GP fundholders. New unitary authorities for local government with social services taking over responsibility for the purchase of places for clients in nursing and residential homes for those admitted after 1 April 1993. Significant new institutions of inspection for health and social care have been set up and were established in April 2004. Subsequently the Care Quality Commission has taken over the regulation, inspection and monitoring of all health and social care establishments.

These major structural changes in the organisation of the NHS present significant challenges for the OT. A useful analysis of the impact of organisational change upon the role and future of occupational therapy is given by Chris Lloyd and Robert King.[22] They consider that whilst the scope and complexity of the restructuring of the NHS present considerable challenges, OTs are well placed to meet these. The core values of the profession are congruent with community-focused, client-centred and outcome-oriented models of service delivery. In addition, the emphasis on enablement occupation provides opportunities to add new roles to occupational therapy. OTs have the skills that are consistent with working at the level of case management and in health promotion.

A COT study in April 2003 commissioned Jennifer Creek to identify the components of OT intervention, the defining features of OT and the limits of OT.[23] The Core skills identified by the study are seen in Figure 1.3. The study did not seek to establish the value of OT. The assumption was made from the beginning that OT is of value. The study considered descriptions of Occupational Therapy, the Occupational Therapist and external influences on the OT process.

In the glossary OT was defined (as practised by the OT) as:

An approach to health and social care that focuses on the nature, balance, pattern and context of occupations and activities in the lives of individuals, family groups and communities. OT is concerned with the meaning

---

Figure 1.3   Core skills identified in COT study 2003.

Collaboration with the client
Assessment
Enablement
Problem solving
Using activity as a therapeutic tool
Group work
Environment adaptation
Analysis of thinking skills: clinical reasoning (scientific reasoning, narrative reasoning,
     interactive reasoning, conditional reasoning, pragmatic reasoning and ethical reasoning)
     reflection.

and purpose that people place on occupations and activities and with the impact of illness, disability, social deprivation or economic deprivation on their ability to carry out those occupations and activities. The main aim of OT is to maintain, restore or create a balance, beneficial to the individual, between the abilities of the person, the demands of her/his occupations in the areas of self care, productivity and leisure and the demands of the environment

OT intervention = actions taken by the therapist, on behalf of the client and in collaboration with the client and/or carer, to assist the client to acquire, maintain or regain the adaptive skills required to support his/her life roles and occupations[24]

OT process = a sequence of thought and actions used by the therapist to structure intervention in order to provide services to a client.[25]

Occupational therapy and physiotherapy

Blom-Cooper suggested that consideration should be given to the creation of a united profession of rehabilitation therapist. This idea has not in general found favour but the relationship between occupational therapy and physiotherapy has led to closer communication between the professional associations of OTs and physiotherapists. Whether there is unnecessary duplication of skills between occupational therapists and physiotherapists is considered by Janet Golledge,[26] who emphasises that occupational therapists should be using purposeful activity and occupations as their therapeutic media, with limited use of activity. (These distinctions are explained in earlier articles.)[27] Activities could be used by physiotherapists, but not purposeful activity or occupation. This is where the two professions could see the distinctions in their therapeutic media. She notes however that the enduring concern is whether managers, purchasers and users of healthcare can understand the distinctions sufficiently. The establishment of the Health Professions Council and the greater flexibility that it can give to the recognition of new state registered professions may facilitate closer associations between physiotherapy and occupational therapy.

Client-centred occupational therapy

Thelma Sumsion[28] discusses the definition of client-centred practice that was developed from 67 OTs participating in nine focus groups; 165 components of client-centred practice were generated and analysed to form seven themes. The final definition was:

Client-centred occupational therapy is a partnership between the client and the therapist that empowers the client to engage in functional performance and fulfil his or her occupational roles in a variety of environments. The client participates actively in negotiating goals which are given priority and are at the centre of assessment, intervention and evaluation. Throughout the process the therapist listens to and respects the client's values, adapts the interventions to meet the client's needs and enables the client to make informed decisions.

The author states that if therapists are working according to this definition, they should be able to ensure that clients do feel like valued human beings. See also her edited work *Client-centred practice in occupational therapy*.[29]

From interface to integration strategy

In January 2002 the College of Occupational Therapists published a consultation paper on a strategy for modernising occupational therapy services in local health and social care communities.[30] This considered a new model of a community-based OT practice and sought responses to this concept. The College stated that:

> The development of a new community-based occupational therapy general practitioner model is central to its wish to resolve the problems around the interface between health and social care. We see this as pivotal to an integrated approach that enables services to be developed as a continuum that is focused on, and responsive to, the needs of all service users and their carers.

The COT considered that this model would assist the OT in responding to the current national and country-specific Government policies and priorities including:

- promoting independence (COT prefers the term 'inter-dependence')
- preventing avoidable or unwanted dependence
- addressing social isolation
- reducing waiting lists
- delivering on the objectives and standards in the National Service Frameworks
- working in partnership with individuals and their carers
- working collaboratively
- eliminating duplication
- supporting public health and prevention
- seeking to provide services on an increasingly sound evidence base
- supporting value for money and best value regimes
- promoting recruitment and retention.

The COT published its response to the consultation in 2002.[31] In April 2003 the College of Occupational Therapists commissioned an independent company, PCA Consulting, to review progress towards the integration of services and to investigate different approaches to service integration and models of care. The review showed that the organisational changes being made around the country ranged from small scale and informal developments; semi-formal development such as integrating management structures; through to major organisational redevelopment, incorporating all occupational therapy services under a single employer. It suggested that initiatives in integrating working needed to be governed by some form of clear inter-agency agreement which could be in the form of a service level agreement or some other form of financial or secondment agreement. A briefing paper on integrated occupational therapy services gave examples of different forms of integrated occupational therapy services.[32]

Conclusions on definition of occupational therapy

Edward Duncan[33] analysed in 1999 the core skills required of an OT working in mental health and concluded:

> It is time for the profession to move from its adolescent identity crisis, within which at times it appears to be stuck, to its rightful sense of a coming of age. This step, as painful for a profession as it is for an individual, would allow the fruitless search for a prescriptive definition of what and what is not occupational therapy to end. Studies of occupational therapy and the further development of an understanding of occupational performance could then develop.

A similar attitude is revealed in a light-hearted paper, but dealing with a very serious topic, in which Adam Goren[34] explores the identity of the occupational therapist and concludes that it is still a profession in its youth, unsure of its own identity, sensitive to its own environment, rebelling against its own conformity, (and in need of some direction and boundaries), highly adaptable, creative, curious and impressionable.

He suggests that this youthfulness may also be the key to a more sensitive, nourishing and mature way of working with clients and patients.

The debate on the role and function of occupational therapy may possibly never end. There is perhaps a danger of too much navel gazing, too much worrying about what OTs should call themselves and their work. Perhaps, as Edward Duncan suggests, it is better to move on and provide the service.

The HPC has published proficiencies for each of the professions registered by it. Each registrant has a copy of these proficiencies and it is clearly incumbent upon each person to ensure that they maintain and develop their competence. (See Chapter 5 for further discussion on this.)

From the legal perspective it is clear that any book which attempts to be relevant to all aspects of the role of the OT needs to be comprehensive and far reaching in its coverage, and it is hoped that this book will provide the necessary framework.

Conclusions

The epic work of Ann Wilcock traces the journey of occupational therapy from the earliest times to the present day.[35] Her concluding hopes for the work are that it

> will encourage a greater range of questions, research and initiatives to facilitate the growth and direction based on in-depth and investigative practices.

The two volumes of the history of occupational therapy sponsored by the British Association and College of Occupational Therapy should give OTs a sense of their history and their significance in the field of health and social care. In spite of major changes since 1989, the recommendations of the Blom-Cooper report are still of value, and perhaps another inquiry to establish what now needs to be done in the light of changing circumstances would be an advantage. Major changes to the professional registration machinery and the nature of professional conduct proceedings were introduced in 2002 and these are discussed in Chapter 3. Their impact upon the status and role of the occupational therapist needs to be evaluated. The initiative of the College of Occupational Therapists in developing new core professional standards in 2003 and updated in 2007[36] to define standards for processes that are central to all practising occupational therapists in all settings is ongoing and will foster the unity of the profession and assist in identifying those practices which are central to all occupational therapists. These core standards are supplemented by clinical guidelines or practice guidance which are relevant to a specialist group working in a particular clinical area or care group. Practice guidelines outline the nature and level of intervention that is considered best practice for specific conditions in specific settings. They incorporate or abide by the College's professional standards for OT Practice. Both the core standards and the clinical guidelines will be referred to throughout this book, since they are pertinent to the reasonable standard of professional practice which the law requires of all health professionals. A review of the standards *COT Professional Standards for Occupational Therapy Practice* is due to start later in 2009 and will be published in 2011. It is planned to hold a think tank/workshop at COT in December 2009 to gain feedback from members to help inform the revision of the standards. The development of specialist sections within the College of Occupational Therapists has been an important feature in ensuring high standards in specific clinical areas. The criteria for the approval of new specialist sections[37] facilitate consistency across the whole field of OT activity and support continuing professional development. Email networks for

OTs specialising in learning disabilities, mental health, vocational rehabilitation or condition management and supervised by the professional affairs officer and professional enquiries co-ordinator enable effective communication across the COT membership.

An edited work by Jennifer Creek and Anne Lawson-Porter should prove a useful introduction to an analysis of the contemporary issues in occupational therapy and assist in the debate on the nature, direction and focus of occupational therapy.[38] In an article on professionalism and OT, Teena Clouston and Steven Whitcombe consider the history and identity of OT as a profession and the threats resulting from the modernisation agenda for the NHS and suggest a way forward.[39] The necessity to prove that occupational therapy is a research-based, cost-effective intervention across all fields of health and social care will provide an ongoing challenge both to individual practitioners and to the profession as a whole.

 Questions and exercises

1   How would you define the core work of the OT?
2   How appropriate do you consider the present title of occupational therapy is for the profession? Would an alternative title be more suitable?
3   Do you consider the personal beliefs and philosophies of OTs are relevant to their work? To what extent, if any, should they be taken into account by prospective employers?

References

1   Blom-Cooper, L. (Chair (1989) Report of Commission of Inquiry Occupational Therapy – an emerging profession in health care. Duckworth, London.
2   Quoted by Ann A. Wilcock in *Occupation for Health*, vol. 2: *a Journey from Prescription to Self Health*. British Association and College of Occupational Therapists (2002) page 501.
3   Council for Professions Supplementary to Medicine (1995) *Who we are and what we do*. CPSM, London.
4   College of Occupational Therapists (May 1990) *Statement on Occupational Therapy Definition*, SPP 140. COT, London.
5   College of Occupational Therapists (2000) *A definition of occupational therapy*. College of Occupational Therapists, London.
6   Phillips, N. & Renton, L. (1995) Is assessment of function the core of Occupational Therapy? *British Journal of Occupational Therapy*, **58**(2), 72–3.
7   Jenkins, M. & Brotherton, C. (1995) In search of a theoretical framework for Practice: Part 1. *British Journal of Occupational Therapy*, **58**(7), 280–5.
8   Turner, A., Foster, M. & Johnson, S.E. (eds) (1990) *Occupational Therapy and Physical Dysfunction: principles, skills and practice*, 3rd edn. Churchill Livingstone, Edinburgh.
9   Turner, A., Foster, M. & Johnson, S.E. (eds) (2002) *Occupational Therapy and Physical Dysfunction: principles, skills and practice*, 5th edn. Churchill Livingstone, Edinburgh.
10 Creek, J. (1998) How Occupational Therapists conceptualise and articulate beliefs about the nature and purpose of their professional practice M.Sc Thesis Available in the COT library.
11 College of Occupational Therapists (2004) *Definitions and Core Skills in Occupational Therapy Briefing*. COT, London.
12 Creek, J. (May 2006) A standard terminology for occupational therapy. *British Journal of Occupational Therapy*, **69**(5), 202–8.
13 College of Occupational Therapists (2008) *Value of occupational therapy and its contribution to adult social care users and their families*. COT, London.

14   Wyn Roberts, G. (2001) The Casson Memorial Lecture 2001: A new synthesis – the emergent spirit of higher level practice. *British Journal of Occupational Therapy*, **64**(10), 493–501.

15   Cunliffe, M. (1994) Rights, ethics, and the spirit of occupation. *British Journal of Occupational Therapy*, **57**(12), 481–2. See also letters by Cunliffe, M., Kelly, G. & Williams, J. (1995) *British Journal of Occupational Therapy*, **58**(5), 220–22.

16   Kelly, G. & McFarlane, H. (1991) Zen in the art of occupational therapy. *British Journal of Occupational Therapy*, **54**(3), 95–100 and (4), 130–34.

17   Udell, L. & Chandler, C. (2000) The role of the occupational therapist in addressing the spiritual needs of clients. *British Journal of Occupational Therapy*, **63**(10), 489–94.

18   Barnitt, R. & Mayers, C. (1993) Can occupational therapists be both humanists and christians? *British Journal of Occupational Therapy*, **56**(3), 84–8.

19   Cunliffe, M. (1994) Rights, ethics, and the spirit of occupation. *British Journal of Occupational Therapy*, **57**(12), 481–2.

20   Mayers, C. (1995) Defining and assessing quality of life. *British Journal of Occupational Therapy*, **58**(4), 146–50.

21   Bannigan, K. (2000) Passion is our greatest asset in marketing occupational therapy. *British Journal of Occupational Therapy*, **63**(10), 463.

22   Lloyd, C. & King, R. (2002) *British Journal of Occupational Therapy*, **65**(12), 536–42.

23   Creek, J. (2003) *Occupational Therapy Defined as a Complex Intervention*. COT, London.

24   Creek J. (ed) (2002) *Glossary of Occupational Therapy Terms in OT and Mental Health*, 3rd edition. Churchill Livingstone, Edinburgh.

25   Hagedorn, R. (2001) *Foundations for Practice in OT*, 3rd edn. Churchill Livingstone, Edinburgh.

26   Golledge, J. (1998) Is there unnecessary duplication of skills between occupational therapists and physiotherapists. *British Journal of Occupational Therapy*, **61**(4), 161–2.

27   Golledge, J. (1998) Distinguishing between occupational, purposeful activity and activity, Part 1: Review and explanation. *British Journal of Occupational Therapy*, **61**(3), 100–4; Part 2 Why is the distinction important, **61**(4), 157–60.

28   Sumsion, T. (2000) A revised occupational therapy definition of client-centred practice. *British Journal of Occupational Therapy*, **63**(7), 304–9.

29   Sumsion, T. (ed) (2006) *Client-centred practice in occupational therapy – a guide to implementation*. Churchill, Edinburgh.

30   College of Occupational Therapists (2002) *From Interface to Integration: A strategy of modernising occupational therapy services in local health and social care communities. A consultation*. COT, London.

31   College of Occupational Therapists (2002) *From interface to integration: the response of the Council of the College of Occupational Therapists to its consultation on a strategy for modernising occupational therapy services in local health and social care communities*. COT, London.

32   College of Occupational Therapists (2007) *Integrated Occupational Therapy Services*. Briefing note no 77. COT, London.

33   Duncan, E.A.S. (1999) Occupational therapy in mental health: It is time to recognise that it has come of age. *British Journal of Occupational Therapy*, **62**(11), 521–2.

34   Goren, A. (2002) Occupational therapy and strictly defined areas of doubt and uncertainty. *British Journal of Occupational Therapy*, **65**(10), 476–8.

35   Wilcock, A.A. In *Occupation for Health, vol. 1, A Journey from Self Health to Prescription* (2001); vol 2, *A Journey from Prescription to Self Health* (2002). British Association and College of Occupational Therapists.

36   College of Occupational Therapists (2003 updated 2007). *Professional Standards for Occupational Therapy Practice*. COT, London.

37   College of Occupational Therapy (2006) *Information for Specialist Sections*. Briefing note No 72. COT, London.

38   Creek, J. and Lawson-Porter, A. (eds) (2007) *Contemporary Issues in Occupational Therapy: Reasoning and Reflection*. Wiley, Chichester.

39   Clouston, T.J. & Whitcombe, S.W. (2008) The Professionalisation of Occupational Therapy: a continuing challenge. *British Journal of Occupational Therapy*, **71**(8), 314–20.

2 The Legal System

For the most part, this book describes the law which applies to England and Wales. It also applies to Scotland and Northern Ireland in most respects, but devolution has led to greater differences between the constituent parts of the UK. To those who have never studied the law, it can be perplexing. The jargon, the complexity of answers to the simplest questions, can place a significant barrier between the ordinary health professional and lawyers. However, all health professionals and health service managers have to work within the context of the law and therefore need to know the basic legal principles which constrain or empower them, and also need to have a clear understanding of the point at which it is essential to bring in legal advice and support. Bond Solon Training has published through the College of Occupational Therapists a useful step-by-step guide for OTs involved in court proceedings.[1] This chapter provides an introduction to the basic terms used and a description of the framework within which the law is implemented. The glossary provides an explanation of some of the technical terms used in this book. The following topics are covered in this chapter:

- Sources of law
- European Community Law
- The European Convention of Human Rights
- Civil and criminal law
- Types of civil action
- Public and private law
- Legal personnel
- Procedure in civil courts
- Procedure in criminal courts
- Accusatorial system
- Law and ethics

Sources of law

Law derives from two main sources: statute law and the common law (also known as case law or judge-made law). The sources of law are illustrated in Figure 2.1. The statute law is based on

Legal Aspects of Occupational Therapy, Third Edition By Bridgit Dimond
© 2010 Bridgit Dimond

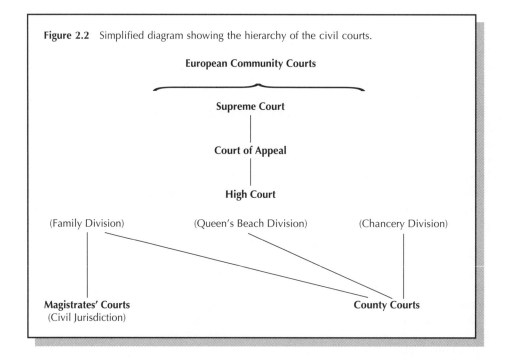

Figure 2.1   Derivation and sources of law.

Statute Law	**Common Law**
EC Regulations	**EC Court rulings**
Acts of Parliament/Statutes	

House of Commons   **Supreme Court** (replacing the House of Lords in 2009)–cases on important points of law

House of Lords   **Court of Appeal**
Royal Assent   **High Court/Crown Court**

Statutory Instruments   Decisions binding on basis of rules of precedent
   made by   relevant Ministry   and hierarchy
          laid before **P**arliament

Statutes and statutory instruments as well as previous cases are interpreted by judges and the decisions become part of the common law

Figure 2.2   Simplified diagram showing the hierarchy of the civil courts.

European Community Courts

Supreme Court

Court of Appeal

High Court

(Family Division)   (Queen's Beach Division)   (Chancery Division)

Magistrates' Courts   **County Courts**
(Civil Jurisdiction)

legislation passed through the agreed constitutional process. Legislation of the European Community (EC) now takes precedence over the Acts of Parliament of the UK Government (see below). Statutory instruments drawn up on the basis of powers delegated to ministers and others supplement the Acts of Parliament. Decisions by judges in courts create what is known as the common law. A recognised hierarchy of the courts determines which previous decisions are binding on courts hearing similar cases. Figure 2.2 shows the civil court system and Figure 2.3 shows the criminal court system.

A recognised system of reporting of judges' decisions ensures certainty over what was stated and the facts of the cases. It may be possible for judges to 'distinguish' previous cases and not follow

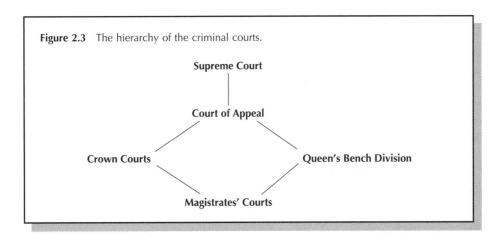

Figure 2.3   The hierarchy of the criminal courts.

them on the grounds that the facts are significantly different. For example, before the Occupiers' Liability Act 1984, which defined the liability of the occupier towards trespassers, such liability was based on decisions made by judges on particular facts. In one case the House of Lords (now replaced by the Supreme Court) held that cases which involved harm to children, where the occupier had been held liable, were not binding on a judge hearing a case involving an adult so that the occupier was not liable to the adult trespasser. The earlier cases relating to children were 'distinguished' .[2]

Judges are, however, bound by statutes and, if the result is an unsatisfactory situation, this may only be remedied by new amending legislation. The registration of OTs is governed by the Health Care Professions Order which was passed under the Health Act 1999 which in turn amended the Professions Supplementary to Medicine Act 1960. Following these changes the Health Professions Council replaced the Council for Professions Supplementary to Medicine in April 2002. The regulations have to be interpreted by judges in court cases if disputes in relation to the meaning of the legislation arise. Thus law develops through a mix of statutory promulgation and common law decision making.

European Community law

Since its signing of the Treaty of Rome, the UK has accepted that it is bound by the legislation of the European Community. It must therefore observe the Treaties of the European Community, and is bound by regulations made by the European Council and the European Commission. The regulations have direct application to member states, unlike the European Directives, which must be incorporated into UK law by the passing of regulations to be effective. (This does not apply to their application to state authorities.) Appeals can be made to the European Court of Justice on issues relating to EC law. It is also possible for the UK courts to refer an issue to the European Court of Justice for a specific point on the interpretation of EC law to be determined.

The European Convention on Human Rights

The European Convention on Human Rights provides protection for the fundamental rights and freedoms of all people. It is enforced through the European Court on Human Rights in Strasbourg.

The decisions of the court are binding on all countries which are signatories to the Convention, of which the UK is one.

The UK, although a signatory, has only recently incorporated the Convention into UK law as a consequence of the Human Rights Act 1998. The Act came into force on 2 October 2000 in England, Wales and Northern Ireland, and in Scotland on devolution. As a consequence of the Human Rights Act applicants who allege a breach of the articles by a public authority or by an organisation exercising functions of a public nature, can take their case to the courts in the UK as well as to the European Court of Human Rights in Strasbourg. The Articles of the European Convention of Human Rights can be found in the Appendix 1 of this book. The rights of the client are discussed in Chapter 6. The articles of the Convention also apply to those employed by public authorities and organisations exercising functions of a public nature. The implications of this for employees are considered in Chapter 19.

Civil and criminal law

The civil law governs disputes between private citizens (including corporate bodies) or between citizens and the state. Thus contract law and the law of torts (civil wrongs which are not breach of contract), rights over property, marital disputes and the wrongful exercise of power by a statutory authority all come under the civil law. Actions are brought in the civil courts in relation to an alleged civil wrong by a claimant (formerly known as the plaintiff) who sues a defendant. The person bringing the action has to prove the defendant's liability on a balance of probabilities.

Criminal law relates to actions which can be followed by criminal proceedings in which an accused is prosecuted. The sources of criminal law are both statutory and the common law; thus the definition of murder derives from a decision of the courts in the seventeenth century whereas theft is defined by an Act of Parliament of 1968 as amended by subsequent legislation. A prosecution is brought in relation to a charge of a criminal offence and heard in the criminal courts, where those prosecuting have to prove beyond reasonable doubt that the accused is guilty. In the magistrates court, the magistrates decide if, on the facts, guilt has been established and if so they sentence the accused. They also have the power to commit the accused to the crown court for sentencing by the crown court judge (in cases where the crime demands a greater punishment than the magistrates have power to give; (certain offences can only be heard in the crown court and are known as indictable only offences). In the crown court, the jury decide if the accused is guilty, and if so the judge sentences. Some of the principal differences between a civil case and a criminal case are shown in Figure 2.4. A child under 10 years old is incapable of being guilty of a crime (doli incapax). For children between 10 and 14 there had been a presumption that the child is incapable of being guilty but this presumption could be rebutted by proof that he had known that something that he was doing was wrong but this presumption was repealed by section 34 of the Crime and Disorder Act 1998 which the House of Lords (now replaced by the Supreme Court) held also implicitly repealed the defence of doli incapax for a 12-year-old charged under the Sexual Offences Act 2003.[3]

There is an overlap between civil and criminal wrongs. Thus touching a person without his consent may be a civil wrong, known as trespass to the person; it may also be a crime, a criminal assault or battery. Similarly, driving a car carelessly may lead to criminal proceedings for driving without due care and attention and also lead to civil proceedings for negligence if it can be established that the driver was in breach of a duty of care owed to a person who was injured as a result. Gross negligence by a health professional, which causes the death of a patient, can lead to criminal prosecutions for manslaughter. Thus in one case[4] an anaesthetist failed to realise that a tube had

Figure 2.4   Differences between civil and criminal hearings.

	Criminal hearings	Civil hearings
basis of action	a charge of a criminal offence	an alleged wrong by one person against another
action brought by	Crown Prosecution Service (CPS) – occasionally a private prosecution	the person wronged (the claimant) or if a child, a person on his/her behalf
standard of proof	beyond reasonable doubt	balance of probabilities
facts decided by	Magistrates Courts – the magistrate(s) Crown Court – the jury	the judge
law applied by	Magistrates Courts – the magistrate(s) (lay magistrates advised by legally qualified clerk) Crown Court – the judge	the judge(s)

become disconnected and he was prosecuted in the criminal courts and convicted of manslaughter. There would also be civil liability for compensation in the civil courts. The anaesthetist would be personally liable for the negligence which caused the death of the patient but in practice compensation to the family would be paid by his employer because of its vicarious liability for negligence by employees in the course of their employment (see Chapter 10 on negligence and vicarious liability). In a recent case the Court of Appeal held that where a person had created a state of affairs which he knew or ought to have known had become life-threatening, then there was a consequent duty to act by taking reasonable steps to save the other's life.[5] The circumstances of the case were that the mother and her daughter who was the half sister of a woman who had self-injected with heroin and suffered from overdose symptoms, had decided not to seek medical assistance (because they feared they would put themselves and her into trouble) but put her to bed hoping that she would recover spontaneously. The following morning she was dead. The court held that the duty to act in such circumstances were not confined to situations where there was a familial or professional relationship between the defendant and the deceased.

A doctor was convicted of manslaughter when she gave an injection of adrenalin against the advice of her colleagues. She received a six month suspended sentence.[6]

Following recommendations by the Law Commission[7] that the law should be changed to enable it to be made easier for corporations and statutory bodies to be prosecuted for manslaughter, the Corporate Manslaughter and Corporate Homicide Act 2007 was passed to ensure that organisations responsible for such deaths were held criminally responsible.

The Corporate Manslaughter and Corporate Homicide Act 2007

The Act abolishes the common law offence of corporate manslaughter by gross negligence by an organisation and replaces it with statutory offences which can be committed by specified organisations if its activities are managed or organised in a way which (a) causes a person's death, and (b) amounts to a gross breach of a relevant duty of care owed by the organisation to the deceased. An organisation is guilty of an offence under this section only if the way in which its activities are managed or organised by its senior management is a substantial element in the breach of the duty of care. The organisations specified include 'corporations' and also the Department of Health. The duty of care is defined widely and includes duties to a detained patient, but excludes any duty of care owed by a public authority in respect of a decision as to matters of public policy (including in particular the allocation of public resources or the weighing of competing public interests). Duty of care also excludes emergency responses carried out by an NHS body or ambulance service. The jury determines if there has been a gross breach of the duty of care beyond reasonable doubt. On conviction the organisation can be fined, subjected to remedial order and required to publish details of the offence, the fine and the remedial action ordered. A prosecution under health and safety laws can proceed at the same time as a prosecution for corporate manslaughter. Individuals cannot be prosecuted under the Act, but they are liable to a common law prosecution for manslaughter and if gross negligence which caused the death is established can be convicted of manslaughter (see the case of the anaesthetist above).[8] Following conviction a company could be given an unlimited fine. The first case of a prosecution under the Corporate Manslaughter and Corporate Homicide Act was that of a Peter Eaton, a director of Cotswold Geotechnical Holdings who was accused of gross negligence leading to the death of a geologist who died whilst taking soil samples when the pit he was working on collapsed on him.[9]

Both criminal proceedings and civil proceedings can arise from the same set of facts or incident.

Types of civil action

Figure 2.5 illustrates some of the kinds of civil action which may be brought. In this book we are principally concerned with the law relating to negligence, breach of statutory duty and trespass to the person. The OT should be aware, however, of the civil law relating to defamation and nuisance.

Public and private law

Another distinction in the classification of laws is that of public and private law. Figure 2.6 illustrates the differences between the two.

Public law deals with those areas of law which are seen to be of public concern and where society intervenes in the actions of individuals. In contrast, private law is concerned with the behaviour of individuals or corporate bodies to each other, without interference of the state. The Children Act 1989 covers both private law and public law relating to children. Care proceedings, protection orders and child assessment orders are part of the public law; orders in relation to children made following

---

Figure 2.5   Types of civil action.

- Negligence
- Nuisance
- Defamation
- Breach of statutory duty
- Trespass (to the person, goods or land)
- Breach of contract

Figure 2.6   Differences between public and private law.

Public Law
Matter of public concern e.g.

- protection of children
- public nuisance
- how statutory duties are carried out

Private Law
Matter arising between individuals (people or organisations) e.g.

- purchasing a house
- suing for personal injury
- suing for breach of contract

divorce, such as with whom the child is to live, are part of the private law. Thus the report by Lord Laming into the death of Victoria Climbié[10] was concerned with the public law – the duty of the Social Services Department to take action to protect children. In contrast, a dispute over whether consent has been given for a child to have treatment would be part of private law. Remedies differ according to whether the matter is seen as a question of public law or of private law.

Public and private law overlap where individuals feel aggrieved by decisions taken by a public body directly affecting them. Such an individual can challenge the decision-making authority or tribunal by a process known as 'judicial review'. Thus if a person detained under the Mental Health Act 1983 were to appeal unsuccessfully to a Mental Health Review Tribunal (MHRT) and considered that the decision not to discharge him was based upon a failure to apply the correct law, he could apply to the High Court, Queen's Bench Division for the decision of the MHRT to be reviewed.[11] However, this course is not recommended where an Act of Parliament lays down a procedure for challenging the decision of a statutory body. For example, in the case of *Gossington v Ealing Borough Council* 1985, Mr Gossington applied for judicial review of the decision of London Borough of Ealing to provide him with five hours of home help per week instead of the original ten hours. The judge held that the Act provided for an application to the Secretary of State if the local authority had failed to carry out its statutory functions. The Secretary of State could, after any necessary inquiry, make an order declaring the local authority to be in default. The applicant had not exhausted the other available routes open to him to remedy the wrong he felt that he had suffered and therefore his application for judicial review was refused.

Legal personnel

If patients believe they have a claim for compensation because of the actions or omissions of health professionals, after possibly seeking advice from their local patient advocacy and liaison service (PALS). (In Wales Community Health Councils have been retained – see Chapter 14), they could ask a solicitor to take the case. A solicitor is a professionally qualified person (usually a law degree or the Common Professional Examination followed by the Law Society's professional examinations and completion of a legal practice course) who tends to have direct contact with the client.

The solicitor may seek the opinion of a barrister (known as counsel) on liability and the amount of compensation. A barrister will usually have a law degree (or the Common Professional Examination) and must complete the examinations set by the Council for Legal Education. The barrister must be a member of an Inn of Court and complete a term of apprenticeship, for a year, known as pupillage. Traditionally the barrister has had the role of conducting the case in court and preparing the documents, known as pleadings, which are exchanged between the parties in the run up to the court hearing. However, increasingly the right of solicitors to represent the client in court has been extended until it is now possible for solicitors with special training and recognition to undertake the work formerly undertaken by barristers alone. Eventually these developments may lead to a single profession.

Procedure in civil courts

Lord Woolf conducted an *inquiry*[12] to determine how access to justice could be simplified and speeded up with the judge having more control in its early stages. Significant changes were brought into effect on 1 April 1999 to implement the changes recommended by Lord Woolf. These are considered in more detail in Chapter 13. The procedures in the County Courts follow a similar pattern.

Procedure in criminal courts

Magistrates, who are either lay people known as justices of the peace (JPs) sitting in threes (the bench) or legally qualified persons known as stipendiary magistrates (who sit alone), can only hear charges which relate to minor offences known as summary offences or offences such as theft which can be heard either as summary offences or on indictment triable either way. Only the crown court (with judge and jury) can hear charges of offences which can only be made on indictment (indictable only offences). Such offences are the most serious, e.g. murder, rape, grievous bodily harm, and other offences against the person. The magistrates, however, have a limited gate-keeping role in relation to these offences. If the magistrates decide that an 'either way' offence (i.e. one which could be heard in the magistrates or in the crown court) should be tried in the Crown Court trial it will be sent there directly and a date for the Plea and Case Management Hearing agreed. Indictable only cases are transferred to the Crown Court immediately (i.e. at first appearance before the magistrates), and sometimes before witness statements are taken. At this preliminary hearing a timetable will be set for the service of the prosecution evidence, service of defence statements and a date for the Plea and Case Management hearing (PCMH). In criminal cases the Crown Prosecution Service (CPS) has the responsibility for preparing the case, including statements, witnesses, etc., for the prosecution in criminal cases. In criminal cases, the Crown Prosecution Service (CPS) has the responsibility for preparing the case, including statements, witnesses, etc. for the prosecution. Reforms to limit jury trial, to enable an accused to be charged with the same offence after an earlier acquittal and to allow evidence of previous convictions to be made known to the jury, were enacted in the Criminal Justice Act 2003.

Accusatorial system

A feature of the legal system in this country is that one side has the responsibility of proving that the other side is guilty, liable or at fault of the wrong or crime alleged. This is known as an 'accusatorial' system (or sometimes 'adversarial') and applies to both civil and criminal proceedings. In civil proceedings the claimant, i.e. the person bringing the action, has to establish on a balance of probability that there is negligence, trespass, nuisance or whatever civil wrong is alleged. In civil cases (apart from defamation) there is no jury and the judge has the responsibility of making a decision on disputed facts and of determining whether the claimant has succeeded in law in establishing the civil wrong.

This system, where one party to a case confronts the other party, also applies in criminal cases where the prosecution attempt to show beyond all reasonable doubt that the accused is guilty of the offence with which the defendant is charged. The magistrates, or the jury in the crown court, determine the facts and whether the prosecution has succeeded in establishing the guilt of the accused, who is presumed innocent until proved guilty. The role of the judge in the Crown Court is to chair the proceedings, intervening where necessary in the interests of justice, and advising on points of law and procedure. (The Health and Social Care Act 2008 requires the use of the civil standard of proof, instead of the criminal standard, to be used in fitness to practise proceedings held by the regulatory bodies and therefore the HPC (see Chapter 3).)

The accusatorial system contrasts with a system of law known as 'inquisitorial' where the judge plays a far more active role in determining the outcome. An example of an inquisitorial system in the UK is the coroner's court. Here the coroner is responsible for deciding which witnesses would be relevant to the answers to the questions which are placed before him by statute (i.e. the identity of the deceased and how, when and where he came to die). The coroner asks the witnesses questions in court and decides who else can ask questions and what they can ask. As a result of this 'inquisition' the coroner, or a jury if one is used, determines the cause of death.

Some may feel that an inquisitorial system of justice is fairer since the outcome of the accusatorial system may depend heavily upon the ability of the barristers representing the party in court. However, the strengths of the accusatorial system probably outweigh the weaknesses. There are after all many challenges to the decisions of coroners. The case management approach implemented as a result of Lord Woolf's reforms keeps the adversarial system but ensures that, where appropriate, expert witnesses have a responsibility to the court. These reforms are considered in Chapters 10 (negligence) and 13 (giving evidence in court).

Law and ethics

Law is both wider and narrower than the field of ethics. On the one hand the law covers areas of practice which may not be considered to give rise to any ethical issue, other than the one as to whether the law should be obeyed. For example, to park in a 'no parking' area would not appear to raise many ethical issues other than the decision to obey or to ignore the law. On the other hand, there are major areas of healthcare which raise significant ethical questions where there appears to be little law. For example, a chaplain visiting a patient in hospital might appear to raise solely ethical issues, but the Information Commissioner has ruled that a chaplain is not a health professional and therefore has no right to be notified of patients belonging to that religion without the consent of the patient. The elective ventilation of a corpse in order to keep the organs alive for transplant purposes raises considerable ethical issues for health professionals and relatives, but, provided the requirements of the Human Tissue Act and the Transplant Acts were satisfied, there were no legal issues but considerable ethical ones. The legal situation has now been changed however by section 47 of the Human Tissue Act 2004 which enables a person to take steps for the purpose of preserving the part for use for transplantation. At any time, of course, a practice which is considered to be contrary to ethical principles can be challenged in court and the judge will make a determination, on the basis of any existing statute law or decided cases, of what the legal position is.

Situations may arise where health professionals consider the law to be wrong and contrary to their own ethical principles. In such a case they have personally to decide what action to take, in full awareness that they could face the effects of the criminal law, civil action, disciplinary procedures by their employers and professional proceedings by their registration body.

In certain cases, however, the law itself provides for conscientious objection. Thus no one can be compelled to participate in an abortion unless it is an emergency situation to save the life or to prevent grave permanent injury to the physical or mental health of a pregnant woman (Abortion Act 1967 section 4(2)). Similar provisions apply to activities in relation to human fertilisation and embryology where the Human Fertilisation and Embryology Act 1990 provides a statutory protection clause.

A health professional may have strong ethical views about the need to save the life of a mentally competent adult who is refusing a life-saving blood transfusion, but the law does not permit the overrule of a refusal made when an adult is mentally competent and a health professional who provided treatment contrary to the wishes of a mentally competent person or contrary to a valid and applicable advance decision could face criminal, civil, disciplinary and professional conduct proceedings. It is inevitable that any discussion of the function of occupational therapy should be concerned with the ethical or philosophical beliefs of the therapist who is providing the treatment and this is considered in Chapter 1. One issue which would appear to have ethical rather than legal dimensions (though legal issues could arise, particularly if the OT was charged with theft,) is the ethical problem of an OT accepting gifts. This is considered by Jani Grisbrooke and Rosemary Barnitt.[13] They conclude that the offer of a gift can be ambiguous, but guidance that gifts should never be accepted is difficult to operate in practice and the OT needs to use ethical reasoning skills in taking the appropriate action.

The Code of Ethics and Professional Conduct[14] for Occupational Therapists (see Chapter 4 for discussion of this) is an example of ethical principles being required of registered practitioners. At the time of writing a new edition of the Code is being drafted.

Reference should be made to the list of recommended further reading for books on ethics. Students must be aware of both legal and ethical dimensions to their practice. This book is concerned with providing the reader with the necessary legal knowledge and understanding of the legal framework within which practice takes place.

 Questions and exercises

1   A client has consulted you about the possibility of bringing a claim for compensation. What advice would you give on the procedure which would be followed and the steps which should be taken?
2   Draw up a diagram which illustrates the difference between civil and criminal procedure.
3   Turn to the glossary and study the definitions of legal terms included there.
4   In what ways do you consider that a conflict between an ethical belief and the law should be resolved?

References

1   Bond Solon Training (2006) *The Occupational Therapist and the Court: A step by step guide for occupational therapists and their staff*. COT, London.
2   *British Railway Board v Herrington* [1972] AC 877; [1972] 1 All ER 749.
3   *R v JTB (on appeal from R v T)* The Times Law Report 4 May 2009 HL.
4   *R v Adomako* [1994] 3 All ER 79 HL.
5   *R v Evans (Gemma)* The Times Law Report 7 April 2009 CA.

6   Smyth, C. Doctor gave fatal injection against colleagues' advice. The Times 7 February 2009.
7   Law Commission (1996) Report on criminal prosecuting. HMSO, London.
8   *R v Adomako* [1995] 1 AC 171; [1994] 3 All ER 79.
9   News item. Manslaughter by negligence case. The Times 24 April 2009.
10   www.victoria-climbie-inquiry.org.uk/
11   *R v Hallstrom, ex parte W*; *R v Gardener, ex parte L* [1986] 2 All ER 306.
12   Lord Woolf (January 1996) *Access to Civil Justice Inquiry*, Consultation Paper. HMSO, London; Lord Woolf (June 1995) *Interim Report on Access to Justice Inquiry*, Lord Chancellor's Office; Lord Woolf (July 1996) Final Report Access to Justice. HMSO, London.
13   Grisbrooke, J. & Barnitt, R. (2002) Accepting gifts: A discussion of ethical issues for occupational therapists. *British Journal of Occupational Therapy*, **65**(12), 559–62.
14   College of Occupational Therapists (2005) *Code of Ethics and Professional Conduct for Occupational Therapists*. COT, London.

3 Registration and the Health Professions Council

In this chapter we consider the statutory basis of the occupational therapist and discuss the provisions for registration and the role of the Health Professions Council (HPC) (which replaced the Council for Professions Supplementary to Medicine (CPSM) in 2002). The following topics are covered:

- Background to the establishment of the HPC
- Health Professions Council (HPC)
  - Fundamental functions
  - Committees
  - Consultation with registrants
- Registration machinery
- Protected titles
- New professional groups
- Non-registered support workers
- Council for Healthcare Regulatory Excellence

Background to the establishment of the HPC

Review of 1960 Act

A review of the Professions Supplementary to Medicine Act 1960 was undertaken by JM Consulting Ltd under a steering group chaired by Professor Sheila McLean. Following a consultation document issued in October 1995, a report was published in July 1996.[1] The report described the weaknesses of the Professions Supplementary to Medicine Act, identifying two broad areas of weakness:

- in the powers provided by the 1960 Act
- in the statutory bodies and working arrangements.

It explored the developments which had taken place since 1960 including:

Legal Aspects of Occupational Therapy, Third Edition By Bridgit Dimond
© 2010 Bridgit Dimond

- the development of primary care
- the introduction of the internal market
- the use of multi-disciplinary teams and the possibility of non-state registered professionals being employed in the NHS by GPs
- the growth of private sector provision
- the changes which have taken place within the professions including strong professional associations with regulations for discipline.

The inappropriateness of the term 'Professions Supplementary to Medicine' was also considered. Other changes included:

- the new professions who have sought state registered status
- developments within higher education and degree status for many professions, and education provision being made outside the NHS
- changing attitudes in society and public expectations.

The recommendations included the establishment of a Council for Health Professionals and Statutory Committees with a panel of professional advisers.

Implementing the proposals

The Government accepted the recommendations of JM Consulting Ltd and in the Health Act 1999 took the preliminary steps to implement the new system for registration and professional control. A consultation paper was published in August 2000,[2] inviting comments within three months on the legislative proposals. It stated that modernising professional self-regulation should be seen as a component part of a wider strategy to modernise the whole of the NHS to help deliver better health and faster, fairer care. A draft order was published in April 2001[3] and was issued as a statutory instrument in 2002.[4]

The new scheme

In April 2002 a new Health Professions Council replaced the Council for Professions Supplementary to Medicine and its twelve boards, and currently regulates 120,000 health professionals. The key objectives of the reorganisation were:

- to reform ways of working, by requiring the Council to:
  - treat the health and welfare of patients as paramount
  - collaborate and consult with key stakeholders
  - be open and proactive in accounting to the public and the profession for its work
- to reform structure and functions by:
  - giving wider powers to deal effectively with individuals who present unacceptable risks to patients
  - creating a smaller Council, comprising directly elected practitioners and a strong lay input
  - linking registration with evidence of continuing professional development
  - providing stronger protection of professional titles
  - enabling the extension of regulation to new groups.

The Council is charged with the strategic responsibility for setting and monitoring standards of professional training, performance and conduct.

The consultation paper quoted from the NHS Plan that the key tests for regulatory bodies are that they must be:

- smaller, with much greater patient and public representation
- have faster, more transparent procedures
- develop meaningful accountability to the public and the health service.

The consultation paper stated that the GMC had been asked to explore the introduction of a civil burden of proof and other reforms. It recommended that the procedures adopted by the new HPC would need to be consistent with those agreed for doctors.

The consultation paper also stated that there needed to be formal co-ordination between the health regulatory bodies, and therefore a UK council of health regulators was to be established (see below). Its initial task would be to help co-ordinate and act as a forum in which common approaches across the professions could be developed for dealing with matters such as complaints against practitioners.

Health Professions Council (HPC)

The Government proposed that the HPC should initially consist of 23 members (12 practitioners, i.e. one from each of the professions covered) and 11 lay members (who may or may not be members of other professions, not covered by the HPC). In addition there are 12 alternate Registrant members who attend instead of Registrant members when they are absent. The emphasis is on a smaller more effective body. In February 2008 the HPC recommended to the DH that the number of members on the HPC Council should be 20 including the President and that there should be an equal representation of registrant and lay members. On 3 July the Council agreed the criteria which would be used to appoint the Chair and members of the restructured Council and the new Council commenced on 1 July 2009.[5]

Fundamental functions of the HPC

These are set out in Schedule 3, para. 8(2), to the 1999 Health Act and are not transferable by Order to another body:

- keeping the Register of members admitted to practise
- determining standards of education and training for admission to practise
- giving advice about standards of conduct and performance
- administering procedures (including making rules) relating to misconduct, unfitness to practise and similar matters.

Section 60 of the Health Act 1999 enables an Order in Council to make provision for:

- modifying the regulation of any profession 'so far as appears to be necessary or expedient for the purpose of securing or improving the regulation of the profession or the services which the profession provides or to which it contributes'
- 'regulating any other profession which appears to be concerned (wholly or partly) with the physical or mental health of individuals and to require regulation in pursuance of the section.'

There is also an overarching duty of the HPC to:

treat the health and wellbeing of persons using or needing services, as well as to work in partnership with employers, educators and other regulatory bodies. (Article 3)

The HPC statutory committees

There are four committees of the Council, known as the statutory committees:

- Education and Training Committee
- Investigating Committee
- Conduct and Competence Committee
- Health Committee.

The last three of these are also referred to as the Practice Committees (see Chapters 4 and 5 for the work of these Practice Committees).

All committees are chaired by a member of Council and each Committee has at least one lay member. They make recommendations and decisions in consultation with the Council.

Flexibility is built in so that the Council may establish other committees to discharge its functions and can establish professional advisory committees whose function is to advise the Council and its statutory committees on matters affecting any of the relevant professions.

The HPC non-statutory committees

The HPC has established the following as non-statutory committees:

- Communications Committee
- Finance and Resources Committee
- Audit Committee
- Registration Committee.

Consultation with registrants

The Council shall inform and educate registrants and the public about its work.

Before establishing any standards or giving guidance the Council must consult representatives of any group of persons it considers appropriate, including:

- Representatives of registrants or classes of registrants
- Employers of registrants
- Users of the services of registrants
- Persons providing, assessing or funding education or training for registrants and potential registrants.

The Council shall publish any standards it establishes and any guidance it gives.

Registration machinery

One of the main functions of the Council is to establish and maintain a register of members of the relevant professions. This entails establishing from time to time the standards of proficiency necessary to be admitted to the different parts of the Register, being standards the Council considers necessary for safe and effective practice under that part of the Register. The standards of proficiency required for the registration of an occupational therapist can be seen on the HPC website[6] (see also Chapter 5). They cover professional autonomy and accountability, skills required for the application of practice and knowledge, understanding and skills.

The Register shows, in relation to each registrant, such address and other details as the Council prescribes. The required details prescribed by Council were set out in the rules which came into force on 9 July 2003.[7] These include:

- the full name of the registrant
- his registration number
- his last known home address (but this shall not be included in any published version of the register without his consent)
- any qualification of the registrant which has led to his registration.

The Registrar may also enter on the Register any other information which is material to a registrant's registration. The Registrar is required to keep the Register in a form and manner which guards against falsification and shall take all reasonable steps to ensure that only he and such persons as have been authorised by him in writing for the purpose shall be able to amend the register or have access to the version of the register which contains entries not included in the published version.

To be effective and enable practitioners to progress in their profession, there shall be one or more designated titles for each part of the Register indicative of different qualifications and different kinds of training, and a registered professional is entitled to use whichever of those titles is appropriate in his case in accordance with set criteria.

The Council, having consulted the Education and Training Committee, can make rules in connection with registration, the register and the payment of fees.

The Council shall make the register available for inspection by members of the public at all reasonable times and shall publish the register in such manner and at such times as it considers appropriate. Rules relating to parts of entries in the Register came into force on 9 July 2003.[8] Schedule 1 sets out the different parts. Occupational therapists are registered in Part 6 of the Register.

Application to be registered

A person seeking admission to a part of the register shall be registered if the application is made in the prescribed form and manner and she:

- satisfies the Education and Training Committee that she holds an approved qualification awarded:
  - less than five years ago
  - more than five years ago, but she has met specified requirements as to additional education, training, and experience
- satisfies the Education and Training Committee that she meets the Council's prescribed requirements as to safe and effective practice
- has paid the prescribed fee.

Provisions for renewal of registration and readmission require the applicant to meet any set requirements for continuing professional development within the specified time.

The Rules cover the procedure to be followed in applications for registration and provisions for amendments to the register and for renewal of registration. Rules also cover the circumstances in which a registered professional's name may be removed from the register on her own application or after the expiry of a prescribed period.

Provision is made for definition of approved qualifications and European Economic Area qualifications.

The Registration period for those who were initially registered under the Council of the Professions Supplementary to Medicine is the date on which her last renewal of registration under the 1960 Act would have expired. Otherwise a person's first registration period begins on the day she is first registered and ends in the second calendar year after the year in which she was registered, on the date shown in column 2 of Schedule 5. For occupational therapists the date is 31 October 2003.

Character and health references

The HPC requires each applicant for registration, or registrant for re-registration, to provide a statement of good character and good health. The Rules which came into force on 9 July 2003 require the applicant to provide a character reference by a person who is not a relative and is a person of standing in the community, such as a registered professional, doctor, solicitor, accountant, bank manager, JP, head of the educational college or religious official. (A Character Reference Form is provided under Schedule 3 to the Rules.) The applicant must also provide a reference as to their physical and mental health from their doctor, unless that doctor is a relative. (A Health Reference Form is provided under Schedule 4 to the Rules.) Alternative arrangements are laid down where these requirements are not possible. The HPC published guidance relating to the health reference in 2007 for prospective registrants and doctors. The HPC also issued in 2007 guidance for potential registrants and admission officers on a disabled person becoming a registered health professional. The HPC states that

> We do not want to have a definite list which might prevent some people from registering. We want to make sure that decisions are made about individuals based on that individual's ability to meet our standards and practise safely.

Examples of situations involving different disabilities are considered in the guidance.

Further information about who would be eligible to provide such references is obtainable from the HPC website (www.hpc-uk.org).

Appeals

Appeals can be made under Article 37 against the decisions of the Education and Training Committee where an application for registration, readmission or renewal or the inclusion of an additional entry has been refused or where specific conditions have been imposed on an applicant. There is also a right of appeal if the name of a registered professional has been removed on the grounds that she is in breach of a condition in respect of continuing education. The appeal lies to the Council.

Under Article 38 an appeal can be made from any decision of a Practice Committee or any decision of the Council under Article 37 to the appropriate court. Proposals for a Health Professions Independent Appeals Tribunal were not included in the final statutory instrument (Health Professions Order 2001 SI 2002/254). Rules relating to appeals on registration matters came into force on 9 July 2003.[9] These cover the service of documents, the period during which an appeal can be made, the notice of appeal, acknowledgement by the Council of the appeal notice, notice of hearing and the duties of parties and representatives to inform Council if they intend to attend. The Council can hear the appeal itself (with a quorum of 7 with registrants and lay members but the registrants cannot exceed the number of lay members by more than one) or appoint an appeal panel (with at least three persons, one of which must be registered in the same part of the Register as the appellant, one of which must not be a registrant under the HPC or GMC, and (where the health of the professional is in issue) a registered medical practitioner). A preliminary meeting can be held in private with the parties. The appeal panel can determine an appeal without an oral hearing and may take into account written representations. A hearing can take place without the presence of the appellant provided that the appeal panel is satisfied that all reasonable steps have been taken to give notice of the hearing to the appellant. The hearing should be held in public unless the appeal panel is satisfied that, in the interests of justice or for the protection of the private life of the health professional, the complainant, any person giving evidence or any patient or client, the public should be excluded from all or part of the hearing. The Rules cover the order of the proceedings and the procedure to be followed.

Offences

It is an offence to:

- falsely claim registration with intent to deceive
- use a title to which one is not entitled
- falsely represent oneself to possess qualifications in a relevant profession.

It is also an offence fraudulently to procure registration or after registration fail to comply with any requirement imposed by the Council or a Practice Committee.

Protected titles

The consultation paper recommended that a registrant should be entitled to use the designated title corresponding to the part or parts of the Register in which he is registered, whether alone or prefixed by the word registered, and that no other person should be so entitled. The consultation paper noted that this provision could be unfair to non-state registered practitioners who practise lawfully and safely and suggested 'grandparenting' arrangements to enable the registration of those who can show that they have practised lawfully, safely and effectively for a number of years, and if appropriate pass a test of competence for that purpose. Alternatively, such persons could be required to undertake some additional training or experience before admission to the Register. To pass oneself off as registered is an offence under Article 39. The offence is committed whether such representation is express or implied.

The HPC, following consultation, agreed on a list of titles which it asked the Privy Council to protect. Occupational therapist is included in the list.

Grandparenting

In accordance with the above recommendations, in preparation for a time when the title 'occupational therapist' became a legally protected title and those using that title had to be registered with the HPC, interim arrangements were set in place to enable those who had not followed an approved course to take advantage of the HPC grandparenting arrangements which provided advice for their becoming recognised as registered professionals. A helpline was set up by the HPC.[10]

Employment within the NHS and by local authorities

Occupational therapists and the other professions registered under the Health Professions Council must be registered to be employed by NHS organisations and local authorities. Directions were issued to NHS trusts, primary care trusts and special health authorities[11] and to local authorities;[12] these came into force on 1 August 2003. Department of Health guidance was provided on the directions and interim arrangements for non-registered staff[13] and these also apply to staff used by contractors and to self-employed persons.

New professional groups

New groups of health professionals, including complementary or alternative therapies, can be added to the jurisdiction of the HPC. On 3 April 2003 the HPC voted to recommend to the Secretary of State that the operating department practitioners should be the first new profession to be regulated by the HPC. The HPC has published guidelines setting criteria on opening new parts of the Register.[14] It has stated that an occupation will only be eligible for regulation if it involves invasive procedure, clinical intervention with the potential for harm, or the exercise of judgment by unsupervised professionals which can substantially impact on patient health or welfare. Occupations where these activities are already regulated by other means will be ineligible. Once the Council has approved an application, an HPC recommendation and an accompanying report to regulate the profession are submitted to the Secretary of State. If the Secretary of State agrees with the application, an Order will be drawn up under section 60 of the Health Act 1999, submitted for consultation, if necessary amended and then placed before Parliament.

For non-registered support workers see below and Chapter 5.

Council for Healthcare Regulatory Excellence (CHRE) (Formerly the Council for the Regulation of Healthcare Professions)

As a result of the NHS Reform and Health Care Professions Act 2002 (sections 25–29 and Schedule 7) a Council for the Regulation of Health Care Professionals was set up. The Council is a corporate body with the following functions:

- to promote the interests of patients and other members of the public in relation to the performance of their functions by the GMC, GDC, NMC, HPC and other health professional registration bodies
- to promote best practice in the performance of those functions
- to formulate principles relating to good professional self-regulation, and to encourage regulatory bodies to conform to them
- to promote co-operation between regulatory bodies; and between them, or any of them, and other bodies performing corresponding functions.

Powers of the Council

The Council has the powers to do anything which appears to it to be necessary or expedient for the purpose of, or connection with, the performance of its functions. Examples are given in the Act as to what this could include:

- investigate and report on the performance by each regulatory body of its functions
- recommend changes to the way in which the regulatory body performs any of its functions.

The Council will not, however, be able to do anything in relation to a case of any individual who is the subject of proceedings before a regulatory body or about whom an allegation has been made to the regulatory body.

Schedule 7 of the NHS Act and subsequent regulations[15] make provision for the finer detail of the Council such as its membership, appointment and procedure. Reforms were made under the Health and Social Care Act 2008 to strengthen the Council and to confirm the change in its name to the Council for Healthcare Regulatory Excellence (section 113). In a new section (2A) of section 25 of the 2002 Act (which established the Council) the main objective of the Council in exercising its functions under subsection (2)(b) to (d) is to promote the health, safety and well-being of patients and other members of the public.

The Health and Social Care Act 2008 changed the composition of the CHRE's governing Council which became smaller and there is no longer respresentation from the regulators on the Council. A new paragraph 4 to Schedule 7 of the 2002 Act is as follows:

The Council is to consist of:

(a) a chair appointed by the Privy Council,
(b) one non-executive member appointed by the Scottish Ministers,
(c) one non-executive member appointed by the Welsh Ministers,
(d) one non-executive member appointed by the Department of Health, Social Services and Public Safety in Northern Ireland,
(e) three non-executive members appointed by the Secretary of State, and
(f) two executive members appointed in accordance with paragraph 11.

Paragraph 11 (1) states the Council may appoint the executive members referred to in paragraph 4(f) on such terms and conditions as the Council may determine.

11(2) The executive members must be employees of the Council.
11(3) Any decision of the Council under sub-paragraph (1) must be taken by the members appointed under paragraph 4(a) to (e).
11(4) The Council may appoint such other employees as it considers appropriate on such terms and conditions as it may determine.

The new provisions for the constitution of the Council mean that health profession regulators no longer sit on the Council.

A new section 26A (1) enables the Secretary of State, the Welsh Ministers, the Scottish Ministers or the relevant Northern Ireland department to request the Council for advice on any matter connected with a profession appearing to the person making the request to be a healthcare profession; and the Council must comply with such a request. Under section 26A(2) these same ministers may require the Council to investigate and report on a particular matter in respect of which the Council's functions are exercisable.

A new section 26B places upon the Council a duty to inform and consult the public:

(1) For the purpose of ensuring that members of the public are informed about the Council and the exercise by it of its functions, the Council must publish or provide in such manner as it thinks fit information about the Council and the exercise of its functions.

(2) Nothing in subsection (1) authorises or requires the publication or provision of information if the publication or provision of that information—

    (a)   is prohibited by any enactment, or

    (b)   would constitute or be punishable as a contempt of court.

(3) In subsection (2) 'enactment' has the same meaning as in Part 2 of the Health and Social Care Act 2008.

(4) The Council must from time to time seek the views of—

    (a)   members of the public, and

    (b)   bodies which appear to the Council to represent the interests of patients, on matters relevant to the exercise by it of its functions."

The Act also gives the CHRE new responsibilities such as auditing the early stages of regulators' fitness to practise procedures. The CHRE can investigate particular cases with a view to making general reports on the performance by the regulatory body of its functions or making general recommendations to the regulatory body affecting future cases.

Directions to a regulatory body

Each regulatory body must co-operate with the Council. The Council may direct a regulatory body to make rules, if it considers that desirable for the protection of members of the public. Rules made under these directions must be approved by the Privy Council or by the Department of Health before coming into force. The regulatory body must comply with the directions of the Council. From January 2009 the CHRE has audit powers over the activities of the regulators and must report to Parliament annually on whether patient safety interests have been properly considered in the decisions and operations of the regulators on fitness to practise cases.

Investigation of complaints about a regulatory body

Regulations may also be made by the Secretary of State on how the Council can investigate complaints made to it about the way in which a regulatory body has exercised any of its functions. These regulations may cover: who is entitled to complain, the nature of complaints which the Council must or need not investigate, matters which are excluded from the investigation, requirements to be complied with by the complainant, making of recommendations and reports by the Council, confidentiality of information supplied to or obtained by the Council, the use which the Council may make of such information, payments to persons in connection with investigations and privilege in relation to any matter published by the Council in the exercise of its functions under the regulations. The regulations can also cover powers to be given to the Council requiring persons to attend before it, give evidence or produce documents and the admissibility of evidence in accordance with the rules of civil proceedings in the High Court.

Referral of professional conduct decision to High Court

Where the Council is of the view that a decision by the regulatory body in professional misconduct proceedings as specified in the Act is unduly lenient or a relevant decision should not have been made, and it would be desirable for the protection of members of the public for the Council to take action, the Council may refer the case to the High Court (or Court of Session in Scotland). The High Court has the power to dismiss the case, allow the appeal and quash the relevant decision, substitute any other decision for the decision of the committee or person concerned, or remit the case to the committee or other person concerned to dispose of the case in accordance with directions from the court. Some of the decisions of professional conduct committee on which the CHRE has appealed to the High Court are considered in the next chapter.

The High Court held on 29 March 2004 that the Council for the Regulation of Healthcare Professions had the right to refer cases to court even after an acquittal by the appropriate regulatory body. The GMC had challenged the CRHCP's (now the CHRE's) right to refer the case of Dr Ruscillo to the court. This judgment applies to all those health registration bodies under the CRHCP, including the HPC. The Health and Social Care Act 2008 extended the CHRE's remit to review fitness to prac- tise cases where the health of the registrant was in issue.

The impact of the Council for Healthcare Regulatory Excellence upon the HPC and the other regulatory bodies

The existence of the overarching Council will inevitably lead to greater uniformity in standards, professional practice, discipline and other procedures across all registered health professions. Each year it publishes an annual review of the regulatory bodies over which it has jurisdiction. In its performance review for 2007/8 of health profession regulators published in August 2008 the CHRE reviewed each of the registration bodies against the standards it had set and made recommendations for future changes. In its review of the HPC it stated that:

> The Health Professions Council is an effective, publicly accountable regulator which has good communica-
> tions with registrants and the public. It regulates a larger number and a wider range of health professions
> than the other regulators. This brings particular challenges, especially in finding the right balance between
> generic and profession-specific regulation. In this context the HPC has well-founded and thought through
> policies and practice.
>   The HPC is a well-organised regulator and is clearly committed to constantly improving the efficiency of
> its performance.

The CHRE commended many areas of good practice, including its decision not to specify continuing professional development in terms of hours or points which the CHRE considered to be reasonable in the circumstances as it allows for the difference between the professions being regulated and it had an effective sampling system to monitor and check CPD in practice. From 2009 the CHRE's performance reviews are part of its statutory report to Parliament.

Future regulation of the health professions

A review of non-medical regulators was published in 2004 (Foster review).[16] The White Paper Trust, Assurance and Safety – the Regulation of Health Professionals in the 21st century[17] set out provisions for reforms to the regulation of health professions. Many of its recommendations were included in the Health and Social Care Act 2008. The Act contains the following provisions:

- the establishment of a new regulator for hospitals, care homes and social services to be known as the Care Quality Commission (This is considered in Chapter 17)

- reforms of the system of professional regulation to ensure it earns and sustains the confidence of patients, professionals and Parliament.
- all healthcare professional regulatory bodies to use the civil, rather than criminal, standard of proof (see below)
- the creation of an independent adjudicator to undertake independent and objective formal adjudication for the professional regulatory bodies
- the appointment by all healthcare organisations employing or contracting with doctors of a 'responsible officer' to work with the GMC to identify and handle cases of poor professional performance by doctors
- amendments to the Public Health (Control of Disease) Act 1984 with the aim of providing a more effective and proportionate response to infectious disease (see Chapter 11)
- provisions in relation to pregnant employees (see Chapter 17).

Civil standard of proof

One of the more significant changes contained in the Health and Social Care Act was the introduction of the civil standard of proof of a balance of probabilities into the procedures of healthcare regulatory bodies instead of the criminal standard of beyond reasonable doubt. The effect of this is to make it easier to achieve a finding of unfitness to practice of a registrant and thus provide greater protection for the public.

Non-registered support workers

The registered practitioner is increasingly expected to work with support from non-registered practitioners known variously as health support workers, care assistants, occupational therapy assistants and other titles. There have been discussions taking place over recent years on the possibility of bringing these support workers under the umbrella of one of the registration bodies such as the Nursing and Midwifery Council or the Health Professions Council. In its White Paper[18] the Department of Health looked at research in Scotland on the regulation of support workers and made the following comments:

> The Scottish model is that induction standards focus on generic public protection concepts such as confidentiality, dignity, advocacy, and similar core concepts and values apply to all HCSWs employed in the NHS, regardless of their role. The Government in England and will evaluate the results of the Scottish pilot study and consider the way forward with stakeholders. The Government will consider whether there is sufficient demand for the introduction of statutory regulation for any assistant practitioner roles at levels 3 and 4 on the Skills for Health Career Framework. This will be subject to the same mechanisms for determining need, suitability and readiness as for the other emerging professions.

The Department of Health published a consultation document on the registration of healthcare assistants.[19] The timetable envisaged that regulatory provisions would be in place by early 2007. This has not been met.

The Green Paper Shaping the Future of Care Together published in 2009[20] envisages the development of a National Care Service that is fair, simple and affordable and which will be underpinned by rights and entitlements, which support a high-quality service. The National Care Service will also support those who work in the care services and the Government intends to develop an action plan to look at how the workforce will need to develop in the medium and long term and is to set up an independent body to provide advice on what works best and is best value for money in care and support.

The COT published an Occupational Therapy Support Worker Framework in order to provide a resource that can be used by any support worker in occupational therapy (OT) to plan their career and chart their development within the field of OT.[21] Delegation to support workers is considered in Chapter 10.

Future Developments

The Better Regulation Task force is an independent body which advises the Government on professional regulation. In 2003 it revised its Report Principles of Good Regulation and identified the following 5 principles:

Proportionality: Regulators should only intervene when necessary. Remedies should be appropriate to the risks posed, and costs identified and minimised.
Accountability: Regulators must be able to justify decisions, and be subject to public scrutiny.
Consistency: Government rules and standards must be joined up and implemented fairly.
Transparency: Regulators should be open, and keep regulations simple and user-friendly.
Targeting: Regulation should be focused on the problem, and minimise side effects.

Following the White Paper Trust, Assurance and Safety – the Regulation of Health Professionals in the 21st century[22] and the consequential changes in the Health and Social Care Act 2008, the Department of Health published two reports: Tackling concerns nationally: establishing the Office of the Health Professions Adjudicator and Tackling Concerns locally: Report of the working group. Both reports are available from the DH publications website. Tackling concerns nationally sets out recommendations in relation to the Office of Health Professions Adjudicator which will look at cases brought forward assessing fitness to practice for healthcare professionals. The Office will be independent of existing regulators, the Government and healthcare professions to ensure independence. It will initially take on cases concerning doctors and then expand to other professions.

Tackling concerns locally sets out recommendations and principles of best practice to strengthen local NHS arrangements for identifying poor performance among healthcare workers and taking effective action. Local implementation will be supported by more detailed operational guidance and by regulations which the DH will introduce later this year.

Conclusions

It is now 7 years since the HPC came into force and it still has a mammoth agenda to ensure effective regulation and the protection of the public from dangerous health practitioners. It published in April 2002 its strategic intent which covered the purpose, working, function, structure and development of the HPC. It has defined the six guiding principles under which it will operate as: transparency; communication and responsiveness; value for money and audit; protecting the public; working collaboratively; and providing a high quality service. It can be contacted on its website.[23] The HPC now comes under the aegis of the CHRE whose remit and powers have been extended and strengthened by the 2008 Act. Over the next few years it is likely that there will be increasing pressures to ensure high standards of professional practice across all healthcare professions.

Questions and exercises

1   To what extent do you consider that the HPC and its constitution protects the public from professional misconduct and unfitness to practice?
2   The title 'occupational therapist' is now a protected title. What does this mean and what is the effect of the law on protected title?
3   A patient states that her son wishes to become an occupational therapist. What advice would you give her?

References

1   *The Regulation of Health Professions:* Report of a review of the Professions Supplementary to Medicine Act 1960 with recommendations for new legislation. Conducted and published by JM Consulting Ltd, July 1996.
2   NHS Executive (2000) *Modernising Regulation – The New Health Professions Council:* A consultation document. Department of Health.
3   Department of Health (2001) *Establishing the new Health Professions Council.* DH.
4   Health Professions Order 2001, SI 2002/254, Article 3.
5   The Health Professions Council (Constitution) Order SI 2009/1345.
6   www.hpc-uk.org/education/docs/HPC_occupational therapists
7   The Health Professions Council (Registration and Fees) Rules, Order of Council 2003, SI 2003, No. 1572.
8   The Health Professions Council (Parts of and Entries in the Register) Rules, Order of Council 2003, SI 2003, No. 1571.
9   The Health Professions Council (Registration Appeals) Rules, Order of Council 2003, SI 2003, No. 1579.
10   Grandparenting information line 0845 300 4720.
11   National Health Service (Employment of Health Professionals) (England) Directions 2003.
12   Local Government (Employment of Health Professionals) (England) Directions 2003.
13   HSC 2003/008; LAC (2003)19 Employment of Health Professionals by NHS Trusts, Primary Care Trusts and Local Authorities.
14   www.hpc-uk.org/professions/newprofessions.htm
15   The Council for Healthcare Regulatory Excellence (Appointment, Procedure etc.) Regulations 2008 SI 2927.
16   Department of Health (2006) Healthcare Professional Regulation: public consultation on proposals for change DH Leeds.
17   White Paper Trust, Assurance and Safety – the Regulation of Health Professionals in the 21st century February 2007 Cmnd 7013.
18   White Paper Trust, Assurance and Safety – the Regulation of Health Professionals in the 21st century February 2007 Cmnd 7013.
19   Department of Health Regulation of Healthcare staff in England and Wales: Consultation. 2004.
20   Department of Health (2009) Green Paper Shaping the Future of Care Together Cm 7673 DH, London.
21   College of Occupational Therapists (2009) Occupational Therapy Support Worker Framework. COT, London.
22   White Paper Trust, Assurance and Safety – the Regulation of Health Professionals in the 21st century February 2007 Cmnd 7013.
23   www.hpc-uk.org/

4 Professional Conduct Proceedings

In Chapter 3 we considered the law relating to the statutory bodies set up to control entry on to the Register and the functions and constitutions of the machinery for professional regulation set up under the Health Professions Council (HPC). In this chapter we consider the regulation of professional discipline and the role of the College of Occupational Therapists and British Association of Occupational Therapists in maintaining professional standards. The following topics are covered:

- Health Professions Council
  - Disciplinary machinery
  - The committees
- Role of the College of Occupational Therapists (COT)
- Code of Practice

Health Professions Council

Duties in respect of conduct and fitness to practise

Part V of the Order establishing the HPC[1] sets out the provisions for Fitness to Practice procedures for health professionals registered under the HPC. The Health Professions Council is required to establish three Practice Committees: an Investigating Committee, the Conduct and Competence Committee and the Health Committee. In relation to Fitness to Practice, the Order requires the Health Professions Council to:

- establish and keep under review the standards of conduct, performance and ethics expected of registrants and prospective registrants and give them such guidance on these matters as it sees fit
- establish and keep under review effective arrangements to protect the public from persons whose fitness to practise is impaired.

Legal Aspects of Occupational Therapy, Third Edition By Bridgit Dimond
© 2010 Bridgit Dimond

Rules relating to the constitution of Practice Committees came into force on 23 May 2003.[2] and were replaced by new rules in 2009.[3] These relate to the appointment of the members and chairman, tenure of the members, vacancies, standards for members and meetings.

Allegations

A procedure is laid down for dealing with allegations made against a registered person to the effect that her fitness to practice is impaired by reason of:

- Misconduct
- Lack of competence
- A conviction or caution in the UK for a criminal offence (or a conviction elsewhere for what would also be a crime in England or Wales)
- Her physical or mental health
- A determination by a UK statutory body responsible for a health or social care profession that she is unfit to practise that profession (or a determination by a licensing body elsewhere to the same effect).

Civil standard of proof

As a consequence of section 112 of the Health and Social Care Act 2008 the civil standard of proof is now used in fitness to practice proceedings of the regulatory bodies. This means that evidence of misconduct has to be established on a balance of probabilities rather than beyond reasonable doubt.

Screeners

Allegations can be referred to a panel of screeners and at least two of them (one lay person and one registrant from the professional field of the person under scrutiny) shall consider whether the allegation is well founded. The Council has made rules relating to the appointment and functions of the screeners; these came into force on 9 July 2003.[4] Under these rules, where a panel comprises two screeners a case may only be closed if made by a unanimous decision, but where a panel comprises more than two screeners it may be made by a majority verdict. A Practice Committee may request screeners to mediate in a case and a panel shall then undertake mediation with the aim of dealing with an allegation without it being necessary for the case to reach the stage at which the Health Committee or Conduct and Competence Committee would arrange a hearing. There is no set procedure for the mediation.

Investigating Committee

The Investigating Committee (Article 26) investigates any allegation referred to it following a set procedure. If the Committee considers that there is a case to answer, it must notify in writing the registered professional concerned and the person making the allegation, giving reasons. It has powers, where it concludes that there is a case to answer, to undertake mediation or to refer the case to screeners for them to undertake mediation, or to the Health Committee or the Conduct and Competence Committee.

Rules of procedure for the Investigating Committee came into force on 9 July 2003[5] and were amended in 2005,[6] including provisions for vulnerable witnesses. Where an allegation is referred to the Committee it shall, at the same time that it sends the notice to the health professional, send her a copy of the standards of conduct, performance and ethics. The Investigating Committee can seek such advice or assistance as it thinks fit, but cannot interview the health professional unless she consents, or take account of any document or other material which the health professional has not had the opportunity to comment upon.

Conduct and Competence Committee

The Conduct and Competence Committee, after consultation with the other Practice Committees, shall consider:

- any allegation referred to it by the Council, screeners or the Investigating Committee of the Health Committee
- any application for restoration referred to it by the Registrar.

Procedure rules for the Conduct and Competence Committee came into force on 9 July 2003.[7](as amended by the Health Professions Council (Practice Committees and Registration) (Amendment) Rules 2005). The Conduct and Competence Committee can refer any allegation to the Health Committee (see below) where it appears to the Committee that an allegation which it is considering would be better dealt with by the Health Committee. The Rules cover the possibility of preliminary meetings in private with the parties concerned, and further investigations carried out by the Committee including:

- asking the health professional to provide a written description of his practice
- inspecting a sample of the health professional's patient or client records (this can only be carried out with the consent of the patient or client, unless the records are provided in a form from which the patient or client cannot be identified)
- inviting the health professional to take a test of competence
- interviewing the complainant, the health professional and any person nominated by the health professional.

Where the Committee has found that the health professional has failed to comply with the standards of conduct, performance and ethics established by the Council,[8] the Committee may take that failure into account, but such failure shall not be taken of itself to establish that the fitness to practise of the health professional is impaired.

The rules include the following provisions:

- The proceedings of the Conduct and Competence Committee shall be held in public unless the Committee is satisfied that, in the interests of justice or for the protection of the private life of the health professional, the complainant, any person giving evidence or of any patient or client, the public should be excluded from all or part of the hearing.
- The rules of admissibility of evidence in civil proceedings apply unless the Committee is satisfied that the admission of evidence is necessary in order to protect members of the public.
- Where the health professional has been convicted of a criminal offence, a certified copy of the certificate of conviction is admissible as proof of that conviction.

- The Committee may require evidence to be given on oath or affirmation.
- The Committee may adjourn the proceedings from time to time as it thinks fit and
- The Committee may exclude from the hearing any person whose conduct, in its opinion, is likely to disrupt the orderly conduct of the proceedings.
- The Committee may require any person (other than the health professional) to attend a hearing and give evidence or produce documents.
- The chairman shall explain the order of proceedings to the parties, and unless it is decided to the contrary, the following is the usual procedure:
  - The chairman invites the Presenting Officer to present the case against the health professional and to give the evidence in support of that case.
  - Any witnesses are called by the Presenting Officer, examined by him, cross-examined by the health professional or her representative, and may be re-examined by the solicitor and may be questioned by the Committee.
  - The health professional may address the Committee and give evidence on her fitness to practise.
  - Witnesses may be called by the health professional, examined in chief by the health professional or her representative, cross-examined by the solicitor, and re-examined by the health professional or her representative and may be questioned by the Committee.
  - The Presenting Officer may address the Committee again.
  - The health professional or her representative may address the Committee.
- Where the health professional is neither present nor represented at a hearing, the Committee may nevertheless proceed with the hearing if it is satisfied that all reasonable steps have been taken to serve the notice of hearing.
- The Committee is required to notify the health professional and complainant of its decision and the reasons for reaching that decision and shall inform the health professional of her right to appeal.
- Proceedings for hearing applications for restoration to the Register are also established.

In 2005 the rules were amended to include provision for the protection of vulnerable witnesses, i.e.:

(a) any witness under the age of 17 at the time of the hearing;
(b) any witness with a mental disorder within the meaning of the Mental Health Act 1983;
(c) any witness who is significantly impaired in relation to intelligence and social functioning;
(d) any witness with physical disabilities who requires assistance to give evidence;
(e) any witness, where the allegation against the practitioner is of a sexual nature and the witness was the alleged victim; and
(f) any witness who complains of intimidation.

The Committee, after consulting the legal assessor, may adopt such measures as it considers desirable to enable it to receive evidence from a vulnerable witness. The measures adopted by the Committee may include, but shall not be limited to:

(a) use of video links;
(b) use of pre-recorded evidence as the evidence-in-chief of a witness, provided that the witness is available at the hearing for cross-examination and questioning by the Committee;
(c) use of interpreters (including signers and translators) or intermediaries;
(d) use of screens or such other measures as the Committee consider necessary in the circumstances, in order to prevent—
    (i)   the identity of the witness being revealed to the press or the general public; or
    (ii) access to the witness by the health professional; and
(e) the hearing of evidence by the Committee in private.

(4)   Where—
 (a)   the allegation against a health professional is based on facts which are sexual in nature;
 (b)   a witness is an alleged victim; and
 (c)   the health professional is acting in person,
 the health professional shall only be allowed to cross-examine the witness in person with the written consent of the witness.

(5)   If, in the circumstances set out in paragraph (4) a witness does not provide written consent, the health professional shall, not less than seven days before the hearing, appoint a legally qualified person to cross-examine the witness on his behalf and, in default, the Council shall appoint such a person on behalf of the health professional.

Health Committee

The Health Committee shall consider any allegation referred to it by the Council, screeners, the Investigating Committee or the Conduct and Competence Committee and also any application for restoration referred to it by the Registrar; Article 29 sets out the procedure to be followed. Procedural rules for the Health Committee have been established by Order in Council and came into force on 9 July 2003.[9] Amendments were made in 2005 which came into force in January 2006.[10] These rules cover the service of documents, the power of the Health Committee to refer a case to the Conduct and Competence Committee, and the action to be taken by the Health Committee if an allegation is referred to it. Its powers are similar to that of the Conduct and Competence Committee (see above) but in addition it can invite the health professional to undergo a medical examination by a registered medical practitioner nominated by the Health Committee. The usual order of proceedings of the Health Committee is similar to that of the Conduct and Competence Committee. The Health Committee can also hear the case in the absence of the health professional if it is satisfied that all reasonable steps have been taken to serve notice on the health professional. A similar procedure is established for the Health Committee to hear applications for restoration to the Register. New rules for dealing with vulnerable witnesses (see above) also apply to the Health Committee.

Guidance for Practice Committees

The HPC's Practice Committees have issued a series of practice notes providing guidance on specific topics. These include:

- Unrepresented Parties
- Self-referrals
- Production of Information and Documents and Summonsing witnesses
- Proceeding in the Absence of the Registrant
- Joinder
- Finding that Fitness to Practise is Impaired
- Conducting Hearings in Private
- Allegations and the Standard of Acceptance for Allegations
- Concurrent Court Proceedings
- Case to answer
- Cross-Examination in Cases of a Sexual Nature
- Disposal of Cases via Consent
- Hearing locations

- Case management and directions
- Service of documents
- Use of Welsh in Fitness to Practise Proceedings
- Postponement and Adjournment of Proceedings
- Mediation
- Interim orders
- Preliminary hearings
- Powers to Require the Disclosure of Information
- Assessors and expert witnesses
- Restoration to the Register
- Indicative Sanctions Policy

Assessors

Articles 30–35 cover further procedural details, including the appointment of legal assessors who have the general function of giving advice to screeners, the statutory committees or the Registrar on questions of law. Rules relating to legal assessors came into force on 9 July 2003.[11] These require any advice given by the legal assessor to be given in the presence of every party, or person representing a party, in attendance at the hearing, unless the Council or Committee has begun to deliberate on its decisions and considers that it would be prejudicial to the discharge of its functions for the advice to be tendered in the presence of the parties or their representatives. In this latter case, as soon as possible after completion of the deliberations, the legal assessor is required to inform the parties of the advice he gave and subsequently record that advice in writing. Where the Council fails to accept the advice of the legal assessor, a record shall be made of the advice and a copy of that given to the parties.

Medical assessors can also be appointed to give relevant advice. Additional rules relating to the functions of assessors came into force on 9 July 2003[12] and these enable legal and medical assessors to be present at any Part V hearing by a Practice Committee or at any appeal hearing held by the Council. The legal assessor, if present, can inform the Practice Committee or Council of any irregularity in its consideration of the matter or in the conduct of the proceedings; the medical assessor, if present, can advise if it appears to him that, without his advice, a mistake may be made in judging the medical significance of information or the absence of information.

Appeals

An appeal from any decision of a Practice Committee lies to an appropriate court. Earlier proposals for the establishment of a Health Professions Independent Appeals Tribunal were not contained in the final order.

Fitness to practise

This is defined by the HPC as involving more than just competence in a registrant's chosen profession. It also includes health and character as well as the necessary skills and knowledge to do their job safely and effectively. Registrants must also be trusted to do their job legally.[13] Impairment of fitness to practise may include: misconduct, lack of competence, a conviction or caution for a criminal offence, the physical or mental health of the registrant and a decision reached by another regulatory responsible for healthcare. Anonymous complaints may be considered if they relate to serious and credible concerns about a registrant's fitness to practise and the HPC considers that it is appropriate to take further action. Information has been provided by the HPC for employers on the Fitness to Practise process.[14]

In the Annual Fitness Report of the HPC for 2007/8 there were 45 allegations against occupational therapists 11% of the total allegations made to the HPC. There were 28,006 number of OT registrants which formed 16% of total number on the HPC register. Complaints may come from a variety of sources including members of the public, other registrants, patients and their families, employers, managers and the police. The figures for OTs in the report for 2007/8 were 23 allegations came from the public; 12 from the employer; 2 from the police; 4 from anonymous sources ; 0 from a professional body and 4 from other sources.

The full details of the cases can be seen on the HPC website. Here are a few examples of cases heard in the past few years.

One Scottish OT was suspended by the HPC following an investigation into the following allegations:

1. poor communication skills, in that she:
    a) was unable to give concise patient reports to nursing staff;
    b) struggled to provide information to other health professionals about patients she had assessed;
    c) failed to request sufficient information of patients and other health professionals to effectively prioritise her case load;
    d) failed to ask questions or seek feedback of her supervisor to improve her understanding of occupational therapy practises; and
    e) gave poor explanations to patients regarding:
        (i)   diagnosis of their condition; and
        (ii) the reason(s) for conducting an assessment.
2. a lack of awareness regarding the importance of:
    a) identifying patients who were almost ready for discharge;
    b) timely referral of patients to outside agencies; and
    c) patient education in:
        (i)   the use of dressing aids; and
        (ii) safety.
3. poor clinical practise, in that she:
    a) was unable to correctly highlight hip precautions to patients;
    b) required prompting and instruction to understand the referral process; and
    c) experienced difficulty in modifying standard treatment plans to suit the needs of complex patients.
4. poor record keeping skills, in that:
    a) she often recorded incomplete personal information of her patients (for example, failing to record DOB, next of kin, address);
    b) she often failed to record the patient's medical history;
    c) her reports were often unrepresentative of the assessments she had carried out; and
    d) her reports often:
        (i)   omitted important information;
        (ii) contained no apparent conclusions; and
        (iii) contained no treatment plan.
5. poor understanding of:
    a) basic physiological terminology; and
    b) the theoretical concepts underpinning occupational therapy.
6. poor time management in regards to:

a) the time taken to complete patient notes;
b) prioritisation of her case load;

The case was heard in her absence as permitted according to the rules, the OT being represented by her parents, since she was abroad.

Not all allegations are established and in one case where allegations were made against an OT that she used inappropriate methods of intervention with a patient, by using: (i) unnecessary administration of medication; and (ii) inappropriate restraint in spraying water over the patient with a hose; and addressed the patient and her colleagues using inappropriate language, the Committee found that the allegations were not well-founded.

In May 2009 the Investigating Committee removed a registrant's name from the register on the grounds that the registrant's UK course was not an approved course for entry on to the register, which was made in error. Her application should have been considered as an International application.

A conditions of practice order was made against an OT whose fitness to practise as a registered health professional was impaired by reason of her physical and/or mental health in that she had an alcohol dependence condition.

An OT who worked in London was struck off the register in January 2009 on the basis of the following allegations, which were established and held to be evidence of impaired fitness to practise by virtue of his misconduct and or lack of competence in that:

1. At all material times he was employed as an occupational therapist by Enfield Council and in the course of this employment.
2. His documentation keeping was below the standard expected of registered occupational therapist in that he:
   (a) did not update his files with all relevant documentation
   (b) did not keep movement sheets and diary entries up to date.
3. His clinical reasoning was below the standard expected of registered occupational therapist in that he:
   (a) in relation to Service User 1, used overly vague sentences to describe her needs
   (b) in relation to Service User 5, did not adequately identify the service user's abilities and difficulties
   (c) in relation to Service User 16, failed to describe how the service user managed on a day-to-day basis
   (d) in relation to Service User 37, failed to accurately record the service user's medical needs.
4. His implementation of identified areas of intervention was below the standard expected of registered occupational therapist in that he:
   (a) in relation to Service User 2, did not adequately follow up the service user's need for a grab-rail
   (b) in relation to Service User 5, took no action with regards to the service user's identified toileting difficulties.

In its discussion in its annual report for 2007/8 on registrants who had been struck off, the HPC noted that the original panel in the case of an occupational therapist determined that the Registrant's fitness to practise was impaired because of her police cautions for shoplifting.

The registrant had not provided the review panel with information to show that she had addressed any of the issues that had lead to her suspension. It was therefore considered that striking off was the appropriate sanction. In the case of another occupational therapist the original panel suspended her following her two convictions for driving a motor vehicle with excess alcohol. Both incidents involved a collision and the second offence was committed whilst being disqualified from driving. Since the original order of suspension the Registrant had made no contact with the HPC. As a result of this there was no evidence that the registrant had addressed the situation and taken any steps towards rehabilitation and she was struck off.

In April 2008 an OT was struck off for failure to report that a patient had reported that she had been subjected to sexual assault by another patient and she also had breached patient confidentiality by telling a patient about another patient crying when they visited the supermarket as part of an assessment. The panel found that she also deliberately and wilfully failed to engage in supervision from the start to the end of her employment with the trust. This is a breach of the standards of proficiency for occupational therapists as well as the HPC's Standards of conduct, performance and ethics. Eventually her failure to engage led to her being removed from her clinical duties. She did not attend the hearing and was not represented. The panel decided the appropriate sanction was to strike her name from the Register.

In January 2008 an OT was suspended for a year. The panel had received verbal and written evidence from four witnesses concerning the registrant's competency in documentation. The evidence demonstrated an inadequacy in recording ability affecting timeliness, accuracy, completeness, lack of clarity and brevity observed in a wide range of documentation types. The panel was also presented with considerable verbal and written evidence of the registrant's lack of clinical reasoning, time management and communication skills.

In October 2008 an OT who was on gardening leave from the Trust was suspended from practising for one year for attempting to make contact with patients while under the influence of alcohol.

Council for Healthcare Regulatory Excellence (CHRE)

The HPC is obliged to inform the Council for Healthcare Regulatory Excellence (CHRE) (see Chapter 3) about cases which have been considered by the panels of the CCC not to be well founded. The CHRE has the power to refer to the High Court those cases in which it considers that the regulatory body has dealt unduly leniently with an allegation of unfitness to practise. For example the Conduct and Competence Committee of the HPC had cautioned a locum physiotherapist who had behaved inappropriately with a female and also smelt of alcohol. The CHRE referred the case to the High Court under S 29 of the NHS Reform and Healthcare Professions Act 2002 on the grounds that the sanction imposed was unduly lenient and did not protect the public interest.[15] It was agreed that the caution would be quashed and the case remitted to the Conduct and Competence Committee for further reconsideration and a redetermination of the sanction. There was then a dispute over costs which the CHRE won. In contrast where the CHRE appealed in a case where a paediatric nurse was given a caution for accessing sexually explicit and/or offensive websites whilst at work, arguing that the sanction was unduly lenient and did not protect the public interest, it was held that the court would not interfere with the penalty ordered.[16] The CHRE also lost a case brought against the GMC following the suspension of a doctor for misconduct of a sexual nature. The High Court held that the Panel had reached a conclusion which was open to it and the doctor would have to satisfy the next Panel that he may properly be restored to the Register, with or without conditions, and the Panel has imposed quite stringent requirements in that regard as to what is to be expected at that review.[17] The CHRE also appealed the decision by the professional conduct committee (PCC) of the GMC in relation to misconduct of Dr Southall, a paediatrician who had given evidence in the case brought against Sally Clarke who was convicted of murdering her two children.[18] The Court held that to impose conditions upon Professor Southall's registration was not unduly lenient. Striking off the register was not required. However the PCC did show undue leniency in the form of the condition and in failing to give an intimation in accordance with Rule 31(5) and the case was remitted to the PCC to impose appropriate conditions.

Interim orders

If the investigating panel feels that the allegation is serious enough that the public might need some type of immediate protection, the panel might make an application for an interim order. A hearing will then take place often at short notice. The panel will consist of a chair person, a person in the same profession as the registrant under investigation, and a lay person and a legal assessor. In hearings of the health committee, a registered doctor will also be on the panel. The solicitor for the HPC will present the case calling witnesses to support the allegation. The registrant or their representative may cross-examine the witnesses. The panel may ask questions. The registrant will then present his or her case calling witnesses and/or making statements to the panel. If the allegation is considered to be proven the panel will declare it to be well-founded.

Sanctions available

- No further action to be taken.
- Mediation. (A consensual process appropriate where issues between the health professionals are unresolved. Only available if the alternative would be no further action.)
- Caution order (can last for between 1 to 5 years).
- Conditions of practice order. (For a specific period not exceeding 3 years. It could require supervised practice and/or further training.)
- Suspend registration (for a specified period, up to a year).
- Striking off order. (Only imposed in very serious circumstances in order to protect the public. It may not be made in respect of an allegation relating to competence or health unless the registrant has been continuously suspended, or subject to a conditions of practice order, for a period of two years at the date of the decision to strike off. Striking off is a sanction of last resort for serious, deliberate or reckless acts involving abuse of trust such as sexual abuse, dishonesty or persistent clinical failure. Striking off should be used where there is no other way to protect the public, for example, where there is a lack of insight, continuing problems or denial.)

Guidance for panel members on the sanctions to be imposed was given by the HPC in September 2007[19] and updated in December 2008.[20] The HPC emphasises that the sanctions are not intended to be punitive. Panels must give appropriate weight to the wider public interest considerations, which include:

- the deterrent effect to other health professionals
- the reputation of the profession concerned and
- public confidence in the regulatory process.

In deciding what, if any, sanction to impose, Panels should apply the principle of proportionality, balancing the interests of the public with those of the registrant.

Review of Conditions of practice or suspension order

These orders will be reviewed shortly before they are due to end. In the case of a conditions or practice order, the review panel will look for evidence that the registrant has met the conditions such as a report from a supervisor or evidence that the registrant has received further training. In the case of a suspension order, the review panel will look for evidence that the problems which led to the suspension have now been dealt with. The panel must be satisfied that the public is adequately protected. If they are not satisfied they could continue the conditions of practice or suspension order or they could replace the suspension order with a conditions of practice order. If they feel that a registrant has not met the terms of a conditions of practice order, they could replace it by a suspension order or by a striking off order. The following list summarises the action which the review panel can take.

- confirm the order
- extend the period for which the order has effect (but a conditions of practice order may not be extended by more than three years at a time or a suspension order by more than one year at a time)
- replace the order with one it could have made at the time it made the order being reviewed
- make a conditions of practice order which takes effect when a suspension order expires
- reduce the duration of an order (but a caution order may not be reduced to a duration of less than one year)
- revoke or vary any condition imposed by the order
- revoke the order.

Review of striking off order and restoration on the register

Article 33(2) of the Health Professions Order 2001 specifies that, unless new evidence comes to light, an application for restoration to the register may not be made within 5 years of the date of the order.

The HPC and Employers

The HPC would expect co-operation from employers in relation to the fitness to practice of registered professionals and it has provided information for employers on the Fitness to Practise process.[21] Employers would be expected to inform the HPC if disciplinary proceedings are being taken against a registrant and there is evidence to suggest that a person's ability to practice their profession may be impaired. Other registrants have a duty under the HPC Standards of Conduct, Performance and Ethics to bring concerns about a fellow registrant to the attention of the HPC. The HPC would seek to work with employers on a collaborative, case by case basis. The HPC has statutory powers to compel those involved (other than the registrant) to provide information and it is a criminal offence to refuse to do so. It is therefore able to pursue lines of inquiry which may not be open to an employer.[22]

Code of ethics and professional practice

Health Professions Council standards of conduct, performance and ethics

The HPC published standards of conduct, performance and ethics for its registered practitioners in 2003. In 2006 it decided to review the standards to ensure they continued to be fit for purpose and that they conformed to the expectations of the public, registrants and other stakeholders. A consultation document was published on the revised standards which had been drawn up on the basis of the following broad principles that the standards should:

- focus where possible on providing guidance to registrants based on our expectations of their behaviour;
- be based on over-arching principles with some further detail on key points (with more detailed guidance available elsewhere, if necessary);
- be applicable to all registrants (as far as possible) including those engaged in research, clinical practice, education and roles in industry; and
- be written in broad terms to accommodate changes in best practice, technology, legislation and in wider society.

Following the consultation a revised standards of conduct, performance and ethics came into force in July 2008.[23] The new standards expand on 14 duties of the registrant which are:

1. You must act in the best interests of service users.
2. You must respect the confidentiality of service users.
3. You must keep high standards of personal conduct.
4. You must provide (to us and to any other relevant statutory regulator) any important information about conduct and competence.
5. You must keep your professional knowledge and skills up-to-date.
6. You must act within the limits of your knowledge, skills and experience and, if necessary, refer the matter to another practitioner.
7. You must communicate properly and effectively with service users and other practitioners.
8. You must effectively supervise tasks that you have asked others to carry out.
9. You must get informed consent to give treatment (except in an emergency).
10. You must keep accurate records.
11. You must deal fairly and safely with the risks of infection.
12. You must limit your work or stop practising if your performance or judgment is affected by your health.
13. You must behave with honesty and integrity and make sure that your behaviour does not damage the public's confidence in you and your profession.
14. You must make sure that any advertising is accurate.

These standards of conduct, performance and ethics are accompanied by standards of proficiency published by the HPC and also available on its website.

British Association of Occupational Therapists (BAOT) and College of Occupational Therapists (COT)

The British Association of Occupational Therapists (BAOT) is the central organisation for OTs throughout the UK. The College of Occupational Therapists (COT) is the subsidiary organisation, with delegated responsibility for the promotion of good practice and the prevention of malpractice. The COT has an important role to play both in the setting and maintenance of educational standards which is discussed in the next chapter, and in the preparation of standards on professional practice and ethics. Its Code of Ethics and Professional Conduct is considered below. In 2002 the COT started the task of reviewing its publications that support excellence in practice.

Professional Standards for Occupational Therapy Practice were revised in 2007[24] and together with the standard statements[25] are seen as central to all practising occupational therapists. The Standards are usable as an audit tool and are worded in terminology that is in keeping with the social model of disability and the World Health Organisation's International Classification of Functioning, Disability and Health. They cover the following topics:

- referral
- consent
- assessment and goal setting
- intervention and evaluation
- discharge, closure or transfer of care
- record keeping
- service quality and governance
- professional development/lifelong learning
- practice placements
- safe working practice
- research ethics.

These standards are supplemented by clinical guidelines or practice guidance for a particular clinical area or care group but used at national level. They are at the time of writing being reviewed and a think tank/workshop at COT was held in December 2009 to gain feedback from Members to help inform the revision of the standards. The finalised standards are due to be published in 2011.

Clinical guidelines will outline the nature and level of intervention that is considered best practice for specific conditions in specific settings and would be systematically developed, evidence-based statements that assist occupational therapists and service users in making decisions about appropriate health and social interventions for a specific condition or population, incorporating and abiding by the Core Professional Standards.[26] The COT assists the specialist groups in the development of clinical guidelines and has set criteria for the establishment of these specialist groups.

Practice guidance is intended to guide the practitioner as to best practice, but does not meet the strict criteria of clinical guidelines. Information briefings, statements and fact sheets are also published by the COT to enable OTs to remain informed and aware of changes and developments as they occur. Local information, such as care pathways, has also been developed, published and implemented. Many of these publications are referred to in the relevant chapters of this book.

Code of Ethics and Professional Conduct for OTs

A new Code of Ethics and Professional Conduct for OTs was produced in 2000 and revised in 2005[27] by the College of Occupational Therapists on behalf of the British Association of Occupational Therapists. The COT has delegated responsibility from the BAOT for the promotion of good practice and the prevention of malpractice. Work has started on the review of the Code of Ethics and this will be published in 2010. At the time of writing a first draft is being drawn up for discussion at the next reference group meeting in November 2009. Following this a consultation draft will be available in Jan 2010.

Contents of the Code

The Code covers the topics set out in Figure 4.1.

Status of the Code

The Code is not law in the sense that a breach of its provisions would lead to criminal or civil proceedings, but it could be used in evidence in conduct and competence hearings or other proceedings

---

Figure 4.1   Contents of the Code of Ethics and Professional Conduct.

Section 1   Introduction

Section 2   Client Autonomy and Welfare: Respecting the autonomy of the client; Duty of care to the client; Confidentiality and Protecting clients

Section 3   Services to the Client: Referral of clients; Provision of services to clients and Record keeping

Section 4   Personal/Professional Integrity: Personal and professional integrity; Professional demeanour; Fitness to practise; Substance misuse; Personal profit or gain; Advertising and Information and representation

Section 5   Professional Competence and Standards: Professional competence; Delegation; Collaborative working; Lifelong learning; Occupational therapy student education and Research and service development

---

where the activities of an OT were in question. It is stated that any action which is in breach of the purpose and intent of the Code shall be considered unethical. It is recommended that employers should incorporate the Code in the contracts of employment of OTs (Para. 1.2). This means that should the OT become involved in disciplinary proceedings with her employer as a result of her attempt to follow and implement the Code, it will be recognised that she had a professional and a contractual duty to take that course of action. Such a contract term may also lead to the employer's recognition of the professional duties which the OT must observe.

Post-registration control and supervision

Once OTs are qualified and registered they are professionally accountable for their actions and are not subject to any system of professional supervision such as that which applies to midwifery. They are expected to provide the reasonable standard of care the patient is entitled to (see Chapter 10) and it would be no defence for them to argue that they were only recently qualified and that was why negligence occurred. In practice, of course, senior colleagues provide support for junior staff and would ensure that some form of supervision and training were in place. It is, however, more difficult in those work areas where an OT is working on her own. The Code of Ethics and Professional Conduct places a duty upon OTs:

> Occupational Therapists shall achieve and continuously maintain high standards of competence in their knowledge, skills and behaviour (Para. 5.1.1)

To fulfil this duty:

> each member of the occupational therapy profession has a duty to maintain their level of professional competence and to work to current legislation, guidance and standards relevant to their practice. This includes compliance with the HPC's current *Standards of Proficiency – Occupational Therapists.* (5.1.2).

Under Paragraph 5.1.5

> Occupational therapy personnel seeking to work in areas with which they are unfamiliar or in which their experience has not been recent, shall ensure that adequate self-directed learning takes place as well as other relevant training and supervision.

Clinical supervision is considered in Chapter 26. Schemes for continuing education and training are considered in Chapter 5.

Off Duty

There has been uncertainty over whether the provisions of the Codes of Practice apply when health-care professionals are off duty. The HPC has answered any such uncertainties very emphatically when it held that an off duty paramedic was guilty of misconduct when he refused to assist a man with a broken back. The HPC did not however strike him off because his fitness to practise was not compromised.[28]

Sexual boundaries

The Council for Healthcare Regulatory Excellence published in January 2008 guidance on Clear sexual boundaries between healthcare professionals and patients: responsibilities of healthcare professionals which can be down loaded from its website. It explains why the guidance is necessary; how breaches of sexual boundaries can be avoided; reporting problems and good practice in maintaining healthcare professional/patient relationships. An appendix gives examples of sexualised behaviour by healthcare professionals towards patients or their carers. The HPC summaries the guidance as follows:

> Healthcare professionals must not display sexualised behaviour towards patients or their carers, because doing so can cause significant and enduring harm. The healthcare professional/patient relationship depends on confidence and trust. A healthcare professional who displays sexualised behaviour towards a patient breaches that trust, acts unprofessionally, and may, additionally, be committing a criminal act. Breaches of sexual boundaries by health professionals can damage confidence in healthcare professionals generally and leads to a diminution in trust between patients, their families and healthcare professionals.

In addition, as seen in the cases before the Conduct and Competence Committee, failure to maintain appropriate sexual barriers could be evidence of lack of fitness to practise.

Receiving gifts

Client may frequently wish to show their appreciation of OT services by presenting personal gifts to the OT, who may feel it offensive to refuse. However this is a minefield of potential problems. Paragraph 4.5 of the Code of Ethics and Professional Conduct of the COT (2005) covers personal profit or gain and advises that

> Occupational therapy personnel shall not accept tokens such as favours, gifts or hospitality from clients, their families or commercial organisations when this might be construed as seeking to obtain preferential treatment.

The duty of care to the client should not be influenced by any commercial or other interest that conflicts with this duty (see also Chapter 10 and the law relating to property).

The HPC Code[29] requires the registered practitioner or the prospective registrant under principle 3 to keep high standards of personal conduct; under principle 14 to behave with integrity and honesty and under principle 17 to make sure that her behaviour does not damage her profession's reputation – all of which could relate to the unauthorised receipt of gifts.

OTS should be aware of any policy prepared by their employer on the acceptance of gifts and other forms of appreciation. If a patient indicates that he or she wished to make a bequest in a will, the solicitors of the trust should be involved to ensure that there is no question of undue influence and that the patient receives independent advice.

Insurance and indemnity

It is essential that any OT should ensure that she is covered in relation to the possibility of claims for compensation. If she is employed she will be covered by the vicarious liability (see Chapter 10) of the employer, provided that the harm occurs while she is working in the course of employment. However, where she works outside the course of employment or as a self-employed OT, she would be personally responsible for the payment of any compensation (see further Chapter 10 on negligence and Chapter 28 on independent practice).

For details on education reference should be made to Chapter 5 and for the law relating to teaching and research, Chapter 26. The scope of professional practice and the legal implications are considered in chapter 10.

Conclusions

Standards of professional practice are constantly being raised and the onus is on the professional personally to ensure that her competence is maintained and that she upholds the reasonable standards of professional practice. She therefore has the responsibility of ensuring that she obtains the necessary training and instruction to remain competent and to develop safely in new areas of practice. Re-registration will require evidence on ongoing professional development. High standards of professional practice are central to the Government's plan for the NHS.[30] As a consequence of the Health and Social Care Act 2008 an Office of Health Professions Adjudicator will be established with power to set up Fitness to Practice panels. This major reform may eventually be applied to the registration bodies for other healthcare professions.

 Questions and exercises

1 A colleague tells you that she has been reported to the HPC for professional misconduct. Advise her on the procedure that will be followed and how she could defend herself.
2 Do you consider that the following conduct by a registered OT should be the subject of conduct and competence proceedings:
   ● accepting a gift from a client
   ● a parking fine
   ● an offence of shop-lifting
   ● being cited in a divorce as an adulterer
   ● being found guilty of a breach of the peace following a New Year's Eve party?
3 Explain the legal situation in relation to insurance cover for an employed and a self-employed OT (see also Chapters 10 and 28).

References

1   Health Professions Council Order 2001, 2002/254.
2   The Health Professions Council (Practice Committees) (Constitution) Rules, Order of Council 2003, SI 2003/1209.
3   The Health Professions Council (Practice Committees (Constitution) and Miscellaneous Amendments) Rules 2009 SI 1355.
4   The Health Professions Council (Screeners) Rules, Order of Council 2003, SI 2003/1573.
5   The Health Professions Council (Investigating Committee) (Procedure) Rules, Order of Council 2003, SI 2003/1574.
6   The Health Professions Council (Practice Committees and Registration) (Amendment) Rules 2005, SI. 2005/1625.
7   The Health Professions Council (Conduct and Competence Committee) (Procedure) Rules, Order of Council 2003, SI 2003/1575.
8   Health Professions Council (2004 revised 2007) Standards of conduct, performance and ethics. HPC, London.
9   The Health Professions Council (Health Committee) (Procedure) Rules, Order of Council 2003, SI 2003/1576.
10   The Health Professions Council (Practice Committees and Registration) (Amendment) Rules 2005, SI.2005/1625.
11   The Health Professions Council (Legal Assessors) Rules, Order of Council 2003, SI 2003/1578.
12   The Health Professions Council (Functions of Assessors) Rules, Order of Council 2003, SI 2003/1577.
13   www.hpc-uk.org/complaints
14   The Health Professions Council (2007) The Fitness to Practise Process. HPC, London.
15   *R (on the application of Council for the Regulation of Healthcare Professionals) v Health Professions Council & Anor* [2006] EWHC 890 (Admin) (30 March 2006).
16   *Council for the Regulation of Healthcare Professionals v Nursing and Midwifery Council* [2004] EWHC 585 (Admin) (31 March 2004).
17   *R (on the application of Council for the Regulation of Healthcare Professionals) v General Medical Council & Anor* [2009] EWHC 596 (Admin) (02 March 2009).
18   *Council for the Regulation of Healthcare Professionals v General Medical Council & Anor* [2005] EWHC 579 (Admin) (14 April 2005).
19   Health Professions Council (2007) Indicative Sanctions Policy. HPC, London.
20   Health Professions Council (2008) *Practice Note: Indicative Sanctions Policy.*
21   Health Professions Council (2007) *Fitness to Practice Process.* HPC, London.
22   www.hpc-uk.org/complaints/
23   Health Professions Council (2008) Standards of conduct, performance and ethics. HPC, London.
24   College of Occupational Therapists (2007) *Professional Standards for Occupational Therapy Practice.* COT, London.
25   College of Occupational Therapists (2007) *Standard Statements.* COT, London.
26   College of Occupational Therapists (2002) *Information and Resources in Support of Excellence in Practice.* COT, London.
27   College of Occupational Therapists (2005) *Code of Ethics and Professional Conduct for Occupational Therapists.* COT, London.
28   News item. Paramedic disciplined. The Times 27 February 2009.
29   Health Professions Council (2008) Standards of conduct, performance and ethics. HPC, London.
30   Department of Health (2000) *NHS Plan.* DH, London.

5 Education and Training

This chapter is concerned with the statutory provisions for controlling the education of the occupational therapist (OT) both pre and post-registration. The following topics are covered:

- Health Professions Council
- Quality Assurance Agency Higher Education (QAA)
- Role of the College of Occupational Therapists

Health Professions Council

The Health Professions Council was launched in April 2002 replacing the Council for Professions Supplementary to Medicine and its Professional Boards (see Chapter 3). The year April 2002–3 was a transitional year while the new regulatory arrangements were put in place. Under the Health Act 1999 one of the statutory duties of the HPC that is not transferable by Order to another body is the determining of standards of education and training for admission to practice.

Education and Training Committee

One of the statutory committees which must be set up by the Health Professions Council is an Education and Training Committee. This advises the Council on the performance of the Council's functions in relation to:

- establishing standards of proficiency
- establishing standards and requirements in respect of education and training for both registration and continuing professional development (CPD)
- giving guidance on education and training standards to registrants, employers and others.

Legal Aspects of Occupational Therapy, Third Edition By Bridgit Dimond
© 2010 Bridgit Dimond

The Council is required to establish from time to time:

- the standards of education and training necessary to achieve the standards of proficiency it has established
- the requirements to be satisfied for admission to such education and training, which may include requirements as to good health and good character.

The Education and Training Committee shall ensure that universities and other institutions are notified of the standards and requirements, and shall take appropriate steps to satisfy itself that those standards and requirements are met. The Education and Training Committee can approve courses of education or training, qualifications, institutions, and such tests of professional competence, education, training and experience as would lead to the award of additional qualifications which would be recorded in the register. The Council is required to publish a statement of the criteria that will be taken into account in deciding whether to give approval. The Council is also required to maintain and publish a list of the courses of education or training, qualifications and institutions which are or were approved under the Order.

The HPC has set out the standards it considers necessary for safe and effective practice under each part of the HPC Register. The standards of proficiency required for the registration of an occupational therapist can be seen in full on the HPC website.[1] The foreword to the standards of proficiency states that they are:

> A vital tool for the Council as it seeks to protect the public by ensuring that its registrants are safe and effective in their practice.

The Standards of Proficiency for the occupational therapist distinguish between generic standards which are written in black and profession-specific standards which are written in blue. In brief they cover the following areas:

1. Professional autonomy and accountability. The OT must:
   - (a) (1) be able to practise within the legal and ethical boundaries of their profession
     - (2) be able to practise in a non-discriminatory manner
     - (3) be able to maintain confidentiality and obtain informed consent
     - (4) be able to exercise a professional duty of care
     - (5) know the limits of their practice and when to seek advice
     - (6) recognise the need for effective self-management of workload and be able to practise accordingly
     - (7) understand the obligation to maintain fitness to practice
     - (8) understand the need for career-long self-directed learning.
   - (b) Professional relationships:
     - (1) know the professional and personal scope of their practice and be able to make referrals
     - (2) be able to work, where appropriate, in partnership with other professionals, support staff, patients, clients and users and their relatives and carers
     - (3) be able to contribute effectively to work undertaken as part of a multi-disciplinary team
     - (4) be able to demonstrate effective and appropriate skills in communicating information, advice, instruction and professional opinion to colleagues, patients, clients, users, their relatives and carers
     - (5) understand the need for effective communication throughout the care of the patient, client or user.

2. Skills required for the application of practice. The OT must:
   (a) (1) be able to gather information
       (2) be able to use appropriate assessment techniques
       (3) be able to undertake or arrange clinical investigations as appropriate
       (4) be able to analyse and evaluate the information collected.
   (b) Formulation and delivery of plans and strategies for meeting health and social care needs:
       (1) be able to use research, reasoning and problem-solving skills (and in the case of clinical scientists, conduct fundamental research)
       (2) be able to draw on appropriate knowledge and skills in order to make professional judgements
       (3) be able to formulate specific and appropriate management plans including the setting of time-scales
       (4) be able to conduct appropriate diagnostic or monitoring procedures, treatment therapy or other actions safely and skilfully
       (5) be able to maintain records appropriately.
   (c) Critical evaluation of the impact of, or response to, the registrant's actions:
       (1) be able to monitor and review the ongoing effectiveness of planned activity and modify it accordingly
       (2) be able to audit, reflect on and review practice.
3. Knowledge, understanding and skills. The OT must:
   (a) (1) know the key concepts of the biological, physical, social, psychological and clinical sciences which are relevant to their profession-specific practice
       (2) know how professional principles are expressed and translated into action through a number of different approaches to practice and how to select or modify approaches to meet the needs of an individual
       (3) understand the need to establish and maintain a safe practice environment.

The HPC has developed a general framework for standards for education and training for all professions registered under it. These were approved following a consultation exercise which began in March 2004 and ended on 31 May 2004. Each registered profession is expected to develop more specific education and training standards fitting in with the general framework. The HPC published its Standards of Education and Training guidance in 2009 which is available on its website. It describes these standards (SET) as being provided to give more information about how it will assess and monitor programmes against its standards. It is written for education providers who are preparing for an approval visit, for the major change process, or for its annual monitoring process. This document will also be useful for practice placement providers who education providers work with.
   The Standards cover the following topics

SET 1. Level of qualification for entry to the register
SET 2. Programme admissions
SET 3. Programme management and resources
SET 4. Curriculum
SET 5. Practice Placements
SET 6. Assessment

The HPC has also published supplementary information for education providers on annual monitoring.[2] This provides a flow chart, explains the monitoring process, provides assistance in completing the annual monitoring declaration form and the audit form.

In June 2009 the HPC published supplementary information for education providers on the approval process.[3] It sets out the detail of the process including pre-visit, visit and post visit information. All these HPC documents are available on its website.

The College of Occupational Therapists has published in 2004 a Curriculum Framework for Pre-Registration Education; Guidance on Disability and Learning in 2005; Accreditation of prior learning in 2006 and Pre-registration Education Standards in 2008 (see below).

Visitors

The Council may appoint persons, known as visitors, to visit any place or institution which gives or proposes to give a relevant course of education, examination or test of competence. A visitor cannot exercise these functions at any institution with which he has a significant connection, but could be a member of the Council or its committees, but not an employee of the Council. Visitors are to be selected with due regard to the profession they are to report on and at least one of the visitors shall be registered in the part of the Register which relates to that profession.

Any institution must give to the Education and Training Committee or Council

such information and assistance as the Committee may reasonably require in connection with the exercise of its functions under this Order.

Withdrawing approval

The Committee can refuse or withdraw approval of courses, qualifications and institutions. Where approval is withdrawn the Committee has to use its best endeavours to secure that any person who is undertaking the education or training concerned or studying for the qualification concerned is given the opportunity to follow the approved education or training or to study for an approved qualification at an approved institution. The procedures are designed to maintain standards but not disadvantage individuals who have the misfortune to be studying on a course or at an institution where approval is withdrawn.

Post-registration training

The Health Professions Council may make rules requiring registered professionals to undertake such continuing professional development (CPD) as it shall specify. The HPC defines CPD as

a range of learning activities through which health professionals maintain and develop throughout their career to ensure that they retain their capacity to practice safely, effectively and legally within their evolving scope of practice[4]

The HPC has published standards for CPD which are available from its website and monitors compliance with these standards through audit. From 1 July 2006 all registrants are required to engage in CPD and must record their activities in their portfolio and if selected for audit must complete the CPD profile which will then be assessed by CPD assessors.

The HPC decided in advance of its consultation on CPD that continuing professional development should:

- avoid monitoring registrants' compliance based simply on the number of hours undertaken each year
- be linked to national standards

- take account of the work of others, such as the Allied Health Professions' (AHP) project on demonstrating competence through CPD that is already being undertaken
- take account of the needs of part-time and self-employed registrants
- require individual registrants to commit themselves to CPD.

The HPC published in 2008 for its registrants 2 documents "Continuing professional development and your registration" and "Your guide to our standards for continuing professional development". The publication sets 5 CPD standards which are as follows:
    A registrant must:

1. maintain a continuous, up-to-date and accurate record of their CPD activities;
2. demonstrate that their CPD activities are a mixture of learning activities relevant to current or future practice;
3. seek to ensure that their CPD has contributed to the quality of their practice and service delivery;
4. seek to ensure that their CPD benefits the service user; and
5. present a written profile containing evidence of their CPD upon request.

The first audit for CPD by OTs was in August 2009 and it is the HPC intention to audit each profession every two years. The guidance gives examples of work-based activity, professional activities, formal/educational activities self-directed learning and other activities which it would see as constituting CPD.
    In April 2007 the COT joined together with several health professional associations to publish a joint statement on continuing professional development for health and social care practitioners.[5] The aim of the joint statement was to influence health and social care policymakers, commissioners and employers to provide enhanced CPD support for health and social care practitioners. The document expected that a minimum 6 days (45 hours) per year for protected CPD time should be granted, above existing statutory and mandatory training and formal study leave arrangements. The time for CPD includes time for the documentation of learning outcomes, alongside direct involvement in CPD activities. The HPC and the COT published a CPD profile for an occupational therapist which is available online. It sets out the information which should be included in a profile.
    The COT published, following its position statement in 2002,[6] a strategic vision and action plan for lifelong learning in 2004 which stated that a commitment to support a culture of lifelong learning as being a continuum within academic, work and social environments.[7] In November 2006 it published a Post Qualifying Framework: a resource for occupational therapists which provides guidance for OTs on lifelong learning which includes interprofessional learning, and team-based learning and development and recognises the need to enable new and creative ways of working to develop.

Wales

The National Assembly for Wales is empowered to create or designate a body with whom the Council may enter into any arrangements for the approval of pre-registration courses etc. and the standards for continuing professional development under articles 16(5) and 20(4) respectively.

Quality Assurance Agency for Higher Education (QAA)

The QAA was set up in 1997 as an independent body funded by the universities and colleges of higher education, and through contracts with education funding bodies.[8] The QAA undertakes both institutional audits, developmental engagements to test out an organisation's internal review procedures and academic reviews at subject level. In addition it undertakes major reviews of NHS-funded healthcare programmes in England. It has issued a Code of Practice for the guidance of educational institutions on the management of academic standards and quality. The QAA published benchmark statements for occupational therapy in 2001 as part of a series of health subjects with a common professional framework.[9]

Approval of education providers and programmes

The Education Department of the HPC has since September 2004 been carrying out approval visits to education providers and programmes throughout the UK. A panel from the HPC consisting of one education executive and two visitors – at least one of whom is from the same part of the Register as the professional with which the programme is concerned. Following the visit the panel may recommend a programme to the Education and Training Committee for one of the following:

- to approve the programme
- to set conditions on the programme, all of which must be met before the programme can be approved
- to not approve the programme
- to withdraw approval of the programme.

In the event of either of the last two recommendations being made, the graduates of the programme will not be entitled to register with the HPC and as such will not be able to practise in the UK using one of the titles protected by the HPC.

A new approvals process has been introduced to allow an independent review of programmes for regulatory purposes and ensure rigour surrounding the outcomes of the approvals event. The HPC Visitors need to be satisfied that the education provider and its programmes meet the HPC Standards of Education and Training to ensure that graduates meet the HPC Standards of Proficiency to allow eligibility for registration with the HPC. The main areas where the new approvals process differs form the previous systems are:

- That, as far as possible, the new procedures will align with and build upon existing approval and quality assurance processes already used by education providers.
- Programmes will be approved on an open-ended basis subject to satisfactory annual monitoring returns. (The HPC reserves the right to visit a programme when problems are apparent.)
- The introduction of a unified approach to allow multiple-professional approvals to be incorporated into a single approvals event.
- Where required formal approval of new education providers will now be achieved at the same time as programme approval.
- Annual monitoring will adopt a lighter touch by reporting by exception and according to an education providers own annual monitoring timetable, using their own documentation where available.
- Following feedback from the HPC consultation process, Annual Monitoring Review will be extended to include Cyclical Review, which will take place according to the education providers own internal programme review timetable. No Annual Monitoring Report will be required in a year where Cyclical Review occurs.
- The HPC will no longer visit clinical/practice placements. Quality assurance of such placements will be the responsibility of the education provider, to be evidenced by the inclusion into an

education provider's own quality assurance mechanisms for QA systems which ensure that the HPC Standards of Education and Training and Standards of Proficiency are being met within clinical/practice placements. The HPC reserves the right to visit clinical/practice placements.

- The HPC will no longer approve the appointment of external examiners. Instead its Visitors will look for evidence that at least one external examiner is from the relevant part of the Register.

Higher Education Funding Council and Quality Assurance Agency

The Higher Education Funding Council which has the responsibility of providing public funds for teaching provision to colleges is also legally responsible for ensuring that the quality of education is assessed in the universities and colleges it funds. It therefore contracts with the Quality Assurance Agency on an annual basis to devise and implement quality assurance methods. The QAA reviews the quality of all publicly funded higher education teaching provision in England. The QAA carries out 2 methods of quality assurance: institutional audit in higher education institutions and an integrated Quality and Enhancement review of higher education delivered in further education colleges.

Department of Health

The Workforce Development Confederation of the Department of Health is responsible for undertaking and negotiating contracts for training within the NHS. Information on local Workforce Development Confederation (WDC) contacts can be obtained from the website.[10] The Quality Assurance Unit within the Department of Health works with the WDCs, regulatory and professional bodies and education providers to establish a shared framework for the quality assurance of healthcare education. The DH QA (education) team is initially focusing on NHS-funded professional education, nursing midwifery and allied health professional programmes.

The NHS Knowledge and Skills Framework and the Development Review Process

The NHS Knowledge and Skills Framework and the Development Review Process (NHS KSF)[11] was published in 2004. It defines and describes the knowledge and skills which NHS staff need to apply in their work in order to deliver quality services. It provides a single, consistent, comprehensive and explicit framework on which to base the review and development for all staff. It is at the heart of the career and pay progression strand of the Agenda for Change (see Chapter 19) It is made up of 6 core dimensions: communication; personal and people development; health, safety and security; service improvement; quality and equality and diversity. The other 24 dimensions are specific and are grouped under health and wellbeing; estates and facilities; information and technology and general. The purposes of the NHS KSF is to facilitate the development of services so that they better meet the needs of users and the public; support effective learning and development of individuals and teams; and promote equality for and diversity of all staff. A COT/BAOT briefing note no 31 provides guidance on the Knowledge and Skills framework for OT staff (February 2006) and briefing note no 108.[12]

Role of the College of Occupational Therapists (COT)

The Council of the COT prescribes qualifications for membership and approves the pre-registration courses which grant professional qualification. It maintains a register of institutions suitable for education and training in occupational therapy. It can also grant worldwide recognition of a course via the World Federation of Occupational Therapists (WFOT). In 2002 the WFOT published revised minimum standards for the education of occupational therapists.[13] These standards have four distinct but inter-related purposes, relating to societal, professional and educational purposes and for membership of the WFOT.

In the past when the approval of institutions to provide pre-registration courses for OTs was being considered a tripartite evaluation occurred, those taking part being representatives of the COT, the validating panel of the degree-awarding institution offering the course, and the HPC. The Joint Validation Committee (JVC) no longer operates but universities invite the COT to participate in the accreditation process so that successful completion of an approved course leads to eligibility for full membership of the COT/British Association of Occupational Therapists (BAOT), membership of the WFOT and registered status on the register maintained by the HPC.

The British Association of Occupational Therapists (BAOT)

The BAOT, of which the COT is the educational offshoot, is a professional, educational and trade union organisation for OTs and occupational therapy support staff in the UK. It has an agreement with UNISON, which undertakes industrial relations on its behalf. UNISON therefore negotiates improvements to pay and/or terms and conditions of employment locally and nationally on behalf of OTs and support workers.

The BAOT has a Council of elected members and a regional framework. It represents the views of its membership to Government, purchasers, other professional bodies, voluntary organisations and consumers. It also works closely through the WFOT and the Committee for Occupational Therapists in the European Community. The BAOT has also established a Disability Information and Study Centre (DISC) which provides post-registration clinical, management and research information and a database reference service.

Syllabus content, accreditation and quality assurance

Whilst the HPC has set pre-registration standards for pre-registration for all its registered professions, the COT has also published and continues to publish documents relating to standards of education. The statement on lifelong learning[14] produced by the College as well as setting minimum standards for pre-registration education, also sets standards for continuing professional development. A strategic vision and action plan for lifelong learning was published by the COT in 2004. The principles of the LifeLong Learning Statement have been incorporated into the Standards for Education: Preregistration Education (College of Occupational Therapists, June 2003 which were revised in 2008[15]). These set standards on:

1. programme management and resources standards
2. curriculum standards
3. learning, teaching and assessment standards
4. Quality Assurance and monitoring standards.

The Accreditation of pre-registration programmes in occupational therapy was published in 2005. A Curriculum Framework Document for Occupational Therapy Education initially published in 1998 was revised 2004 and again in 2009. The 2009 edition covers requirements relating to the European network for OT. Sustaining a high quality workforce is the subject of a joint publication of the COT and the DH.[16]

External placement for clinical training

Whilst the theoretical content of the training and education will take place largely within universities or colleges of higher education, it is necessary for the colleges to agree placements for clinical training and instruction with NHS trusts and social services departments (SSDs). A memorandum of agreement will be drawn up to set down the basic principles behind the placement. It should cover:

- the number of students to be taken by the trust/SSD
- the liability for any harm caused by the student
- the liability for any harm caused to the student
- the duties of the clinical instructor.

Some agreements may now include payment for the clinical placements from the college to the trust/SSD, or even from the trust to the college – third year students may be valuable members of the multi-disciplinary team. Similar agreements could be established between the college and other locations suitable for clinical placements, such as charitable organisations.

Supervision and mentoring

It cannot be assumed that only full time clinical teachers have responsibilities in education and training. Increasingly, the colleges are looking for practitioners to provide not only clinical supervision for pre-registration students, but also a mentoring role for students and newly qualified registered staff. The responsibilities of the senior practitioner in relation to supervision and delegation cannot, however, be underestimated and reference should be made to Chapter 10 on this topic. In Chapter 26 we consider the legal liability of lecturers and researchers and the law relating to research practice.

Non-registered support workers

Training of support workers is of increasing importance as the ratio of registered OTs to support workers decreases. Increasingly too, such healthcare support workers are likely to be carrying out work delegated from several different health professionals (e.g. physiotherapists and OTs). Jacqueline Ham and Anne Fenech discuss the continuing professional development for OT support workers[17] and conclude that CPD is important for both registered and non-registered staff and should be based upon a development plan that is tailored to personal and service needs but that may also reflect the needs of the profession. The COT has published Standards of Practice on the role and responsibilities of support workers in the delivery of occupational therapy services[18] (see Chapter 10). The COT in conjunction with the Chartered Society of Physiotherapy published a national framework for support worker education and development.[19] The legal aspects relating to the supervision of the activities of non-registered practitioners and delegation to them are considered in Chapter 10 on negligence. Care workers in a wide range of specialisms are now receiving training through the National Vocational Qualifications scheme, which provides a basic training at specified levels. Funding was available from the NHS learning account scheme to help staff who did not have a work-related professional qualification to develop their skills. The NHS learning account provided £150, at the time of writing towards the cost of a learning/training programme. Further information can be obtained from its website.[20] The moneys were administered through the local Workforce Development Confederations. In March 2004 the Department of Health published a consultation document on the registration of healthcare support workers (see Chapter 3).

General Social Care Council (GSCC)

The General Social Care Council (GSCC), which was established under the Care Standards Act 2000, is responsible for codes of practice, the Social Care Register and social work education and training. In September 2002 it issued codes of practice which set out the standards of practice and conduct to be followed by social care workers and employers.[21] In April 2003 it launched a social care register for all social care workers in England. To be able to register, workers must have an appropriate qualification, commit to uphold the Code of Practice for Social Care Workers and be physically fit to do their jobs. The GSCC is also responsible for regulating and supporting social work education and training.

Conclusions

The Health Professions Council has established clear standards for pre-registration and continuing professional development for its registrants and in the case of occupational therapists is receiving strong support from the College of Occupational Therapy. One of the challenges for the future, when many registrants will be trained to undertake activities normally associated with other registered health professions, will be to ensure that individual competence is defined, evaluated and monitored.

 Questions and exercises

1   Define a development plan to ensure your continued professional competence.
2   What improvements do you consider could be made in ensuring the integration of theoretical and clinical training for the pre-registration student?
3   Design a protocol which could be used for those OTs who act as mentors for junior colleagues.

References

1   www.hpc-uk.org/education/docs/HPC_occupational therapists
2   The Health Professions Council (2008) Annual Monitoring. HPC, London.
3   The Health Professions Council (2009) Approval Process. HPC, London.

4   Allied Health Professions (2002) 'Demonstrating competence through CPD' quote in HPC's Your guide to our standards for continuing professional development 2008; www.hpc-uk.org/registrants/cpd/

5   College of Occupational Therapists and others (2007) *Joint statement on continuing professional development for health and social care practitioners.* Royal College of Nursing, London.

6   College of Occupational Therapists (2002) Position Statement on Lifelong Learning. *British Journal of Occupational Therapy* **65**(5), 198–200.

7   College of Occupational Therapists (2004) College of Occupational Therapists: Strategic Vision and Action Plan For Lifelong learning. *British Journal of Occupational Therapy*, **67**(1), 20–28.

8   www.qaa.co.uk/aboutqaa/aboutQAA.htm

9   Quality Assurance Agency for Higher Education (2001) Subject Benchmark Statements, Health care Programmes – Occupational Therapy.

10 www.doh.gov.uk/nhslearningaccount/guide.htm

11 Department of Health (2004) *The NHS Knowledge and Skills Framework and the Development Review Process.* DH, London.

12 College of Occupational Therapists (2008) Knowledge and Skills Framework for OT staff in the NHS Briefing note no 108. COT, London.

13 Hocking, C. & Ness, N.E. (2002) *Revised Minimum Standards for the Education of Occupational Therapists.* World Federation of Occupational Therapists; www.wfot@-multiline.com.au; www.wfot.org

14 College of Occupational Therapists (2002) Position Statement on Lifelong Learning. *British Journal of Occupational Therapy* **65**(5), 198–200.

15 College of Occupational Therapists (2008) *Pre-registration Education Standards*, 3rd edn. COT, London.

16 Riley, J. & Whitcomber, S. (2008) *OT in adult social services in England: sustaining a high quality workforce for the future.* COT and DH, London.

17 Ham, J. & Fenech, A.M. (2002) Continuing professional development for OT support workers. *British Journal of Occupational Therapy*, **65**(5), 227–8.

18 College of Occupational Therapists (2000) *Standards of Practice on the role and responsibilities of support workers in the delivery of occupational therapy services.* COT, London.

19 Chartered Society of Physiotherapy and College of Occupational Therapists (2007) *A National Framework for Support Worker Education and Development.* COT and CSP, London.

20 www.doh.gov.uk/nhslearningaccount/guide.htm

21 www.gscc.org.uk/about.htm

6 Rights of Clients

Chapters 6 to 9 look at the rights of the client. In this chapter we take an overview of the basic statutory and common law rights, Chapter 7 looks at consent to treatment and information to be given to the client and the remaining chapters consider confidentiality and the right of access to health records.

The following topics are covered in this chapter:

- Statutory and common law basis of client's rights
- The Human Rights Act
- Rights to health and social care
- Charters

Statutory and common law basis of the client's rights

In this country the Articles of the European Convention on Human Rights grant specific legal rights to individuals. In addition, rights are recognised by individual Acts of Parliament or Regulations and Directions from the European Community which are binding on this country. The common law – those decisions of judges in the courts which become part of the law through the doctrine of precedent and the hierarchy of the courts (see Chapter 2) – also recognises many rights of the individual.

The Human Rights Act 1998

The Act came into force in England, Wales and Northern Ireland on 2 October 2000 (earlier in Scotland, on devolution) and has three effects:

Legal Aspects of Occupational Therapy, Third Edition By Bridgit Dimond
© 2010 Bridgit Dimond

- It requires public authorities and organisations exercising functions of a public nature to recognise the rights set out in the European Convention on Human Rights and to be found in Schedule 1 of the Human Rights Act 1998 (see Appendix 1 of this book).
- It enables citizens in this country to bring an action in the courts to enforce their rights as set out. Previously, those who felt that the rights set out in the Convention had been breached had to take a case to the European Court of Human Rights in Strasbourg, which could take several years with considerable cost.
- It requires judges to make a declaration of incompatibility in relation to any legislation which they consider is in conflict with the rights set out in the Schedule. In April 2003 the House of Lords made a declaration of incompatibility in relation to English law which stated that a person born male who had undergone a gender reassignment treatment could not enter into a valid marriage with another male.[1] Subsequently the Gender Recognition Act 2004 was passed by Parliament to rectify this injustice, as well as the Civil Partnership Act which gives rights to same sex couples. Both Acts are essential if the human rights of all persons are to be respected.

Who can be sued?

The Human Rights Act permits action to be brought by a person who claims that a public authority has acted (or proposes to act) in a way which is incompatible with a Convention right. The definition of public authority includes a court or tribunal or any 'person certain', i.e. organisation, whose functions are functions of a public nature.

Case law has developed on how organisations with functions of a public nature are defined. In a case brought against the Leonard Cheshire Foundation,[2] the Court of Appeal held that on those particular facts (the redeveloping of the home), the charity had not carried out the functions of a public authority. The House of Lords held,[3] in a majority decision, that private care homes under contract with local authorities for the provision of places were not exercising functions of a public nature for the purposes of the Human Rights Act. This led to an understandable reaction from many charities concerned with the care of vulnerable adults that overriding legislation be passed. As a consequence section 145 of the Health and Social Care Act 2008 provides for the provision of certain social care to be seen as a public function. Section 145 states that:

(1) A person ("P") who provides accommodation, together with nursing or personal care, in a care home for an individual under arrangements made with P under the relevant statutory provisions is to be taken for the purposes of subsection (3)(b) of section 6 of the Human Rights Act 1998 (c. 42) (acts of public authorities) to be exercising a function of a public nature in doing so.
(2) The relevant statutory provisions include:
(a) in relation to England and Wales, sections 21(1)(a) and 26 of the National Assistance Act 1948 (c. 29),
(b) in relation to Scotland, section 12 or 13A of the Social Work (Scotland) Act 1968 (c. 49), and
(c) in relation to Northern Ireland, Articles 15 and 36 of the Health and Personal Social Services (Northern Ireland) Order 1972 (S.I. 1972/1265 (N.I. 14)).

This provision is not retrospective and does not apply to cases prior to the coming into force of section 145.

The High Court held that a housing trust, which was a registered social landlord could be a public body for the purposes of the Human Rights Act 1998.[4] The Court held that the nature of its activities and the context within which it operated was a very different situation from an ordinary commercial business. It was heavily subsidised by the government and played a role in the implementation of government policy.

The Convention

The Convention is set out in Schedule 1 of the Human Rights Act 1998 and can be found in Appendix 1 of this book. Probably the most significant rights in terms of healthcare are in Articles 2, 3, 5, 6, 8 and 14. These will be considered in this chapter, but reference should be made to Appendix 1 for all the rights.

Article 2

> Everyone's right to life shall be protected by law. No one shall be deprived of his life intentionally save in the execution of a sentence of a court following his conviction of a crime for which this penalty is provided by law.

Recent decisions of the courts show how this right is interpreted. For example in one case,[5] parents lost their attempt to ensure that a severely handicapped baby, born prematurely, was resuscitated if necessary. The judge ruled that the hospital should provide him with palliative care to ease his suffering but should not try to revive him as that would cause unnecessary pain.

In another case, the President of the Family Division, Dame Elizabeth Butler-Sloss, held that the withdrawal of life-sustaining medical treatment was not contrary to Article 2 of the Human Rights Convention and the right to life, where the patient was in a persistent vegetative state. The ruling was made on 25 October 2000 in the cases involving Mrs M, 49 years old, who suffered brain damage during an operation abroad in 1997 and was diagnosed as being in a persistent vegetative state (PVS) in October 1998, and Mrs H, aged 36, who fell ill in America as a result of pancreatitis at Christmas 1999.[6]

Article 2 was also invoked in the case involving the separation of Siamese twins, in which the Court of Appeal decided on 22 September 2000 that they could be separated even though this would undoubtedly lead to the death of the one who depended on the heart and the lungs of the other[7] (see Chapter 25 for further details of the case).

More cases are likely to be heard on the issue as to whether there has been an infringement of Article 2 of the European Convention of Human Rights. For example, Article 2 may be used if a person is marked down as NFR (not for resuscitation) and the relatives disagree with the clinicians. In addition, the Article may be relied upon where a patient alleges that failure to provide health services is infringing her right to life. Diana Pretty failed in her attempt to argue that the Suicide Act 1961 was contrary to Article 2 (and other articles) and her right for her husband to assist her in securing a dignified death.[8] In the case of Debbie Purdy[9] the legality of the help given by relatives in accompanying patients to the Dignitas clinic in Switzerland was considered. Both the High Court and the Court of Appeal held that there was no breach of her article 8 rights. However the House of Lords upheld her appeal and required the DPP to formulate a clear policy on the factors to be taken into account when considering prosecution.[10] The DPP published guidelines on 23 September 2009. For more details of these cases and the guidelines see Chapter 25.

The House of Lords has held that the right to life protected by article 2 of the ECHR imposed an operational obligation on medical authorities to do all that could reasonably be expected of them to prevent a patient detained in a mental hospital who was known to be a real and immediate risk of committing suicide from doing so.[11] The health authorities were under an over-arching obligation to protect the lives of patients in their hospitals. In order to fulfil that obligation, and depending on the circumstances, they might be required to fulfil a number of complementary obligations. These included employing competent staff, trained to a high professional standard and ensuring that hospitals adopted systems of work which would protect the lives of patients. Failure to perform those general obligations might result in a violation of Article 2. If they fulfilled these obligations but staff were negligent, then the health authorities could be held vicariously liable and a breach of Article 2 to protect the patient's life.

The House of Lords has also held that Article 2 rights were violated if an independent inquiry was not held into a near suicide in custody where the prisoner was left mentally incapable.[12]

Article 3

No one shall be subjected to torture or to inhuman or degrading treatment or punishment.

Whilst it is hoped that torture does not take place in healthcare, there are evident examples of degrading and inhuman treatment. The patient who is left on a stretcher outside the accident and emergency department while waiting for a bed, could be said to be the victim of inhuman or degrading treatment. Handcuffing a patient to a bed during the delivery of her baby may also be seen as a breach of Article 3. Perhaps some of the treatments and investigations carried out in Occupational Therapy Departments are not always sensitive to the need to treat patients with dignity and mitigate discomfort and distress, but these will seldom be seen as a breach of article 3. A case heard by the European Court of Human Rights ruled that severe corporal punishment by a stepfather to discipline his stepson was a breach of Article 3 of the European Convention on Human Rights.[13] The stepfather had on several occasions beaten the 9-year-old boy with a garden cane. The stepfather had been prosecuted for assault occasioning actual bodily harm, but had been acquitted by the jury who had accepted his defence that the caning had been necessary and reasonable to discipline the boy. The European Court of Human Rights held that ill-treatment must attain a minimum level of severity if it is to fall within the scope of Article 3. It depended on all the circumstances of the case, such as the nature and context of the treatment, its duration, its physical and mental effects and in some instances, the sex, age and state of health of the victim (these factors are known as the reasonable chastisement test). In finding that there had been a breach of Article 3 in this case, it awarded the boy £10 000 against the UK Government, and costs. The events following this case are considered in Chapter 23. In Scotland, legislation to prohibit physical punishment of children under 3 years has been passed.

Article 3 rights cover a wide range of situations as the following cases show. Failure to prosecute following an assault on the grounds that the victim was mentally unstable was held to be a breach of the victim's human rights under article 3.[14] The House of Lords held that a mandatory sentence of life imprisonment without eligibility for parole, which would be imposed on a prisoner convicted of two murders, did not amount to inhuman or degrading punishment so as to justify a refusal to extradite him to the USA to stand trial.[15] In a case involving the protection of a mother and daughter in Northern Ireland in securing safe access to school in an area of bitter religious feuds, the House of Lords held that the duty of the state under article 3 to prevent inhuman and degrading treatment was not an unqualified or absolute one. The duty was to do all that could be reasonably expected of them.[16] The failure of the Home Secretary to investigate allegations of inhuman and degrading treatment of inmates at a privately run immigration detention centre was a breach of article 3.[17] Inmates at Winchester prison were paid £11,400 after it was ruled that denying them drugs such as heroin and substitute substances was a denial of their human rights: expecting them to go 'cold turkey' was inhuman treatment.[18]

Article 5

1. Everyone has the right to liberty and security of person. No-one shall be deprived of his liberty save in the following cases and in accordance with a procedure prescribed by law.

Many situations are then listed including:

e. the lawful detention of persons for the prevention of the spreading of infectious diseases, or persons of unsound mind, alcoholics or drug addicts or vagrants.

The House of Lords decided in the *Bournewood*[19] case that a person who lacked the mental capacity to consent to admission to a psychiatric hospital could be detained there in his best interests without being detained under the Mental Health Act 1983. Although such detention is justified under common law (i.e. judge-made law), statutory provisions to ensure that such de facto detentions are not contrary to Article 5 is essential. However the European Court of Human Rights[20] held that such action was contrary to Article 5 and as a consequence amendments were made to the Mental Capacity Act 2005 to ensure that there were safeguards in place to prevent a breach of Article 5 rights (see Chapter 22). In a case in 2000, the Court of Appeal held that in the absence of statutory provision for mentally incapacitated adults, the court did have an inherent power to hear issues involved in the day-to-day care of such persons and to grant declarations in the best interests of mentally incapable persons.[21] (See Chapter 21 on the mentally ill person and Chapter 22 on the patient with learning disabilities.)

The European Court of Human Rights held that the UK was in breach of Article 5.1 of the ECHR in respect of non-national terrorist suspects since they had not been detained with a view to deportation and the derogating measures permitting their indefinite detention discriminated unjustifiably between nationals and non-nationals.[22] The House of Lords held that crowd control measures used by the police in order to prevent a breach of public order, which resulted in several thousand people being confined within a police cordon for several hours, did not amount to a violation of the right to liberty if the measures were used in good faith, were proportionate and were enforced for no longer than was reasonably necessary.[23]

Article 6

The right to a fair trial:

1. In the determination of his civil rights and obligations or of any criminal charge against him, everyone is entitled to a fair and public hearing within a reasonable time by an independent and impartial tribunal established by law. Judgment shall be pronounced publicly but the press and public may be excluded from all or part of the trial in the interest of morals, public order or national security in a democratic society, where the interests of juveniles or the protection of the private life of the parties so require, or to the extent strictly necessary in the opinion of the court in special circumstances where publicity would prejudice the interests of justice.
2. Everyone charged with a criminal offence shall be presumed innocent until proved guilty according to law.

This right will have significant implications since it applies not just to criminal charges but also to the determination of civil rights and obligations. It would therefore apply to disciplinary actions and other such forums, where at present employees may not have representation and may be in a very weak situation compared with the employer. The new professional conduct and registration machinery for health professions has been drafted with the rights set out in this Article in mind (see

Chapters 3 and 4). The High Court held that the governors' decision to permanently exclude a child from a particular school did not engage the fair trial provisions protected by article 6 of the ECHR.[24] The proceedings of the panel were not classified as criminal under domestic law.

Article 8

1. Everyone has the right to respect for private and family life, his home and his correspondence.
2. There shall be no interference by a public authority with the exercise of the right except such as is in accordance with the law and is necessary in a democratic society in the interests of national security, public safety or the economic well-being of the country, for the prevention of disorder or crime, for the protection of health or morals, or for the protection of the rights and freedoms of others.

This right will require greater sensitivity about patient privacy than has been shown in the past within healthcare. The traditional ward round, where a curtain is seen as a soundproof barrier and all those on the ward can hear the intimate details of a patient's diagnosis, prognosis and treatment, may have to be reviewed. Many other actions may have to be taken in order to ensure that this right of the patient is recognised and protected. The Caldicott Guardians, whose role is considered in Chapter 8, will take on the responsibility for ensuring that there is no breach of Article 8. The respect for family life did not enable a prisoner to utilise artificial insemination to create a family[25] and he lost his appeal in the Court of Appeal.[26] The Court of Appeal, however, accepted that there might be circumstances where to deny a prisoner the opportunity to conceive a child might be a breach of Article 8. In another case it was held that high security restrictions on child visits were valid and not a breach of Article 8.[27] The European Court of Human Rights has held that the monitoring by the prison authorities of medical correspondence between a convicted prisoner and his external specialist doctor violated the prisoner's right for respect for his correspondence as guaranteed by article 8 of the European Convention on Human Rights.[28]

Article 8 has to be interpreted in relation to Article 10 which recognises a right to freedom of expression. Both Articles 8 and 10 are qualified by specified circumstances in which the right is limited, and the courts will balance the one against the other in determining whether there has been a breach of either article. The Court of Appeal overruled a decision of the High Court which found in favour of Naomi Campbell, a model, who sued a newspaper for breach of privacy and confidentiality, and held that the newspaper's report was justified in the public interest, considering that she had courted rather than shunned publicity. Naomi Campbell was faced with a legal costs bill of about £700 000. The House of Lords overruled the Court of Appeal's decision and in a majority verdict found in favour of Naomi Campbell.[29] It held that the publication of information about her drug treatment coupled with a photograph taken of her covertly outside the treatment centre, constituted a violation of her Article 8 rights (see Chapter 8).

The balance between Articles 8 and 10 was also considered by the House of Lords in a case involving a defendant in a rape case where an anonymity order had been made. The defendant had been acquitted and the BBC wished the anonymity order discharged. The House of Lords held that the balance fell in favour of the BBC's right to free expression.[30] In an earlier case the House of Lords held that the Article 10 right of expression by a newspaper prevailed over the Article 8 rights of a child who was the sibling of a child who allegedly died after being poisoned with salt by his mother.[31]

Article 8 rights were linked with Article 14 by pensioners living abroad who had been excluded from the index-linked updating, but the European Court of Human Rights held that they had not established a breach of the ECHR.[32]

Article 14

The enjoyment of the rights and freedoms set forth in this Convention shall be secured without discrimination on any ground such as sex, race, colour, language, religion, political or other opinion, national or social origin, association with a national minority, property, birth or other status.

Article 14 prohibits discrimination in the implementation of the Articles of the European Convention. It will be noted that the list of types of discrimination in Article 14 is preceded by the words 'such as' and they are therefore only examples of kinds of discrimination, and others could be added, such as disability, age or sexual orientation or being travellers, suffering from AIDS or being HIV positive, or being an asylum seeker. Disability discrimination is considered in Chapter 18.

Other significant articles

Whilst the above Articles have been looked at in detail, there are others which have considerable significance for healthcare. Article 2 of the first protocol recognises a right to education which may be significant for staff who are caring for children with long-term illnesses. Parents also have the right to ensure that such education and teaching is in conformity with their own religious and philosophical convictions under Article 9.

Action

There are considerable advantages in each department carrying out an audit to ascertain the extent to which the department is human rights compliant. Many changes may be required, but these may be of a procedural kind rather than ones which require expenditure and building work.

Defences

Many Articles have their own specific defences as can be seen from Appendix 1 in this book. Some rights are absolute, others qualified. With absolute rights there can be no interference (such as Article 3), but there can be disputes over interpretation, e.g. what is meant by 'inhuman or degrading treatment'? Where rights are qualified (such as Article 8), interference is permitted provided that it is justified. Where there is an apparent conflict the courts will have to balance the rights of the individual with the broader interests of society as a whole in order to determine justification. The courts have to apply the concept of proportionality in interpreting the application of those Articles which are not absolute. The concept of proportionality means that there should be a reasonable relation between a decision and its objectives. The means to a particular end should not be more oppressive than they need be to secure those ends.

Further information on the Human Rights Act and cases under it can be obtained from the Ministry of Justice website[33] and from the Equality and Human Rights Commission.[34]

Rights to healthcare and social care

Rights to healthcare and social care derive from the legislation shown in Figure 6.1 and from the common law.

Figure 6.1   Statutes relating to rights to health and social care.

- National Health Service Act 1977 (replacing NHS Act 1946)
- National Assistance Act 1948
- Health Service and Public Health Act 1968
- Children Act 1989
- Chronically Sick and Disabled Persons Act 1970
- Local Authority Social Services Act 1970
- Local Government Act 1972
- Health and Social Services and Social Security Adjudications Act 1983
- Disabled Persons (Services, Consultation and Representation) Act 1986
- Mental Health Act 1983 (as amended by 2007 Act)
- NHS and Community Care Act 1990
- Carers (Recognition and Services) Act 1995
- Health Act 1999
- Carers and Disabled Children Act 2000
- Care Standards Act 2000
- Health and Social Care Act 2001
- NHS Reform and Healthcare Professions Act 2002
- Health and Social Care (Community Health and Standards) Act 2003
- National Health Service Act 2006
- Health and Social Care Act 2008
- Health Act 2009

Some of these Acts are considered in more detail in the Chapters 20–24 covering specific client groups.

Absolute or discretionary rights

It should be noted that very few statutes bestow absolute rights on clients or patients. The National Health Service Act 2006 re-enacted the duty of the Secretary of State to continue to promote in England and Wales a comprehensive health service designed to secure improvement in the physical and mental health of the people of those countries, and in the prevention, diagnosis and treatment of illness. The duty, however, left much to his discretion, as can be seen from Figure 6.2.

The rights recognised by the statutes and common law are summarised in Figure 6.3. These are discussed in the chapters indicated in the figure.

Enforcement of rights

These rights can be enforced by the individual patient in many ways through administrative and judicial machinery. Administrative machinery includes:

- complaint through the set procedure (see Chapter 14)
- inquiry by Secretary of State
- independent inquiry.

Figure 6.2   Discretionary duties of the Secretary of State – National Health Service Act 2006 section 3(1).

The Secretary of State must provide through out England ... to such extent *as he considers necessary* to meet *all reasonable* requirements –

(a)   hospital accommodation;
(b)   other accommodation for the purpose of any service provided under this Act;
(c)   medical, dental, nursing and ambulance services;
(d)   such other facilities for the care of pregnant women, women who are breast feeding and young children *as he considers are appropriate* as part of the health service;
(e)   such other services or facilities for the prevention of illness, the care of persons suffering from illness and the after-care of persons who have suffered from illness *as he considers are appropriate* as part of the health service;
(f)   such other services as are required for the diagnosis and treatment of illness.

Figure 6.3   Summary of client rights in the NHS and under social services.

- To receive care and treatment (not absolute) (see below)
- To receive a reasonable standard of care and treatment (see Chapter 10)
- To give or withhold consent to treatment and/or care (see Chapter 7)
- To confidentiality (see Chapter 8)
- To access health and personal social services records (see Chapter 9)
- To complain (see Chapter 14)

Judicial remedies include:

- an action for negligence, when harm has occurred (see Chapter 10)
- an action for trespass to the person, where treatment has been given without consent (see Chapter 7)
- an action for breach of statutory duty, where it is alleged that a statutory authority has not fulfilled its duties (see specific client groups, Chapters 20–24)
- an action for judicial review of the functions of a statutory authority or other administrative body.

The right to care and treatment

Unenforceable rights

As can be seen from Figure 6.3, there is no absolute right to obtain treatment under the NHS. In the inevitable situation where resources are finite and demand outmatches supply, providers and funders have to weigh priorities. Where individual patients have sought to enforce the statutory duty to provide services, the courts have refused to intervene unless there is evidence that there has been a failure to make a reasonable decision about the allocation of resources.[35] Thus patients who brought an action for breach of statutory duty against the Secretary of State for Health and the relevant regional and area health authorities on the grounds that they had waited too long for hip operations, failed in their claim.

Since then a child (Jamie Bowen) suffering from leukaemia was refused a course of chemotherapy and a second bone marrow transplant on the grounds that there was only a very small chance of the treatment succeeding and therefore it would not be in her best interests for the treatment to proceed. The Court of Appeal[36] upheld the decision of the health authority as they were unable to fault its process of reasoning, and allowed the appeal.

The Master of the Rolls (Sir Thomas Bingham) stated:

> While I have every sympathy with B, I feel bound to regard this as an attempt – wholly understandable, but nevertheless misguided – to involve the court in a field of activity where it is not fitted to make any decision favourable to the patient.

There have however been several cases where the courts have recognised claims brought against health authorities for failures to provide services.

One was in relation to the failure of a health authority to permit a drug for multiple sclerosis to be prescribed in its catchment area.[37] The health authority decided that it would not enable beta interferon to be prescribed for patients in its catchment area, since it was not yet proved to be clinically effective for the treatment of multiple sclerosis. A sufferer from multiple sclerosis challenged this refusal of the health authority and succeeded on the grounds that the health authority had failed to follow the guidance issued by the Department of Health.[38] A declaration was granted that the policy adopted by the health authority was unlawful and an order of mandamus was made requiring the defendants to formulate and implement a policy which took full and proper account of national policy as stated in the circular.

In another a health authority refused to fund treatment for three transsexuals who wished to undergo gender reassignment,[39] on the grounds that it had been assigned a low priority in its lists of procedures considered to be clinically ineffective in terms of health gain. Under this policy, gender reassignment surgery was, among other procedures, listed as a procedure for which no treatment, apart from that provided by the authority's general psychiatric and psychology services, would be commissioned save in the event of overriding clinical need or exceptional circumstances. The transsexuals sought judicial review of the health authority's refusal and the judge granted an order quashing the authority's decision and the policy on which it was based. The health authority then took the case to the Court of Appeal but lost its appeal. The Court of Appeal held that:

(1) Whilst the precise allocation and weighting of priorities is a matter for the judgment of the authority and not for the court, it is vital for an authority:
(a) to assess accurately the nature and seriousness of each type of illness and
(b) to determine the effectiveness of various forms of treatment for it and
(c) to give proper effect to that assessment and that determination in the formulation and individual application of its policy.
(2) The Authority's policy was flawed in two respects:
(a) it did not treat transsexualism as an illness, but as an attitude of mind which did not warrant medical treatment and
(b) the ostensible provision that it made for exceptions in individual cases and its manner of considering them amounted to the operation of a 'blanket policy' against funding treatment for the condition because it did not believe in such treatment.

(3)   The authority were not genuinely applying the policy to the individual exceptions.
(4)   Article 3 and Article 8 of the European Convention on Human Rights (see above and the Appendix) did not did not give a right to free health care and did not apply to this situation, where the challenge is to a health authority's allocation of finite funds. Nor were the patients victims of discrimination on the grounds of sex.

In spite of the decision of the Court of Appeal in this case that the Articles of the European Convention of Human Rights did not apply to the allocation of resources, there are undoubtedly likely to be cases in the future where claimants utilise the Human Rights Act 1998 when facilities and services have not been made available and as a consequence a person has been subjected to inhuman or degrading treatment. Such actions will be assisted where NICE, the Care Quality Commission and National Service Frameworks publish guidance on what they consider are minimal standards of care (see Chapter 17).

A cancer patient obtained a court order that he could be given a drug which had been refused by West Sussex Primary Care Trust on the grounds that it would not be cost-effective. It ruled that he should receive Revlimid as an exceptional case. An emergency injunction was issued on an interim basis pending a further appeal.[40]

The European Court of Justice has set down the principles which apply when a patient is seeking treatment in a member state. In this case[41] Mrs Watts was waiting for a hip replacement operation and went abroad for treatment after being told that she would have to wait a year for the operation on the NHS. She asked her local hospital in Bedford to pay for the trip under the E112 certificate scheme, but Bedford Primary Care Trust refused on the grounds that the wait was within the government's waiting times guidelines. She brought an action for judicial review of the PCT's refusal, claiming that its decision was unlawful and infringed her rights under Articles 3 and 8 of the European Convention on Human Rights.

The judge held, based on Article 49 of the EC Treaty[42] (which prohibited restrictions on freedom to provide services within the Community) that prior authorisation for treatment by an NHS patient in another member state of the European Union at the expense of the NHS could be refused on the ground of lack of medical necessity only if the same or equally effective treatment could be obtained without undue delay at an NHS establishment. He also held that in assessing what amounted to undue delay, regard had to be had to all the circumstances of the specific case, including the patient's medical condition and, where appropriate, the degree of pain and the nature and extent of the patient's disability. Consideration of NHS waiting times and waiting lists were relevant, when having regard to all the circumstances. On the facts of the case, however, the claimant did not recover the money, since the local hospital had offered her an earlier operation. The Court of Appeal referred the case to the European Court of Justice for a preliminary ruling on the application of article 49 and article 22 of Regulation 1408/71.

The European Court of Justice held that:[43]

1.   In order to be entitled to refuse to grant the authorization referred to in Article 22(1)(c)(i) of that regulation on the ground that there is a waiting time for hospital treatment, the competent institution is required to establish that that time does not exceed the period which is acceptable on the basis of an objective medical assessment of the clinical needs of the person concerned in the light of all of the factors characterizing his medical condition at the time when the request for the authorization is made or renewed, as the case may be.
2.   An NHS patient is entitled under Article 49 EC to receive hospital treatment in another Member state at the expense of that national service and refusal of prior authorization cannot be based merely on the existence of waiting lists intended to enable the supply of hospital care to be planned and managed on

the basis of predetermined general clinical priorities, without carrying out an objective medical assessment of the patient's medical condition, the history and probable cause of his illness, the degree of pain he is in and/or the nature of his disability at a time when the request for authorization was made or renewed.

3. Where the delay arising from such waiting lists appears to exceed an acceptable time having regard to an objective medical assessment of the above mentioned circumstances, the competent institution may not refuse the authorisation sought on the grounds of the existence of those waiting lists, an alleged distortion of the normal order of priorities linked to the relative urgency of the cases to be treated, the fact that the hospital treatment provided under the national system in question is free of charge, the obligation to make available specific funds to reimburse the cost of treatment in another Member State and/or a comparison between the cost of that treatment and that of equivalent treatment in the competent Member State.

4. Article 49 EC must be interpreted as meaning that where the legislation of the competent Member State provides that hospital treatment provided under the national health service is to be free of charge, and where the legislation of the Member State in which a patient registered with that service was or should have been authorized to receive hospital treatment at the expense of that service does not provide for the reimbursement in full of the cost of that treatment, the competent institution must reimburse that patient, the difference (if any) between the cost, objectively quantified, of equivalent treatment in a hospital covered by the service in question up to the total amount invoiced for the treatment, provided in the host Member State and the amount which the institution of the latter Member State is required to reimburse under Article 22(1)(c)(i) of Regulation No 1408/71 (as updated) of behalf of the competent institution pursuant to the legislation of that Member State.

5. A patient who is authorized to receive treatment in another Member State or who is refused authorization which is subsequently held to be unfounded, is entitled to receive both the costs of medical treatment and also the ancillary costs associated with cross-border movement for medical purposes provided that the legislation of the competent Member State imposes a corresponding obligation on the national system to reimburse in respect of treatment provided in a local hospital covered by that system.

In July 2008 the EU published a draft directive which would allow patients to seek cross-border healthcare with their countries of residence paying the costs.[44] The draft directive is to be examined by the European Parliament and the Council of Ministers before being finalised. The stated aim of the EC was to lay down a framework on patients' rights to treatment abroad.

Refunding care provided outside the NHS

In a bizarre case a private medical services company, European Surgeries Ltd, arranged for a patient to have a contract operation performed by a German Company. The patient paid European Surgeries Ltd who paid the German Company. European Surgeries Ltd then sought judicial review of the Trust's refusal to reimburse the patient. The judge refused the application noting that the patient had never been in touch with the trust or requested payment, nor had the trust commissioned the service. The fact that the company wished to increase its business by telling customers that the trust would have to reimburse them was not a justiciable claim.[45]

No right to demand treatment contrary to professional judgment

The right of the health professional to use her professional discretion in refusing to provide treatment which she considers to be inappropriate for the patient has been reinforced by a decision of the Court of Appeal in a case where a patient challenged the GMC's guidelines on withholding treatment.

The Burke Case

Leslie Burke, a patient suffering from a degenerative brain condition, brought an action against the General Medical Council arguing that their guidance[46] to doctors on withholding and withdrawing life prolonging treatment: good practice in decision making was illegal. Counsel for the GMC argued that there is no obligation to provide treatment that would enable a patient to survive a life-threatening condition regardless of the suffering involved in the treatment and regardless of the quality of life the patient would experience thereafter. She also stated that no evidence existed that Mr Burke would ever be denied life-prolonging treatment. Withdrawing artificial feeding and hydration in his case would be entirely inappropriate.[47]

Mr Burke won his case before the High Court. The judge granted judicial review holding that once a patient had been admitted to an NHS hospital there was a duty of care to provide and go on providing treatment, whether the patient was competent or incompetent or unconscious. This duty of care, which could not be transferred to anyone else, was to provide that treatment which was in the best interests of the patient. It was for the patient if competent to determine what was in his best interests. If the patient was incompetent and had left no binding and effective advance directive, then it was for the court to decide what was in his best interests. To withdraw ANH at any stage before the claimant finally lapsed into a coma would involve clear breaches of both Article 8 and 3 because he would thereby be exposed to acute mental and physical suffering. The GMC guidelines were therefore in error in emphasising the right of the claimant to refuse treatment, but not his right to require treatment.

The GMC appealed against this ruling and the Court of Appeal's reserved judgment was given on 29 July 2005.[48] The Court of Appeal held that doctors are not obliged to provide patients with treatment that they consider to be futile or harmful, even if the patient demands it. Autonomy and the right of self-determination do not entitle the patient to insist on receiving a particular medical treatment regardless of the nature of the treatment. However where a competent patient says that he or she want to be kept alive by the provision of food and water, doctors must agree to that. Not to do so would result in the doctor not merely being in breach of duty in the law of negligence but guilty of the criminal offence of murder.

Decisions on whether or not treatment should be provided should ideally be informed by information relating to their effectiveness. Unfortunately this is not always so as research carried out in paediatric OT shows.[49] (See also Chapter 25 and the discussion on the extent of the duty to maintain life.)

Topping up NHS care

Considerable controversy took place in 2008 over Department of Health rules that where patients were supplementing their NHS care with medicines or other treatments which the NHS did not supply, then they would be charged for their NHS care. After considerable media coverage the DH in November 2008 announced that patients would not have to pay for their NHS care in such circumstances. Critics have argued that this automatically makes for a two-tier health service since those who could afford to would be able to pay for treatments which NICE had ruled against for the NHS (see Chapter 17).

Enforceable rights

Rights which would be enforceable by the patient include failure to provide a general practitioner and failure to provide appropriate emergency service in an accident and emergency department. Here the claim would be based on the duty to ensure that a reasonable standard of care was provided (see Chapter 10 on negligence).

Charters

There are several international charters or conventions which, unlike the European Convention on Human Rights, do not have direct force in the UK but which are of persuasive authority. For example, the United Nations Convention on the Rights of the Child is implemented through an analysis every other year of the extent of compliance with its terms (see Chapter 23). Conventions covering research standards are considered in Chapter 25.

As well as these international charters, there are now several national charters for patients both in secondary and primary care, and many hospitals, community health services and GP practices have prepared their own charters. These give certain assurances to clients and patients that services will be provided within set times and to a specific quality. In 1999 the Department of Health and the Department of the Environment[50] published a national charter and guidance which suggested standards for local housing, health and social care and recommended the adoption of local charters. The guidance was updated in March 2001,[51] when the Department of Health made it clear that social services departments with their partners in housing and health should have a new charter in place for April 2001 and it should be published by 30 June 2001. A checklist of charter contents is included in the guidance. The aim of the charters is to inform users and carers of what they can expect in terms of health and social care.

However, these charters do not bestow legal rights and the client or patient cannot enforce them unless the declarations are recognised in statute or common law and therefore enforceable through those means.

On the other hand, where the client is receiving independent healthcare under a contract agreed with an occupational therapist (OT) in independent practice, then the charter might be written in as part of the specific contractual agreement and the client would then be able to sue for breach of contract (see Chapter 28).

Statements of Standards on health service care set by the Secretary of State under section 45 of the Health and Social Care Act 2008 are enforceable upon health service bodies and subject to monitoring by the Care Quality Commission. Section 45(2) obliges the Secretary of State to keep the standards under review and enables him to publish amended statements if he considers it appropriate.

NHS Constitution

Whilst NHS Charters and declaration of rights are not legally enforceable unless they repeat existing legal rights a new dimension has been added by the introduction of an NHS Constitution which will be legally enforceable. In 2008 Mr Darzi, a surgeon, was appointed by the Government to report on the NHS. His report includes a draft NHS constitution[52] which can be seen in Appendix 2 of this book. The constitution sets out the 7 key principles which guide the NHS; the rights and responsibilities of patients, the rights and responsibilities of staff and the values underpinning the NHS. It thus attempts to consolidate all the existing legal rights of patients, staff and public in one document and to set down some pledges such as:

> The NHS will strive to provide all staff with personal development, access to appropriate training for their jobs, and line management support to succeed. (pledge)

The NHS Constitution is accompanied by a statement of accountability. All organisations providing NHS services will be obliged by law to take account of the Constitution and its principles and values in their decisions and actions. The legal basis of the NHS Constitution is underpinned by the statutory duties placed on NHS organisations to have regard to the NHS Constitution in the performance of their NHS functions.

The Health Act 2009 sections 1–7 makes provision for the preparation, enforcement, and regular revision of the NHS Constitution. Those bodies which are required to have regard to the NHS Constitution include: Strategic Health Authorities; Primary Care Trusts; National Health Service trusts; Special Health Authorities; NHS foundation trusts; the Independent Regulator of NHS Foundation Trusts; and the Care Quality Commission (see Appendix 3).

A Handbook must also be made available to patients, staff, and members of the public. At least once in any period of 3 years the Secretary of State must carry out a review of the Handbook, with the first review being completed not later than 5 July 2012.

These reforms, which follow the Darzi review, are discussed in more detail in Chapter 29.

Fraudulent or unjustifiable claims for services

Resources within health and social services are limited, and there is a danger that if services are claimed by those lacking justification, then other more deserving patients and clients may have to go without or wait a long time for the service. OTs cannot therefore, as part of sound professional practice, collude with patients whom the OTs know are not justified in demanding a service. This applies both to the decisions about giving out disabled parking badges (see Chapter 16) and to decisions about services required as part of a court report. The requirement for the OT to follow the professional standards of assessment in making reports to be used in court action is considered in Chapter 13 and is equally applicable to these circumstances. It is unfortunate but inevitable that on the one hand the OT must provide a reasonable standard of care for her clients, but on the other she must accept her role as a gate keeper to limited resources which do not match the demands which arise. The ethical conflict which arises from this dual role is examined by Karen Whalley Hammell.[53]

Conclusions

This is a complex area of law, partly because, although rights set out in the European Convention are enforceable in the courts of the UK, there has, until the proposed NHS Constitution, been no attempt to codify the health rights to which a patient/client is entitled, nor has there been an attempt to ensure that such a code is enforceable through the legal system. Any potential litigant has in the past therefore had to first to ascertain if the wrong which he claims to have suffered is one recognised by the common law or statute law or is covered by the Articles of the European Convention on Human Rights, and if so, to consider what are the means of enforcement. The following chapters cover the separate rights which are currently recognised in statute or common law.

Questions and exercises

1   What client rights do you consider that the law should recognise in relation to health and social care?

2   There will never be the resources to meet all demands upon health and social services. What criteria would you draw up to determine priorities to receive occupational therapy services in your area of expertise and how would you involve clients in the process?

3   Consider the articles of the European Convention on Human Rights (see Appendix one) and identify the extent to which your department and working practices respect the rights set out in these articles. If there are shortfalls, what action would be necessary to ensure compliance?

References

1   *Bellinger v Bellinger*. Lord Chancellor intervening. Times Law Report, 11 April 2003.

2   *R (On the application of Heather) v Leonard Cheshire Foundation* [2002] EWCA Civ 366; The Times, 8 April 2002.

3   *YL v Birmingham City Council* [2007] UKHL 22; The Times 21 June 2007.

4   *R (Weaver) v London and Quadrant Housing Trust* The Times Law Report 8 July 2008 QBD.

5   Oliver Wright and Laura Peek, Judge rules boy must be left to die, The Times, 13 July 2000, p. 1; *A National Health Service Trust v D*. Times Law Report, 19 July 2000; [2000] 2 FLR 677; [2000] 2 FCR 577; (2000) 55 BMLR 19; [2000] Fam Law 803.

6   *NHS Trust A v Mrs M and NHS Trust B v Mrs H*, Family Division, The Times, 25 October 2000; [2001] 1 ALL ER 801; [2001] 2 FLR 367. For further discussion on the law relating to palliative care and death, see Dimond, B. (2002) *Legal Aspects of Pain Management and* Dimond, B. (2008) *Legal Aspects of Death*. Quay Publications, Dinton, Wilts.

7   *Re A (minors) (conjoined twins: surgical separation)*. Times Law Report, 10 October 2000; [2001] Fam 147, CA.

8   *R (on the application of Pretty) v DPP* [2001] UKHL 61; [2001] 3 WLR 1598; [2002] 1 All ER 1; *Pretty v UK* ECHR Current Law 380 June 2002.

9   *R (Purdy) v Director of Public Prosecutions* The Times Law Report 24 February 2009.

10   *R (Purdy) v Director of Public Prosecutions* The Times Law Report 31 July 2009 HL.

11   *Savage v South Essex Partnership NHS Foundation Trust* Times Law Report 11 December 2008.

12   *R (JH) (A Youth) v Secretary of State for Justice* The Times Law Report 2 December 2008.

13   *A v The United Kingdom* (100/1997/884/1096) judgment on 23 September 1998.

14   *R (B) v. Director of Public Prosecutions (Equality and Human Rights Commission intervening)* The Times Law Report 24 March 2009 QBD.

15   *R (Wellington) v Secretary of State for the Home Department* Times Law Report 12 December 2008 HL.

16   *E v Chief Constable of the Royal Ulster Constabulary and another* The Times Law Report 19 November 2008.

17   *R (AM and others) v Secretary of State for the Home Department and Another* The Times Law Report 20 March 2009.

18   News item. Inmates receive cold turkey cash. The Times 4 December 2008.

19   *R v Bournewood Community and Mental Health NHS Trust, ex parte L* [1998] 3 All ER 289.

20   *HL v United Kingdom* [2004] ECHR 720 Application No 45508/99 5 October 2004; Times Law Report 19 October 2004.

21   *Re F (Adult: Court's Jurisdiction)* [2000] 2 FLR 512, CA.

22   *A and others v United Kingdom* (Application No 3455/05) The Times Law Report 20 February 2009.

23   *Austin v Commissioner of Police of the Metropolis* The Times Law Report 29 January 2009.

24   *R (V: a child) v Independent appeal panel for Tom Hood School and others* Times Law Report 18 March 2009.

25   *R v Secretary of State for the Home Department ex parte Mellor*, Times Law Report, 31 July 2000; [2000] 2 FLR 951; [2000] 3 FCR 148; [2000] Fam Law 881.

26   *R v Secretary of State for the Home Department ex parte Mellor*, Times Law Report, 1 May 2001, CA; [2001] EWCA Civ 472; [2001] 3 WLR 533; [2001] 2 FLR 1158; [2001] 2 FCR 153.

27   *R v Secretary of State for Health ex parte Lolly*, Times Law Report, 11 October 2000.

28   *Szuluk v United Kingdom* (Application No 36936/05) The Times Law Report 17 June 2009 ECHR.

29   *Campbell v Mirror Group Newspapers plc.* [2004] UKHL 22, [2004] 2 AC 457 HL Times Law Report, 7 May 2004.

30   *In re British Broadcasting Corporation* Attorney-General's Reference (No 3 of 1999) The Times Law Report 18 June 2009 HL.

31   *S (a child)*, Re [2004] UKHL 47 (28 October 2004).

32   *Carson and others v United Kingdom* (Application Number 42184/05) The Times Law Report 20 November 2008.

33   www.justice.gov.uk

34   www.equalityhumanrights.com

35   *R v Secretary of State for Social Services, ex parte Hincks and others*. Solicitors Journal, 29 June 1979, p. 436.

36   *R v Cambridge Health Authority ex parte B* [1995] 2 All ER 129.

37   *R v North Derbyshire Health Authority* [1997] 8 Med LR 327.

38   NHS Executive Letter: EL (95)97.

39   *North West Lancashire Health Authority v A, D, and G* [1999] Lloyds Law Reports Medical, p. 399.

40   Rose, D. Cancer patient with months to live wins court order for last-chance drug on NHS. The Times 11 September 2008.

41   *R (Watts) v Bedford Primary Care Trust and Another* The Times Law Report, 3 October 2003; [2003] EWHC 2228; [2004] EWCA Civ 166.

42   (Previously Article 59) EC Treaty (OJ 1992 C224/6).

43   *Watts v Bedford Primary Care Trust and the Secretary of State for Health* Case C-372/04 May 2006.

44   David Charter. Patients to travel for treatment in Europe and the NHS will pay. The Times 3 July 2008 page 16.

45   *European Surgeries Ltd v Cambridgeshire Primary Care Trust* [2007] EWHC 2758; [2008] P.I.Q.R.P8 QBD.

46   General Medical Council Withholding and withdrawing life prolonging treatment: good practice in decision making GMC 2002.

47   Michael Horsnell. Feeding a terminal patient `is treatment'. The Times 28 February 2004.

48   *R (On the application of Burke) v General Medical Council and Disability Rights Commission and Official Solicitor to the Supreme Court* [2004] EWHC 1879; [2004] Lloyd's Rep. Med 451; [2005] EWCA Civ 1003, 28 July 2005.

49   Kolehmainen, N., Francis, J. & McKee, L. (2008) To provide or not to provide treatment? That is the question. *British Journal of Occupational Therapy*, **71**(12), 510–23.

50   Department of Health/Department of the Environment (1999) *Better Care Higher Standards*: a charter for long term care – guidance for housing, health and social services. DH, London.

51   HSC 2001/006; LAC(2001)006 *Better Care Higher Standards*.

52   Available on the DH website with supporting documents; dh.gov.uk.

53   Hammell, K.W. (2007) Client Centred Practice: Ethical obligation or professional obfuscation. *British Journal of Occupational Therapy*, **70**(6), 264–6.

7 Consent and Information Giving

This chapter covers the legal issues relating to consent to treatment. It will be concerned with those issues which arise in relation to the mentally competent adult, and the provisions of the Mental Capacity Act 2005 which provides a framework for decision making in relation to those over 16 years who lack the requisite capacity to make specific decisions. The laws relating to consent in the case of children, the mentally ill, older people and those with learning disabilities are covered in Chapters 20–24 dealing with those specialist client groups[1] and consent in relation to research is considered in Chapter 26. The College of Occupational Therapists (COT) has set five consent standard statements within its professional standards for OT practice.[2] These statements include the need to obtain consent, record it and regularly confirm it, to ensure that full information is given about the interventions, the right of the service user to refuse or withdraw consent at any time, the duty to respect confidentiality (see Chapter 8) and the legal situation when the client is incapable of giving consent. An addendum has been provided on the need to adhere to the Mental Capacity Act 2005.

The statements are as follows:

Standard 1 Consent to OT should be obtained from the service user, recorded and regularly confirmed

Standard 2 Occupational therapists should ensure that the service user is fully informed about the nature of the occupational therapy generally and the specific nature of the interventions relevant to them. This means that their decisions on consent will be informed

Standard 3 Occupational therapists should accept the service user's decision to refuse or withdraw consent at any time, unless the individual lacks the requisite capacity to make valid decisions.

Standard 4 Occupational therapy staff have a professional and legal obligation to respect the duty of confidentiality, subject to statutory and common-law exceptions to this duty.

Standard 5 Occupational Therapy staff should be aware of the correct legal approach to take when obtaining consent is difficult or impossible.

Each aspect of these standards for practice on consent to treatment is discussed below and in the specialist chapters of the book (Chapters 20–24). The topic of disclosure of information is considered in Chapter 8 on confidentiality. The following topics are covered in this chapter:

Legal Aspects of Occupational Therapy, Third Edition By Bridgit Dimond
© 2010 Bridgit Dimond

- Two distinct issues: Trespass to the person and informed consent
- Trespass to the person
- Determination of competence
- Mental Capacity Act 2005

- Informing the client
- Duty to inform
- Application to OT practice
- Documentation and consent

Two distinct issues: trespass to the person and the duty to inform

There are two distinct aspects of the law relating to consent to treatment. One is the actual giving of consent and the possibility that a trespass to the person has occurred because the patient did not give consent to the treatment. The other is the duty to give information to the patient prior to obtaining consent. The absence of consent could result in the patient suing for trespass to the person. The failure to provide sufficient relevant information could result in an action for negligence. These two different legal actions will be considered separately.

Trespass to the person

A trespass to the person occurs when an individual either apprehends a touching (an assault) or the individual is actually touched (a battery) and has not given consent and there is no other legal justification. The person who has suffered the trespass can sue for compensation in the civil courts (and in criminal cases a prosecution could also be brought).

In the civil cases, the victim has to prove the touching or the apprehension of the touching and that it was a (potentially) direct interference with the person. The victim does not have to show that harm has occurred. This is in contrast with an action for negligence in which the victim must show that harm has resulted from the breach of duty of care (see below in relation to a breach of the duty to inform and also Chapter 10 on the law relating to negligence).

Defences to an action for trespass to the person

The main defence to an action for trespass to the person is that consent was given by a mentally competent person. In addition, there is a defence where justification can be claimed as a result of statutory authorisation, e.g. the Mental Health Act 1983 (as amended by the Mental Health Act 2007) (discussed in Chapter 21) and the Mental Capacity Act 2005 (see below and Chapter 22 in relation to deprivation of liberty safeguards).

Consent

For consent to treatment to be valid, the person giving it must be mentally competent (a child of 16 and 17 has a statutory right to give consent, and a child below 16 has a right recognised at common law, if 'Gillick competent' (see Chapter 23)). There is a presumption (section 1(2) Mental Capacity Act 2005) that a person over 16 years has the capacity to give consent, but this presumption can be rebutted (i.e. removed) if there is evidence to the contrary. The standard of proof to be used to displace the presumption is a balance of probabilities i.e. the civil standard of proof. Consent must be given voluntarily, without any duress or force or deceit. It can be given by word of mouth, in writing or can be implied, i.e. the non-verbal conduct of the person indicates that she is giving consent. All these forms of giving consent are valid but where procedures entail risk and/or where there are likely to be disputes over whether consent was given, or whether specific information was given, it is advisable to obtain evidence in writing that consent was given. It is then easier to establish in a court of law that consent was given and/or the information conveyed.

There are very few situations where the law requires consent to be evidenced in writing. The Human Fertilisation and Embryology Act 1990 requires written consent to be obtained for fertilisation treatment including the retrieval, storage and use of gametes and whilst these stringent requirements of the Act were modified by the 1992 Act, the absence of her late husband's agreement to fertilisation of his sperm prevented Diane Blood obtaining treatment in the UK but did not prevent her using the sperm abroad[3] and the withdrawal of her husband's consent prevented Ms Evans utilising the embryos and the European Court of Human Rights considered did not breach her human rights.[4] In a recent case the family division held that the absence of an effective consent by a husband, now deceased, meant that the court had no power to authorise retrieval or storage of gametes pending a decision of the Human Fertilisation and Embryology Authority.[5] The Human Tissue Act 2004 requires consent to be obtained before a person's organs and tissue can be stored or used for purposes such as research, post-mortem examination and transplantation and also before a deceased person's organs can be removed for specified purposes. Codes of Practice have been issued by the Human Tissue Authority giving guidance on consent and other aspects of the legislation.

The Mental Health Act 1983 (as amended by the Mental Health Act 2007) also stipulates strict provisions over the giving of treatment to detained patients for mental disorder which are covered in Chapter 21.

Consent forms

The Department of Health has provided a reference guide on the law relating to consent, which is available from the department's website.[6] It is intended that this guide should be regularly updated. In addition, practical guidance has been issued on consent to examination and treatment, which includes forms recommended for use by trusts.[7] These new forms, which replace those recommended in 1992, can be used by any health professionals and therefore could be used by an OT for her treatments. Form 1 is for adults, Form 2 for children, Form 3 for use where the patient does not lose consciousness and Form 4 for use where the patient is incapable of giving consent. There are clear advantages in obtaining the patient's consent in writing if there are any risks inherent in the treatment or if there is likely to be a dispute later as to whether consent was actually given. The giving of consent should be seen as part of a process of communication between patient and health professional. It must be emphasised that where consent is recorded in writing, that consent form is evidence that consent has been given: it is not the actual consent. The actual consent is the state of mind of the person agreeing to have the treatment. The Report of the Inquiry into children's heart surgery at the Bristol Royal Infirmary emphasised the importance of openness and trust between health professionals and patients.[8] It also made significant recommendations on obtaining consent which included the following:

- In a patient-centred healthcare service patients must be involved, wherever possible, in decisions about their treatment and care.
- Information should be tailored to the needs, circumstances and wishes of the individual.
- We note and endorse the recent statement on consent produced by the DH reference guide to consent for examination and treatment (DH 2001). It should inform the practice of all healthcare professionals in the NHS and be introduced into practice in all trusts.

- The process of informing the patient, and obtaining consent to a course of treatment, should be regarded as a process and not a one-off event consisting of obtaining a patient's signature on a form.
- The process of consent should apply not only to surgical procedures but also to all clinical procedures and examinations that involve any form of touching. This must not mean more forms: it means more communication.
- As part of the process of obtaining consent, except when they have indicated otherwise, patients should be given sufficient information about what is to take place, the risks, uncertainties, and possible negative consequences of the proposed treatment, about any alternatives and about the likely outcome, to enable them to make a choice about how to proceed.

(see below and the duty to inform).

What if someone wishes to leave hospital or discontinue treatment?

It is a principle of the law on consent that where a person has given consent, the consent can be withdrawn at any time unless there is a contractual reason why this cannot be done. This means that if people wish to leave hospital contrary to their best interests then, unless they lack the capacity to make a valid decision, they are free to go. Clearly there are advantages in obtaining the signature of the patient that the self-discharge or refusal to accept treatment was contrary to clinical advice.

Refusal to consent

The Court of Appeal set out the basic principles of self-determination of the mentally competent adult in the case of *Re T*.[9] However, it also emphasised the importance of the health professional ensuring that any refusal to consent to life-saving treatment and care was valid. In that case a woman had stated that she would not wish to have a blood transfusion. She was very much under the influence of her mother, a Jehovah's Witness. When it became evident that she would need blood to stay alive, the court allowed the cohabitee's and father's application for the blood to be given on the grounds that her refusal was not valid. This decision was confirmed by the Court of Appeal; the refusal was made under the influence of another person and was made at a time when it was not anticipated that a life and death situation could arise. Since this case the Mental Capacity Act 2005 has set down statutory principles to be followed in determining the mental capacity of an individual, in defining mental capacity and in acting in the best interests of the mentally incapacitated person (see below).

Switching off a ventilator

In the case of *Re B*,[10] the President of the Family Division stated that a mentally competent patient could ask for her ventilator to be switched off and that it was a trespass to her person to treat her without her consent.

Case: *Re B*

Miss B suffered a ruptured blood vessel in her neck which damaged her spinal cord. As a consequence she was paralysed from the neck down and was on a ventilator. She was of sound mind and knew that there was no cure for her condition. She asked for the ventilator to be switched off. Her doctors wished her to try out some special rehabilitation to improve the standard of her care and felt that an intensive care ward was not a suitable location for such a decision to be made. They were reluctant to perform such an action as switching off the ventilator without the court's approval. Ms B applied to court for a declaration to be made that the ventilator could be switched off.

The main issue in the case was the mental competence of Miss B. If she were held to be mentally competent, then she could refuse to have life-saving treatment for a good reason, a bad reason or no reason at all. She was interviewed by two psychiatrists who gave evidence to the court that she was mentally competent. The judge therefore held that she was entitled to refuse to be ventilated. The judge, Dame Elizabeth Butler-Sloss, President of the Family Division, held that B possessed the requisite mental capacity to make decisions regarding her treatment and thus the administration of artificial respiration by the trust against her wishes amounted to an unlawful trespass. It was reported on 29 April 2002 that Miss B had died peacefully in her sleep after the ventilator had been switched off.

The sole issue before the Family Court was whether Miss B had the mental capacity to refuse life-saving treatment and care. The President of the Family Division, Dame Elizabeth Butler-Sloss, restated the principles which had been laid down by the Court of Appeal in the case of *St George's Healthcare Trust*:[11]

- There was a presumption that a patient had the mental capacity to make decisions, whether to consent to or refuse medical or surgical treatment offered.
- If mental capacity was not an issue and the patient, having been given the relevant information and offered the available option, chose to refuse that treatment, that decision had to be respected by the doctors; considerations of what the best interests of the patient would involve were irrelevant.
- Concern or doubts about the patient's mental capacity should be resolved as soon as possible by the doctors within the hospital or other normal medical procedures.
- Meanwhile the patient must be cared for in accordance with the judgment of the doctors as to the patient's best interests.
- It was most important that those considering the issue should not confuse the question of mental capacity with the nature of the decision made by the patient, however grave the consequences. Since the view of the patient might reflect a difference in values rather than an absence of competence, the assessment of capacity should be approached with that in mind and doctors should not allow an emotional reaction to, or strong disagreement with, the patient's decision to cloud their judgment in answering the primary question of capacity.
- Where disagreement still existed about competence, it was of the utmost importance that the patient be fully informed, involved and engaged in the process, which could involve obtaining independent outside help, of resolving the disagreement, since the patient's involvement could be crucial to a good outcome.
- If the hospital was faced with a dilemma which doctors did not know how to resolve, that must be recognised and further steps taken as a matter of priority. Those in charge must not allow a situation of deadlock or drift to occur.
- If there was no disagreement about competence, but the doctors were for any reason unable to carry out the patient's wishes, it was their duty to find other doctors who would do so.

Determination of competence

There is a presumption that a person over 16 years of age has the mental capacity to give a valid consent (this is now a statutory principle under the Mental Capacity Act 2005) but this presumption can be rebutted on a balance of probabilities. The existence of a mental illness does not automatically mean that a person is incapable of validly refusing treatment. In the case of *Re C*,[12] a patient who suffered from chronic schizophrenia and was detained in Broadmoor was assessed as requiring a leg amputation as a life-saving necessity. The patient refused to give consent and the issue of the patient's capacity to give a valid refusal came before the court. The judge used the following test to determine his mental capacity:

- Could the patient comprehend and retain the necessary information?
- Was he able to believe it?
- Was he able to weigh the information, balancing risks and needs, so as to arrive at a choice?

After applying these tests to the patient, the judge ordered an injunction to prevent anyone carrying out an amputation of his leg without his consent. (See Chapter 21 for further details of the law of consent and the mentally ill.)

Subsequently the Court of Appeal in the case of *Re MB*[13] set the following definition of competence:

A person lacks the capacity if some impairment or disturbance of mental functioning renders the person unable to make a decision whether to consent to or to refuse treatment. That inability to make a decision will occur when:

(a) The patient is unable to comprehend and retain the information which is material to the decision, especially as to the likely consequences of having or not having the treatment in question
(b) The patient is unable to use the information and weigh it in the balance as part of the process of arriving at the decision.

These definitions in case law have now been replaced by a statutory definition of mental capacity contained in the Mental Capacity Act 2005, most of which provisions came into force in October 2007.

Mental Capacity Act 2005

Definition of Mental Capacity

The Mental Capacity Act (MCA) 2005 provides a statutory definition of capacity to give consent, which is specific to the decision which has to be made (i.e. a person may have the mental capacity to give consent to one decision (e.g. what clothes he should wear), but not to another decision (e.g. whether to have an appendectomy).

Section 1(2) of the MCA recognises as a basic principle that:

A person must be assumed to have capacity unless it is established that he lacks capacity.

This presumption can be rebutted on a balance of probabilities (i.e the civil standard of proof) if there exists an impairment or disturbance in the functioning of the mind or brain and this impairment or disturbance results in an inability to make or communicate decisions. The MCA defines a lack of mental capacity as follows:

A person lacks capacity for the purposes of the MCA in relation to a matter:

if at the material time he is unable to make a decision for himself in relation to the matter because of an impairment of, or a disturbance in the functioning of, the mind or brain.

The impairment or disturbance can be permanent or temporary

The MCA thus requires a two stage test of the lack of mental capacity: the existence of an impairment or functioning in the mind or brain and secondly an inability to make or communicate decisions as a result of this defect.

The MCA section 2(3) states that a lack of capacity cannot be established merely by reference to-
(a) a person's age or appearance, or

(b)   a condition of his, or an aspect of his behaviour, which might lead others to make unjustified assumptions about his capacity.

Superficial assumptions cannot therefore be the basis of a decision on whether a person has the requisite mental capacity.

Under section 3(1) of the MCA a person is unable to make a decision for himself if he is unable:

(a)   to understand the information relevant to the decision,
(b)   to retain that information,
(c)   to use or weigh that information as part of the process of making the decision, or
(d)   to communicate his decision (whether by talking, using sign language or any other means).

This follows closely the definition of mental incapacity used in the case of the Broadmoor patient (see above).[14]

Section 3(2) of the MCA stated that a person is not to be regarded as unable to understand the information relevant to a decision if he is able to understand an explanation of it given to him in a way that is appropriate to his circumstances (using simple language, visual aids or any other means). This requirement could be resource intensive since high technology equipment may be necessary to assist persons with certain types of brain damage to communicate.

Under section 3(3) the fact that a person is able to retain the information relevant to a decision for a short period only does not prevent him from being regarded as able to make the decision.

This would enable persons who have intermittent competence to make decisions during those short times of competence.

What information must the person making the decision be able to understand? This information is defined by the MCA in section 3(4) as including information about the reasonably foreseeable consequences of:

(a)   deciding one way or another, or
(b)   failing to make the decision.

Once an assessment has concluded that a person has the mental capacity to make a specific decision then that person can make a decision for a good reason, a bad reason or no reason at all. The fact that the decision is unwise is not grounds for overruling the person's right to make the decision. However too many unwise decisions may be grounds for reviewing the assessment of capacity in order to confirm that the person has the requisite mental capacity.

On the other hand, if the assessment is that the person lacks the requisite mental capacity, then decisions must be made in that person's best interests and the MCA provides guidance on how these decisions should be made including the appointment of an independent mental capacity advocate. The other provisions of the MCA are considered in later chapters of this book (Lasting Powers of Attorney (Chapter 24); advance decisions/living wills (Chapter 25); the Court of Protection and its deputies and new criminal offence of wilful neglect and ill treatment (Chapter 22)).

A Code of Practice[15] which was prepared by the Department of Constitutional Affairs is available from its successor, the Ministry of Justice, which provides guidance on the implementation of the MCA.[16]

Background to the Mental Capacity Act 2005

The Mental Capacity Act 2005 resulted from over 10 years of discussions and consultations designed to fill the vacuum in statute law on decision making on behalf of a mentally incapacitated adult (i.e. a person over 16 years). The Law Commission had published draft legislation in 1995 in a Mental Incapacity Bill.[17] This was followed by a further consultation document: Who decides?[18] And then by a report setting out proposals for change.[19] A draft Bill was prepared[20] and subjected to scrutiny by a Joint Committee of Parliament.[21] The Mental Capacity Bill received royal assent in April 2005 but was not brought fully into force until October 2007. The Act covers the following subjects:

- basic principles (see below)
- definition of capacity (see above)
- acting in the best interests of an adult lacking mental capacity (see below)
- deprivation of liberty (i.e. Bournewood) safeguards (see Chapter 22)
- independent mental capacity advocates (see Chapter 22)
- lasting powers of attorney (see Chapter 24)
- advance decisions/living wills (see Chapter 25)
- Court of Protection, deputies, visitors, Office of Public Guardian (see Chapter 22)
- criminal offence of wilful neglect and ill treatment (Chapter 22)
- Code of Practice (see below)

Basic Principles

Section 1 of the Mental Capacity Act sets out the basic principles which apply for the purposes of the Act. They are shown in Box 7.1.

These principles would apply to all persons who are likely to be caring for or making decisions on behalf of those who may lack the requisite mental capacity.

Best interests

Where, but only where, the patient lacks the capacity to give consent to treatment, treatment can proceed on the basis that it is in the best interests of that individual. This is laid down by the Mental Capacity Act 2005 which replaces the right at common law (i.e. judge-made law) to act out of

---

Box 7.1   Basic principles of the Mental Capacity Act 2005.

- A person must be assumed to have capacity unless it is established that he lacks capacity.
- A person is not to be treated as unable to make a decision unless all practicable steps to help him to do so have been taken without success.
- A person is not to be treated as unable to make a decision merely because he makes an unwise decision.
- An act done, or decision made, under this Act for or on behalf of a person who lacks capacity must be done, or made, in his best interests.
- Before the act is done, or the decision is made, regard must be had to whether the purpose for which it is needed can be as effectively achieved in a way that is less restrictive of the person's rights and freedom of action.

necessity in the best interests of the mentally incompetent person. Where the health professional acts in the best interests of a person lacking the requisite mental capacity, he or she would not be committing a trespass to the person. The common law ruling was made by the House of Lords in the case of *Re F*.[22] In that case the House of Lords declared that it was lawful for doctors to sterilise a mentally handicapped person who lacked the capacity to give a valid consent provided that they acted in her best interests. The court did, however, require a reference to the court to be made in future cases, and a Practice Direction[23] was issued.

Section 4 of the MCA outlines the steps which must be taken into account in determining the best interests of a person incapable of making a specific decision and is shown in Box 7.2.

Determining the best interests of a person lacking the requisite mental capacity could be a slow and lengthy process and it is helpful if each department has a pro forma to ensure that the correct steps have been taken and full consultation has taken place with those able to give information on the matters listed in section 4(6). As in the assessment of mental capacity, no superficial assumptions should be made on the basis of a person's appearance, so in determining what are a person's best interests, reliance cannot be based solely on a person's age, appearance or behaviour or condition.

Restraint

The MCA (apart from the Deprivation of Liberty (i.e. Bournewood) safeguards – see below and Chapter 22) permits limited restraint to be used but only in specified circumstances. These circumstances are shown in Box 7.3.

If the conditions set out in Box 7.3 are satisfied then limited restraint could be used if it is in a person's best interests.

The deprivation of liberty (*Bournewood*) safeguards

The House of Lords, in the case of *R v Bournewood Community and Mental Health NHS Trust*,[24] held that the common law power to act out of necessity in the best interests of the patient also included the right to admit adult mentally incapacitated patients to psychiatric hospital. It overruled a decision of the Court of Appeal that such patients had to be detained under the Mental Health Act 1983 where this applied. However the European Court of Justice[25] overruled the House of Lords holding that the detention of a person incapable of consenting to admission other than under the Mental Health Act was contrary to their human rights as set out in article 5. The Government was therefore compelled to fill the gap revealed by this decision and did so by amending the Mental Capacity Act 2005 to provide measures which are known as the Bournewood safeguards. These are considered in Chapter 22.

Code of Practice

The MCA (S 42 (1)) places a duty upon the Lord Chancellor to provide a Code or Codes of Practice for the guidance of the following persons or covering certain topics:

a.   persons assessing whether a person has capacity in relation to any matter
b.   persons acting in connection with the care or treatment of another person (see S.5),
c.   donees of lasting powers of attorney
d.   deputies appointed by the court

Box 7.2   Section 4 of the Mental Capacity Act 2005 Acting in the best interests.

4. (1)   In determining for the purposes of this Act what is in a person's best interests, the person making the determination must not make it merely on the basis of—
    (a)   the person's age or appearance, or
    (b)   a condition of his, or an aspect of his behaviour, which might lead others to make unjustified assumptions about what might be in his best interests.
    (2)   The person making the determination must consider all the relevant circumstances and, in particular, take the following steps.
    (3)   He must consider—
    (a)   whether it is likely that the person will at some time have capacity in relation to the matter in question, and
    (b)   if it appears likely that he will, when that is likely to be.
    (4)   He must, so far as reasonably practicable, permit and encourage the person to participate, or to improve his ability to participate, as fully as possible in any act done for him and any decision affecting him.
    (5)   Where the determination relates to life-sustaining treatment he must not, in considering whether the treatment is in the best interests of the person concerned, be motivated by a desire to bring about his death.
    (6)   He must consider, so far as is reasonably ascertainable—
    (a)   the person's past and present wishes and feelings (and, in particular, any relevant written statement made by him when he had capacity),
    (b)   the beliefs and values that would be likely to influence his decision if he had capacity, and
    (c)   the other factors that he would be likely to consider if he were able to do so.
    (7)   He must take into account, if it is practicable and appropriate to consult them, the views of—
    (a)   anyone named by the person as someone to be consulted on the matter in question or on matters of that kind,
    (b)   anyone engaged in caring for the person or interested in his welfare,
    (c)   any donee of a lasting power of attorney granted by the person, and
    (d)   any deputy appointed for the person by the court,
as to what would be in the person's best interests and, in particular, as to the matters mentioned in subsection (6).
    (8)   The duties imposed by subsections (1) to (7) also apply in relation to the exercise of any powers which—
    (a)   are exercisable under a lasting power of attorney, or
    (b)   are exercisable by a person under this Act where he reasonably believes that another person lacks capacity.
    (9)   In the case of an act done, or a decision made, by a person other than the court, there is sufficient compliance with this section if (having complied with the requirements of subsections (1) to (7)) he reasonably believes that what he does or decides is in the best interests of the person concerned.
    (10)   "Life-sustaining treatment" means treatment which in the view of a person providing healthcare for the person concerned is necessary to sustain life.
    (11)   "Relevant circumstances" are those—
    (a)   of which the person making the determination is aware, and
    (b)   which it would be reasonable to regard as relevant.

Box 7.3   Use of restraint and the Mental Capacity Act 2005 section 6: conditions.

The first condition is that D reasonably believes that it is necessary to do the act in order to prevent harm to P.
   The second is that the act is a proportionate response to:
      (a)   the likelihood of P's suffering harm, and
      (b)   the seriousness of that harm.
  (4)   For the purposes of this section D restrains P if he—
      (a)   uses, or threatens to use, force to secure the doing of an act which P resists, or
      (b)   restricts P's liberty of movement, whether or not P resists.

---

e.   persons carrying out research in reliance on any provision made by or under the Act (and otherwise with respect to sections 30–34)
f.   independent mental capacity advocates
fa.   persons exercising functions under Schedule A1 (i.e. the Bournewood safeguards)
fb.   representatives appointed under Part 10 of Schedule A1
g.   with respect of the provisions of sections 24–26 (advance decisions and apparent advance decisions) and
h.   with respect to such other matters concerned with this Act as he thinks fit.

The Code of Practice came into force in April 2007 and has been updated to incorporate guidance on the Deprivation of Liberty (Bournewood) safeguards. It can be accessed online at the Ministry of Justice's website.[26]

Duty to inform

As part of the duty of care owed in the law of negligence, the professional has a duty to inform the patient about the significant risks of substantial harm which could occur if treatment were to proceed.

   If the risk of harm has not been explained to the patient and harm then occurs, the patient could claim that had she known of this possibility she would not have agreed to undergo the treatment. She could then bring an action in negligence. To succeed the patient would have to show that:

- there was a duty of care to give specific information
- the defendant failed to give this information and in so doing was in breach of the reasonable standard of care which should have been provided
- as a result of this failure to inform, the patient agreed to the treatment
- as a consequence the patient suffered the harm.

The leading case is that of Sidaway,[27] where the House of Lords stated that the professional was required in law to provide information to the patient according to the Bolam test, i.e. the standard of the reasonable practitioner following an accepted and approved standard of care.

   To ensure that the patient understands the information which is given, there are considerable advantages in a written handout being provided (checking of course that the patient is literate and does not have visual impairments, and that the handout is kept up to date). This would also assist if there were any dispute over whether the information had been given.

Case: *Chester v Afshar*[28]

The patient suffered from severe back pain and gave consent to an operation for the removal of three intra-vertebral discs. The patient claimed that the neurosurgeon failed to give a warning to her about the slight risk of post-operative paralysis which the patient suffered following the operation. The trial judge held that the doctor was not negligent in his conduct of the operation, but was negligent in failing to warn her of the slight risk of paralysis which she suffered, and gave judgment for damages to be assessed. The defendant appealed to the Court of Appeal against this finding of failing to give the appropriate information to the claimant.

The Court of Appeal held that the purpose of the rule requiring doctors to give appropriate information to their patients was to enable the patient to exercise her right to choose whether or not to have the particular operation to which she was asked to give her consent. The patient had the right to choose what would and would not be done with her body and the doctor should take the care expected of a reasonable doctor in the circumstances in giving her the information relevant to that choice. The law was designed to require doctors properly to inform their patients of the risk attendant on their treatment and to answer questions put to them as to that treatment and its dangers, such answers to be judged in the context of good professional practice, which had tended to a greater degree of frankness over the years, with more respect being given to patient autonomy.

The object was to enable the patient to decide whether or not to run the risks of having that operation at that time. If the doctor's failure to take care resulted in her consenting to an operation to which she would not otherwise have given her consent, the purpose of that rule would be thwarted if he were not to be held responsible when the very risk about which he failed to warn her materialised and caused her an injury.

The outcome in the Court of Appeal therefore was that the appeal by the surgeon against the finding of negligence in not giving information failed and the patient won the case.

The defendant then appealed to the House of Lords which by a majority verdict dismissed his appeal. The House of Lords held that the claimant had shown that had she been notified of the risk of paralysis, which in fact occurred, she would have had to think further about undergoing the surgery and therefore she had established a causal link between the breach and the injury she had sustained and the defendant was liable in damages.

In a High Court case Mrs Birch suffered harm following a catheter angiography, which it was held had been performed without negligence. However, she obtained compensation since the surgeon failed to discuss with her the imaging methods and their comparative risks and was therefore in breach of the duty of care to inform.[29]

Application to OT practice

Trespass to the person

In practice there are many occupational therapy activities and treatments which cannot proceed without the co-operation of the patient, and consent to involvement is often implied from the patient's non-verbal communication. In such cases, therefore, trespass to the person actions are unlikely. The focus is more likely to be on the nature of the information given (see below).

Care should, however, be taken, if it is necessary to examine a patient or have physical contact, to ensure that the patient is consenting to this contact, as merely touching another person without consent is actionable as trespass to the person. Unlike negligence (see Chapter 10), there is no need for the claimant to prove that harm ensued. The OT should also be aware of the dangers of any compromising situation if treating a patient of the opposite sex, and the difficulties of countering false allegations of impropriety if no chaperone is present. (See also the section on sexual harassment in Chapter 11 and the guidance on sexual boundaries issued by the Council for Healthcare Regulatory Excellence and the Health Professions Council discussed in Chapter 4.)

Competence

It has been emphasised that, in order to give a valid consent, an individual must have the competence to do so, and it has also been seen in the case of Re T that the Court of Appeal emphasised the duty of the health professional to ensure that a person refusing necessary treatment had the capacity to do so. The statutory definition of mental capacity as laid down in the Mental Capacity Act 2005 must be applied. Of relevance to the assessment of mental capacity is the work of Fleming and Strong[30] in research on self-awareness of deficits following acquired brain injury and what must be taken into account in rehabilitation. Where there is any doubt about the competence of an individual to give a valid consent there are considerable advantages if that capacity could be checked by a person who is not involved in the treatment which is being recommended. This person should record her actions and observations.

Informing the client

The duty placed upon the OT is that she should ensure that the patient is given information about the significant risks of substantial harm which could arise from treatment and questions raised by the patient should be answered honestly and correctly. The OT would be judged by the standard of the reasonable occupational therapist in that situation with that specific patient (The Bolam test is used to determine the standard which should apply and is discussed in Chapter 10). This requires the OT to ensure that she maintains her competence and knowledge about current issues and research.

Documentation and consent

It will be noted from the above that many occupational therapy treatments will be given without any written evidence of consent. Where, however, it is feared that there may be significant risks of substantial harm or there is likely to be any dispute as to whether consent was given, it is advisable for consent to be evidenced in writing.

The forms issued by the Department of Health can be used by any health professional and could be adapted for specific OT treatment where it is considered that there are certain risks. Their use should ensure that all the requisite information is recorded. Form 4 can be used where an adult lacks mental capacity to give consent to treatment, and care is provided in the absence of consent under the provisions of the Mental Capacity Act 2005. Barbara Steward[31] in an editorial suggests that now may be the time for OTs to consider how and when clients should give informed choice or consent and how this should be recorded and monitored. The adaptation of the DH forms for specific OT activities could be part of this review process.

Written information provided about treatments must be regularly updated. For example after scientists criticised the leaflets used for breast cancer screenings on the grounds that the information was inadequate and manipulative, the DH stated that it was preparing new leaflets following a formal review.[32]

The COT's Standard for Practice on consent to treatment[33] gives advice on the information which should be recorded. This includes:

- the fact that consent was given and how it was given
- that the OT was satisfied as to the client having the requisite level of mental capacity
- the proposed course of action
- the points of discussion about substantial risks that preceded written consent being obtained
- the points of discussion about recordings of an audio, photograph, or video which preceded written consent being obtained
- the client's agreement if intervention was to be made by a student.

Recording this information should ensure that other occupational therapists and other health professionals caring for the patient are aware of what the patient has been told. There are also advantages in arranging for specific information to be provided in writing to the patient, ensuring that any such leaflets are kept up to date.

Conclusion

The law recognises the autonomy of the mentally competent adult to decide whether or not to participate in treatment activities. The onus is on the health professional to inform the patient fully about the benefits and risks of the treatment. The implementation of the Mental Capacity Act 2005 means that there is now in place a statutory framework for decision making on behalf of those who lack the requisite mental capacity. Each department should have a copy of the Code of Practice on the MCA to assist individual practitioners in the determination of capacity and the assessment of the individual's best interests. The GMC has updated its guidance on consent after collaborating with National Theatre actors who performed scenes which raised the issues of patients, carers and doctors. The guidance reflects the changing relationship between doctors and patients, with the decline in deference and demands for more information.[34] It expands on the guidance in *Good Medical Practice*,[35] which requires doctors to be satisfied that they have consent from a patient, or other valid authority, before undertaking any examination or investigation, providing treatment, or involving patients in teaching and research. The guidance, which is available on the GMC website,[36] would be of value to occupational therapists.

   Questions and exercises

1   Obtain copies of the Department of Health's guidance on consent to examination and treatment. In the light of this information, analyse your practice in obtaining consent from the patient and decide if it could be improved.
2   In the light of the Department of Health forms on consent to examination and treatment, draw up a form for consent to specific occupational therapy treatments.
3   Prepare a handout for the client/patient giving information about the nature of any specific treatment you provide setting out any inherent risks.
4   How does the Mental Capacity Act 2005 affect your practice as an OT?

References

1   For further details on the law relating to consent, see Dimond, B. (2009) *Legal Aspects of Consent*, 2nd edn. Quay Books, Dinton, Salisbury.

2   College of Occupational Therapists (2003 revised 2007) *Professional Standards for Occupational Therapy Practice*. COT, London.

3   *R v Human Fertilisation and Embryology Authority ex parte Blood* (1999) Fam 151.

4   *Evans v United Kingdom* [2007] ECHR 264 No 6339/05.

5   *L v Human Fertilisation and Embryology Authority* The Times Law Report 16 October 2008.

6   Department of Health (2001) *Reference Guide to Consent for Examination or Treatment*; www.doh.gov.uk/consent

7   Department of Health (2001) Good practice in consent implementation guide. DH, London.

8   Bristol Royal Infirmary Inquiry (Kennedy Report), Learning from Bristol: the report of the public inquiry into children's heart surgery at the Bristol Royal Infirmary 1984–1995, Command paper Cm 5207, The Stationery Office, London, 2001.

9   *Re T (Adult: refusal of medical treatment)* [1992] 4 All ER 649.

10 *Re B (Consent to treatment: capacity)*, Times Law Report, 26 March 2002; [2002] 2 All ER 449.

11 *St George's Healthcare NHS Trust v S.* The Times, 8 May 1998; [1999] Fam 26.

12 *Re C (Adult: refusal of medical treatment)* [1994] 1 All ER 819.

13 *Re MB (an adult: medical treatment)* [1997] 2 FLR 426.

14 *C (re) (an adult) (refusal of medical treatment)* FD [1994] 1 All ER 819.

15 Department of Constitutional Affairs Code of Practice 2007; www.justice.gov.uk

16 www.justice.gov.uk

17 Law Commission (1995) *Mental Incapacity*. HMSO, London.

18 Lord Chancellor (1997) *Who Decides?* Lord Chancellor's Office, Stationery Office.

19 Lord Chancellor's Office (1999) *Making Decisions: The Government's proposals for decision making on behalf of mentally incapacitated adults*. Stationery Office, London.

20 Department of Health Draft Mental Incapacity Bill CM 5859 June 2003.

21 House of Lords and House of Commons Joint Committee on the Draft Mental Incapacity Bill Session 2002–3 HL paper 189-1; HC 1083-1.

22 *F v West Berkshire Health Authority and another* [1989] 2 All ER 545.

23 Practice Note [1993] 3 All ER 222 (replaces previous Practice Note issued 1989).

24 *R v Bournewood Community and Mental Health NHS Trust, ex parte L* (HL) [1998] 1 All ER 634.

25 *R v Bournewood Community and Mental Health NHS Trust ex p L* [1998] 3 All ER 289; [1999] AC 458; *L v United Kingdom* (Application No 45508/99) Times Law Report 19 October 2004.

26 www.justice.gov.uk

27 *Sidaway v Bethlem Royal Hospital Governors* [1985] 1 All ER 643.

28 *Chester v Afshar* Times Law Report, 13 June 2002; [2002] 3 All ER 552, CA. Department of Health the NHS Confidentiality Code of Practice DH 2003 available on www.doh.gov.uk/ipu/confiden/protect/ (superseding HSG(96) 18 LASSL (96)5).

29 *Birch v University College London Hospital NHS Foundation Trust* [2008] EWHC 2237 (QB) (29 September 2008).

30 Fleming, J. & Strong, J. (1995) Self-awareness of deficits following acquired brain injury: Considerations for rehabilitation. *British Journal of Occupational Therapy*, **58**(2), 55–60.

31 Steward, B. (2001) Informed consent. *British Journal of Occupational Therapy*, **64**(4), 163.

32 Smyth, C. NHS rips up breast cancer leaflet and starts all over again. The Times 21 February 2009.

33 College of Occupational Therapists (2003) *Standards for Practice Consent for Occupational Therapy*. COT, London.

34 General Medical Council (2008) *Consent: patients and doctors making decisions together*. GMC, London.

35 General Medical Council (2006) *Good Medical Practice*. GMC, London.

36 www.gmc-uk.org

8 The Duty of Confidentiality and Data Protection

All practitioners, whether working in the public or independent sector, have a duty to maintain the confidentiality of information obtained from or about the patient. This chapter explores the source of this obligation and the exceptions to the duty that are recognised in law.[1] The most significant legislation in this field is the Data Protection Act 1998 and this will be considered initially. Regulations on access by persons to their records under the Data Protection Act 1998 and the Freedom of Information Act 2000 will be considered in the next chapter. A useful guide on Data Protection law is provided by Peter Carey[2] The following topics are covered in this chapter:

- Data protection legislation
- Data protection principles
- Rights of data subjects
- Information Commissioner

- Duty of confidentiality
- Exceptions to the duty of confidentiality
- Caldicott Guardians

Data protection legislation

The European Directive on Data Protection[3] was implemented in this country by the Data Protection Act 1998. Member states were required to comply with its provisions by 24 October 1998, although the UK did not meet this target. Under the legislation members had to establish a set of principles with which users of personal information must comply. The legislation also gives individuals the right to gain access to information held about them and provides for a supervisory authority to oversee and enforce the law. Guidance from the Department of Health on the Act for both the NHS and local authorities was provided by a circular in March 2000,[4] and the NHS Information Authority action plan for the NHS, to ensure that the processing of personal data within the organisation is in

Legal Aspects of Occupational Therapy, Third Edition By Bridgit Dimond
© 2010 Bridgit Dimond

compliance with the Act, was available on its website.[5] The NHS Information Authority was abolished in April 2005 and its work undertaken by NHS Connecting for Health.[6] (The Information Security Management: Code of Practice prepared by the DH is considered in Chapter 12.)

There are some significant differences between the Data Protection Act 1984 and the Data Protection Act 1998, the most significant of which is that the 1998 Act applies to manual records (if they form part of a relevant filing system) as well as to computerised records. Some terms are defined slightly differently and there are tighter provisions on the processing of sensitive personal data. The fundamental rights are amended and there are new rules for the transfer of personal data outside the European Community.

The person in charge of Data Protection is known as the Information Commissioner (following the Freedom of Information Act, the same person is responsible for the implementation of both the Data Protection Act 1998 (see below) and the Freedom of Information Act 2000 (see Chapter 9)). Considerable information on both Acts is available from the Information Commissioner's website together with technical briefing notes.[7]

The Data Protection Act 1998 must be read in conjunction with the Human Rights Act 1998 (see Chapter 6). Article 8 of the European Convention of Human Rights, which is set out in Schedule 1 of the Act, (and can be seen in Appendix 1 of this book) recognises an individual's right to private and family life, subject to specific qualifications and this article has been relied upon when breaches of confidentiality have been alleged.

Computerised and manually held records

The Data Protection Act 1984 applied only to computerised records but since the passing of the Data Protection Act 1998 patient records held in a manual form may come under the same rules as those on a computer. Data now includes manually held records if they form part of a relevant filing system. A possible exception to manual records not coming under Data Protection provisions are clinical supervision records in which specific patients are named. These may not come under the provisions of the Data Protection Act since they may not form part of a relevant filing system. The Court of Appeal considered the meaning of relevant filing system in the case of *Durant v Financial Services Authority*[8] and held that the Act intended to cover manual files "only if they are of sufficient sophistication to provide the same or similar ready accessibility as a computerised filing system". It stated that

"a 'relevant filing system' for the purposes of the Act, is limited to a system:

1) in which the files forming part of it are structured or referenced in such a way as to clearly indicate at the outset of the search whether specific information capable of amounting to personal data of an individual requesting it under section 7 is held within the system and, if so, in which file or files it is held; and
2) which has, as part of its own structure or referencing mechanism, a sufficiently sophisticated and detailed means of readily indicating whether and where in an individual file or files specific criteria or information about the applicant can be readily located".

Further explanation of relevant filing system is given by the Information Commissioner in his briefing note on the Durant case in 2006.[9]

Data Protection Act 1998

The main provisions of the Act are shown in Figure 8.1.

Figure 8.1 Data Protection Act 1998.

Part 1 Preliminary: basic interpretative provisions; sensitive personal data; the special purposes; data protection principles; application of Act; Commissioner and Tribunal

Part 2 Rights of Data subjects and others:
Rights of access
Rights to prevent processing likely to cause damage or distress
Rights to prevent processing for direct marketing
Rights in relation to automated decision-taking
Compensation for failure to comply with certain requirements
Rectification, blocking, erasure and destruction

Part 3 Notification to the data controller: duty to notify; register of notifications; offences; preliminary assessment by Commissioner; power to make provision for appointment of data protection supervisors; duty of certain data controllers to make certain information available; functions of Commissioner in relation to making of notification regulations; fees regulations

Part 4 Exemptions:
National Security
Crime and taxation
Health, education and social work
Regulatory activity
Journalism, literature and art
Research, history and statistics
Information available to the public by or under enactment
Disclosure required by law or made in connection with legal proceedings
Domestic purposes
Powers to make further exemptions by order

Part 5 Enforcement

Part 6 Miscellaneous and General: Functions of the Commissioner

Schedule 1 Data Protection Principles
Schedule 2 Conditions for processing any personal data
Schedule 3 Conditions for processing sensitive personal data
Schedule 4 Cases where the 8th principle does not apply
Schedule 5 Data Protection Commissioner and Data Protection Tribunal
Schedule 6 Appeal proceedings
Schedule 7 Miscellaneous exemptions
Schedule 8 Transitional Relief
Schedule 9 Powers of entry and inspection
Schedule 10 Assistance under section 53
Schedule 11 Educational records
Schedule 12 Accessible public records
Schedule 13 Modifications of Act having effect pre 24 October 2007

Terminology

The following are some of the definitions of terms used in the Data Protection Act 1998:

- The Data Subject is 'the individual who is the subject of personal data', but under the 1998 provisions the law applies only to living people and if the information is anonymous, then the person will not be considered to be identifiable, unless it is possible to link together separate items of information to identify an individual. If that is possible, the Act would then apply. Further guidance on the meaning of personal data is given by the ICO in its technical note.[10]

- Processing under the 1998 Act includes any operation involving personal data including the holding of the information.
- The term 'data user' (from the 1984 Act) is replaced by the term 'controller' and is the person who determines the purposes for which and the manner in which any personal data are to be processed.
- Computer bureaux' is replaced by 'processor'.
- The Data Protection Registrar, who is the national officer responsible for the oversight of the implementation of the law, is now to be known as the Information Commissioner, and since the Freedom of Information Act 2000, statutory duties under that statute and the Data Protection Act 1998 are under the control of the Information Commissioner.

Data protection principles

The 1998 Act slightly amends the data protection principles and the new wording is shown in Figure 8.2. Interpretation of the data protection principles is provided in part II of Schedule 1 of the 1998 Act.

Under principle 1 personal data shall be processed fairly and lawfully and, in particular, shall not be processed unless: (a) at least one of the conditions in Schedule 2 is met; and (b) in the case of sensitive personal data, at least one of the conditions in Schedule 3 is also met. In a case on principle 1 an orthopaedic surgeon lost his appeal against the refusal of the High Court to hold that removal

Figure 8.2   Data protection principles 1998, Schedule 1, Part 1.

(1) Personal data shall be processed fairly and lawfully and, in particular, shall not be processed unless:
   (a) at least one of the conditions in Schedule 2 is met; and
   (b) in the case of sensitive personal data, at least one of the conditions in Schedule 3 is also met.
(2) Personal data shall be obtained only for one or more specified and lawful purposes, and shall not be further processed in any manner incompatible with that purpose or those purposes.
(3) Personal data shall be adequate, relevant and not excessive in relation to the purpose or purposes for which they are processed.
(4) Personal data shall be accurate and, where necessary, kept up to date.
(5) Personal data processed for any purpose or purposes shall not be kept for longer than is necessary for that purpose(s).
(6) Personal data shall be processed in accordance with the rights of data subjects under this Act.
(7) Appropriate technical and organisational measures shall be taken against unauthorised or unlawful processing of personal data and against accidental loss or destruction of, or damage to, personal data.
(8) Personal data shall not be transferred to a country or territory outside the European Economic Area unless that country or territory ensures an adequate level of protection for the rights and freedoms of data subjects in relation to the processing of personal data.

of his name from the register of members of the Medical Defence Union breached principle one of the Data Protection Act 1998 in that his personal data was not processed fairly.[11]

Principle 1 refers to Schedule 2 conditions and these include:

- The consent of the data subject
- The processing is necessary:
  - for the performance of a contract to which the data subject is a party
  - for taking steps, at the request of the data subject, to enter a contract.
- The processing is necessary for compliance with a legal obligation of the data subject.
- The processing is necessary to protect the vital interests of the data subject.
- The processing is necessary
  - for the administration of justice
  - the exercise of functions conferred by any enactment
  - the exercise of function of the Crown, Minister or Government department or
  - for the exercise of other functions of a public nature.
- The processing is necessary to meet the legitimate interests of the data controller or a third party.

Clearly patient records are covered by several of these conditions, only one of which is needed to legitimate the processing.

Personal data

Guidance on the meaning of personal data was published by the Information Commissioner in August 2007.[12] It stated that information that is not personal data today may become personal data as technology advances. The Court of Appeal in 2003 in the case brought by Michael Durant against the Financial Services Authority defined personal data narrowly. Subsequently the IC updated its guidance and says that information could count as personal data even if it does not include a person's name. For example:

> There will be circumstances where the data you hold enables you to identify an individual whose name you do not know and you may never intend to discover. Similarly, a combination of data about gender, age, and grade or salary may well enable you to identify a particular employee even without a name or job title.

Sensitive personal data

Sensitive personal data is defined in section 2 (see Figure 8.3). Records relating to physical or mental health come within the definition of sensitive personal data and Schedule 3 conditions for disclosure of such information are shown in Figure 8.4.

Circumstances have been specified in which the data protection principle contained in the Data Protection Act 1998 Schedule 1 para. 1 (which prohibits the processing of sensitive personal data unless one of the specified conditions is met) does not apply.[13] These circumstances include where the processing is in the substantial public interest, is necessary for the purposes of the prevention or detection of any unlawful act and must necessarily be carried out without the explicit consent of the data subject being sought so as not to prejudice those purposes. Subsequent regulations provide an exemption from data protection principle 1 where disclosure of sensitive personal data is made available to elective representatives such as MPs.[14]

Figure 8.3 Sensitive personal data, section 2 of Data Protection Act 1998.

Means personal data consisting of information as to:

- The racial or ethnic origin of the data subject
- His political opinions
- His religious beliefs or other beliefs of a similar nature
- Whether he is a member of a Trade Union
- His physical or mental health or condition
- His sexual life
- The (alleged) commission of any offence by him
- Any proceedings for any (alleged) offence, disposal of such or sentence.

Figure 8.4 Schedule 3 Conditions for disclosure of sensitive personal data.

1. The data subject has given his explicit consent to the processing of personal data
2. (1) The processing is necessary for the purposes of exercising or performing any right or obligation which is conferred or imposed on the data controller in connection with employment
   (2) The Secretary of State may exclude the application of sub-paragraph 1 in such cases as may be specified, or specify further conditions for satisfaction
3. The processing is necessary:
   (a) to protect the vital interests of the data subject or another person, in a case where:
      (i) consent cannot be given by or on behalf of the data subject or
      (ii) the data controller cannot reasonably be expected to obtain the consent of the data subject or
   (b) in order to protect the vital interests of another person, in a case where consent by or on behalf of the data subject has been unreasonably withheld
4. The processing:
   (a) is carried out in the course of its legitimate activities by any body or association which:
      (i) is not established or conducted for profit and
      (ii) exists for political, philosophical, religious or trade union purposes
   (b) is carried out with appropriate safeguards for the rights and freedoms of the data subject
   (c) relates only to individuals who either are members of the body or association or have regular contact with it in connection with its purposes, and
   (d) does not involve disclosure of the personal data to a third party without the consent of the data subject
5. The information contained in the personal data has been made public as a result of steps deliberately taken by the data subject
6. The processing;
   (a) is necessary for the purpose of, or in connection with, any legal proceedings (including prospective legal proceedings)
   (b) is necessary for the purpose of obtaining legal advice, or
   (c) is otherwise necessary for the purposes of establishing, exercising or defending legal rights

continued

Figure 8.4 Continued.

7. (1) The processing is necessary:
     (a) for the administration of justice
     (b) for the exercise of any functions conferred on any person by or under an enactment or
     (c) for the exercise of any functions of the Crown, Minister of the Crown or a Government department
   (2) The Secretary of State may by order:
     (a) exclude the application of sub-paragraph (1) in such cases as may be specified, or
     (b) provide that, in such cases as may be specified, the condition in subparagraph (1) is not to be regarded as satisfied unless such further conditions as may be specified in the order are also satisfied
8. (1) The processing is for medical purposes and is undertaken by:
     (a) a health professional, or
     (b) a person who in the circumstances owes a duty of confidentiality which is equivalent to that which would arise if that person were a health professional
   (2) In this paragraph, 'medical purposes' includes the purposes of preventative medicine, medical diagnosis, medical research, the provision of care and treatment and the management of healthcare services.
9. (1) The processing;
     (a) Is of sensitive personal data consisting of information as to racial or ethnic origin.
     (b) Is necessary for the purpose of identifying or keeping under review the existence or absence of equality of opportunity or treatment between persons of different racial or ethnic origins, with a view to enabling such equality to be promoted or maintained, and
     (c) Is carried out with appropriate safeguards for the rights and freedoms of data subjects
   (2) The Secretary of State may by order specify circumstances in which processing falling within subparagraphs (I)(a), and (b) is, or is not, to be taken for the purposes of sub-paragraph (I)(c) to be carried out with appropriate safeguards for the rights and freedoms of data subjects
10. The personal data are processed in circumstances specified in an order made by the Secretary of State for the purposes of this paragraph.

Consent

Schedule 2 requires the consent of the data subject or one of the other conditions to be satisfied for processing to be carried on.

Schedule 3 requires that one of the conditions set out in the Schedule must be satisfied before processing of sensitive data can comply with the first principle. Consent is not required under condition 3, where processing is necessary to protect the data subject's vital interests and consent cannot be given by or on behalf of the data subject, or the data controller cannot be reasonably expected to obtain the consent of the data subject. This situation would obviously cover records relating to the mentally incapacitated adult and children. Another condition of Schedule 3 is that the processing is necessary for medical purposes (including the purposes of preventative medicine, medical

> **Figure 8.5**   Rights of the data subject under the 1998 Act.
>
> 1. Right of subject access (section 7 to 9)
> 2. Right to prevent processing likely to cause damage or distress (section 10)
> 3. Right to prevent processing for the purposes of direct marketing (section 11)
> 4. Right in relation to automated decision taking (section 12)
> 5. Right to take action for compensation if the individual suffers damage by any contravention of the Act by the data controller (section 13)
> 6. Right to take action to rectify, block, erase or destroy inaccurate data (section 14)
> 7. Right to make a request to the Commissioner for an assessment to be made as to whether any provision of the Act has been contravened (section 42)

diagnosis, medical research, the provision of care and treatment and the management of healthcare services) and is undertaken by a health professional or a person who owes a duty of confidentiality which is equivalent to that which would arise if that person were a health professional. Satisfaction of this condition would obviate the need to obtain the explicit consent of every patient, in order for their health records to be processed.

Rights of the data subject

The rights of the individual under the Data Protection Act 1998 are shown in Figure 8.5.

Section 7 Right of access to personal data

Section 7, which enables an individual to be informed of data held about him and to access that data, is considered in Chapter 9.

Section 30 Health education and social work

Section 30 enables the Secretary of State to draw up specific provisions setting exemptions from the statutory rights of access in relation to health, education and social work records. Statutory Instruments have been enacted setting out details of the restrictions on access to these records[15] and these are considered in Chapter 9 on access.

Information Commissioner (formerly Data Protection Commissioner)

The Information Commissioner has the responsibility for promoting good practice and observance of the laws, providing an information service and encouraging the development of Codes of Practice. He has considerable powers of enforcement under Parts 3 and 5 of the Act. These include the power to serve enforcement notices and powers of entry and inspection. Information is available from the Commissioner's office free of charge.[16] An explanatory guide to the legislation is available.[17] The

Figure 8.6   Offences under the Data Protection Act 1998.

1.   Offences relating to failure to notify the Commissioner or comply with his requests
2.   Unlawfully obtaining personal data
3.   Unlawful selling of personal data
4.   Forcing a person to compel access
5.   Unlawful disclosure of information by the commissioner/staff or agent

website is www.ico.gov.uk. An application for judicial review by the Secretary of State of an information tribunal decision which had quashed a ministerial certificate claiming exemption from providing subject access on grounds of national security failed. The High Court held that the Information Commissioner had the power to check whether an exemption was properly claimed.[18]

Offences under the Act are shown in Figure 8.6.

Guidance from the NHS Executive

The NHS Executive has published guidelines on the protection and use of patient information to support the implementation of the Data Protection Act.[19] It stated that a working group at the Department of Health was developing national guidance to assist NHS bodies and local authorities on the principles and practical issues involved in sharing client/patient records for service delivery and of using such aggregated data for planning, commissioning, managing and monitoring. This group was working under the aegis of the Information Policy Unit of the Department of Health, which can be accessed via its website.[20]

DNA information

DNA databases

A recent case came before the European Court of Human Rights concerning the National DNA database. Two men from Sheffield, Michael Marper and S. brought the case because they were arrested in 2001 and had their fingerprints and DNA samples taken. They were not convicted of any crime and argued that the samples should have been destroyed. Their case was rejected by the British courts and in February 2008 the ECHR gave permission for the case to proceed.[21] The ECHR subsequently held that storage of DNA profiles of suspects who were not convicted was a breach of Article 8 and constituted a disproportionate interference with the applicants' right to privacy.[22] The ECHR considered that the blanket and indiscriminate nature of the powers given to the police could not be regarded as necessary in a democratic society. As a consequence of this judgment more than 1.6 million DNA and fingerprint samples must be destroyed from police databases.[23]

The Information Tribunal held that police were breaking rules on the holding of personal details and that they should remove information about minor crimes from their records because storing it breached data protection laws.[24]

Duty of confidentiality

The duty to respect confidentiality arises from a variety of sources which are set out in Figure 8.7, for the employed health professional. The Department of Health has prepared a Code of Practice on confidentiality.[25] Those who work as self-employed professionals do not have an obligation to an employer but they do have a contract for services with their patients, which may impose conditions relating to confidentiality. Should the self-employed health professional be in breach of these contractual conditions, then the patient could bring an action in the civil courts and have the usual remedies for breach of contract. In addition, a self-employed professional is bound by the Data Protection Act 1998. A nurse who secretly filmed the neglect of elderly patients for a television documentary was struck off the nursing register by the NMC. The fact that she was a whistle blower reporting on abuse of the elderly was not seen as justification for her admitted breach of patient confidentiality. The chair of the NMC fitness to practice panel said that she had given priority to the filming over her professional duties.[26] The decision was not without controversy.[27] The NMC subsequently substituted a 12 month caution for the striking off.

Anonymous data

The duty of confidentiality applies if persons can be identified from the information, or from that and other information. There is no breach of confidentiality if the confider's identity is protected. This was the decision in a case where the Department of Health attempted to prevent a firm collecting data on the prescribing habits of general practitioners, which it planned to sell to pharmaceutical companies so that they could market their products more effectively. The company believed the information would be useful to drug companies and would provide useful data for those interested in monitoring prescribing patterns. Even though the information would be anonymous, the Department of Health challenged the use of this information as a breach of the guidelines put forward by the Department of Health[28] in 1996. It succeeded before the High Court but the Court of Appeal[29] reversed this decision. It held that GPs and pharmacists providing prescription information that did not identify the patient was not a breach of confidence. Anonymous data did not involve a risk to the patient's privacy, even if, with effort, the patient could be identified.

In 2008 the House of Lords held that data on childhood leukaemia could be released if it was anonymised. The facts are given below.

Figure 8.7   Sources of the obligation to respect the confidentiality of patient information.

a.   Duty set out in the Code of Professional Conduct
b.   Duty in the contract of employment
c.   Duty as part of the duty of care owed to the patient in the law of negligence
d.   Duty set out in specific statutes, especially the Data Protection Act 1998 and Human Rights Act 1998
e.   Duty as part of the trust obligation between health professional and patient

Case: *Common Services Agency v Scottish Information Commissioner* Times 2008[30]

A researcher acting on behalf of a member of the Scottish Parliament asked the Common Services Agency which collected and disseminated epidemiological information for details of all incidents of childhood leukaemia for all the Dumfries and Galloway postal areas by census ward. The agency refused the researcher's request. There was a danger of indirect identification of living individuals because of the low numbers involved. The data was personal data within the meaning of the 1998 Act and was exempt from disclosure under the Freedom of Information (Scotland) Act 2002. The researcher appealed to the Scottish Information Commissioner who decided that the information could be disclosed if it had undergone a process known as Barnardisation which rendered the data anonymous and more difficult to identify individuals. The effect of this process could mean that the data was no longer "personal" The House of Lords declared that the researcher should reapply to the Commissioner so that he could consider whether the process of Barnardisation had resulted in the data being anonymised and therefore no long personal data, or whether disclosure by the Agency would be in accordance with Schedules 1, 2 and 3 of the Data Protection Act 1998.

Duty in the Code of Professional Conduct

Each registered health professional has certain professional obligations which are enforceable through the professional conduct machinery set up under the Health Professions Council. Clause 2 of the HPC Standards of conduct, performance and ethics.[31] This requires its registrants to:

Respect the confidentiality of your patients, clients and users.

It amplifies this by requiring the registrant:

to treat information about patients, clients or users as confidential and use it only for the purpose for which it was given. You must not knowingly release any personal or confidential information to anyone who is not entitled to it, and you should check that people who ask for information are entitled to it.
   You must only use information about a service user:

To continue to care for that person; or
For purposes where that person has given you specific permission to use the information.

You must also keep to the conditions of any relevant data protection legislation and always follow best practice for handling confidential information. Best practice is likely to change over time, and you must stay up to date.

The HPC published a consultation document on confidentiality guidance for registrants in June 2007. The final guidance was published in 2008 and is available on the HPC website.[32] The HPC describes its guidance as not being designed to replace local procedures and not being meant to cover every situation where problems can come up.

However, it is meant to act as a 'toolkit' which you can use to make informed and reasonable decisions relating to issues of confidentiality, in line with our standards.

The guidance sets the following principles for registrants:

You should:

- take all reasonable steps to keep information about service users safe;
- get the service user's informed consent if you are passing on their information, and get express consent, in writing, if you are using the information for reasons which are not related to providing care or services for the service user;
- only disclose identifiable information if it is absolutely necessary, and, when it is necessary, only disclose the minimum amount necessary;

- tell service users when you have disclosed their information (if this is practical and possible);
- keep appropriate records of disclosure;
- keep up to date with relevant law and good practice;
- if appropriate, ask for advice from colleagues, professional bodies, unions, legal professionals or us; and
- make your own informed decisions about disclosure and be able to justify them.

The Guidance covers: confidentiality and the law; identifiable information and anonymised information; keeping information safe; disclosing information; disclosing information without consent; disclosing information by law; and confidentiality and accountability.

Duty in the contract of employment

The employed health professional also has an obligation enforceable by the employer, which derives from the contract of employment, to observe the confidentiality of patient information. This will usually be set out expressly in the contract of employment, but even if the contract is silent on the topic, the courts may imply into the contract such a term. Should the health professional be in breach of this expressed or implied term, then the employer can take appropriate action through the disciplinary machinery. This may be simply counselling or an oral warning, or any of the stages in the disciplinary procedure may be invoked, depending on the circumstances. In serious cases, the employer may be considered justified in dismissing the employee. In such a case, if the employee has the necessary continuous service requirement (see Chapter 19) the employee could challenge the dismissal by an application to an employment tribunal for unfair dismissal. In a recent case, the House of Lords required a newspaper to disclose the name of its informant who had provided information about one of the patients at Ashworth Special Hospital[33] (see below). The employer would therefore be able to discipline the employee.

Duty in the law of negligence

The health professional owes a duty to the patient to retain information given to her in confidence. Should the health professional be in breach of this duty, then the patient could bring an action against the employer of the health professional on the basis of its vicarious liability for the actions of an employee acting in course of employment. In the New Zealand case of *Furniss v Fitchett*,[34] the court upheld an action for damages in the tort of negligence for breach of confidence. A doctor treating the claimant had given to the patient's husband a letter about the patient's mental state, which was used by the husband's solicitor in matrimonial proceedings. The doctor was held to be in breach of the duty of care which he owed to the patient, in those particular circumstances. The court did not express an opinion on whether such disclosure would always be a breach of the duty of care.

One weakness with the patient's right of action in the law of negligence is that the patient has to prove harm. Following unauthorised disclosure, harm may eventually arise, but until it does the patient cannot obtain compensation. He could, however, obtain an injunction to prevent disclosure (see the Case of *X v Y* below).

Case of *X v Y*[35]

Two general practitioners were diagnosed as having contracted AIDS. They received counselling in a local hospital, but continued their medical practice. A journalist heard of the situation from an employee of the health authority and wrote an article for a national newspaper. The health authority sought an injunction to prevent any further disclosure of the information obtained from the patients' records. The judge granted the injunction on the grounds that the records of hospital patients, particularly those suffering from this appalling condition, should be as confidential as the courts can properly make them in order that the claimants may be free from suspicion that they are harbouring disloyal employees. He rejected the defendant's argument that it was in the public interest for the identity of these doctors to be known.

The court ordered an injunction to be issued to prevent the disclosure by the press of the identity of doctors suffering from AIDS. The judge did not, however, agree to the health authority's application for the name of the employee who had disclosed the information to the journalist. He held that the exceptions under section 10 of the Contempt of Court Act 1981 to the principle that the court cannot require disclosure from a journalist did not apply to the situation and the journalist was entitled to protect his source.

In a more recent case, the House of Lords ordered a newspaper to disclose its source of confidential information.[36] An employee in Ashworth Hospital gave verbatim extracts of the medical records of convicted murderer Ian Brady, a patient at the hospital, to a national newspaper. The court ordered the publisher to identify the employee and the name of the intermediary person who was involved in the publisher acquiring possession of the records. The Court of Appeal dismissed the publisher's appeal. The publisher appealed to the House of Lords, arguing that the order for disclosure was not justified: it was not itself a wrongdoer and disclosure was limited to cases where such disclosure was required in order to enable the claimant to bring procedures against the wrongdoer; and the order for disclosure was neither proportionate nor necessary. The House of Lords held that a disclosure order did not require that the person should be an actual wrongdoer. It was sufficient if he had become involved in the wrongdoing. Nor was it necessary that there should be an intention to bring civil proceedings against the wrongdoer. This was an exceptional situation where disclosure of sources was justified. The care of the patients at the special hospital was fraught with difficulty and danger and it was essential that the source should be identified and punished in order to deter the same or similar wrongdoing in future. The order to disclose was therefore necessary, proportionate and justified. In a subsequent case brought by the journalist the Court of Appeal held that the protection of journalistic sources was one of the basic conditions of press freedom and the hospital had to establish an overriding public interest amounting to a pressing social need to which the need to keep press sources confidential should give way. The current case was different from the original MGN case, since as a journalist he was entitled to present different evidential material from a different perspective. The passage of time since the original case meant that there was no cloud of suspicion that was still blighting activity at the hospital and there had been no breach of confidentiality.[37] On 27 July 2007 the House of Lords refused leave to appeal against the Court of Appeal decision. Robin Ackroyd was thus not forced to disclose the source of his information.

Duty in specific statutes

Figure 8.8 identifies the statutes which make it an offence to disclose specified information.

Article 8 of the Human Rights Act 1998 states that everyone has the right to respect for private and family life, his home and his correspondence. This came into effect on 2 October 2000 in terms of enforcement in England, Wales and Northern Ireland (it came into force in Scotland on devolution), but before then any violation of the European Convention on Human Rights could be taken to European Court of Human Rights in Strasbourg (see Chapter 6). It would appear from recent court decisions that this right to privacy has strengthened the duty of confidentiality.

In one case involving internationally famous film stars, the Court of Appeal[38] held that the concept of privacy accords recognition to the fact that the law has to protect not only those people whose

> **Figure 8.8**   Statutory prohibition against disclosure.
>
> 1.   Abortion Regulations 1991 made under the Abortion Act 1967
> 2.   NHS (Venereal Disease) Regulations 1974
> 3.   Human Fertilisation and Embryology Act 2008
> 4.   Data Protection Act 1998
> 5.   Human Rights Act 1998 Article 8

trust has been abused, but also those who simply find themselves subjected to an unwanted intrusion into their personal lives. The law no longer needs to construct an artificial relationship of confidentiality between intruder and victim; it can recognise privacy itself as a legal principle drawn from the fundamental value of personal autonomy. In the case of Naomi Campbell, the House of Lords in a majority decision held that even though she had brought into the public domain the fact that she was being treated for drug addition, certain information could still be kept confidential, including the time, form and place of the drug therapy and she was therefore entitled to damages against the Mirror Group Newspapers for that breach of confidence.[39] In this respect her right to privacy succeeded against the right to freedom of expression under Article 10. In a case brought by Max Mosley against the New of the World which published accounts of his alleged sado-masochistic sex sessions, the judge decided that there was no evidence of Nazi behaviour and his private rights under Article 8 should be upheld. There was no public interest which justified a breach of Article 8.[40]

The European Court of Human Rights held that secret interception by the Ministry of Defence of the external communications of Liberty were not dealt with adequately under the Interception of Communications Act 1985 with sufficient clarity to give individuals protection and there was therefore a breach of Article 8 rights.[41]

Where information is disclosed in breach of the statutory provisions set out in Figure 8.8, the holder of the records or the patient can initiate the appropriate enforcement machinery. In the case of unauthorised disclosure of information by a person or organisation registered (or who should have been registered) under the Data Protection Act 1998, the Information Commissioner could remove from a data user his right to be registered under the Act and to hold personal information in computerised form (see below).

Duty as part of trust obligation between health professional and patient

This duty was acknowledged by the House of Lords[42] in the case known as the Spycatcher case. It was accepted that as a broad principle a duty of confidence arises:

- if information is confidential; and
- comes to the knowledge of a person where he or she has notice or is held to have agreed, that the information is confidential, with the effect that it would be just that he or she should be precluded from disclosing the information, and
- it is in the public interest that the confidentiality should be protected.

Clearly these principles would apply to information which the practitioner was given by or about a patient. The principles were applied in the case of *Stephens v Avery*.[43]

Case: *Stephens v Avery and Others*: unconscionable disclosure

The plaintiff and first defendant were close friends who freely discussed matters of a personal and private nature on the express basis that what the plaintiff told the first defendant was secret and disclosed in confidence. The first defendant passed on to the second and third defendants, who were the editor and publisher of a newspaper, details of the plaintiffs sexual conduct, including details of the plaintiffs lesbian relationship with a woman who had been killed by her husband. The plaintiff brought an action against the defendants claiming damages on the grounds that the information was confidential and was knowingly published by the newspaper in breach of the duty of confidence owed by the first defendant to the plaintiff. In an action by the defendants to strike out the claim as disclosing no reasonable cause of action, the defendants failed and appealed to the Chancery Division. They lost on the grounds that although the courts would not enforce a duty of confidence relating to matters which had a grossly immoral tendency, information relating to sexual conduct could be the subject of a legally enforceable duty of confidence if it would be unconscionable for a person who had received information on the express basis that it was confidential subsequently to reveal that information to another.

Exceptions to the duty of confidentiality

All the sources of law which recognise that there is a duty of confidentiality also recognise that there will be exceptions where it is lawful to disclose confidential information. The main exceptions to the duty of confidentiality are shown in Figure 8.9.

Consent of the patient

The duty of confidentiality is in the interest of the patient, and the patient therefore can give consent to disclosure which without that consent would be unlawful. The patient should be competent to give consent. In the case of a mentally incompetent adult, consent to disclosure could be given on the patient's behalf in the patient's best interests by a representative guardian or carer of the patient in accordance with the principles and provisions set out in the Mental Capacity Act 2005. Where the patient is a child under 16 years, then the principles of the Gillick case (see Chapter 23) would apply and a mature competent child under 16 could give consent to disclosure of confidential information. In the Axon case[44] a mother of teenage daughters applied for judicial review of DH guidelines on advice and treatment of young people under 16 years on contraception, sexual and reproductive health which was based on the Gillick judgment. She claimed that she should have been told that her daughter had given consent to an abortion. The High Court dismissed her application and the

---

Figure 8.9   Exceptions to the duty of confidentiality.

- Consent of the patient
- Disclosure in the clinical care or in the interests of the patient
- Court order or pre-trial order
- Statutory duty to disclose
- Disclosure in the public interest

Court of Appeal dismissed her appeal, upholding the guidance laid down by Lord Fraser in the Gillick case.

The consent of the patient or his representative would be a defence against any potential proceedings being brought against the health professional. It is essential that evidence is available that consent has been given. There are therefore considerable advantages in obtaining this information in writing. The patient has the right to withdraw consent unless the terms of the disclosure are contrary to this. For example, a patient may agree that a video could be made about his care and treatment. Considerable expense may then be incurred for the video to be produced. The patient may then decide that he does not wish the video to be shown. Whether or not this can be prevented will depend upon the terms on which his agreement to the disclosure was obtained.

Where the patient specifically refuses to give his consent to the disclosure of his diagnosis to others, such as his relatives, this request should as far as possible be respected under the duty of confidentiality and only if a specific exception to the duty applies could the information be passed on.

In the clinical care or in the interests of the patient

Health professionals working in a multi-disciplinary setting need to share information about the patient in order to fulfil their duty of care to the patient. Indeed, it could be said that if relevant information were not passed to professionals caring for the patient and harm were to occur to the patient as a result of that failure, then the professional and her employer could be answerable to the patient in a negligence action for failure to communicate significant information.

Situation: a justifiable disclosure

An occupational therapist is told by the patient that she has unexplained bouts of feeling faint. However, she did not want any fuss made. The occupational therapist informed the doctor who recommended that the patient should cease to drive a car until this fainting has been investigated. The patient complained about the disclosure of this information to the doctor.

In the above situation the OT should be able to defend herself against any complaint of breach of confidentiality on the grounds that the doctor was a member of the multi-disciplinary team caring for the patient, and the information was passed on in the interests of the patient. In fact failure to pass on significant information which could affect the patient's treatment could be a breach of the duty of care owed to the patient. In practice, the OT would have been wise to ensure that the patient was notified in advance that this information would have to be passed on.

Where information is disclosed to colleagues as part of the duty of care to the patient, care should be taken to ensure that it is relevant to and necessary for their responsibilities, and documented.

Court order

The court has the right to require that information relevant to an issue being decided at a hearing is made available to the court in the interests of justice. Both criminal and civil courts therefore have the right to issue a subpoena for the necessary information to be produced before it. Other quasi judicial proceedings such as inquiries may also have a right to subpoena information depending upon the statutory provisions under which they were established.

Where a court requires information, a health professional cannot refuse to comply on the grounds that the information was received in professional confidence. The courts do not recognise any privilege from disclosure attaching to the doctor or other health professional, or even a priest. The only exceptions recognised by the courts to their right to order disclosure are: legal professional privilege and privilege on grounds of the public interest (e.g. national security) (see below). If a health professional refused to answer questions in court on the grounds that answers would lead to a breach of confidentiality, the judge has the right to require the questions to be answered and has the power to send the witness who refuses to answer to prison for contempt of court.

Disclosure can also be ordered under the Supreme Court Act 1981, either in advance of litigation for personal injuries commencing by a party involved in the case, or after the claim form has been issued for disclosure by a third party not involved in the case. One of the effects of the Woolf reforms to civil procedures is that parties to litigation are required to disclose information relevant to the proceedings to the other party as soon as possible. The rules on civil procedure are considered in Chapter 13.

Exceptions to court order: legal professional privilege

This covers communications between clients and their legal advisers. The judge cannot order disclosure of such communications. The reason is that it is in the interests of justice for a client to be able to confide fully with legal advisers without fear that such communications would be ordered to be disclosed in court. Reports to legal advisers are also privileged from disclosure if the principal purpose for which they were written is in contemplation of litigation.[45] The court held in March 2008 that the mention of a document in a written statement did not constitute an automatic waiver of legal professional privilege so as to entitle the other party to inspect it.[46] A person could agree to a partial waiver of the right to legal professional privilege without having to lose the right entirely.[47]

The House of Lords held in March 2009 that covert surveillance of communications between clients and their lawyers was permitted under the Regulation of Investigatory Powers Act 2000 and not protected by legal professional privilege notwithstanding any statutory rights of persons in custody to consult their lawyers in private.[48]

Under section 42 of the Freedom of Information Act 2000 information which comes under the heading of legal professional privilege is categorised as exempt information which is subject to a public interest test before disclosure can be required (see Figure 9.1).

Exceptions to court order: public interest immunity

The other exception to the right of the judge to order disclosure of any document relevant to an issue before him, is that of public interest immunity. This covers such interests as the national security. The privilege from disclosure is given under the sworn affidavit of a Minister and can be overruled by the judge. Public interest immunity was considered by the Scott inquiry, which investigated the background to the Matrix Churchill prosecutions in the sale of weapons. The inquiry recommended that immunity certificates should not be issued in criminal proceedings, if the liberty of the subject was at stake.

Statutory duty to disclose

Several statutes require disclosure to be made, whether or not the patient gives consent. These are shown in Figure 8.10.

Figure 8.10   Statutory provisions requiring disclosure to be made.

Notifications of Communicable Diseases
Public Health Act 1936
Public Health (Infectious Diseases) Regulations 1988 (SI 1988 No. 1546)
Public Health (Control of Disease) Act 1984

Notifications of Abortions
Abortion Act 1967, section 2
Abortion Regulations 1991 (SI 1991 No. 499)

Notification of Births and Deaths
National Health Service Act 1977, section 124
National Health Service (Notification of Births and Deaths) Regulations 1982
  (SI 1982 No. 286)

Notification of Poisonings and Health and Safety matters
Health and Safety at Work etc. Act 1974
Reporting of Injuries, Diseases and Dangerous Occurrences Regulations 1995
  (SI 1995 No. 3163)

Disclosure for Civil Justice
Supreme Court Act 1981, sections 33 and 34

Disclosure for Criminal Justice
Police and Criminal Evidence Act 1984
Prevention of Terrorism Acts
Road Traffic Act 1988, section 172

Where the Acts shown in Figure 8.10 are relevant to the work of the practitioner, care should be taken to ensure that he or she is fully conversant with the statutory requirements on disclosure and ensure that any disclosure which is made can be justified in law.

Disclosure in public interest

This is the most difficult exception to the duty of confidentiality. Professional registration bodies all recognise that in certain circumstances, disclosure without the patient's consent and contrary to his wishes may be justified. Disclosure in the 'public interest' would include situations where there were reasonable fears for the safety of the patient or of other persons. The most obvious example would be concern about child abuse. This is considered in Chapter 23.

In one decided case (*W. v Egdel*[49]), on the issue of disclosure in the public interest, the Court of Appeal held that it was permissible for a psychiatrist who had been asked for a report by a patient who was seeking his discharge from detention under the Mental Health Act 1983, to send his report to the Mental Health Review Tribunal and the hospital without the consent of the patient. The public interest in ensuring the disclosure of this report outweighed the public interest in protecting the patient's confidentiality.

Other situations where disclosure in the public interest would be justified, would include a situation where harm is occurring or likely to occur to a child or another person, as this situation illustrates.

Situation: disclosure in the public interest

A patient has suffered a stroke and is receiving OT as part of her rehabilitation. She has been instructed that she is not yet fit to drive. However the OT sees her arrive at the OT clinic in a car driven by herself. What action should the OT take?

In this situation the patient must be reminded that she is committing a criminal offence contrary to road traffic legislation in driving when she has been assessed as medically unfit to drive, as well as putting herself and other road users at risk. There would be justification in the OT telling the patient that she could be reported to the Driving and Vehicle Licensing Authority if she continued to drive while unfit.

Statutory provision for disclosure of patient information

Under section 60(1) of the Health and Social Care Act 2001 the Secretary of State has power to make regulations to require or regulate the processing of prescribed patient information for medical purposes as he considers necessary or expedient:

1. in the interests of improving patient care or
2. in the public interest.

Subsections 2 and 3 of section 60 set out the details of what these regulations can include and enable patient information to be disclosed by health service bodies. Specific restrictions on these powers include prohibiting such processing if it would be reasonably practicable to achieve that purpose by other means. Under section 61, the Secretary of State had to establish a Patient Information Advisory Group whose advice had to be sought before any regulations were laid before Parliament. Sections 60 and 61 came into force on the passing of the Act (11 May 2001). The Patient Information Advisory Group has subsequently been replaced by the National Information Governance Board for Health and Social Care (see below).

Under section 60(3), regulations may *not* make provision requiring the processing of confidential patient information for any purpose if it would be reasonably practicable to achieve that purpose otherwise than pursuant to such regulations, having regard to the cost and/or the technology. Under section 60(5), regulations may not make provision for requiring the processing of confidential patient information solely or principally for the purpose of determining the care and treatment to be given to particular individuals. Under section 60(6), regulations under this section may not make provision for or in connection with the processing of prescribed patient information in a manner inconsistent with any provision made by or under the Data Protection Act 1998.

Under section 60(7) before making any regulations, the Secretary of State shall consult such bodies appearing to him to represent the interests of those likely to be affected by the regulations as he considers appropriate. Under section 61(2) the Secretary of State had to consult the patient information advisory group before making any regulations. (The PIAG has now been replaced by the National Information Governance Board for Health and Social Care – see below)

Regulations passed under the Act[50] have enabled Cancer Registers to receive confidential patient information, and communicable diseases and other risks to public health can also be passed on under Regulation 3. Regulation 4 states that:

Anything done by a person that is necessary for the purpose of processing confidential patient information in accordance with these regulations shall be taken to be lawfully done despite any obligation of confidence owed by that person in respect of it.

This provides protection from any potential breach of confidentiality action if the Regulations have been complied with.

Regulation 5 and the Schedule to the Regulations enable confidential information to be processed for medical purposes provided that the processing has been approved, in the case of medical research, by the Secretary of State and a research ethics committee, and in any other case by the Secretary of State. The Schedule defines the circumstances in which this processing can take place.

National Information Governance Board for Health and Social Care (NIGB)

The National Information and Governance Board for Health and Social Care (www.nigb.nhs.uk) has been established under section 157 of the Health and Social Care Act 2008 and replaces the Patient Information Advisory Group. The NIGB website hosts the NHS Care Record Guarantee.[51] Its overall role is to support improvements to information governance practice in health and social care.

The functions of the new Board include:

(a) to monitor the practice followed by relevant bodies in relation to the processing of relevant information,

(b) to keep the Secretary of State, and such bodies as the Secretary of State may designate by direction, informed about the practice being followed by relevant bodies in relation to the processing of relevant information,

(c) to publish guidance on the practice to be followed in relation to the processing of relevant information,

(d) to advise the Secretary of State on particular matters relating to the processing of relevant information by any person, and

(e) to advise persons who process relevant information on such matters relating to the processing of relevant information by them as the Secretary of State may from time to time designate by direction.

(3) The Board must, in exercising its functions, seek to improve the practice followed by relevant bodies in relation to the processing of relevant information.

'Relevant information' is defined as:

(a) patient information
(b) any other information obtained or generated in the course of the provision of the health service and
(c) any information obtained or generated in the course of the exercise by a local social services authority in England of its adult social services functions.

'Patient information' means:

(a) information (however recorded) which relates to the physical or mental health or condition of an individual ("P"), to the diagnosis of P's condition or to P's care or treatment, and
(b) information (however recorded) which is to any extent derived directly or indirectly, from that information whether or not the identity of the individual in question is ascertainable from the information.

The Ethics and Confidentiality Committee (ECC) has been established to undertake the responsibilities of the NIGB under section 251 of the NHS Act 2006 and to consider and advise on ethical issues relating to the processing of health or social care information as referred to it by the NIGB. Section 251 of the NHS Act 2006 (originally enacted under section 60 of the Health and Social Care Act 2001), allows the common law duty of confidentiality to be set aside in specific circumstances where anonymised information is not sufficient and where patient consent is not practicable. Applications for approval to use section 251 support were previously considered by the Patient Information Advisory Group (PIAG) but are now be considered by the ECC.

Figure 8.11   Checklist for good practice in maintaining confidentiality.

- Are the records securely stored with restricted access?
- If access to the records or information is requested, who is making the request?
- What are their reasons for the request?
- What relationship do they have with the patient?
- Has the patient given consent?
- If not, why not?
- Is the patient under the care of a consultant?
- Has he or she been asked to permit disclosure?
- Is there a duty in law to disclose?
- If so, under what category does the duty arise?
- What part, if any, of the information should be released to the person making the request?
- What should be recorded about the request and the response?

Implications for the practitioner

A procedure is necessary for the practitioner to ensure that the confidential nature of information about the patient is preserved. This would also include safe storage of the records which she keeps and should also cover any sharing of records on a multi-disciplinary team basis. In addition, the exceptions to the duty should be clarified so that the practitioner can be confident that she is acting within the law and retains the trust of the patient.

Figure 8.11 shows a checklist for ensuring that precautions are taken against any unauthorised disclosure.

Caldicott Guardians

The Government appointed a committee chaired by Dame Fiona Caldicott to make recommendations on how to improve the way in which the NHS managed patient confidentiality. It reported in December 1997 and included in its recommendations the need to raise awareness of confidentiality requirements, and specifically recommended the establishment of a network of Caldicott Guardians of patient information throughout the NHS. Subsequently a steering group was set up to oversee the implementation of the report's recommendations. Following a consultation period the NHS executive issued a circular on the establishment of Caldicott Guardians,[52] giving advice on the appointment of the Guardians, the programme of work for the first year for improving the way each organisation handles confidential patient information, and identifying the resources, training and other support for the Guardians.

Each health authority, special health authority, NHS trust and primary care group was required to appoint a Caldicott Guardian by 31 March 1999. Ideally the Guardian should be at board level, be a senior health professional and have responsibility for promoting clinical governance within the organisation. The name and address of the Guardian was to be notified to the NHS Executive.[53] The Guardian was expected to liaise closely with others involved in patient information, such as information management and technology (IM&T) security officers and data protection officers. In making the appointment and defining the role of the Guardian, the duties which are not to be delegated should be clarified. Guardians are responsible for agreeing and reviewing internal protocols governing the protection and use of patient-identifiable information by the staff of their organisation, and must be satisfied that these proposals address the requirements for national guidance/policy and law. The operation of these policies must also be monitored. Policies for inter-agency disclosure of patient information must also be agreed and reviewed, to facilitate cross-boundary working.

In 2000 the Department of Health issued guidance to Caldicott Guardians on the method by which information flows should be reviewed in NHS organisations.[54] It provided a manual which covers the mapping of information flows, the prioritising of mapped flows for review purposes and a rolling programme of review. The specific areas which are considered include commissioning flows, clinical audit and coding, medical records and patient care services. Guidance on the implementing of Caldicott standards into social care was given by the Department of Health in January 2002.[55] The guidance includes a timetable for the implementation of Caldicott standards and also a management audit organisational profile set at three levels to determine the compliance in 18 audit areas. Details of an electronic Caldicott toolkit are also provided as part of a training and educational pack. Further information for Caldicott Guardians is available from the Information Policy Unit of the Department of Health.[56]

If issues on confidentiality arise, a healthcare practitioner can raise these with the Caldicott Guardian, who in turn can access the legal advisers to the trust.

Information Commissioner

The management of information between the Data Protection Act and the Freedom of Information Act is facilitated by the fact that under the Freedom of Information Act an Information Commission[57] is appointed and this post incorporates the duties of the former Data Protection Commissioner as well as those under the Freedom of Information Act (see Chapter 9). The website of the ICO provides useful guidance on both the Data Protection Act and the Freedom of Information Act.

Conclusion

The Data Protection Act 1998 has strengthened provisions on access to and disclosure of personal information, putting more pressure on the decisions of the individual practitioner. However, the absence of a statutory definition of 'the public interest' makes it difficult to determine whether this exception to the duty of confidentiality applies. Each individual practitioner is personally and professionally accountable for any disclosure. The Human Rights Act, in enabling persons to bring actions against public authorities who have failed to uphold a person's right to respect for private and family life as set out in Article 8, has led to more litigation where patients claim that their right to confidentiality and privacy has not been respected. The effect of the powers given to the National Information Governance Board for Health and Social Care cannot yet be evaluated. The Information Commissioner has notified the Department of Health that the NHS is not complying fully with the laws of confidentiality, and some disclosures of personal information are taking place without the proper consent of the patient. The Information Commissioner is taking a proactive role in ensuring that the principles of confidentiality are respected and stronger criminal sanctions have been called for as a result of recent losses of unencrypted data by the Child Support Agency, the Driving Standards Agency, the Revenue and Customs, the Ministry of Works and Pensions and the Ministry of Defence in 2007 and 2008. A cross-party Commons Justice Committee called for stronger criminal sanctions where personal data is lost.[58] There have also been protests that a new child database known as Contact Point covering all 11 million children living in England will be accessed by over 400,000 persons and there are therefore considerable fears about its security.[59] In March 2009 the Department for Children, Schools and Families announced that security flaws have halted work on the Contact Point database. It had uncovered problems in the system for shielding details of an estimated 55,00 vulnerable children.[60]

The Information Commissioner expressed concern that clause 152 of the Coroners and Justice Bill would enable the transfer of health and tax records to private companies such as insurance firms and medical researchers. He considered that data sharing should only be allowed in carefully defined circumstances such as law enforcement, improving public services and for research.[61] The clause on information sharing was deleted from the final bill.

These concerns about protecting confidentiality when vast databases are being created as well as concerns about the security of the information itself when passed within and between organisations are at the forefront of the Information Commissioner's agenda. Access under the Freedom of Information Act by Pulse (The GP journal) revealed that NHS trusts are failing to take action against staff who lose personal records, breach patient confidentiality or access patient records without authorisation. PCTs, NHS Trusts and health authorities followed up only 14 of the 263 incidents with formal disciplinary action. The figures suggest that confidentiality of patient data is not a high priority within the NHS, a fact that might lead to the down fall of the NHS electronic system which is discussed in Chapter 12. Section 76 of the Health and Social Care Act 2008 creates a criminal offence in relation to the unauthorised disclosure of confidential personal information held by the CQC.

 Questions and exercises

1 Examine your practice in relation to passing on confidential information. What faults would you see in it?
2 To what extent can an employer enforce the duty of confidentiality among employees? Prepare a procedure for this.
3 What exceptions have you relied on in passing on confidential information?

References

1 Dimond, B. (2010) *The Legal Aspects of Patient Confidentiality*, 2nd edn. Quay Publications, Dinton, Salisbury.
2 Carey, P. (2004) *Data Protection: a Practical Guide to UK and EU Law*, 2nd edn. Oxford University Press, Oxford.
3 European Directive of Data Protection 95/46/EC.
4 NHS Executive. Data Protection Act 1998, HSC 2000/009; LASSL(2000)2 Data Protection Act 1998: Guidance.
5 www.standards.nhsia.nhs.uk/sdp
6 www.connectingforhealth.nhs.uk/
7 www.ico.gov.uk
8 *Michael John Durant v Financial Services Authority* [2003] EWCA Civ 1746, Court of Appeal (Civil Division) www.courtservice.gov.uk
9 Information Commissioner (2006) The 'Durant' Case and its impact on the interpretation of the Data Protection Act 1998.

10   Information Commissioner (2007) Data Protection Technical Guidance Determining what is personal data.

11   *Johnson v Medical Defence Union* [2007] EWCA 262.

12   www.ico.gov.uk

13   Data Protection (Processing of Sensitive Personal Data) Order 2000, SI 2000/417.

14   Data Protection (Processing of Sensitive Personal Data) (Elected Representatives) Order 2002, SI 2002/2905.

15   Data Protection (Subject Access Modification) (Health) Order 2000/413; Data Protection (Subject Access Modification) (Education) Order 2000, SI 2000/414; Data Protection (Subject Access Modification) (Social Work) Order 2000, SI 2000/415.

16   Data Protection Commissioner (Registrar), Wycliffe House, Water Lane, Wilmslow, Cheshire SK9 5AF. Information line: 01625 545745; Switchboard: 01625 545700; Fax 01625 524510.

17   Data Protection Registrar (1998) The Data Protection Act 1998: an introduction. Office of Data Protection Registrar.

18   *R (on the application for the Secretary of State for the Home Department) v Information Tribunal (Information Commissioner, interested party)* [2006] EWHC 2958 Admin, [2007] 2 All ER 703.

19   NHS Executive. Data Protection Act: Protection and Use of Patient Information; HSC 2000/009.

20   www.doh.gov.uk/ipu/

21   *Marper v UK* [2007] EHCR 110; application nos 30562/04 and 30566/04 .

22   *S and Marper v UK* (Application Nos 30562/04 and 30566/04 ECHR [2008] The Times 8 December 2008 [2008] ECHR 1581.

23   Richard Ford. Police are ordered to destroy all DNA samples taken from innocent people. The Times 5 December 2008 page 16.

24   Richard Ford. Ruling could wipe out criminal records. The Times 22 July 2008 page 5.

25   Department of Health (2003) *The NHS Confidentiality Code of Practice* (superseding HSG(96) 18 LASSL (96(5)), available on www.doh.gov.uk/ipu/confiden/protect/

26   Rose David. Nurse who filmed hospital neglect for BBC struck off. The Times 17 April 2009.

27   Peter Lindon. Jeeny McCoy letter to the editor. The Times 20 April 2009.

28   Department of Health HSG (1996) 18, *Protection and Use of Patient Information*. DH circular, March 1996 (superseded by Department of Health, NHS Confidentiality Code of Practice, DH, 2003 available on www.dh.gov.uk/ipu/confiden/protect/)

29   *R v Department of Health ex p Source Informatics Ltd* [2000] TLR 17, [2000] 1 All ER 786 CA.

30   *Common Services Agency v Scottish Information Commissioner* Times Law Report 14 July 2008 HL.

31   Health Professions Council (2003 revised 2008) *Standards of conduct, performance and ethics*. HPC, London.

32   www.hpc-uk.org

33   *Ashworth Hospital v MGN* [2002] 4 All ER 193.

34   *Furniss v Fitchett* [1958] NZLR 396.

35   *X v Y* [1988] 2 All ER 648.

36   *Ashworth Hospital Authority v MGN Ltd* [2001] 1 All ER 991; *Ashworth Hospital v MGN* [2002] 4 All ER 193.

37   *Mersey Care NHS Trust v Ackroyd* [2007] EWCA 101.

38   *Douglas and others v Hello! Ltd* [2001] 2 All ER 289.

39   *Campbell v MGN Ltd* [2004] UKHL 22, [2004] 2 AC 457 HL.

40   *Mosely v News Group Newspapers* [2008] EWHC 1777.

41   *Liberty and others v United Kingdom* The Times Law Report 11 July 2008.

42   *Attorney General v Guardian Newspaper Ltd (No 2)* [1988] 3 All ER 545.

43   *Stephens v Avery and others* [1988] 2 All ER 477.

44   *R (On the application of Axon) v Secretary of State for Health* [2006] EWCA 37 Admin; [2006] 2 W.L.R. 1130.

45   *Waugh v British Railway Board* [1980] AC 521.

46   *Expandable Ltd and others v Rubin* The Times Law Report 10 March 2008.

47   *Fulham Leisure Holdings Ltd v Nicholson Graham and Jones (a firm)* [2006] EWHC 158 Ch, [2006] 2 All ER 599.

48   *McE v Prison Services of Northern Ireland and Another; C and A v Chief Constable of the Police Service of Northern Ireland; M v Same* The Times 12 March 2009.

49   *W v Egdell* [1989] 1 All ER 1089, CA; The Times, 20 November 1989.

50   SI 2002/1438.
51   www.nigb.nhs.uk/guarantee
52   NHS Executive HSC 1999/012, Caldicott Guardians, 31 January 1999.
53   Raj Kaur, NHS Executive, 3E58 Quarry House, Leeds LS2 7UE, Fax 0113 254 6114.
54   Department of Health (2000) *Protection and using patient information: A manual for Caldicott Guardians.*
55   HSC 2002/003; LAC(2002)2 Implementing the Caldicott Standard into Social Care.
56   www.doh.gov.uk/ipu/confiden/index.htm
57   Information Commissioner, Wycliff House, Water Lane, Wilmslow, Cheshire SK9 5 AF; Tel. 01625 545700; email: data@dataprotection.gov.uk; www.dataprotection.gov.uk
58   Greg Hurst. Whitehall should be prosecuted over data loss, say MPs in call for new law. The Times 3 January 2008.
59   Bennett Rosemary & Frean Alexandra. Parents alarmed over security of child database. The Times 27 January 2009.
60   Frean Alexandra. Child database halted as safeguards fail. The Times 24 March 2009.
61   Mostrous Alexi and Ford Richard. Too far and too fast – the laws that make everyone a suspect. The Times 27 February 2009.

9 Access to Records and Information

Patients have a statutory right to see their health records, whether they are held in computer or manual form, and subject only to a few exceptions. The definition of health records includes records kept by the occupational therapist (OT). The statutory right of access also applies to records held by health professionals working in independent practice, but here access might also be subject to conditions agreed in the contract between therapist and private patient. The contractual conditions could not, however, limit the statutory right. Separate statutory provisions cover the records held by those who work for social services departments (SSDs).

An OT's records may also become relevant to reports written by the patient's doctor for insurance or employment purposes and therefore come under the rules relating to disclosure of such reports.

In addition to the statutory rights of access to health records and personal files kept by SSDs, there is also a right at common law for the patient to receive, as part of the duty of care owed by the health professional to the patient, information which is relevant to decisions which the patient may be required to consider in relation to her treatment and care. The rights at common law for the patient to be given information are set out in the leading case of Sidaway[1] and are considered in Chapter 7 on consent and information giving.

The following topics are covered in this chapter:

- Data Protection Act 1998
- Right of subject access (under section 7 of Data Protection Act 1998)
- Procedures for access
- Requests on behalf of children or mentally incapacitated adults
- Rights of the data subject
- Exceptions to the right of access
- Serious harm
- Identification of third party
- Non-statutory rights of access
- Access and the occupational therapist
- Instructions to withhold information
- Freedom of Information Act 2000

Legal Aspects of Occupational Therapy, Third Edition By Bridgit Dimond
© 2010 Bridgit Dimond

Statutory rights

The legislation giving statutory rights is as follows:

- Data Protection Act 1998 Act
- Access to Medical Reports Act 1988
- Access to Health Records Act 1990 (for the records of deceased persons)
- Data Protection (Subject Access Modification) (Health) Order 2000
- Data Protection (Subject Access Modification) (Social Work) Order 2000
- Data Protection (Subject Access Modification) (Education) Order 2000
- Education (Pupil Information)(England) Regulations 2005
- Freedom of Information Act 2000

Data Protection Act 1998

The Data Protection Act 1998 gives rights of access to both automated processed and manually held personal health information subject to the conditions laid down by statutory instrument.[2] The Access to Health Records Act 1990 has been repealed except for provisions dealing with health records of dead people (see later in this chapter). Clarification of the statutory provisions is given by the Department of Health.[3] The guidance also provides examples of forms which could be used to seek access. The Data Protection Act 1998 covers only those records which consist of information relating to a living individual who can be identified from that information (or from other information in the possession of the data user) and includes any expression of opinion (section 1(3)).

Provisions on access

The data subject, i.e. the person about whom the information is recorded, has a right of access under section 7 of the 1998 Act. The request must be made in writing to the data controller with the appropriate fee. The controller must have sufficient information to be able to satisfy himself about the identity of the person making the request and the location of the information. Unless the exclusion provisions discussed below apply, the data controller must comply with the request within 40 days (or other prescribed period) of the application with all the necessary information being received. Recent guidance, changed as a result of a Parliamentary debate,[4] when Ministers gave a commitment to Parliament that the 21 day period would be retained for the NHS and extended to all requests; not just those where the record has been recently amended.[5]

Rights of data subject

Under the access provisions of the 1998 Act, the data subject can have:

- a description of the data being processed
- a description of the purposes for which it is being processed
- a description of any potential recipients of his data
- any information as to the source of his data where this is available.

Under the 1984 Act, the data subject was only entitled to have a copy of any data processed with reference to him.

Duty to consult

The data controller who is not a health professional (see definition below) cannot withhold information until he has consulted the person who appears to the data controller to be the appropriate health professional on the question whether or not the exemption applies with respect to the information. A data controller who is not a health professional cannot communicate information unless he has consulted the appropriate health professional on whether the exemption applies.

This duty to consult does not apply where the data subject has already seen or knows about the information which is the subject of the request, nor in certain circumstances where consultation has been carried out prior to the request being made.

Under the Act an 'appropriate health professional' means:

(a) the health professional who is currently or was most recently responsible for the clinical care of the data subject in connection with the matters to which the information which is the subject of the request relates or

(b) Where there is more than one such health professional, the health professional who is most suitable to advise on the matters to which the information which is the subject of the request relates or

(c) Where:
  (i) there is no health professional available falling within paragraph (a) or (b), or
  (ii) the data controller is the Secretary of State in his functions under the child support or social security legislation,
  a health professional who has the necessary experience and qualification to advise on the matters to which the information which is the subject of the request relates.

If the information supplied to the data subject is inaccurate he or she can request that the information is rectified or erased and has the right to enforce this in the court. If the inaccuracy causes distress to the data subject, then he or she has the right to claim compensation for the harm suffered. The data user has a defence if the inaccurate information was received from the patient or a third person or if the data user took such care as was reasonably required in the circumstances to ensure the accuracy of the data at the material time. If the data subject is refused the information, he or she can either make an application to the County or High Court or to the Information Commissioner for the enforcement of the statutory rights. One of the working groups of the National Information Governance Board for Health and Social Care (see Chapter 8) has produced draft guidance for patients, service users and health and social care professionals on how requests to amend the content of medical and social care records should be handled, and the reasons for this. The report can be downloaded from the NIGB website (www.nigb.nhs.uk).

Requests on behalf of children or mentally incapacitated adults

Children have the right of access if they have the maturity to make a valid application. The concept of being 'Gillick competent' would apply (see Chapter 23).

Where a request is made on behalf of a child by a person with parental responsibility for a child or on behalf of a person who is incapable of managing his own affairs by a person who has been appointed by a court to manage those affairs, if such a person has a right under any law to make the request, they cannot have access to:

- information provided by the data subject in the expectation that it would not be disclosed to the person making the request

- information obtained as a result of any examination or investigation to which the data subject consented in the expectation that the information would not be so disclosed; or
- information which the data subject has expressly indicated should not be so disclosed.

The first two exceptions do not apply if the data subject has expressly indicated that he no longer has the expectation referred to.

The Act provides for regulations to be made to enable those who are responsible for the management of the affairs of an incompetent adult to have access. The Mental Capacity Act 2005 now provides a legal framework for decision making on behalf of the mentally incapacitated adult (see Chapter 7) and this would include access to the records of a person lacking the requisite capacity to give consent. Guidance has been provided by the Department of Health on access to health records, including answers to frequently asked questions.[6] The ICO has issued a good practice note on how the Data Protection Act applies to professional opinion.[7] It gives several examples where patients have disagreed with the opinion expressed by the health professional and as a result of a request by the patient, a comment to the effect that the patient did not agree with the opinion is added to the notes. The advice is considered in Chapter 12.

Exceptions to the right of access to personal data

Under section 30 of the Data Protection Act 1998 the Secretary of State is given the power to exempt from the subject access information provisions, personal data consisting of information as to the physical or mental health or condition of the data subject. Under this power the Statutory Instruments have been drawn up which modify the right of subject access to health records and to social services records under section 7.[8]

Exemptions from subject access to health records

Personal data processed by a court

This relates to information supplied in a report or other evidence given to a court by a local authority, Health and Social Services Board, Health and Social Services Trust, probation officer, or other person in the course of any proceedings under specified legislation dealing with children.

Serious harm

Also exempted from the subject access provisions is personal data:

> in any case to the extent to which the application of section 7 would be likely to cause serious harm to the physical or mental health or condition of the data subject or any other person.

The meaning of serious harm was considered in the case of *R (on the application of Lord) v Secretary of State for the Home Department*,[9] which involved an application for judicial review of a decision to disclose only the gist of a category A prisoner's annual security classification report. The judge held that

> In my judgment 'likely' in section 29(1) connotes a degree of probability where there is a very significant and weighty chance of prejudice to the identified public interests. The degree of risk must be such that there 'may very well' be prejudice to those interests, even if the risk falls short of being more probable than not.

This ruling was applied in the case of *Clive Roberts v Nottinghamshire Healthcare NHS Trust*[10] where a patient sought access to his medical report under the Data Protection Access provisions. He failed in his attempt. The Judge found that the defendants had clear and compelling reasons not to disclose the report and the claimant's suggestion, that the report could be disclosed to his solicitors on the basis that they would not show it to him, had no basis in law and his legal representatives would have no grounds for withholding it from him.

Third party identification

Under the access provisions of section 7, access can be withheld if another individual would be identified by the information disclosed. This does not apply where:

- the individual has consented to the disclosure or
- where it is reasonable in all the circumstances to comply with the request for access, without the consent or
- where the other individual is a health professional who has contributed to the health record or has been involved in the care of the data subject in his capacity as a health professional. (This does not apply if it would be the health professional who would suffer serious harm to his physical or mental health or condition by the giving of access.)

The circumstances in the second point above include the following:

- any duty of confidentiality owed to that individual
- any steps taken by the data controller with a view to seeking the consent of the other individual
- whether the other individual is capable of giving consent
- any express refusal of consent by the other individual.

Access should be given to any other information which can be disclosed without identifying the third party.

Situation: third party protection

June, a patient who had been discharged from mental hospital, was required to take medication. A neighbour noticed that June appeared to becoming increasingly disturbed and believed that she was not taking her medication. She therefore phoned the hospital to recommend that June was visited by a community psychiatric nurse, but asked that her identity should not be revealed to June.

In the above situation the identity of the neighbour should be protected and whilst there should be a record of the telephone call in the patient's records, it should be clearly indicated that this information is not to be disclosed to the patient.

Exemptions from subject access to social service records

Similar exemptions to subject access to health records have been set by statutory instrument.[11] These provisions cover access to social services records, local education authority records, special hospital records and other records specified in the Schedule to the statutory instrument.

Prejudice to the carrying out of social work

Access is not permitted:

> In any case to the extent to which the application … would be likely to prejudice the carrying out of social work by reason of the fact that serious harm to the physical or mental health or condition of the data subject of any other person would be likely to be caused.

Access to Health Records Act 1990

The only provisions of the Access to Health Records Act 1990 which remain are those relating to records of dead people. Under section 3(l)(f) of the 1990 Act, where the patient has died, the patient's personal representative and any person who may have a claim arising out of the patient's death, may apply for access to the patient's health records. However, under section 4(3), where an application is made in such circumstances, access shall not be given if the record includes a note, made at the patient's request, that he did not wish access to be given on such an application. In addition, under section 5(4) access shall not be given to any part of the record which, in the opinion of the holder of the record, would disclose information which is not relevant to any claim which may arise out of the patient's death.

Access to Medical Reports Act 1988

This Act enables a patient to see and if necessary suggest corrections where an insurance company or employer requests a medical report from the patient's own doctor for insurance or employment purposes. The records to which the doctor might refer may include information received from OTs.

The right of access can be withheld in similar circumstances to those stated in the section above. Therefore, in the unlikely circumstances that the OT is concerned that any information is likely to cause serious harm to the physical or mental health of the patient or identify a third person who has requested not to be identified, she should ensure that the information which she passes to the doctor is suitably annotated with the words that it is not to be disclosed to the patient, with the reasons for this.

A life insurance company may seek information in order to decide whether to make a payment under a life assurance policy and require doctors to give information about the cause of death. Doctors could release information in accordance with the Access to Health Records Act 1990.

The Information Tribunal ruled that a dead woman's medical records should not be released because a duty of confidentiality survives her death when this was challenged by the mother of the deceased.[12] (see below) The BMA has provided guidance on access to medical reports which was revised in June 2007.[13]

Education (Pupil Information)(England) Regulations 2005[14]

These regulations which revoke and reenact with modifications the Regulations of 2000 enable education records on pupils held by maintained and special schools to be open to access on specified conditions.

Under Regulation 5(3), the governing body must provide a copy of a pupil's educational record to the parent, on payment of a specified fee, within 15 days of receipt of the parent's written request for access to that record. This regulation is subject to the conditions, that the record may not be made available for inspection or a copy provided if:

1. it could not lawfully be disclosed to the pupil himself under the Data Protection Act 1998 or
2. the pupil would have no right of access to it under the Data Protection Act 1998 or under any regulations made under the Act.

Regulations under the Data Protection Act[15] set out similar exclusions from the right of access to those under the Access to health records, including those cases where access would be likely to cause serious harm to the physical or mental health or condition of the data subject or any other person. There is also an exclusion from access where the data subject is or may be at risk of child abuse and access would not be in the best interests of the data subject. This latter exemption from access applies where the data subject is a child and the applicant has parental responsibility for the data subject or the data subject is incapable of managing his own affairs. Child abuse includes physical injury (other than accidental injury) to, and physical and emotional neglect, ill-treatment and sexual abuse of, a child.

Non-statutory rights of access

Evidence suggests that there are few formal applications made under the statutory provisions, which indicates that health professionals are disclosing the records without requiring the patient to make a formal application. It should be remembered that the existence of statutory rights of access for the patient does not mean that the patient necessarily has to apply formally for access. There may be many reasons why the health professional agrees to informal access of the patient to his records and this could then be arranged. There is the possibility that greater openness over access to records and information may make patients less suspicious and there will be even fewer formal applications for access under the statutory provisions.

However, a decision by the Court of Appeal[16] has established that, even if the statutory provisions do not apply, the patient does not have an absolute right of access at common law. This decision must now be reviewed in the light of Article 8 of the European Convention of Human Rights (see Chapter 6 and Appendix 1). This Article gives a right to respect for privacy and family life and has been interpreted by the European Court of Human Rights in Strasbourg as giving a right to access information held about oneself. For example, in the Gaskin case[17] the claimant sought access to his social services records held by Liverpool City Council covering the time when he had been in its care during his childhood. As a result of the intervention of the Attorney General, the Council stated that it would only provide the records if the consent of those who had prepared them – doctors, foster parents, and social workers – were obtained. Mr Gaskin then took his case to the Court of Human Rights in Strasbourg under Articles 8 and 10. He claimed that the failure of the state to provide access to his records was a breach of his right to private life. The court held that under Article 8 he was entitled to the records of his childhood from the public authority charged with his care, but that where such information related to others it could be withheld. (Provisions relating to third parties are considered above.)

Access and the occupational therapist

It is seldom that secrecy of information from the patient can be justified in the case of the treatment provided by the OT. There are very few situations where the OT would feel that serious harm could arise to the physical or mental health or condition of the patient or another person if access were to be permitted.

Instructions to withhold information

Sometimes, however, the problems which can arise are not of the OT's making as the following situation illustrates.

Situation: forbidden information

> A consultant physician treating a patient has diagnosed multiple sclerosis. It is his view that the patient could not yet cope with this diagnosis and he therefore instructs the multi-disciplinary team caring for the patient that she should not be told. The OT takes part in a pre-discharge assessment of the patient and accompanies her home to decide if she could cope with living on her own. During the visit the patient raises with the OT her concerns about her illness and asks the OT directly if she has multiple sclerosis. What is the legal situation?

Although the OT is a personally accountable registered professional who should use her own discretion in making health decisions, she is also part of a multi-disciplinary team usually headed by the consultant responsible for the care and treatment of the patient. In this case her concerns about openness and disclosure to the patient should have been raised as soon as she was aware of the restrictions ordered by the consultant and she should have taken this up with him. In the situation which occurs she has the following options:

- To refuse to say, and suggest that the patient should have an appointment to discuss with the consultant her diagnosis and treatment.
- To answer the patient honestly and ignore the consultant's orders.
- To lie to the patient.

It would be hoped that the third option would be unacceptable to all health and social services professionals. The first option would probably be appropriate in most cases. The second option may be justified in exceptional circumstances. If the OT follows the second option, however, then she must be prepared to justify her actions:

- before disciplinary proceedings should the consultant report her to her managers and they decide to take such action
- in civil litigation, if the patient reacts to this information by attempting to take (or succeeding in taking) her own life and the employer of the OT is sued for its vicarious liability for the harm caused by her
- in professional conduct proceedings if it is decided that she is guilty of professional misconduct as a registered professional.

It may be that before all three forms of hearing she is able to justify her actions as being in the best interests of the patient. She should ensure that her records are comprehensive and explain clearly why she took the decisions she did. In deciding whether it is appropriate to ignore the consultant's direction that the patient should not be told, the OT should be mindful of the fact that there is no absolute duty to disclose everything to the patient; under the statutory provisions there is a right of exclusion from access which the holder of records can exercise on the basis of the advice of the health professional concerned. At common law, the House of Lords in the Sidaway case[18] recognised the right of therapeutic privilege to withhold information from the patient in circumstances when it is justified as being in the best interests of that patient. The OT should discuss the issue of withholding information from the patient with the multi-disciplinary team and seek the advice of the Caldicott Guardian and her own professional association.

The GMC has advised registered medical practitioners that they should ensure that patients are given full information about their condition and that those who fail to tell patients the truth about their treatment risk being struck off. The new guidelines were issued in the updated *Good Medical Practice* booklet issued by the GMC (revised again in 2006).[19]

A distinction may have to be made for OTs who work for social services, where the patient may not be directly under a consultant and the general practitioner is therefore the lead medical practitioner responsible for the clinical care of the patient.

Truth telling

'Truth telling in occupational therapy'[20] by Rosemary Barnitt is an excellent analysis of the ethical issues which arise in deciding whether or not the patient should be given full information. It shows the difficulties which can arise in a multi-disciplinary team over who controls the truth telling. She concludes that there is a clear need for simple policies and procedures to be established around truth telling in healthcare settings, and for these to be made available to all participants in the treatment transaction. Her research was based on a postal questionnaire across England and Wales. As shown above, there is a right recognised both by statute and at common law for information to be withheld from the patient in exceptional circumstances if it would cause serious harm to the mental or physical condition of the patient. The Report of the Bristol Inquiry[21] recommended that there should be openness and honesty and a partnership between health professionals and patients. This philosophy is also present in the new NHS Redress Scheme which was set up for obtaining compensation for clinical negligence (see Chapter 13).

Diagnosis not given to the OT

A variant of the situation discussed above is the situation where the OT herself is not told the diagnosis of the patient. Problems can then arise for the OT when she does not know the medical condition of a referral – how for example can she decide on priorities? Can the doctor be forced to disclose? What happens if a patient does not want the OT to get in touch with the doctor?

In such a situation each case would have to be treated on its own particular circumstances and many different legal principles apply. The duty in relation to confidentiality is discussed in Chapter 8 where it is noted that providing personal patient information to the multi-disciplinary team is a justifiable exception to that duty since it would be in the interests of the patient.

Another issue which arises in the situation where the doctor is refusing to give the OT patient information, is that of the standard of care to be provided by the OT. If she is kept in ignorance of certain information about the patient's condition, she may make some grave errors of judgment which could cause harm to the patient. Her right to have the relevant information to care appropriately for the patient would be clear and she should bring up any such issue with the multi-disciplinary team. It is more difficult in the community, where an OT working for social services may not be a member of such a team and it may be the GP who is refusing to give the necessary information. It might have to be explained by senior management that unless specific information is made available priorities cannot be set reasonably or the appropriate care given.

Access by others

Statutory rights of persons other than the patient under the 1990 Act are discussed above. Other rights of access including those of the courts and where certain statutes require information to be disclosed are considered in Chapter 8 on confidentiality. Access to anonymous data is also considered in Chapter 8.

Freedom of Information Act 2000

The Freedom of Information Act was given royal assent on 30 November 2000 and was brought fully into force by January 2005. The Act gives a general right of access to information held by public authorities, but this right is subject to significant exceptions.

The main exemptions from the duty are set out in Part 2 of the Act. Some of the exemptions are subject to a public interest test and these are shown in Figure 9.1. Others are absolute exemptions and these are shown in Figure 9.2. In addition to the exemptions shown in Figures 9.1 and 9.2, under section 14 a request that is vexatious or where the public authority has already complied with the request, does not have to be complied with. For the exemptions listed in Figure 9.1 a public interest test applies. This means that a public authority must consider whether the public interest in withholding the exempt information outweighs the public interest in releasing it. The majority of exemptions fall into this category. For those exemptions listed in Figure 9.2, there is no requirement for the public authority to consider the public interest. OTs might find the manual on the right to know developed by Dilys Jones and Christina Gifford of assistance on the Freedom of Information Act.[22]

Figure 9.1   Exempt Information where the public interest test applies.

- Information intended for future publication
- National security
- Defence
- International relations
- Relations within the UK
- The economy
- Investigations and proceedings conducted by public authorities
- Law enforcement
- Audit functions
- Formulation of government policy
- Prejudice to effective conduct of public affairs
- Communication with Her Majesty, etc. and honours
- Health and safety
- Environmental information
- Personal information
- Legal professional privilege
- Commercial interests

Figure 9.2   Absolute exemptions.

- Information accessible to the applicant by other means
- Information supplied by or relating to bodies dealing with security matters
- Court records
- Parliamentary privilege
- Prejudice to effective conduct of public affairs
- Personal information where the applicant is the subject of the information
- Information provided in confidence
- Prohibitions on disclosure where a disclosure is prohibited by an enactment or would constitute contempt of court

Data protection and freedom of information legislation

From Figure 9.2 it will be noted that personal information where the applicant is the subject of the information is absolutely exempt from the Freedom of Information Act. Section 40 states that:

> any information to which a request for information relates is exempt information if it constitutes personal data of which the applicant is the data subject.

If a data subject wants access to personal information, then the route for that application is the Data Protection Act 1998, and in general the Freedom of Information Act 2000 tries to prevent an overlap between the two Acts (see Chapter 8 for the Data Protection Act).

The House of Lords held in a majority judgment that whilst the BBC was regarded as a public authority under the 2000 Act and information held for the purposes of art, journalism or literature was exempt from disclosure, all requests for information were subject to the jurisdiction of the Information Commissioner and on appeal to the jurisdiction of the Information Tribunal and the BBC was obliged to disclose its internal report on Middle East coverage.[23]

Publication schemes

Section 19 of the Freedom of Information Act requires every public authority:

(a) to adopt and maintain a scheme which relates to the publication of information by the authority and is approved by the Commissioner
(b) to publish information in accordance with its publication scheme
(c) from time to time to review its publication scheme.

The publication scheme must specify classes of information which the public authority publishes or intends to publish, specify the manner in which information of each class is intended to be published, and specify whether the material is to be made available to the public free of charge or on payment. The public authority must have regard to the public interest in adopting or reviewing a publication scheme, by allowing public access to information held by the authority, and in the publication of reasons for decisions by the authority. The Commissioner can revoke approval to a publication scheme after giving six months' notice to the authority. The Commissioner must give reasons to the authority for refusing to approve a scheme or for revoking approval.

The Department of Health has in accordance with the statutory requirements set out a Publication Scheme which aims at explaining what information the Department of Health makes available to the public, and wherever possible providing an easy method of accessing the information. Most of the information listed is available free on the DH website.[24]

Individual request for information

Since January 2005 individuals have been able to exercise their general rights of access to information, given by the Freedom of Information Act 2000. The procedure to be followed is for a person to request in writing (or by email) the required information, giving full details of the information sought. The public authority has a duty to notify the applicant if the information is held by that authority and, unless an exemption applies, to give the applicant the information or allow the applicant to inspect the information. The public authority must respond to the request within 20 working days of the fee being paid. If the application is refused, then the applicant can appeal to the Information Commissioner and from his refusal to the Information Tribunal. Many cases in recent years relate to applications for further information relating to the deaths in hospital, where the NHS trust has refused to provide the information on grounds of legal professional privilege.[25] One case related to an application under the Freedom of Information Act for information relating to the withdrawal of treatment from the applicant, and the policy under which the treatment was withheld. The Tribunal held that the trust was in breach of its obligations.[26] In one case a widow whose husband had died following a fall from a hospital bed was given a report of the Trust's inquiry but she asked for the witness statements, which were refused. The Commissioner upheld the Trust's decision that they were exempt from FOIA under sections 31 and 36 and her appeal to the Tribunal failed.[27] In another case the Information Tribunal held that a parent was not entitled to see parts of a letter sent by the headmaster to the local authority to request additional funding to enable the school to provide additional teaching support that the son required, since it was exempt under S 40 of the FOIA in that personal information would have been disclosed.[28]

Dispute between Health Professions Council and the Information Commissioner

Sue Lee[29] applied to the Health Professions Council for information relating to her complaint. The HPC refused her request and she then applied to the ICO under section 50 of the FOI Act. The ICO issued an information notice requesting sight of the information which the HPC had refused to disclose. HPC appealed the Information Notice under section 57(2) of FOIA. The Tribunal upheld the Information Notice and dismissed the appeal. The HPC had argued that it had a duty of confidentiality to its registrants, that its procedures in protecting the public would be jeopardised by such disclosure. However the Tribunal was of the view that the HPC would be able to revise its procedures to ensure that those providing information were accurately forewarned that the HPC's dealing with this information would be subject to its duties under FOIA and the DPA. If registrants enquired further they could be provided with a number of reassurances.

In another case[30] Ms Fortune's baby daughter Sherin died in the Paediatric Intensive Care Unit of the Hull Royal Infirmary on 7 January 2003. The circumstances were logged as a critical incident and Dr Klonin the consultant in paediatric intensive care, stated in a letter to the Chief Executive of the hospital that she wished to report the incident to the National Patient Safety Agency (NPSA). It appeared that in the course of litigation against the hospital a copy of this letter was disclosed to Ms Fortune. On 21 January 2007 Ms Fortune made a request under the Freedom of Information Act

2000 to the NPSA for a copy of the report sent to them by Dr Klonin about the critical incident. The NPSA responded to Ms Fortune's request by denying that the information she had requested was held by them. They advised her that such information would normally be collated within the National Reporting and Learning System (NRLS) but that this system was not operational until November 2003. Ms Fortune complained to the Information Commissioner but, having sought detailed explanations from the NPSA, he concluded on the balance of probabilities that they did not hold the information requested. She appealed to the Tribunal against the Commissioner's decision. The Tribunal, in deciding whether the Information Commissioner was correct in coming to this conclusion, concluded that on the balance of probabilities that the NPSA did not hold the information.

Her appeal failed.

Restriction on Freedom of Information

Mother of deceased woman refused access to her daughter's records

The mother of a girl who had died in hospital appealed against the decision of the Information Commissioner to refuse her access to her daughter's records.[31] The trust was unwilling to release the records without the consent of the daughter's husband as her next of kin. The hospital had admitted liability for the daughter's death and had reached a settlement with the husband involving payment of substantial compensation. The mother contended that the records did not fall within the exception for confidential information under the Freedom of Information Act 2000 S 41, since the trust would have the following defences to any breach of confidence claim arising from the disclosure:

1. the public interest in the disclosure of information in cases where a hospital had been negligent in its treatment of a patient, leading to the patient's death, outweighed the public interest in maintaining confidence
2. neither the daughter nor her estate would suffer any detriment as a result of the disclosure
3. a cause of action in breach of confidence could not survive the death of the person to whom the duty of confidence was owed and
4. even if the cause of action did survive, the deceased's personal representative would not be entitled to bring an action to enforce the deceased's right to confidentiality in relation to medical records.

The Judge refused the application:

1. The public interest ensuring that patients retained trust in confidentiality of information they gave to doctors outweighed, by some way, the countervailing public interest in disclosure of a deceased's medical records.
2. If disclosure would be contrary to an individual's reasonable expectation of maintaining the confidentiality of his or her private information, then the absence of detriment in the sense contemplated by the mother was not a necessary ingredient of the cause of action.
3. The duty of confidence was capable of surviving the death of the confider
4. The trust would be in breach of confidence owed to the daughter if it disclosed her medical records other than under the terms of the Act, and the breach would be actionable by the daughter's personal representatives. Her records were exempt information under S 41 and should not be disclosed.

5.   The rights of the next-of-kin had to prevail where the rights and wishes of family members differed.

Codes of practice

Codes of practice giving practical guidance to public authorities on the discharge of their duties under the Act have been issued by the Lord Chancellor as required under section 45 of the Act[32] (referred to as the section 45 Code of Practice). In December 2003 a model action plan for preparation for the implementation of the Freedom of Information Act 2000 was published.[33] While this model action plan was not compulsory, it was intended as a tool to disseminate ideas and best practice and to assist public authorities in creating a structure path towards full implementation of the Act in 2005. Freedom of Information Act Awareness Guidance leaflets are available from the Information Commissioner's website.[34]

Conclusions

A Health Records and Data Protection Review Group (HRDG) was set up to advise the Government on helping people gain access to their health records.[35] It published its report in June 2003.[36] Forms are included which could be adapted for use by patients wishing to access their health records. The HRDG will continue to meet to provide guidance on charges, the use of the NHS number and other relevant topics.[37] More and more applications are being made under the Freedom of Information Act and the Information Commissioner has assisted in clarifying the role of public authorities.

   Questions and exercises

1   A client asks for sight of the clinical records you are keeping on her. What action do you take and what considerations do you take into account?
2   Explain to a colleague the legal procedure under the access provisions to health records of the Data Protection Act 1998 and the statutory regulations, which enable a patient to have sight of her records.
3   In what circumstances do you consider that it would cause serious harm to the physical or mental health of the patient to see his or her records?
4   What are the implications of the Freedom of Information Act 2000 for an Occupational Therapy Department?

References

1   *Sidaway v Bethlem Royal Hospital Governors* [1985] 2 WLR 480; [1985] 1 All ER 643.
2   Data Protection (Subject Access Modification) (Health) Order 2000/413.
3   Department of Health (2002) *Guidance for access to health records requests under the Data Protection Act 1998*; www.doh.gov.uk/ipu/ahr/
4   www.parliament.uk/hansard/hansard.cfm 25/10/2000, col. 464.

5   Department of Health (2003) *Guidance for Access to Health Records Requests under the Data Protection Act 1998*.

6   www.doh.gov.uk/ipu/confiden/faq.htm

7   Information Commissioner's Office (2006) *Data Protection Good Practice Note: How Does the Data Protection Act apply to professional opinions?* ICO, London.

8   Data Protection (Subject Access Modification) (Health) Order 2000/413; Data Protection (Subject Access Modification) (Social Work) Order 2000/415.

9   *R (on the application of Lord) v Secretary of State for the Home Department* [2003] EWHC 2073 (Admin); [2004] Prison L.R. 65.

10 *Clive Roberts v Nottinghamshire Healthcare NHS Trust* [2008] EWHC 1934 (QB) Case No: IHQ/08/0528.

11 Data Protection (Subject Access Modification) (Social Work) Order SI 2000/415.

12 *Bluck v Information Commissioner* (2007) 98 B.M.L.R. 1.

13 British Medical Association (2007) *Guidelines on Access to Medical Reports*. BMA, London.

14 Education (Pupil Information)(England) Regulations 2005 SI No 1437.

15 The Data Protection (Subject Access Modification) (Education) Order 2000 (SI 2000/414).

16 *R v Mid Glamorgan Family Health Services Authority, ex parte Martin* (1993) 137 SJ 153; (QBD) Times Law Report, 2 June 1993, upheld by CA Times Law Report, 16 August 1994; [1994] 5 Med LR 383.

17 *Gaskin v United Kingdom* [1990] 167 1 FLR (Case no 2/1988/146/200); [1990] 12 EHRR 36.

18 *Sidaway v Bethlem Royal Hospital Governors* [1985] 1 All ER 643.

19 General Medical Council (1998 revised 2006) Good Medical Practice. GMC, London.

20 Barnitt, R. (1994) Truth telling in occupational therapy. *British Journal of Occupational Therapy*, **57**(9), 334–40.

21 Learning from Bristol: the report of the public inquiry into children's heart surgery at the Bristol Royal Infirmary 1984–1995 (Kennedy Report). Command paper CM 5207.

22 Jones Dilys and Gifford Christina (2003) *The right to know: manual to support your delivery of the Freedom of Information Act 2000*. Pavilion Publishers, Brighton.

23 *British Broadcasting Corporation v Sugar and another* The Times Law Report 12 February 2009.

24 www.doh.gov.uk/freedom of information/

25 *Francis v Information Commissioner* [2008]UKIT EA_2007_0091 (21 July 2008).

26 *Brigden v Information Commissioner* [2007] UKIT EA_2006_0034 (05 April 2007).

27 *Galloway v IC* [2009] UKIT EA_2008_0036 (20 March 2009).

28 *A v The Information Commissioner* [2006] UKIT EA_2006_0012 (11 July 2006).

29 *Health Professions Council v the Information Commissioner* [2008] UKIT EA/2007/0116 14 March 2008.

30 *Fortune v Information Commissioner and National Patient Safety Agency* [2008] UKIT EA/2008/0004 (16 April 2008).

31 *Bluck v Information Commissioner* (2007) 98 B.M.L.R. 1.

32 Lord Chancellor, Code of Practice on the Discharge of Public Authorities' Functions under Part 1 of the Freedom of Information Act 2000; Lord Chancellor, Code of Practice on the Management of Records (Section 46 Code of Practice); www.dataprotection.gov.uk

33 www.dca.gov.uk/foi/map/modactplan.htm

34 www.ico.gov.uk

35 www.doh.gov.uk/ipu/ahr/pressrelease.htm

36 Department of Health (2003) *Guidance for Access to Health Records Requests under the Data Protection Act 1998*. DH, London.

37 www.doh.gov.uk/ipu/ahr/tor.htm

10 Negligence

Litigation is increasing as the expectations of clients in relation to healthcare grow and the publicity about awards of compensation raises hopes of vast settlements. In September 2007 it was revealed that current claims against the NHS for negligence handled by the NHS Litigation Authority amounted to almost £4.5 billion, of which £3.3 billion related to incidents alleging oxygen starvation at birth. In the decade ending in 2008 there were 1,179 clinical negligence claims relating to cancer treatment leading to £47 million paid out in compensation and claims of £50 million still outstanding.[1] The fact that more than 1 in 4 NHS trusts are paying out more in legal costs than in damages is leading to concerns that the present system of no win no fee is not working and lawyers are exploiting the NHS[2] (see Chapter 13). The employed practitioner is unlikely to be sued personally, because the employer is indirectly responsible in law for the wrongful acts of his employee while the employee is acting in the course of employment. This is known as the vicarious liability of the employer and is explained further below. The employed practitioner might however be held personally liable for 'Samaritan' acts, if harm is caused, in a situation where the employer might argue that it is not vicariously liable because the employee was not acting in the course of employment. Even if the practitioner is an employee, she still needs to have an understanding of the law relating to negligence so that she is appropriately prepared to defend any allegations against her.

The following topics are covered:

- Civil actions
- Principles of negligence
  - Duty of care
  - Breach of the duty of care and standards of care
  - Causation
  - Harm
- Vicarious and personal liability distinguished
- Defences to an action for negligence
- Calculation of compensation (quantum)
- Situations involving OTs
- Liability for student or unregistered assistance: delegation and supervision
- Scope of professional practice
- Volunteers
- Care of property
- Proof of the facts and documentation
- Litigation in the NHS
- NHS Redress Scheme

Legal Aspects of Occupational Therapy, Third Edition By Bridgit Dimond
© 2010 Bridgit Dimond

Civil actions

Civil actions include those actions brought in the civil courts by an individual or organisation, usually with the aim of obtaining compensation or other remedy which the court is able to order. The main group of civil actions is called torts, i.e. civil wrongs excluding breach of contract. Within the group of civil actions called torts are negligence, trespass, breach of statutory duty, defamation, nuisance and others. In each case the burden will usually be upon the person bringing the action (known as the claimant, but prior to April 1999 referred to as the plaintiff) to establish on a balance of probabilities the existence of each of the elements which make up each cause of action. Thus in an action for trespass to the person (see Chapter 7) the claimant must show that there was a direct interference or touching of her person without her consent or other lawful justification. It should also be noted that in serious cases gross negligence may amount to the criminal offence of manslaughter. This is considered in Chapter 2 and Chapter 25. Other criminal offences may also be committed as a result of negligence. For example two ambulance men who decided that a dying man was not worth saving and whose conversation was heard by ambulance control since the telephone line was still open were arrested and could face charges of wilfully neglecting to perform a duty in public office contrary to the common law.[3]

Principles of negligence

Negligence is the most common civil action, brought in situations where the claimant alleges that there has been personal injury, death, or damage or loss of property. Compensation is sought for the loss which has occurred. To succeed in the action, the claimant has to show the following elements:

- that the defendant owed to the person harmed a duty of care
- that the defendant was in breach of that duty
- that the breach of duty caused reasonably foreseeable harm
- that harm was caused to the claimant.

These four elements – duty, breach, causation, and harm –are discussed below.

Duty of care

The law recognises that a duty of care will exist where one person can reasonably foresee that his or her actions and omissions could cause reasonably foreseeable harm to another person. A duty of care will always exist between the health professional and the patient, but it might not always be easy to identify what it includes. Where there is no pre-existing duty to a person, the usual legal principle is that there is no duty to volunteer services. There may, however, be a professional duty to volunteer help in certain circumstances.

In the case of Donoghue and Stevenson[4] the House of Lords defined the duty of care owed at common law (i.e. judge made law) as being:

> You must take reasonable care to avoid acts or omissions which you can reasonably foresee would be likely to injure your neighbour. Who then in law is my neighbour? The answer seems to be persons who are so closely and directly affected by my act that I ought reasonably to have them in contemplation as being so affected when I am directing my mind to the acts or omissions which are called in question.

In a case involving the escape of Borstal boys who caused serious damage to a yacht,[5] the House of Lords held that a duty of care was owed by the Home Office to any persons who were injured or whose property was damaged as a result of failure to keep the boys under proper control.

No duty of care of police and fire service

The Court of Appeal decided that the police did not owe a duty of care to the victims of crime in deciding whether or not to prosecute a suspected offender, even where the decision took into account the interests of the victim.[6] V and her sisters alleged that the police had failed to investigate allegations of indecent assault and cruelty and to prosecute. The Court of Appeal held that there were policy reasons for the general rule that the police owed no duty of care to investigate allegations of crime victims, in particular the diversion of resources and that police investigations might be carried out defensively. Their claim was struck out. The ruling in the cases of *Hill v Chief Constable of West Yorkshire Police*[7] and the case of *Brooks v Commissioner of Police of the Metropolis*[8] was applied. The Court of Appeal held that a fire brigade did not owe a duty of care to an owner or occupier merely by attending a fire.[9]

The case of Hill was followed by the House of Lords (in a majority judgment) in two cases where the existence of a duty of care by victims of a crime was debated.[10] In a dissenting judgement Lord Bingham argued in favour of the recognition of "a liability principle" in the following circumstances:

> If a member of the public (A) furnishes a police officer (B) with apparently credible evidence that a third party whose identity and whereabouts are known presents a specific and imminent threat to his life or physical safety, B owes A a duty to take reasonable steps to assess such threat and, if appropriate, take reasonable steps to prevent it being executed.

This was not accepted by his colleagues, who held that the police did not owe a duty of care to the victims.

Duty of care and local authority

In the case of *X(1) and Y(2) v London Borough of Hounslow* the High Court[11] held that a duty of care is owed by a local authority when a couple with learning disabilities were being assaulted and victimised by a gang of youths. The Court of Appeal however allowed the appeal by the local authority.[12] The case is discussed in Chapter 22.

The House of Lords held that local housing authority landlords were under no duty of care to notify a neighbour over an eviction warning. The neighbour had received death threats from an abusive tenant and was not told that a meeting had been arranged at which the tenant was warned that he would be evicted unless his behaviour improved. Afterwards the tenant inflicted fatal injuries on the neighbour.[13]

In contrast the House of Lords held that the duty of care owed by a local authority's children's services to look after a homeless child could not be fulfilled by referring the child to the homeless persons unit.[14]

The local authority was held to be in breach of its duty of care when it failed to ensure that a child who was abused, beaten burnt and tortured was not taken into care. Jake Pierce was awarded £25,000 against Doncaster Metropolitan Borough Council in 2008 and in December 2008 the Court of Appeal rejected the local authority's appeal against the award, returning the case to the trial court on the issue of the judge's discretion over time limits.[15] He was supported with legal aid from the Legal Services Commission.

Duty of care and the OT

A frequent concern of the OT is when does the duty of care start – when a referral is received or when the client is placed on a waiting list or when the client is placed on an OT's caseload? The answer that a duty of care begins as soon as there is a referral, but at each stage the duty of care is different in nature. When the OT receives a referral, she would have a duty to act according to the reasonable practice in relation to that referral, by ensuring that all the necessary information had been sent and by ensuring that any immediate action which could be reasonably expected of an OT was taken. She would then have a duty to assess the priority of that referral against other referrals and to assess priorities at regular intervals and if she is informed of a change of circumstances. When the client becomes part of the OT's case load then she would have to provide the reasonable standard of care of an OT to that client. Similar considerations would take place in determining when the duty of care ended. Discharge from hospital may not end the OT's duty it depends upon the nature of after-care. The hospital OT may simply have the responsibility of ensuring that social services are notified of the discharge and are given necessary information. Does an OT have a duty of care in relation to 'inactive' cases? The answer of course does depend upon the definition of 'inactive'. If these refer to clients who are no longer receiving OT input, then before the decision was made to cease OT, a determination should have been made on whether the situation should be reviewed by the OT and when or whether the client would notify the OT if circumstances changed. The duty of care in relation to equipment is considered in Chapter 15.

Breach of duty

Determining the standard of care

In order to determine whether there has been a breach of the duty of care, it will first be necessary to establish the required standard. The courts have used what has become known as the Bolam Test to determine the standard of care required by a professional. In the case from which the test took its name,[16] the court laid down the following principle to determine the standard of care which should be followed:

> The standard of care expected is 'the standard of the ordinary skilled man exercising and professing to have that special skill' (Judge McNair, p. 121)

The Bolam test was applied by the House of Lords in a case where negligence by an obstetrician in delivering a child by forceps was alleged:[17]

> When you get a situation which involves the use of some special skill or competence, then the test as to whether there has been negligence or not ... is the standard of the ordinary skilled man exercising and professing to have that special skill. If a surgeon failed to measure up to that in any respect (clinical judgement or otherwise) he had been negligent and should be so adjudged.

The House of Lords found that the surgeon was not liable in negligence and held that an error of judgement may or may not be negligence. It depends on the circumstances.

This standard of the reasonable professional man following the accepted approved standard of care can be used to apply to any professional person – architect, lawyer and accountant as well as any health professional. The standard of care which a practitioner should have provided would be judged in this way. Expert witnesses would give evidence to the court on the standard of care they would expect to have found in the circumstances before the court. These experts would be respected members of the profession of occupational therapy, possibly a head of department or training college, and lawyers would look to the leading organisations of individual professional groups to obtain recommended names. The experts would be expected to place themselves in the situation of the practitioners at the time the alleged negligent act took place, and give their opinion on the standard of care that they would have expected to have been followed at that time (see Chapter 13 for the expert witness).

In a civil action, the judge would decide in the light of the evidence given to the court, what standard should have been followed. The standards at the time of the alleged negligence apply, not the standards at the time of the court hearing. This is significant, since many cases take several years to come to court, in which time standards may have changed.

Experts can of course differ and a case may arise where the expert giving evidence for the claimant states that the accepted approved standard of care was not followed by the defendant or its employees. In contrast, the expert evidence for the defendant states that the defendant or his employees followed the reasonable standard of care. Where such a conflict arises the House of Lords (in the Maynard case[18]) has laid down the following principle:

> It was not sufficient to establish negligence for the plaintiff (i.e. claimant) to show that there was a body of competent professional opinion that considered the decision was wrong, if there was also a body of equally competent professional opinion that supported the decision as having been reasonable in the circumstances.

The determination of the reasonable standard of care has been considered by the House of Lords in the case of *Bolitho v City and Hackney Health Authority*.[19] In this case the House of Lords stated that:

> The court had to be satisfied that the exponents of the body of opinion relied on can demonstrate that such opinion has a logical basis. In particular in cases involving, as they often do, the weighing of risks against benefits, the judge, before accepting a body of opinion as being responsible, reasonable or respectable, will need to be satisfied that, in forming their views, the experts had directed their minds to the question of comparative risks and benefits and had reached a defensible conclusion on the matter.
>
> The use of the adjectives "responsible, reasonable and respectable" (in the *Bolam* case) all showed that the court had to be satisfied that the exponents of the body of opinion relied upon could demonstrate that such opinion had a logical basis.
>
> It would seldom be right for a judge to reach the conclusion that views held by a competent medical expert were unreasonable.

Following the Woolf Reforms (see Chapter 13) parties to personal injury litigation are expected to agree on an expert witness.

It follows from the *Bolitho* judgment that there will be exceptional cases where a judge decides that expert opinion given by a defendant is not reasonable. This occurred in the following case.

Case: *Marriott v West Midlands Health Authority*[20]

The claimant fell downstairs at his home, suffered a head injury and was unconscious for 20–30 minutes. He was admitted to hospital and following X-rays and neurological observations he was discharged the next day. He remained lethargic with no appetite and had headaches. He called the GP who was informed of the history, gave him neurological tests but found no abnormality. He told the claimant's wife to call him if the condition deteriorated and advised him to take pain killers for his headache. Four days later his condition suddenly deteriorated and he became unconscious and was returned to hospital. A massive left extradural haematoma was operated upon. A linear fracture of the skull was discovered. The claimant was left with hemiplegia, dysarthria and was severely disabled.

The claimant sued the health authorities and the GP. There was disputed expert evidence over the correct course which should have been followed by the GP. The trial judge found against the GP on the basis of 'the only reasonable prudent course in any case where a GP remains of the view that there is a risk of an intracranial lesion such as to warrant the carrying out of neurological testing and the giving of further head injury instructions, then the only prudent course judged from the point of view of the patient is to re-admit for further testing and observation'.

The GP appealed against this decision. The Court of Appeal held that the judge was entitled to subject a body of opinion to analysis to see whether it can properly be regarded as reasonable. The judge was entitled to find it could not be a reasonable exercise of a GP's discretion to leave a patient at home.

The White Paper[21] on the NHS and the Health Act 1999, which are discussed in Chapter 17, has led to increasing emphasis on standard setting on the basis of evidence-based research: The National Institute for Health and Clinical Excellence (NICE), the Care Quality Commission (replacing the Healthcare Commission and other bodies) and the National Service Frameworks are leading to more guidance on standards to be achieved in all departments of a hospital and community care. In addition, the power given to the Secretary of State to set standards legally binding on NHS organisations under the Health and Social Care (Community Health and Standards) Act 2003, reenacted in the Health and Social Care Act 2008 may have a significant effect on standards being followed. It is anticipated that these standards will be incorporated into the Bolam test of reasonable professional practice. Practitioners will be expected to follow the results of clinical effectiveness research in their treatment and care of the patients, unless the specific circumstances of the patient should otherwise indicate. Patients are able to use these national guidelines to argue that inadequate care has been provided. For example, in January 2001 the Government published its national standards for cancer services[22] (see Chapter 17 for National Service Frameworks). If a hospital fails to meet these standards and a claimant can show that he or she has suffered consequential harm, then this failure could be used as evidence in a claim for compensation for negligence. In addition to showing that there has been vicarious liability by a trust, the claimant may also be able to establish a failure in the direct liability of the trust for the inadequate services. Thus if a stroke victim were to bring a case alleging a breach of the duty of care, he could refer to the NSF for older people which envisaged that everyone who had a stroke would have access to a specialist stroke service by 2004. He could also refer to the second edition of the National Clinical Guidelines for stroke published in 2004 by the Royal College of Physicians and the Physiotherapy Concise Guide for Stroke published by the CSP and the Royal College of Physicians in 2006. The COT has also published a manual giving practical advice on the development of clinical guidelines.[23]

NICE Clinical guideline for Parkinson's Disease was published in June 2006. The NICE guideline for multiple sclerosis was published in 2003 and the NSF for long-term conditions in 2005 and in 2009 the MS Society in conjunction with the COT published a guide for OTs.[24] This provides a valuable practical tool for OTs to ensure that they understand and implement the official guidance. Each guideline of NICE and the NSF is considered in relation to key reflections and audit statements by the OT.

A decision of the Court of Appeal has emphasised that the highest standards are not those which have to be implemented in the law of negligence. The Court of Appeal suggested that where there was more than one acceptable standard, competence should be gauged by the lowest of them.[25] The Bolam test applied where there was a conscious choice of available courses made by a trained professional. It was inappropriate where the alleged neglect lay in an oversight.

Other organisations are involved with NICE in determining the appropriate standards for different clinical areas. (The College of Occupational therapists has set out its involvement as a NICE stakeholder[26]) Once standards are finalised (though subject always to review), it is likely that they will have considerable weight in determining the Bolam test of approved accepted practice.

Legal significance of guidelines

It should be emphasised that the publication of national guidelines will never remove the need for individual professional discretion to be exercised to ensure that the specific circumstances of the patient are taken into account in determining what would be the reasonable standard of care. On some occasions it may be negligence to fail to follow guidelines, on others it may be negligence to follow them. Brian Hurwitz[27] points out the complexities of the legal status of clinical guidelines.

The Court of Appeal held in a case,[28] where it was alleged that cervical screening had not been properly carried out, that the Bolam test is not always the appropriate test to use for negligence. It held that the Bolam test was appropriate where the exercise of skill and judgment of the screener was being questioned. In the case before it, however, the Bolam test did not apply since the screeners were not expected to exercise judgment.

NICE describes its clinical guidelines in the following terms:

> The guidelines look at the most up-to-date clinical evidence as well as the needs of patients and their families. Clinical guidelines also take into account the cost-effectiveness of the various methods of treating and managing a condition. The guidelines are advisory rather than compulsory, although healthcare professionals must consider the guidelines when deciding on the best possible treatment for their patient.

The COT has published an information guide on producing clinical guidelines for occupational therapy practice.[29] It gives a step-by-step outline description of how to produce, test and apply clinical guidelines to OT practice and complements two other OT publications on clinical audit information pack and using evidence base.[30] In addition, the COT has published details on how college documents on position statements, standards for practice and clinical guidelines should be produced.[31] The COT has also provided a briefing on integrated care pathways (ICPs).[32] The briefing emphasises that, 'The ICP is not cast in stone and should be used as a guideline to ensure that the most appropriate care is provided. It should not be followed blindly and clinical judgement should be used at all times.'

The standards and standard statements for OT practice developed in 2007[33] would be used to determine the reasonable standards of OT practice in any litigation. The statements cover: referral, consent, assessment and goal setting, intervention and evaluation, discharge, closure or transfer of care, record keeping, service quality and governance, professional development/lifelong learning, practice placements, safe working practice and research ethics (see Chapter 4 on professional practice).

Has there been a breach of the duty of care?

Once it has been established in court what the reasonable standard of care should have been, the next stage is to decide whether what took place was in accordance with the reasonable standard, i.e. has there been a breach of the duty of care? Gross negligence which results in death could be followed by criminal proceedings (see Chapter 2). In the civil courts evidence will be given by witnesses of fact as to what actually took place. The role of witnesses is considered in Chapter 13.

The Bolam test applies to the standards of care which should have been provided at the time the alleged negligence took place. Clearly by the time the case is actually heard, standards may well have improved. For example, in the care of stroke victims, ideas on rehabilitation may well have changed in recent years but it would be the standards which applied at the time of the alleged negligence which would be applied in determining whether compensation was payable.

The standard of care required of a child was considered by the Court of Appeal when a child ran into a playground supervisor causing her serious brain damage leading to partial paralysis and balance problems.[34] The Court of Appeal held that the primary question was whether the conduct of the child was culpable i.e. whether it had fallen below the standard that should objectively be expected of a child of that age. For a child to be culpable the conduct must be careless to a very high degree, and where a child aged 13 was participating in a game in a play area, was not breaking any rules and was not acting to any significant degree beyond the norms of that game he would not be held culpable. The play ground supervisor lost her case.

Causation

The claimant must show that not only was there a breach of the duty of care, but that this breach of duty caused actual and reasonably foreseeable harm to the claimant. This requires:

- factual causation to be shown
- evidence that the type of harm which occurred was reasonably foreseeable
- no intervening cause which breaks the chain of causation.

Factual causation

There may be a breach of the duty of care and harm but there may be no link between them. In the classic case of *Barnett v Chelsea HMC*[35] a casualty doctor failed to examine patients who came in vomiting severely. The widow of one failed to obtain compensation, since the patient would have died anyway. There was no factual causation between the failure to examine and the death of the patient.

The onus is on the claimant to establish that there is this causal link between the breach of the duty of care and the harm which occurred. In the following case, the plaintiffs failed to establish causation and the House of Lords ordered a new hearing on the issue of causation. The parties then agreed to a settlement.

Case: excess oxygen – *Wilsher v Essex Area Health Authority*[36]

A premature baby was being treated with oxygen therapy. A junior doctor mistakenly inserted the catheter to monitor the oxygen intake into the vein rather than an artery. A senior registrar when being asked to check what had been done failed to notice the error. The baby was given excess oxygen. The parents claimed compensation for the retrolentalfibroplasia that the baby suffered, but failed to prove that it was the excess oxygen which had caused the harm. They therefore failed in their claim. It was agreed that there were several different factors which could have caused the child to become blind and the negligence was only one of them. It could not been presumed that it was the defendant's negligence which had caused the harm.

It has also been difficult for claimants to establish causation when suing for compensation for harm which it is claimed has resulted from vaccine damage.

Case: vaccine damage – *Loveday v Renton*[37]

A case was brought against the Welcome Foundation who made vaccine against whooping cough and against the doctor who administered it, seeking compensation for brain damage which was alleged to have been caused by the vaccine. The case failed because the judge held that the claimant had not established on a balance of probabilities that the pertussis vaccine had caused the brain damage.

That case contrasts with the following Irish case in which causation was established.

Case: successful action for vaccine damage – *Best v Welcome Foundation*[38]

The High Court had dismissed the claimant's claim because of the lack of proof of causation. However the Irish Supreme Court held that the Welcome Foundation was liable for the negligent manufacture and release of a particular batch of triple vaccine and that the brain damage was caused as a result. It referred the case back to the High Court on the amount of compensation. On 11 May 1993 the High Court approved an award of £2.75 million as compensation for the brain damage sustained in September 1969.

Reasonably foreseeable harm

The harm which might arise may not be within the reasonable contemplation of the defendant so that even though there is a breach of duty and there is harm, the defendant is not liable. What can be reasonably contemplated depends on the circumstances. For example, in the case of *Jolley v Sutton London Borough Council*[39] (where a boy of 14 was paralysed when a boat that had been jacked up fell on him), the House of Lords held that even though the exact type of mischief carried out by children could not be foreseen, the Council were liable, subject to a reduction of 25% contributory negligence. The risk which should have been contemplated was that if children meddle with a rotten boat, then injuries are likely to occur (see Chapter 11 for further discussion of Occupier's Liability).

No intervening cause which breaks the chain of causation (novus actus interveniens)

It may happen that any causal link between the plaintiff's breach of duty and the harm suffered by the client is interrupted by an intervening event.

Situation: intervening act

An OT fails to check that a hoist delivered to a home is properly installed. The patient falls to the floor while being hoisted and suffers a cardiac arrest. There is no suggestion that the wrong installation caused the cardiac arrest.

In this situation the negligence of the practitioner has not caused the death of the patient so her employer would not be vicariously liable. There may, however, be subsequent disciplinary and even professional misconduct proceedings taken against the practitioner because of her failure to carry out a proper check on the installation.

Loss of a chance

Case: *Hotson v E Berks HA*[40]

A 13-year-old boy fell out of a tree and suffered a slipped femoral epiphysis. He attended the A&E department, but the doctor failed to carry out an X-ray of the hip. The boy suffered considerable pain and returned to hospital five days later, when the fracture was diagnosed. He developed avascular necrosis of the femoral head which medical evidence suggested occurred in 75% of patients. Expert evidence for the claimant was that as a result of the delay in diagnosis he lost a 25% chance of avoiding this complication. The judge awarded the boy £150 damages for the pain suffered by him for the 5 days, which he would have been spared by prompt diagnosis and treatment. In addition the boy was awarded 25% of the damages which would have been awarded if the entire injury had been attributable to negligence (i.e. 25% of £45 000), for the loss of the chance of recovery.

The House of Lords allowed the health authority's appeal, holding that the claimant had not established that the defendant's negligence had caused the avascular necrosis. The question of causation was to be determined on the balance of probabilities with the onus on the claimant.

Harm

To succeed in an action for negligence the claimant or her representative must establish that she has suffered harm which the court recognises as being subject to compensation. Thus personal injury, death and loss or damage to property are the main areas of recognisable harm. In addition, the courts have ruled that nervous shock (now known as post traumatic stress syndrome), where an identifiable medical condition exists, can be the subject of compensation within strict limits of liability. A test of proximity to the defendant's negligent action or omission has been set by the House of Lords in the case of *Alcock v Chief Constable of South Yorkshire* [1992] [41] This test of proximity can be used to argue that the harm is not subject to compensation or that no duty of care is owed in the circumstances (see cases above under Duty of Care).

In one case[42] where a mother claimed compensation for post traumatic stress the defendants argued that since the events took place over a period of time it was not simply one horrifying event.

Case: *North Glamorgan NHS Trust v Walters* 2003

A 10-month-old boy was admitted to hospital suspected of suffering from hepatitis. The doctors failed to diagnose that this was acute and accepted that had it been properly diagnosed and treated by means of a liver transplant, he may have lived. During the night he suffered a fit and the mother was told by the nurse that it was unlikely that he had suffered any brain damage. In fact, there had been a major epileptic seizure that led to a coma and irreparable brain damage. A scan was carried out and the mother was told incorrectly that it showed no brain damage. He was transferred to a London hospital where he was placed on a life support machine. A further scan showed that he had suffered severe brain damage and the parents agreed that it was in the boy's best interests for the life support to be turned off. He died in his mother's arms. She was subsequently told that had he been transferred earlier he would have had a far better chance of survival.

It was agreed that the mother was suffering from a pathological grief reaction, which was a result of witnessing, experiencing and participating in the events described. The judge found that the mother was a secondary victim and her psychiatric injury was caused by sight and sound of a horrifying event that had covered a period of time. The defendants appealed to the Court of Appeal on the grounds that the 36-hour period could not be regarded in law as one horrifying event, but the claimant's appreciation was not sudden. The Court of Appeal held that the 36-hour period could be viewed as a single horrifying event and the judge was correct to find that the claimant's appreciation of the events was sudden as opposed to an accumulation of gradual assaults on her mind.

A similar decision is seen in another Court of Appeal case[43] where the claimant suffered post-traumatic stress syndrome after her daughter was killed in a road accident when a car mounted the pavement. The claimant rushed to the scene of the accident, which was cordoned off, and she was prevented from crossing the tape. She was told that her daughter was dead and she screamed hysterically and collapsed to the ground. Subsequently at the mortuary, while the worst of the injuries on the girl's lower part were covered by a blanket, the mother saw that the daughter's face and head were disfigured. She cradled the daughter saying she was cold. She lost her case on the grounds that the judge could not accept that what happened in the mortuary could be said to be part of the aftermath. The shock from which she suffered was a result of what she had been told by the police. The Court of Appeal allowed the claimant's appeal holding that the immediate aftermath extended from the moment of the accident until the moment that the claimant left the mortuary. The judge had artificially separated out the mortuary visit from what was an uninterrupted sequence of events.

A victim of the Ladbrooke Grove rail crash who suffered depression which led to his killing someone, was unable to recover damages for the loss of his earnings after the manslaughter from the defendants who admitted liability for negligence up to the date of the manslaughter.[44] Whilst his physical injuries were minor the accident had a major psychological impact on him. He suffered post traumatic stress disorder with a marked depressive component and a significant personality change. In August 2001 he stabbed a stranger to death. The Court of Appeal held that his claim was not founded on an illegal act. The manslaughter was not inextricably bound up with the claim for loss of earnings before and after the manslaughter, which resulted from the defendant's negligence. It was for the court to determine to what extent the manslaughter was the claimant's fault and therefore could be viewed as contributory negligence under the 1945 Act (see below). However the House of Lords allowed the defendant's appeal and held that the claimant could not recover damages for loss of earnings following his detention in prison and in mental hospital following the killing on the basis that a person cannot benefit from his own wrong (ex turpi causa non oritur actio). The defendants had accepted liability in negligence up to the date the claimant had committed the manslaughter.[45]

Vicarious and personal liability distinguished

As stated above, it is unlikely that an employee will be sued personally since the employer would be vicariously liable for her actions. To establish the vicarious liability of the employer the claimant must show:

- the employee
- was negligent or was guilty of another wrong
- while acting in the course of employment.

An independent practitioner would have to accept personal and professional liability for her actions but she may also be vicariously liable for the harm caused during the course of employment, by any one she employs. A practitioner who is an employee but who also works as an independent practitioner would have to have indemnity cover in respect of the independent practice. The COT has published guidance on professional indemnity in a briefing note.[46]

An employer is not liable for the acts of his independent contractors, i.e. self-employed persons who are working for him on a contract for services, unless he is at fault in selecting or instructing them.

The employer may challenge whether the actions were performed in the course of employment. For example, an OT may have undertaken training in a complementary medicine such as acupuncture. If she decided to use these new skills while at work without the agreement, express or implied, of the employer and through her use of the remedies caused harm to the client, the employer might refuse to accept vicarious liability on the grounds that the employee was not acting in the course of employment. (Complementary therapies are considered in Chapter 27.)

The House of Lords has widened the scope of vicarious liability. It ruled that the owners of a boarding school were vicariously liable for sexual abuse carried out by a warden.[47] The council had been responsible for the care of vulnerable children and employed the deputy headmaster to carry out that duty on its behalf. The sexual abuse had taken place while the employee had been engaged in duties at the very time and place demanded by his employment. The warden's wrongs were so closely connected with his employment that it would be fair and just to hold the defendants vicariously liable.

In a recent case the Court of Appeal had to decide whether throwing a punch in a rugby match could be considered to be in the course of employment so as to make the Club vicariously liable.[48] The player punched a member of the opposing team on the field and caused a fracture which required reconstructive orbital surgery. The player had a contract with Redruth Rugby Football Club by which it employed him to play rugby for it. The Court of Appeal held that the employer was vicariously liable for the acts of its employees committed whilst in the course of employment. There was a close connection between the punch and his employment. He was employed to play rugby and that was what he was doing at the time. There was a melee going on of the kind which frequently took place during rugby matches. The melee was part of the game. It was just the kind of thing that both clubs would have expected to occur. Unfortunately the throwing of punches was not uncommon in such situations. The player was acting in the course of employment when he punched the claimant and the Club was therefore vicariously liable for his actions.

A trust may also be criminally responsible as a result of its vicarious liability for the actions of an employee. For example an NHS trust was fined because of failures of employees to comply with the Medicines Act 1968 in supplying a medical product not of a nature or quality specified in a prescription. The Court of Appeal, however, felt that the £75,000 fine imposed by the Crown court failed to give adequate recognition to the fact that this was a case of vicarious liability for the acts of two employees whose work had been properly delegated and who had been properly trained. The fine was reduced to £15,000.[49]

The self-employed practitioner

Where a practitioner is self-employed, she must ensure that she takes out public indemnity cover for any alleged negligence, since she would be personally liable for any harm caused by her negligence and there would be no employer who would be vicariously liable. Practitioners working in the independent sector should check to ascertain whether they are under a contract for services, in which case they are self-employed professionals and would have to have their own personal insurance cover, or whether they have a contract of service, in which case they are employees for whom the employer would be vicariously liable (see Chapter 28).

Defences to an action

The main defences to an action for negligence are:

- dispute allegations
- deny that all the elements of negligence are established
- contributory negligence
- exemption from liability
- limitation of time
- voluntary assumption of risk.

Dispute allegations

Many cases will be resolved entirely on what facts can be shown to exist. Thus the effectiveness of the witnesses for both parties in establishing the facts of what did or did not occur will be the determining factor in who wins the case. Reference should be made to Chapter 12 on record keeping and to Chapter 13 on witnesses in court, for further discussion on the nature of evidence and the role of the witnesses. In theory, it might appear before the court hearing that one party has a particularly strong case, but unless the facts on which its case rests can be proved in court, the actual outcome of the case might be that the opponent wins.

All elements of negligence established

The claimant must establish, on a balance of probabilities, that all elements required to prove negligence are present, i.e. duty, breach, causation and harm. If one or more of these cannot be established then the defendant will win the case.

Contributory negligence

If the claimant is partly to blame for the harm which has occurred, then there may still be liability on the part of the professional but the compensation payable might be reduced in proportion to the claimant's fault. In extreme cases, such a claim by the defendant of contributory negligence may be a complete defence, if 100% contributory negligence is claimed. In determining the level of contributory negligence, the physical and mental health and the age of the claimant would be taken into account.

Situation: contributory negligence

An OT is undertaking rehabilitation work with a patient who has suffered a stroke. She warns the patient that she should not attempt to use the kettle, but the OT would obtain details of a different model for her to use safely. The OT fails to obtain these details and the patient uses the kettle and suffers a serious scald. There is a clear breach of duty by the OT, but the patient is also at fault and this would be taken into account in assessing any compensation payable.

The Law Reform (Contributory Negligence) Act 1945 enables an apportionment of responsibility for the harm which has been caused which may result in a reduction of damages payable. The court can reduce the damages

to such extent as it thinks just and equitable having regard to the claimant's share in the responsibility for the damage. (section 1(1))

The defences of contributory negligence, *volenti non fit injuria* (see below) and novus acto interveniens (see above) were all used by the defendant in a case brought against the Commissioner for the Metropolitan police[50] The administratrix of L who had committed suicide whilst in police custody sued the police for breach of its duty of care to the prisoner, who was known to be a suicide risk. The trial judge found that there was a breach of the duty of care by the police since they had left the hatch of his cell door open and this had been used in the suicide. However he held that this breach of duty had not caused the death on the basis of either *volenti non fit injuria* or novus actus interveniens, the sole cause of death was L's deliberate act in killing himself. The Court of Appeal allowed the claimant's appeal holding that neither *volenti non fit injuria* nor novus actus interveniens applied where the act which caused the death was the act which the defendant was under a duty to prevent. It awarded £8,690 compensation. The defendant appealed and the House of Lords held that there was a duty of care owed to L and it was self-contradictory to say that breach of that duty could not have been a cause of harm because the victim had caused it to himself. The police was in breach of its duty of care and caused the death, but so did L cause his own death. However L was in sound mind and therefore he must be considered to have some responsibility for his death. Applying the 1945 Act compensation was reduced by 50% to allow for L's responsibility for the death. (For contributory negligence by a child see Chapter 23.)

Exemption from liability

It is possible for a person to exempt herself from liability for harm arising from her negligence but the effects of the Unfair Contract Terms Act 1977 mean that this exemption only applies to loss or damage to property. A defendant cannot exclude liability from negligence which results in personal damage or death either by contract or by a notice.

Where exemption from liability for loss or damage to property is claimed by the defendant, it must be shown by the defendant that it is reasonable to rely upon the term or notice which purported to exclude liability. The provisions of the Unfair Contract Terms Act 1977 are shown in Figure 10.1.

Reasonableness in relation to a notice not having contractual effect, means that 'it should be fair and reasonable to allow reliance on it, having regard to all the circumstances obtaining when the liability arose or (but for the notice) would have arisen' (section 11(3)). 'It is for those claiming that a contract term or notice satisfies the requirements of reasonableness to show that it does' (section 11(5)).

The effect of this legislation is that notices which purport to exempt a person or an organisation from liability for negligence are invalid if that negligence leads to personal injury or death. However,

Figure 10.1   Unfair Contract Terms Act 1977 – section 2.

2(1)   A person cannot by reference to any contract term or to a notice given to persons generally or to particular persons exclude or restrict his liability for death or personal injury resulting from negligence.

2(2)   In the case of other loss or damage, a person cannot so exclude or restrict his liability for negligence except in so far as the term or notice satisfies the requirement of reasonableness.

a notice which excludes liability for loss or damage to property may be valid if it is reasonable for the negligent person or organisation to rely upon it.

Limitation of time

Actions for personal injury or death should normally be commenced within three years of the date of the event which gave rise to the harm, or three years from the date on which the person had the necessary knowledge of the harm and the fact that it arose from the defendant's actions or omissions. The Court of Appeal held that the cause of action accrues when the injury is suffered.[51] There are, however, some major qualifications to this three year time limit and these are shown in Figure 10.2.

The implication of the rules relating to limitation of time is that in those cases which might come under one of the exceptions to the three-year time limit, records should be kept and not destroyed. This is particularly important in the case of children and those with learning disabilities. For example, in the case of *Bull v Wakeham*[52] the case was brought 18 years after the birth. In a news report in 1995[53] a man then 33 obtained compensation of £1.25 million because of a failure to diagnose severe dehydration a few weeks after birth.

The definition of knowledge[54] for the purposes of the limitation of time is that a person must have knowledge of the following facts:

- that the injury in question was significant
- that the injury was attributable in whole or in part to the act or omission which is alleged to constitute the negligence, nuisance or breach of duty
- the identity of the defendant
- if it is alleged that the act or omission was that of a person other than the defendant, the identity of that person and the additional facts supporting the bringing of an action against the defendant.

Knowledge that any acts or omissions did or did not, as a matter of law, involve negligence, nuisance or breach of duty is irrelevant. A person is not fixed with knowledge of a fact ascertainable only with the help of expert advice so long as he has taken all reasonable steps to obtain, and where appropriate to act on, that advice.

In a significant decision the House of Lords[55] ruled in January 2008 that claims could be brought by the victims of rape and sexual assault outside the time limit, if the judge ruled that the personal characteristics of the claimant might have prevented him or her acting as a reasonable person. Three

---

Figure 10.2   Situations where the limitation of time can be extended.

- Those suffering from a disability:
  - ○ Children under 18 years – the time does not start to run until the child is 18 years.
  - ○ Mental disability – time does not start to run until the disability ends. In the case of those who are suffering from severe learning disabilities or brain damage this may not be until death.
- Discretion of the judge – The judge has a statutory power to extend the time within which a claimant (plaintiff) can bring an action for personal injuries or death, if it is just and equitable to do so.

of the cases were remitted to High Court for reconsideration in the light of the House of Lords ruling. It overruled its previous decision in the case of *Stubbings v Webb*[56] and allowed time barred appeals in cases which involved a rape victim, whose rapist had subsequently won the lottery, and several victims of sexual assault by council employees in council run schools or residential homes. The consequence of the decision is that many thousands of victims of indecent assault may pursue claims against the councils and churches. The High Court also held that claims by former servicemen for radiation injury resulting from nuclear tests from 1950's could go ahead and were not to be struck out on grounds that they were time barred or had no reasonable prospect of success.[57]

Voluntary assumption of risk

Volenti non fit injuria is the latin name for the defence that a person willingly undertook the risk of being harmed. It is unlikely to succeed as a defence in an action for professional negligence since the professional cannot exempt herself from liability where harm occurs as a result of her negligence. (See the Unfair Contract Terms Act which is considered above.) The defence of *volenti non fit injuria* would not be available to an employer as a defence against an OT who argued that she had been exposed to violent patients as a result of her work. The employers have a duty of care to ensure that reasonable care is taken to prevent reasonably foreseeable risks from dangerous patients (see Chapter 11) and it cannot be argued successfully that an OT working in mental health accepts a risk of being injured by patients as an occupational hazard. This can be contrasted with a case involving injury to a rugby player who was held to have willingly accepted the risk of playing on the field, which complied with the regulations relating to sports fields and sports activities.[58]

Calculation of compensation, i.e. quantum (how much?)

In some cases of negligence, liability might be accepted by the defendant, but there might be disagreement between the parties over the amount of compensation. In other cases, there might be agreement over the amount of compensation but liability alone may be in dispute. In others, both liability and quantum might be in dispute.

Social security payments received have to be paid out of the compensation awarded. The court in its calculation of compensation takes into account the fact that the award is being made at once and therefore the claimant is benefiting from the ability to obtain interest on the lump sum. Calculations are made as to what interest can be expected.

In one case the House of Lords ruled that in awarding compensation, victims should not be expected to speculate on the stock market and therefore lower levels of return based on index-linked government securities can be used as the basis of calculation.[59] The effect of this ruling is to increase the capital amount awarded to victims. In the case itself, James Thomas, a cerebral palsy victim as a result of negligence at birth, was awarded £1285 000 by the High Court judge, but this was reduced by the Court of Appeal by £300 000 on the basis that the capital could be invested in the higher returns (but more risky) equities. The House of Lords restored the original amount.

The Court of Appeal held in January 2008 that where compensation was being awarded in the case of catastrophic injury, then in calculating the future cost of the wages of carers, the court should use the annual earnings survey published for care assistants and home carers rather than the retail price index.[60]

The Court of Appeal held that a girl who had suffered severe disabilities as a result of the failure of the defendants to ensure her mother received a rubella vaccination was entitled to opt for receiving the full cost of care and accommodation and was not bound to be dependent on the state. Since her affairs were dealt with by the Court of Protection there was no danger of double recovery of the compensation.[61]

Occupational therapists may be involved as witnesses of fact or expert witnesses (see Chapter 13) in giving assessments of compensation in personal injuries case. For example in one case[62] the Court of Appeal was not prepared to reject the trial judge's acceptance of the assessment by an occupational therapist of future care costs.

Occupational therapists may also be claimants in their own right. In one case where the compensation awarded was disputed the claimant was a senior occupational therapist in the defendant's hospital in Brighton and she sustained an accident when attempting to open a window. Liability was not in dispute the appeal was over what damages should have been awarded in relation to her loss of prospects of earnings as a piano teacher which was always something which was a sideline in her possible future development. She was awarded £10,000 in relation to the loss of prospects as a piano teacher and challenged this figure, but lost on the grounds that the Court of Appeal were not prepared to disturb the findings of the trial judge.[63]

Compensation following death

Where a claim is brought under the Fatal Accidents Acts in respect of a death caused by negligence, the statutory payment for bereavement for deaths after 1 January 2008 is £11,800.[64] Dependants of the deceased can sue for the income and support which the deceased provided and which they have lost as a consequence of the death.

Under the Law Reform Miscellaneous Provisions Act 1934 the estate of the dead person is able to continue certain legal actions as though the person were still alive. The personal representative acts on behalf of the estate and can continue actions which have already commenced or begin those which the deceased was entitled to bring but died before being able to do so. This includes the right to sue those responsible for bringing about the death of the deceased.

Situations involving OTs

Failures in communication

Crucial to the reasonable standard of care of the patient is the communication between different departments within the trust and with the patient. Communication between health and social services professionals is essential in ensuring that the client receives the appropriate standard of care. This is particularly important where one person is designated as the key worker on behalf of the multi-disciplinary team. However, the Court of Appeal[65] has stated that the courts do not recognise a concept of team liability and it is therefore for each individual professional to ensure that her practice is according to the approved standard of care. Nor should a professional take instructions from another professional which she knows would be contrary to the standard of care which her profession would require.

Communications with the patient

Policies are necessary to ensure that 'bad news' is communicated in an appropriate way.

Case: Notifying persons that they had been treated by an HIV positive health worker[66]

It was alleged by 114 of the patients who had been notified that the two defendant health authorities were negligent in choosing to inform patients by letter as opposed to face-to-face and that the facilities offered by the letter were not properly provided. The High Court judge found in favour of the claimants on the grounds that the health authorities did not exercise due care in that they should have realised that the best method of communicating the news was face-to-face and that there was a foreseeable risk that some vulnerable individuals might suffer psychiatric injury going beyond shock and distress. The health authorities appealed and the Court of Appeal found for the defendants. The Exeter model should not have been adopted by the judge without consideration of the different circumstances in this case. There was a duty on the defendants to take such steps as were reasonable to inform the patients, having regard to the possibility of psychiatric injury. However, there was no evidence of negligence in fulfilling this duty.

Subsequently policy has changed and the Department of Health has updated its guidance on the management of infected healthcare workers and patient notification.[67] It states that it is no longer necessary to notify every patient who has undergone an exposure prone procedure by an HIV infected heath care worker because of the low risk of transmission and the anxiety caused to patients and the wider public.

An OT may fail to ensure that a carer knows how to use a hoist. In the event of harm arising to the client, as a result of the carer's ignorance, the OT could be held at fault and her employer vicariously liable. Where certain information is regularly given to patients and clients, there are considerable advantages in ensuring that the information is communicated in writing as well as by word of mouth.

Interprofessional communication

Communication between health and social services professionals is essential in ensuring that the client receives the appropriate standard of care. This is particularly important where one person is designated as the key worker on behalf of the multi-disciplinary team (see below). However the Court of Appeal[68] has stated that the courts do not recognise a concept of team liability and it is therefore for each individual professional to ensure that her practice is according to the approved standard of care (See below under scope of professional practice). Nor should a professional take instructions from another professional which she knows would be contrary to the standard of care which her profession would require. The occupational therapist is entitled to refuse to act contrary to her professional judgment and this would include refusing to take instructions from the patient where these are inappropriate as the case of *R (on the application of Burke) v GMC*[69] shows (see Chapter 6).

Negligent advice

There can be liability for negligence in giving advice but the claimant would have to show that it was clear to the defendant that the claimant would rely on the advice and in so doing had suffered reasonably foreseeable loss or harm.[70]

References

If a reference is written negligently then liability can arise both to the recipient of the reference, if in reliance upon that reference she has suffered harm, and also to the person who is the subject of the reference.[71] Every care should be taken to ensure that it is written accurately in the light of the facts available.

Liability for student or unregistered assistant: supervision and delegation

Because of the shortage of registered staff and also as part of strategic planning by the DH, more and more activities are being delegated to healthcare assistants who are at present unregistered. In addition, many OTs will be required to supervise students as part of their professional activities. Exactly the same principles apply to the delegation and supervision of tasks as to the carrying out of professional activities. The professional delegating a task should only do so if she is reasonably sure that the person to whom the task is delegated is reasonably competent and experienced to undertake that activity safely for the care of the patient. At the same time, she must ensure that the person undertaking that activity has the level of supervision which is sufficient to ensure that the delegated activity can be carried out reasonably safely. Should harm befall a client because an activity was carried out by a junior member of staff, a student or an assistant, it is no defence to the client to argue that the harm occurred because that person did not have the ability, competence or experience to carry out that task reasonably safely.[72]

It is essential that delegation is on a personal basis and takes into account the individual assistant's personal knowledge, experience, skill and training. The College of Occupational Therapists set standards for practice for the role and responsibilities of the work of support workers[73] in 2000 and subsequently in conjunction with the Chartered Society of Physiotherapy prepared a National Framework for support worker education and development.[74] This covers the political context and support workers both in the NHS and in social care, education and development learning opportunities. The professional standards of the COT cover the scope of the duty, accountability, supervision and education and training. Reference would clearly be made to these standards if it were alleged that an OT failed to follow reasonable standards of practice in delegating and supervising particular activities. If the activity were appropriately delegated and supervised but the assistant is at fault and causes harm, the registered OT should not be held personally to blame, but the assistant could be disciplined and held to account, the employer being held vicariously liable in respect of any compensation due. In the case of a student, a memorandum of agreement with the training institute should establish which organisation (provider of the clinical placement or teaching institution) should be held liable for the harm caused by the student – see Chapter 26).

Generic support workers

Increasingly support workers are likely to be shared between different health professionals so that one support worker may provide input of OT activities, physiotherapy activities and speech therapist activities for a single patient. This is acceptable provided that the support worker has the competence to carry out those particular activities, and works within the limits of her competence. It is also essential that those delegating the activities are clearly identified and the chain of accountability clearly spelt out.

Situation: mixed delegation

Mohammad is a healthcare worker who has had training to carry out both physiotherapy and occupational therapy in the care of older people. He is asked to provide OT interventions for an older man who has been discharged following a stroke and also carry out some basic physiotherapy exercises with the patient. Unfortunately he fails to carry out the correct physiotherapy exercises and causes harm to the patient. An investigation is carried out following a complaint from the patient, and it is found that the healthcare worker did not have the appropriate supervision from a registered physiotherapist.

In a situation such as this it is essential that there is supervision of the healthcare assistant or support worker from all registered professionals who have delegated activities to him or her. A registered therapist should perhaps be identified as the lead therapist to ensure that other registered professionals are involved in the supervision of such staff. Supervision, accountability and delegation of activities to support workers – a guide was published jointly by the CSP, RCN, Royal College of Speech and Language Therapists and the British Dietitic Association in 2006 for registered practitioner and support workers.[75] Plans to introduce registration for support workers are considered in Chapter 3.

Significant input of non-registered or more junior staff

There is a danger that the real contribution which can be made to the care planning and multidisciplinary decision making by persons such as assistants, technicians and support workers may not be recognised or may be treated dismissively. Many support workers may develop a close rapport with clients and it is essential that any relevant information which they possess should be made known to the team and listened to. In Chapter 4 of the Report of the Inquiry about the homicides by Jason Mitchell[76] there is a discussion of the assessments made of Jason by professional staff in disciplines other than psychiatry and nursing. The report points out that:

> They contained observations and insights into Jason Mitchell's thoughts and feelings which were rarely recorded in the medical and nursing notes and which could present a different perspective on his case. They tended to be recorded in detail, but were marginalised.

Attention is drawn in the Report to the contribution of a technical instructor in the occupational therapy department at West Park Hospital whose report on Jason Mitchell is given in full as an addendum to the chapter. The Inquiry noted that her report was not included in the Mental Health Review Tribunal papers. In general her report tended to be ignored or discounted by the doctors central to the care and treatment of Jason Mitchell. In the Inquiry's view:

> the material in her report ought to have prompted at least an assessment, if not a further therapeutic involvement, with a qualified and experienced clinician, possibly a psychologist.

The Inquiry concluded that:

> Jason Mitchell's case illustrates how contributions from an unqualified member of staff were disregarded, and consequently how important data were put out of sight and mind. Nothing relevant to the assessment and treatment of a patient should be ignored, whatever its origins.

Scope of professional practice

The White Paper[77] on the NHS and the subsequent NHS Plan[78] envisaged changes in the scope of professional practice so that the traditional boundaries between different registered professionals were removed. This policy presented challenges as well as dangers for the registered OT. The following are some of the basic legal principles which apply to the scope of professional practice.

No team liability

The Court of Appeal has held that the courts do not recognise the existence of team liability.[79] Each individual practitioner is personally and professionally accountable for his or her own actions and cannot blame the team or team instructions for negligence which has led to harm.

No defence of inexperience

The Court of Appeal has also held that the patient is entitled to the reasonable standard of care whoever provides the treatment. A junior practitioner will be expected to provide the reasonable standard of care which a more senior person would provide. It is no defence to a claimant to argue that a young inexperienced person carried out a particular activity and that is why it was performed negligently.[80] In practice of course the junior member of staff, even though a registered practitioner, should receive supervision from more senior practitioners who should ensure that she has some support for responsibilities which require more experience than she has obtained. It follows from what has been said that where a practitioner takes on responsibilities which would normally be undertaken by another professional, the same standard of care would be expected of that practitioner as would have been provided by the other. Thus it would be no defence to argue that an OT carrying out an expanded role normally carried out by a doctor could follow a lower standard of care than would have been provided by a doctor who in the past normally performed that activity. Each individual practitioner is personally and professionally accountable for her or his actions.

Determination of competence

One of the most difficult areas for the individual practitioner in expanding her role is to know whether she is competent. In the past, competency in an individual task was evidenced by a certificate following a training course. Now, however, the tendency is to move away from such task-based professional development and certificates are not relied on. Other forms of competence determination are required. This could include assessment by competent colleagues or external assessors.

Refusal to undertake activities outside scope of competence

It follows from what has been written above that no OT should undertake activities which are outside the scope of her professional practice. She should ensure that she has the training, supervised practice, experience and knowledge necessary to undertake the new activity safely. She should have the assertion skills to refuse to perform those activities she is not competent to perform. Where she is incapable of undertaking expanded role activities it would be reasonable to refuse to obey the employer's instructions to perform them.

The COT published a briefing note no 14 on extended scope practice in 2006 which was revised in 2009.[81] It defined extended scope as:

working outside or beyond the recognised elements of occupational therapy practice, using skills and techniques that are:

- Not included in the defined core skills of an OT
- Not included in the qualifying professional education curriculum.

The briefing note sets out the factors which an OT should consider before taking on an extended scope activity. These include checking that it is legal to take on the task, role or responsibility; ensuring the employer recognises and supports the inclusion of the task, role, responsibility formally; ensuring they have adequate knowledge skills and experience to render them competent and confident to fulfil the task; ensuring that the employer has appropriate insurance cover and ensuring that an increase in responsibility, specialist skills etc. is recognised and suitably rewarded by the employer. The person carrying out the extended scope activity will require supervision and support. Examples of activities are given in the briefing note: Prescription, administration and supply of medicines, requesting and interpreting X-rays; complementary therapies.

Briefing note no 21 considers the role of the Consultant OT (May 2004 revised in 2007) which is structured around 4 core functions: expert clinical practice; professional leadership; practice and service development research and evaluation and education and professional development. It considers these roles within the context of OT and presents answers to frequently asked questions about the new role. Briefing note no 23 which was revised in 2006 defines the core skills of the Occupational therapist. For prescribing and the OT see Chapter 15.

Volunteers

Considerable encouragement[82] is given to the use of volunteers within both health and social services and assistance provided by voluntary organisations and charities. However, by definition a volunteer is not an employee and therefore the principle of vicarious liability does not apply to the organisation which is using a volunteer who causes harm to other people. There are considerable benefits to both the general public and the volunteer if the organisation using their services accepts indirect responsibility for any harm caused. Those working for voluntary organisations should check to ensure that the organisation is covered in respect of liability for any harm caused by the volunteer and also for any harm caused to the volunteer. Guidance on the use of volunteers was given in 1999.[83] In 2004 a Promotion of Volunteering Bill was introduced into Parliament which would, if enacted, enable a statement of inherent risk to be given to the volunteer.

Care of property

Failure to look after another person's property could lead to criminal prosecution, e.g. theft, civil action for trespass to the person, or negligence in causing harm to property. In an action for negligence, the person who has suffered the loss or damage of property must establish the same four elements as must be shown in a claim for compensation for personal injury, i.e. duty, breach, causation and harm.

Where, however, property is left in the care of a person (the bailee) then, should the property be lost or damaged, the burden would be on the bailee to establish how that occurred without fault on his or her part. It should be noted that liability for loss or damage to property can be excluded if such an exclusion is reasonable (see the Unfair Contract Terms Act above).

The Court of Appeal has held that a sample of sperm from a person undergoing chemotherapy, which a hospital stored in case he became infertile after treatment, was that person's property and its loss or damage was capable of establishing a claim in negligence.[84] The court held that there was a bailment of the sperm to the trust capable of rendering it liable under the law of bailment.

Proof of the facts and documentation

Factual evidence over what actually occurred may often be the main point in a legal dispute. Absence of documentation or low standards in record keeping may lead to cases being lost. In every area of professional practice, it is essential to ensure that comprehensive clear records are kept in the interests of patient care and also for the defence of the practitioner in the event of any dispute or complaint. Reference should be made to Chapter 12 on record keeping.

Often the exact circumstances of a case are unknown to the claimant, who may be able to obtain some information through the disclosure of records and other information during the stages leading up to a hearing. Sometimes a claimant might be assisted by the application of a legal doctrine known as *res ipsa loquitur*. This literally means the thing speaks for itself. It applies where the claimant is able to show that:

- what has occurred would not usually occur if reasonable care were taken
- the circumstances were entirely under the control of the defendants
- the defendants have not offered any explanation of what occurred.

If these elements can be shown by the claimant, then he has made out a prima facie case that there is evidence of negligence by the defendants. The burden of proof, however, remains with the claimant to satisfy on a balance of probabilities.[85]

An obvious example of where the doctrine might apply would be the amputation of the wrong limb, or leaving a swab in the patient after an operation, or using the incorrect dye in a diagnostic test.

Litigation in the NHS

Clinical Negligence Scheme for Trusts (CNST)

The Clinical Negligence Scheme for Trusts (CNST)[86] was established by the NHS Executive in 1994, to provide a means for trusts to fund the cost of clinical negligence litigation and to encourage and support effective management of claims and risk. The scheme covers claims arising from incidents on or after 1 April 1995. The NHS Litigation Authority (NHSLA), a Special Health Authority, administers the scheme (see below). Membership is voluntary and open to all NHS trusts in England. Each trust can choose its own level of self-retention, and the scheme will contribute to the cost of claims in excess of this figure. Funding is on a 'pay as you go' non-profit basis. Actuaries appointed by the NHSLA analyse the available data and predict the total amount expected to be paid to the member trusts in respect of damages, costs and other expenses which will be incurred in the ensuing financial year. This amount is then apportioned between the member trusts. Individual trust contributions are based on a range of criteria, such as activities, budget, numbers of doctors by discipline, nurses and other professionals. These contributions can be reduced if a trust meets certain risk management criteria (the CNST Risk Management Standards).

Standards of CNST

The assessment is based on nine core standards. In addition, there are separate standards for maternity care, mental health and ambulance services, which are applicable only to trusts which provide such services. There are three levels of criteria: level one criteria represent the basic elements of a clinical risk management framework; levels two and three are more demanding. Many are concerned with the implementation and integration into practice of policies and procedures, monitoring them and acting on the results. The NHS Litigation Authority (NHSLA) has set risk management standards for acute trusts, which were revised in 2008.[87] These replace the general clinical risk management standards prepared by the Clinical Negligence Scheme for Trusts (CNST).

Advice on the standards and general aspects of risk management is given in *NHSLA Review*, and at workshops and seminars.

NHS litigation authority (NHSLA)

A litigation authority was set up for the NHS.[88] The NHSLA exercises functions in connection with the establishment and the administration of the scheme for meeting liabilities of health service bodies to third parties for loss, damage or injury arising out of the exercise of their functions. Membership and claims issues of the CNST are dealt with by the NHSLA.

Guidance on NHS indemnity for clinical negligence claims has been issued by the NHS Executive.[89]

The Law Commission recommended changes to the present system relating to the quantifying of damages for personal injury[90] in 1996 and suggested, among other recommendations, that the NHS should be able to recover the costs arising from the treatment of road traffic and other accident victims. It was estimated that this could bring in £120 million to the NHS. Further radical measures are being considered to make a significant reduction in the present costs of the NHS.

Litigation in local authorities

Each local authority handles its own litigation using its own legal department or contracting with outside solicitors. The local authority is required by law to take out public indemnity insurance cover and the insurers can be effective in monitoring standards.

No-fault liability

The Royal Commission[91] which reported in 1978 recommended that the UK should on the whole retain its present system of liability by establishing fault, except in some specific circumstances (e.g. vaccine damage, volunteers in medical research). Weaknesses in the pre-April 1999 system of obtaining compensation for personal injury have led to suggestions that a system of no-fault liability should be introduced and it was part of the consultation process under the Chief Medical Officer of Health (see below). However, the consultation document *Making Amends*[92] (see below) did not recommend that the NHS Redress Scheme should set up a system of no-fault liability. There were, however, elements of no-fault liability in the scheme for compensation for brain damaged babies and in settling smaller claims. In a scheme for no-fault liability, following an arrangement (usually) between insurance companies, employers and the state, a compensation fund is set up from which payment is made to the person who was injured. Countries such as Sweden, Finland and New Zealand have adopted no-fault liability systems. In such schemes, it is not necessary to prove that the defendant (or his employees) has been at fault, but that something which had not been anticipated has occurred which has caused harm to an individual. The Pearson Report which considered reforms in 1978 did not recommend no-fault liability in the case of medical negligence.

Mediation or alternative dispute resolution

The Department of Health consultation report *Making Amends* also recommended that mediation should be seriously considered before litigation for the majority of claims which do not fall within the proposed NHS Redress Scheme. The introduction of an alternative form of dispute resolution such as mediation or arbitration would have the advantage of a cheaper, speedier resolution and there is much to recommend any system which ensures that any money paid out is to the benefit of the person who has suffered the harm, rather than to the benefit of the lawyers. The Woolf Reforms have recommended that mediation should become an essential part of the litigation process.

NHS redress scheme

The costs of compensation resulting from clinical negligence in the NHS have been constantly growing. The Department of Health announced in July 2001[93] that it was setting up a committee under the chairmanship of the Chief Medical Officer of Health to consider a new scheme for compensation for clinical negligence. A consultation paper was published in July 2001. This was followed, on 30 June 2003, by a further consultation document 'Making Amends'.[94] 'Making Amends' provided a comprehensive account of the background to the present situation. It looked at the present system of medical negligence litigation and its costs. It analysed public attitudes and concerns and the earlier reviews of the negligence system by the Pearson Commission,[95] the Woolf Report on Access to Justice[96] and the National Audit Office Report in 2001.[97] It considered recent action taken to reform civil court procedures, claims handling by the NHS Litigation Authority and the use of alternative dispute resolution. It analysed systems of no-fault liability in Denmark, Finland, France, New Zealand, Norway and Sweden and discussed no-fault liability as an option along with continued reform of the present tort process, a tariff-based national tribunal or a composite option drawing on all three. The scheme eventually recommended in 'Making Amends'[98] was a composite package of reform drawing on the best elements of the three options. It included suggestions for the care and compensation for severely neurologically impaired babies; for the NHS redress scheme to be part of the system for handling complaints; for the retention of right to pursue litigation through the courts and changes to existing scheme for civil proceedings; and for a duty of candour to be placed on healthcare professionals and managers to inform patients where they become aware of a possible negligent action or omission.

NHS Redress Act 2006

The NHS Redress Act which was eventually agreed was a very much less radical scheme than that proposed in the consultation paper *Making Amends*. It gives power to the Secretary of State to establish a scheme for the purpose of enabling redress to be provided without recourse to civil proceedings. Regulations are to be drawn up giving the details. The scheme can cover services provided by the Secretary of State, a Primary Care Trust or a designated Strategic Health Authority or an organisation or person providing services under an arrangement with these bodies. Excluded from the redress scheme are primary dental services, primary medical services, general ophthalmic services and pharmaceutical services. A scheme does not apply in relation to a liability that is or has been the subject of civil proceedings (S.2(2)). Ordinarily the scheme will provide for the following redress:

1. an offer of compensation in satisfaction of any right to bring civil proceedings
2. giving an explanation

3. giving an apology
4. giving a report on the action which has been or will be taken to prevent similar cases arising.

The scheme may make provision for compensation to take the form of entry into a contract to provide care or treatment or of financial compensation or both. It can also detail the circumstances in which different forms of compensation may be offered. The scheme can set the upper limit on the amount of financial compensation to be offered and if it does not do so, it must specify an upper limit on the amount of financial compensation that may be included in such an offer in respect of pain and suffering. The scheme may not specify any other limit on what may be included in such an offer by way of financial compensation. The scheme can detail the following provisions relating to the commencement of proceedings:

1. who may commence proceedings
2. how proceedings are commenced
3. time limits for commencing
4. circumstances precluding proceedings being commenced
5. proceedings being commenced in specified circumstances
6. notification of the commencement of proceedings in specified circumstances

The scheme may also make provision for proceedings under the scheme including details of the investigation of cases, decisions about the application of the scheme, the time limits within which an offer can be accepted, certain settlements in specified cases to be subject to approval by the court and the termination of proceedings under the scheme.

The scheme must make provision for the findings of an investigation of a case to be recorded in a report and make provision for a copy of the report to be provided on request to the individual seeking redress. However no copy of an investigation report need be provided before an offer is made under the scheme or proceedings are terminated or in other specified circumstances. A settlement agreement must include a waiver of the right to bring civil proceedings in respect of the liability to which the settlement relates and the scheme must also provide for the termination of proceedings under the scheme if the liability to which the proceedings related becomes the subject of civil proceedings. The scheme must also provide for the suspension of the limitation period under the Limitation Act 1980.

The provision of legal advice (from a specified list of persons) without charge to individuals seeking redress may be specified under the scheme. The scheme may also include the provision of other services including the services of medical experts who must be instructed jointly by the scheme authority and the individual seeking redress. The Secretary of State also has a duty to arrange, to such extent as he considers necessary to meet all reasonable requirements, for the provision of assistance (by way of representation or otherwise) to those seeking redress. (S.9(1)). Payments may be made to any person under these arrangements, who should be independent of any person to whose conduct the case related or who is involved in dealing with the case. The Secretary of State can make provision about the membership of the scheme and the functions of members. Section 10 sets out the members responsibilities, including the duty to publish an annual report. The Secretary of State may also make provision for the scheme authority i.e. the special health authority to have specified functions. The scheme must include provision requiring the scheme authority and the members of the scheme, in carrying out their functions under the scheme, to have regard in particular to the desirability of redress being provided without recourse to civil proceedings (S.12). Section 13 specifies a general duty of co-operation between the scheme authority and the Commission for Healthcare Audit and Inspection (now the CQC), and between the scheme authority and the National Patient Safety Agency. Regulations may determine provisions about complaints on the handling and consideration of complaints relating to the scheme (S.14) and the remit of the Health Service Commissioner is extended to include complaints about the exercise of functions under a scheme established under the NHS Redress Act 2006. This Act is not yet in force.

Conclusions

Litigation will always be a concern for the occupational therapist, even though the employed professional may not be personally sued. The employer may face proceedings as a result of the concept of vicarious liability. The effect of the NHS Redress Scheme in reducing litigation through the civil courts cannot yet be calculated. Identifying reasonable standards of care and monitoring their implementation must be a constant concern for the occupational therapist.

 Questions and exercises

1   Explain the difference between vicarious liability and personal liability.
2   Take any situation where harm nearly occurred to a patient, and work out what the patient would have had to prove to obtain compensation if he had suffered an injury.
3   How would you define the reasonable standard of care in relation to any chosen treatment or investigation provided by yourself?
4   Prepare a protocol to ensure safe delegation to and safe supervision of a healthcare assistant.
5   To what extent do you consider that a system of no-fault liability combined with mediation could replace the current system of liability for personal injury in health cases?
6   Examine the provisions of the NHS Redress Act 2006 and consider the extent to which it could impact upon your practice.

References

1   David Rose. £100 million payouts for cancer negligence. The Times 10 March 2008.
2   Ungoed-Thomas Jon. Lawyers use NHS as £100m cash cow. Sunday Times 22 March 2009.
3   Fresco Adam. Ambulancemen decided dying man not worth saving. The Times 31 December 2008.
4   *Donoghue and Stevenson* [1932] AC 562.
5   *Home Office v Dorset Yacht Co Ltd* [1970] 2 All ER 294, HL.
6   *Victoria v Commissioner of Police of the Metropolis* [2007] EWCA Civ 1361; The Times Law Report 4 January 2008 CA.
7   *Hill v Chief Constable of West Yorkshire Police* [1989] AC 53.
8   *Brooks v Commissioner of Police of the Metropolis* [2005] 1 WLR 1495; [2005] UKHL 24.
9   *Capital & Countries plc v Hampshire County Council* (CA) [1997] WLR 331.
10   *Hertfordshire Police v Van Colle and Smith v Chief Constable of Sussex Police* [2008] UKHL 50.
11   *X and Y v London Borough of Hounslow* [2008] EWHC 1168 (QB) 23 June 2008.
12   *X and Y v London Borough of Hounslow* [2009] EWCA Civ 286.
13   *Mitchell and another v Glasgow City Council* The Times Law Report 26 February 2009 HL.
14   *R (G) v Southwark London Borough Council* The Times Law Report 4 June 2009.
15   *Pierce v Doncaster LA* [2008] EWCA Civ 1416.
16   *Bolam v Friern Hospital Management Committee* [1957] 1 WLR 582.
17   *Whitehouse v Jordan* [1981] 1 All ER 267.
18   *Maynard v W Midlands Regional Health Authority* [1985] 1 All ER 635, HL.
19   *Bolitho v City and Hackney Health Authority* [1997] 3 WLR 1151.
20   *Marriott v West Midlands Health Authority* [1999] Lloyds Reports Medical, p. 23.

21   White Paper *The New NHS – Modern Dependable* (1997) Department of Health. HMSO, London.
22   Department of Health (2001) *The Manual of Cancer Service Standards*. DH, London.
23   College of Occupational Therapists (2004) Practice guidelines development manual. COT, London.
24   College of Occupational Therapists (2009) Translating the NICE and NSF guidance into practice. COT, London.
25   *Michael Hyde & Associates Ltd v J.D. Williams & Co Ltd* Times Law Report, 4 August 2000.
26   College of Occupational Therapists (2007) NICE COT stakeholder involvement Briefing note no 38. COT, London.
27   Hurwitz, B. (1998) *Clinical Guidelines and the Law*. Radcliffe Medical Press, Oxford.
28   *Penney, Palmer & Cannon v East Kent Health Authority* [2000] Lloyds Reports Medical, p. 41, CA.
29   Sealey, C. (2000) *Guide Producing Clinical Guidelines for Occupational Therapy Practice*. COT, London.
30   Sealey, C. (1998) Clinical Audit Information Pack. COT, London; Mountain & Lepley (1998) *Finding and Using the Evidence Base*. COT, London.
31   College of Occupational Therapists (2000) *Information Guide Production of College Documents*. COT, London.
32   College of Occupational Therapists (2003 updated 2005) *Briefings Integrated Care Pathways*. COT/BAOT.
33   College of Occupational Therapists (2007) Professional Standards for Occupational Therapy Practice: Standard statements. COT, London.
34   *Orchard v Lee* The Times Law Report 14 April 2009 .
35   *Barnett v Chelsea HMC* [1968] 1 All ER 1068.
36   *Wilsher v Essex Health Authority* [1986] 3 All ER 801.
37   *Loveday v Renton* The Times 31 March 1988; [1990] 1 Med LR 117.
38   *Best v Welcome Foundation, Dr O'Keefe, the Southern Health Board, the Minister for Health of Ireland and the Attorney General* [1994] 5 Med LR 81 and discussed in Medico Legal Journal vol. 61, part 3, 1993, p. 178.
39   *Jolley v Sutton London Borough Council* Times Law Report, 23 June 1998, CA.
40   *Hotson v E Berks HA* [1987] AC 750.
41   *Alcock v Chief Constable of South Yorkshire* (HL) [1992] 1 AC 310.
42   *North Glamorgan NHS Trust v Walters*, Lloyd's Rep Med 2 [2003] 49 CA.
43   *Giullietta Galli-Atkinson v Sudhaker Seghal*, Lloyd's Rep Med 6 [2003] 285.
44   *Gray v Thames Trains Ltd and another* The Times Law Report 9 July 2008 CA; [2008] EWCA Civ 713.
45   *Gray v Thames Trains Ltd and another* The Times Law Report 10 June 2009 HL; [2009] UKHL 33.
46   College of Occupational Therapy (2007) Professional indemnity insurance for BAOT members Briefing note no 66. COT, London.
47   *Lister and others v Hesley Hall Ltd* Times Law Reports, 10 May 2001, HL.
48   *Gravil v Carroll and Another* Times Law Report 22 July 2008.
49   R. Guy's and St Thomas's NHS Trust The Times Law Report 10 October 2008.
50   *Reeves v Commissioner of Police for the Metropolis* [1999] ll ER (D) 793.
51   *Spencer v Secretary of State for Work and Pensions; Moore v Secretary of State for Transport and Another* The Times Law Report 24 July 2008.
52   *Bull v Wakeham* Transcript 2 February 1989.
53   Jeremy Laurance, Man handicapped as a baby 33 years ago wins £1.25 m. *The Times*, 15 November 1995, p. 5.
54   Section 14, Limitation Act 1980.
55   *A v Hoare; X and Another v Wandsworth LBC; C.v. Middlesbrough Council; H v Suffolk CC; Young v Catholic Care (Diocese of Leeds) and Another* The Times Law Report 31 January 2008.
56   *Stubbings v Webb* 1993 AC 498.
57   *AB and others v Ministry of Defence* The Times Law Report 10 June 2009.
58   *Simms v Leigh Rugby Football Club Ltd* [1969] 2 All ER 923.
59   *Wells v Wells* [1998] AC 345.
60   *Thompstone v Tameside and Glossop Acute Services NHS Trust (and other cases)* The Times Law Report 30 January 2008 CA.
61   *Peters v East Midlands Strategic Health Authority and Another* The Times Law Report 16 March 2009.
62   *Monteith v Aqua Gas Manufacturing Ltd* [1998] EWCA Civ 402.

63   *Chamberlain v South Downs Health NHS* [2001] EWCA Civ 881.
64   Damages for bereavement (Variation of Sum) (England and Wales) SI 2007/3489.
65   *Wilsher v Essex Area Health Authority* [1986] 3 All ER 801, CA.
66   *AB and others v Tameside & Glossop HA* [1997] 8 Med LR 91.
67   Department of Health, AIDS/HIV Infected Health Care Workers: guidance on the management of infected health care workers and patient notification, DH, London, 1999 updated July 2005.
68   *Wilsher v Essex Area Health Authority* (CA) [1986] 3 All ER 801.
69   *R (On the application of Burke) v General Medical Council and Disability Rights Commission and Official Solicitor to the Supreme Court* [2004] EWHC 1879; [2004] Lloyd's Rep. Med 451; [2005] EWCA Civ 1003, 28 July 2005.
70   *Hedley Byrne & Co Ltd v Heller & Partners Ltd* [1963] 2 All ER 575, HL.
71   *Spring v Guardian Assurance PLC and others* Times Law Report, 8 July 1994.
72   *Wilsher v Essex Area Health Authority* [1986] 3 All ER 801, CA.
73   College of Occupational Therapists (2000) Standards for Practice: The Role and Responsibilities of support workers in the delivery of occupational therapy services. COT, London.
74   Chartered Society of Physiotherapy and College of Occupational Therapists (2005) A National Framework for Support Worker Education and Development. CSP and COT, London.
75   RCN, CSP, and others Supervision, accountability and delegation of activities to support workers – a guide for registered practitioner and support workers 2006.
76   Blom-Cooper et al. (1996) *The Case of Jason Mitchell: Report of the Independent Panel of Inquiry.* Duckworth, London.
77   DoH (1997) *The New NHS – modern – dependable.* Stationery Office, London.
78   DoH (2000) *The NHS Plan.* Stationery Office, London.
79   *Wilsher v Essex Area Health Authority* [1986] 3 All ER 801.
80   *Nettleship v Weston* [1971] 2 QB 691.
81   College of Occupational Therapists (2009) Extended Scope Practice Briefing note no.14. COT, London.
82   HSC 1999/023; LAC(99)(6) Promoting Volunteering and Relations with the Voluntary Sector in the NHS and Social care.
83   HSC 1999/023; LAC(99)(6) Promoting Volunteering and Relations with the Voluntary Sector in the NHS and Social care.
84   *Yearworth and others v North Bristol NHS Trust* The Times Law Report 10 February 2009 CA.
85   *Ratcliffe v Plymouth & Torbay Health Authority, Exeter and Devon HA* [1998] Lloyd's Rep Medi 162, CA.
86   A disc setting out standards information is available from the CNST: helpline 0845 300 12230.
87   www.nhsla.co/RiskManagement/
88   National Health Service Litigation Authority (Establishment and Constitution) Order 1995 SI No. 2800.
89   HSG(96)48 NHS Indemnity: Arrangements for Clinical Negligence Claims in the NHS.
90   Law Commission (1996) Damages for Personal Injury: medical, nursing and other expenses. Stationery Office, London.
91   Pearson Report (1978) Royal Commission on Civil Liability and Compensation for Personal Injury. HMSO, London.
92   Department of Health, Making Amends: a consultation paper setting out proposals for reforming the approach to clinical negligence in the NHS, CMO, June 2003.
93   Department of Health press release 2001/0313, New clinical compensation scheme for the NHS, 20 July 2001.
94   Department of Health, Making Amends: a consultation paper setting out proposals for reforming the approach to clinical negligence in the NHS, CMO, June 2003.
95   Pearson Report, Royal Commission on Civil Liability and Compensation for Personal Injury, HMSO, London, 1978.
96   Lord Woolf, Final Report: Access to Justice, HMSO, London, July 1996.
97   National Audit Office, Handling Clinical Negligence Claims in England, Report of the Comptroller and Auditor General, HC 403 Session 2000–2001, 3 May 2001.
98   Department of Health, Making Amends: a consultation paper setting out proposals for reforming the approach to clinical negligence in the NHS, CMO, June 2003.

11 Health and Safety

The occupational therapist (OT) works in a potentially dangerous environment, whether in a domestic setting or in hospital therapy centres and workshops. This chapter covers the basic principles of law relating to health and safety at work, both statutory provisions and common law duties, taking examples from occupational therapy practice. The following topics are covered:

- The Health and Safety at Work etc. (HASAW) 1974
- Regulations under HASAW
- The Management of Health and Safety at Work Regulations 1999
- Risk Management and the OT
- Manual Handling Regulations
- Reporting of Injuries, Diseases and Dangerous Occurrences Regulations 1995
- National Patient Safety Agency
- The Occupiers' Liability Act 1957
- The Occupiers' Liability Act 1984

- Control of Substances Hazardous to Health Regulations (COSHH) 1988
- The Employers' Liability (Defective Equipment) Act 1969
- Employers' Liability (Compulsory Insurance) Act 1969
- Common law duty implied in the contract of employment
- Special areas: cross-infection, animals, violence, stress and bullying, sexual harassment
- Staff health

Laws relating to medical devices and the Consumer Protection Act 1987 are considered in Chapter 15 on equipment and those relating to transport in Chapter 16.

Legal Aspects of Occupational Therapy, Third Edition By Bridgit Dimond
© 2010 Bridgit Dimond

The Health and Safety at Work etc. Act 1974 (HASAW)

The Health and Safety at Work etc. Act 1974 (HASAW) is enforced through the criminal courts by the Health and Safety Executive (HSE) and its Inspectorate, which has the power to prosecute for offences under the Act and the Regulations, and which also has powers of inspection and can issue enforcement or prohibition notices. Since the abolition of the Crown's immunity in relation to the health and safety laws (by the National Health Service (Amendment) Act 1986) prosecutions and notices can be brought against health authorities. Trusts do not enjoy any immunity from prosecution under health and safety legislation. Social services departments can also be prosecuted.

The basic duty on the employer is set out in Figure 11.1.

Section 2(2) of the 1974 Act gives examples of the various duties which must be carried out, but these do not detract from the width and comprehensiveness of the general duty. The Act also places a specific responsibility upon the employee. This is shown in Figure 11.2. Under section 3 of HASAW the employer owes a wider duty to persons not in his employment. In the following case the Court of Appeal had to determine whether a particular risk was part of everyday life or an offence under section 3 of HASW.

Case: *R v Porter 2008*[1]

The headmaster of a private school was prosecuted under section 3 following an accident to a child of 3 years. The boy jumped down some steps in the playground. He fell and suffered a head injury. He was taken to hospital and subsequently died after contracting MRSA. In the crown court the headmaster was convicted of failing to ensure the health and safety of persons not in this employment contrary to section 3(1) of the Health and Safety at Work Act 1974. His appeal to the Court of Appeal succeeded. The Court of Appeal held that the risk which the prosecution had to prove was a real risk as opposed to a fanciful or hypothetical risk. The fact that risk was a part of everyday life went to the issue of whether the injured person was exposed to that risk by the conduct of the operation in question. The evidence suggested that there was no real risk

---

Figure 11.1   Duty under HASAW.

Section 2(1) It shall be the duty of every employer to ensure, so far as is reasonably practicable, the health, safety and welfare at work of all his employees.

Figure 11.2   Employee's statutory duty under section 7 of HASAW.

It shall be the duty of every employee while at work –

(a)   to take reasonable care for the health and safety of himself and of other persons who may be affected by his acts or omissions at work; and

(b)   as regards any duty or requirements imposed on his employer or any other person ...,
to co-operate with him so far as is necessary to enable that duty or requirement to be performed or complied with.

of the kind statutorily contemplated. Unless it could be said that the child was exposed to a real risk by the conduct of the school, no question as to the reasonably practicable measures taken to meet risk arose.

The House of Lords has held that in criminal prosecutions against an employer following an accident at work, it was sufficient for the prosecution to prove merely a risk of injury arising from a state of affairs at work, without identifying and proving specific breaches of duty by the employer. Once that was done, a prima facie case of breach was established. The onus then passed to the employer to make good the defence of reasonable practicability.[2]

It is also a criminal offence for an employee to interfere with health and safety measures. See Figure 11.3.

Regulations under HASAW

Regulations came into force on 1 January 1993 as a result of European Directives. These are shown in Figure 11.4.

The Management of Health and Safety at Work Regulations 1999

Of the regulations that came into force in 1993, the Management of Health and Safety at Work Regulations, which were updated in 1999, are the most far reaching and apply to all work environments and both employers and the self-employed. Figure 11.5 shows the areas covered by these Regulations.

Figure 11.3   HASAW – section 8.

No person shall intentionally or recklessly interfere with or misuse anything provided in the interests of health, safety or welfare in pursuance of any of the relevant statutory provisions.

Figure 11.4   Health and Safety Regulations.

- Management of Health and Safety at Work Regulations 1992 (SI No. 2051) (re-enacted 1999, SI 1999/3242)
- Provision and Use of Work Equipment Regulations (SI 1992/2932) (re-enacted 1998, SI 1998/2306)
- Manual Handling Operations Regulations 1992 (SI 1992/2793) (considered in detail below)
- Workplace (Health, Safety and Welfare) Regulations 1992 (SI No. 3004) (amended by SI 1999/2024)
- Personal Protective Equipment at Work Regulations 1992 (SI No. 2966) (amended in relation to ionising indications by the Ionising Radiations Regulations 1999, SI 1999/3232)
- Health and Safety (Display Screen Equipment) Regulations 1992 (SI No. 2792)

Figure 11.5   Regulations relating to the Management of Health and Safety at Work.

The regulations include the following areas:

- The general principles and purpose of risk assessment
- Principles of prevention to be applied
- Health and safety arrangements
- Health surveillance
- Procedures for serious and imminent danger and for danger areas
- Contacts with external services
- Information for employees
- Co-operation and co-ordination
- Capabilities and training
- Employees' duties
- Risk assessment, certificate and notification, in respect of new or expectant mothers
- Protection of young persons

The Approved Code of Practice (ACOP)

An Approved Code of Practice has been issued in conjunction with these regulations.[3] This is described in the foreword as giving advice that has a special legal status:

> The Code has special legal status. If you are prosecuted for breach of health and safety law, and it is proved that you did not follow the relevant provisions of the Code, you will need to show that you have complied with the law in some other way or a court will find you at fault.

In addition there is general guidance, that does not have this special status, on ways of complying with the law.

Risk assessment

Not all the provisions in the Management of Health and Safety at Work Regulations can be covered in detail in a book like this, but Regulation 3 on risk assessment will be looked at in detail.

The law

Figure 11.6 sets out the basic requirement as specified in Regulation 3(1). The duty also applies to the self-employed OT in independent practice under Regulation 3(2). Figure 11.7 sets out Regulation 3(2).

There is a duty under Regulation 3(3) to review the assessment when there is reason to suspect that it is no longer valid or if there has been a significant change in the matters to which it relates.

Under Regulation 3(4) an employer shall not employ a young person unless he has, in relation to risks to the health and safety of young persons, made or reviewed an assessment in accordance with paragraphs (1) and (5).

Figure 11.6   Regulation 3(1).

Every employer shall make a suitable and sufficient assessment of—

(a)   the risks to the health and safety of his employees to which they are exposed whilst they are at work; and
(b)   the risks to the health and safety of persons not in his employment arising out of or in connection with the conduct by him of his undertaking,

for the purpose of identifying the measures he needs to take to comply with the requirements and prohibitions imposed upon him by or under the relevant statutory provisions.

Figure 11.7   Regulation 3(2).

Every self-employed person shall make a suitable and sufficient assessment of —

(a)   the risks to his own health and safety to which he is exposed whilst he is at work; and
(b)   the risks to the health and safety of persons not in his employment arising out of or in connection with the conduct by him of his undertaking,

for the purposes of identifying the measures he needs to take to comply with the requirements and prohibitions imposed upon him by or under the relevant statutory provisions.

The guidance

The Approved Code of Practice emphasises that risk assessment must be a systematic general examination of all work activity, with a recording of significant findings.

Definition of risk

The definition of risk is the likelihood of potential harm from that hazard being realised. The extent of the risk will depend on:

- the likelihood of that harm occurring
- the potential severity of that harm, i.e. of any resultant injury or adverse health effect
- the population which might be affected by the hazard, i.e. the number of people who might be exposed.

Risk assessment

The aim of risk assessment is to help the employer or self-employed person to determine what measures should be taken to comply with duties under the relevant statutory obligations.

The keywords 'suitable and sufficient' are defined in the Approved Code as being a risk assessment that:

(a)   should identify the significant risks arising out of work ...
(b)   should enable the employer or the self-employed person to take reasonable steps to help themselves identify risks, by looking at appropriate information.
(c)   should be appropriate to the nature of the work and identify the period of time for which it is likely to remain valid.

Practical advice on how the risk assessment should be carried out is given in the Approved Code. Employers are required to identify hazards; identify who might be harmed and how; and evaluate the risk from the identified hazards.

It may be possible for several employers engaged in the same activity to share model risk assessments.

Recording

The record should represent an effective statement of hazards and risks, which then leads management to take the relevant action to protect health and safety. It should be in writing unless in computerised form and should be easily retrievable. It should include:

- a record of the preventive and protective measures in place to control the risk
- what further action, if any, needs to be taken to reduce the risk sufficiently
- proof that a suitable and sufficient assessment has been made.

Preventive and protective measures

Regulation 4 requires employers to introduce preventive and protective measures. Schedule 1 to the Regulations sets out the general principles of prevention as:

- avoiding risks
- evaluating risks which cannot be avoided
- combating risks at source
- adapting work to the individual
- adapting to technical progress
- replacing the dangerous by the non-dangerous or less dangerous
- developing a coherent overall prevention policy which covers technology, organisation of work, working conditions, social relationships and the influence of factors relating to the working environment
- giving collective protective measures priority over individual protective measures
- giving appropriate instructions to employees.

New or expectant mothers and young employees

The 1999 Regulations include new provisions on the health and safety of new and expectant mothers and young people. Specified factors must be taken into account in undertaking risk assessments and preventive measures in relation to their health and safety. The employer may be required to alter her working conditions or hours of work or offer her suitable alternative work or suspend her from work (when she would be entitled to full pay under the Employment Rights Act 1996.) Young people should not be employed for work which is beyond their physical or psychological capacity or in other specified circumstances (unless it is necessary for training, where he is supervised and any risk is reduced to the lowest level that is reasonably practicable.)

The Court of Appeal[4] held that the duty of the employer to provide a suitable and sufficient risk assessment under Regulation 3 of the Management of Health and Safety at Work Regulations 1999[5] and training for its employee under Regulation 9 of the Provisions and Use of Work Equipment Regulations 1998[6] imposed a higher standard that the common law duty which incorporated reasonable foreseeability. The claimant worked for London Underground first as a guard and then as a driver and developed tenosynovitis in her shoulder due to the strain from the prolonged use of the traction brake controller, known as the dead man's handle. The employer had a duty to provide adequate training which included a duty to investigate the risks inherent in its operations taking professional advice where necessary. The right approach to deciding whether the training was adequate for health and safety purposes was to examine whether the risk assessment was suitable and sufficient.

In a case on the Provisions and Use of Work Equipment Regulations 1998 Regulation 4 and 5, the court had to decide if the council was responsible for a ramp.

Case: *Smith (Jean) v Northamptonshire County Council*

The Court of Appeal[7] held that an employer was not liable for a slip on another's ramp. Mrs Smith was employed by the council as carer/driver and collected a client in a wheelchair from her home. When pushing the chair down the ramp, which had been installed by the NHS, she stepped on the edge and it gave way.

The trial judge had held that regulation 5 imposed strict liability on the council for maintaining the ramp as work equipment for use at work and found in favour of Mrs Smith. The Court of Appeal, however, allowed the Council's appeal and held that strict liability should only be imposed by clear language. For someone to have an obligation to maintain something it would normally have to be within his power to do so without obtaining someone else's consent. Strict liability should not flow out of a position in which there was no right and no responsibility to do that thing or insist on doing that thing for which strict liability was being imposed.

The claimant appealed to the House of Lords but lost her appeal.[8] The House of Lords, in a majority judgment, held that the test to be applied was whether the work equipment was incorporated into and adopted as part of the employer's undertaking. It could not be said that the ramp was either incorporated into or adopted as part of the council's undertaking or under their control. They did not provide it or own it or possess it. They did not have any responsibility or indeed any right without more to repair it.

The House of Lords[9] held that a door-closing device could be work equipment for the purposes of Regulation 2 of the Provision and Use of Work Equipment Regulations[10] so that a mechanic who was injured whilst repairing such a device could bring proceedings against his employer.

The Court of Appeal has held that earlier good industrial practice is no defence and whether a work place was in fact made and kept safe was to be judged objectively without reference to what might earlier had been thought to be good practice.[11] The claimants held that they had suffered hearing loss in a knitwear factory.

The Workplace (Health, Safety and Welfare) Regulations (SI 1992 No 3004) were breached by an employer when an accident occurred when a school caretaker pushing a trolley hit a protruded paving slab. The council was held liable in damages since it was in breach of the regulations. The council could not plead as a defence that it was a freak accident.[12]

Risk management and the OT

For the most part, the OT would share common health and safety hazards with other hospital, community or social services-based employees and so models of risk assessment and management which apply to occupational therapy would also apply to other health professionals. Thus hazards relating to the safety of equipment, cross-infection risks, safe working practices or to violence at work would all apply to OTs, who should be involved in the system of the assessment of risk. Each OT should therefore be able to carry out a risk assessment of health and safety hazards in relation to both colleagues, clients, carers and the general public. An information guide on risk management has been published by the College of Occupational Therapists (COT).[13] It covers the regulation context and risk assessment and management and what happens if risks become reality. It also provides useful details of information resources. Reference could also be made to the user guide on risk management provided by Channine Clarke,[14] which gives practical examples of the application of risk management to common examples of risk in occupational therapy.

Manual handling

Back injuries have been recognised as a major reason for sickness and staff retiring early on grounds of ill health. Whilst there are no reported cases of claims brought by OTs, they are vulnerable to the possibility of back injury because of the work which they undertake in the movement of clients and the lifting of equipment. It is essential, therefore, that they should have a good understanding of the regulations relating to manual handling and the duties of the employer and of themselves. Sue Hignett considered manual handling risk assessments in occupational therapy,[15] looking at the risk assessments which arise across three areas: treatment handling, interagency communication and non-hospital property. She concluded that there will always be an element of unpredictability for manual handling activities involving human beings, but suggested a process of reducing risks by using a qualitative research study within an ergonomic framework.

The Manual Handling Regulations and guidelines

Figure 11.8 sets out the content of the Regulations.

Figure 11.8   The Manual Handling Regulations 1992.

(4)   Duties of employers
    (1)   (a)   Avoidance of manual handling
        (b)   (i)   Assessment of risk
            (ii)   Reducing the risk of injury
            (iii)   The load – additional information
    (2)   Reviewing the assessment
(5)   Duty of employees
(6)   Exemption certificates

Schedule 1: Factors to which the employer must have regard and questions he must consider when making an assessment of manual handling operations.

The list shown in Figure 11.8 constitutes the Regulations which have been enacted under HASAW. In addition, guidance is offered by the Health and Safety Executive.[16] The guidelines are not themselves law and the booklet advises that they 'should not be regarded as precise recommendations. They should be applied with caution. Where doubt remains a more detailed assessment should be made.' A working group set up by the Health and Safety Commission has produced a booklet *Guidance on Manual Handling of Loads in the Health Services*,[17] which is described as 'an authoritative document which will be used by health and safety inspectors in describing reliable and fully acceptable methods of achieving health and safety in the workplace.' Part of this health services specific guidance material relates to staff working in the community. Subsequently the HSE has provided a short guide for employers called Getting to grips with manual handling.[18] The guide includes a table on making an assessment which looks at the problems to be considered in making an assessment and the corresponding ways of reducing the risk of injury. It lists the factors to be taken into account in good handling technique for lifting and for pushing and pulling.

The COT has also provided guidance in 2006 on the Manual Handling Regulations.[19] This covers the law, risk assessment, safer handling policies, delegation and guidance to others, providing manual handling equipment and training. See also a two-part article on disability equipment and the law by Michael Mandelstam.[20] Backcare (formerly the National Back Pain Association) has published Safer Handling of People in the Community which considers the legal aspects, principles of safer handling, risk assessment, training and equipment amongst other issues[21] and also a guide to the handling of people edited by Jacqui Smith.[22]

Duties under the Regulations

The duty under the regulations can be summed up as:

- If possible avoid hazardous manual handling.
- Make a suitable and sufficient assessment of any hazardous manual handling which cannot be avoided.
- Reduce the risk of injury from this handling so far as is reasonably practicable.
- Give both general indications of risk and precise information on the weight of each load; and indicate the heaviest side of any load where the centre of gravity is not positioned centrally.
- Review the assessment.

Avoiding the risk

By Regulation 4(l)(a), each employer shall:

> so far as is reasonably practicable, avoid the need for his employees to undertake any manual handling operations at work which involve a risk of their being injured.

The guidance asks the question, as an example of this, 'whether a treatment can be brought to a patient rather than taking the patient to the treatment'. It may be that in the case of occupational therapy it would be very difficult to remove the risk of injury entirely without reducing patient choice to unacceptable levels.

Carrying out the assessment

By Regulation 4(l)(b) each employer shall:

Figure 11.9   Schedule 1 of the Manual Handling Regulations 1992.

Factors to which the employer must have regard and questions he must consider when making an assessment of manual handling operations.

Column 1	Column 2
Factors	*Questions*
1. The tasks	e.g. do they involve holding or manipulating loads at a distance from trunk, etc.
2. The loads	e.g. are they: heavy, bulky or unwieldy, etc.?
3. The working environment	e.g. are there space constraints preventing good posture; uneven, slippery or unstable floors, etc.?
4. Individual capability	Does the job require unusual strength, height, etc.?
5. Other factors	Is movement or posture hindered by personal protective equipment or by clothing?

where it is not reasonably practicable to avoid the need for his employees to undertake any manual handling operations at work which involve a risk of their being injured ... make a suitable and sufficient assessment of all such manual handling operations to be undertaken by them, having regard to the factors which are specified in column 1 of Schedule 1 to these Regulations and considering the questions which are specified in the corresponding entry in column 2 of that Schedule.

Schedule 1 is set out in Figure 11.9.

Appendix 2 of the Regulations gives an example of an assessment checklist:

- Section A covering the preliminary stages
- Section B considering the more detailed assessment where necessary
- Section C identifying the remedial action which should be taken.

Amendments to the manual handling regulations[23] tighten up on the nature of the risk assessment:

In determining for the purposes of this regulation whether manual handling operations at work involve a risk of injury and in determining the appropriate steps to reduce that risk, regard shall be had in particular to:

(a)   the physical suitability of the employee to carry out the operations
(b)   the clothing, footwear or other personal effects he is wearing
(c)   his knowledge and training
(d)   the results of any relevant risk assessment carried out pursuant to Regulation 3 of the Management of Health and Safety at Work Regulations 1999
(e)   whether the employee is within a group of employees identified by that assessment as being especially at risk
(f)   the results of any health surveillance provided pursuant to Regulation 6 of the Management of Health and Safety Regulations 1999.

Taking appropriate steps to reduce risk

By Regulation 4(l)(b)(ii), where it is not practicable to avoid manual handling operations involving a risk of employees being injured, each employer shall take appropriate steps to reduce the risk of injury to those employees arising out of their undertaking any such manual handling operations to the lowest level reasonably practicable.

For example, in carrying out the assessment of risk and deciding how to minimise the risk, it could be decided, in the circumstances of that particular case, to install a hoist. This might include the possibility of installing a hoist for a domiciliary confinement, even though temporarily. The Court of Appeal has held that where a hospital employee was injured using a mechanical hoist to move a patient, the burden was on the employer to prove that it had taken appropriate steps to reduce any risk to the lowest reasonably practicable level.[24] The facts of the case are given below.

A nurse had been injured when a mechanical hoist that she had been using to transport a patient into a bath had stopped suddenly when the hoists wheels jambed. No risk assessment had been carried out by the trust and the trust was found to be in breach of regulation 4(l)(b)(ii) of the Manual Handling Operations Regulations 1992 (SI 2793) and the Work Equipment Regulations (1998 SI 2306). The nurse was found to be 50% contributorily negligent.

Giving general and specific information

By Regulation 4(l)(b)(iii), where it is not practicable to avoid the need to undertake manual handling:

Each employer shall … [t]ake appropriate steps to provide any of those employees who are undertaking any such manual handling operations … , where it is reasonably practicable to do so, [with] precise information on:

(aa)   the weight of each load, and
(bb)   the heaviest side of any load whose centre of gravity is not positioned centrally.

OTs are obviously at risk. Awkward equipment should be clearly marked and employers are under a duty to get information for their staff on how much patients weigh. It is necessary to ensure that information is accurate and regularly updated and that it is passed on to new staff.

Review

Regulation 4(2) requires the employer to review the assessment:

(a)   if there is reason to suspect that it is no longer valid; or
(b)   there has been a significant change in the manual handling operations to which it relates; and where as a result of any such review changes to an assessment are required, the relevant employer shall make them.

It is in the interests of all OTs to ensure that the employer is reminded when a review becomes necessary under the above provisions.

Lifting Operations and Lifting Equipment Regulations 1998 (LOLER 1998)

These regulations came into force for all lifting equipment on 5 December 1998, as a result of the lifting provisions of the Amending Directive to the Use of Work Equipment Directive (AUWED 95/63/EC). They are to be read in conjunction with the Provision and Use of Work Equipment Regulations 1998 (PUWER). They apply to all equipment including second-hand or leased equipment, old and new equipment. The duty holders have to comply with all the requirements from 5 December 1998 (HSC 1998). Some of the pertinent LOLER regulations for health professionals are discussed below.

The definitions make it clear that 'lifting equipment' means work equipment for lifting or lowering loads and includes its attachments used for anchoring, fixing or supporting it. 'Load' includes a person. Paragraph 29 of the guidance on LOLER gives examples of the types of equipment and operations covered by the regulations and includes (e) a bath hoist lifting a resident into a bath in a nursing home. Equipment used by many health professionals would therefore come within the regulations. Paragraph 47 of the guidance explains how the guidance applies to hoists:

> As hoists used to lift patients e.g. from beds and baths, in hospitals and residential homes are provided for use at work and are lifting equipment to which LOLER applies, the duty holder, e.g. the NHS Trust running the hospital or the owner of the residential home must satisfy their duties under LOLER.

In practice, of course, the NHS trust would delegate the day-to-day responsibilities under the Regulations to the head of each clinical department.

Duties under the Regulations

Regulation 4: every employer shall ensure that:

(a) lifting equipment is of adequate strength and stability for each load, having regard in particular to the stress induced at its mounting or fixing point;
(b) every part of a load and anything attached to it and used in lifting it is of adequate strength.

The Code of Practice in paragraph 117 states that where the lifting equipment is used on rails it should be fitted with suitable devices, for example to remove loose material from the rails to minimise the risks of the equipment being derailed.

Regulation 5 covering lifting equipment used for lifting persons is set out in Figure 11.10.

Figure 11.10   Regulation 5 of LOLER.

(1)   Every employer shall ensure that lifting equipment for lifting persons
    (a)   subject to subpara (b) is such as to prevent a person using it being crushed, trapped or struck or falling from the carrier.
    (b)   is such as to prevent, so far as is reasonably practicable, a person using it, while carrying out activities from the carrier, being crushed, trapped or struck or falling from the carrier;
    (c)   subject to paragraph (2) has suitable devices to prevent the risk of a carrier falling:
    (d)   is such that a person trapped in any carrier is not thereby exposed to danger and can be freed.
(2)   Every employer shall ensure that if the risk described in paragraph (c) cannot be prevented for reasons inherent in the site and height differences:
    (a)   the carrier has an enhanced safety coefficient suspension rope or chain; and
    (b)   the rope or chain is inspected by a competent person every working day.

Regulation 6:

(1) Every employer shall ensure that lifting equipment is positioned or installed in such a way as to reduce as low as is reasonably practicable the risk:
  (a) of the equipment or a load striking a person; or
  (b) from a load:
    (i)   drifting
    (ii)   falling freely; or
    (iii) being released unintentionally;
  and is otherwise safe.
(2) Every employer shall ensure that there are suitable devices to prevent a person from falling down a shaft or hoistway.'

Regulation 7 requires machinery and accessories for lifting loads to be clearly marked to indicate their safe working loads. Lifting equipment which is designed for lifting persons should be appropriately and clearly marked to this effect and lifting equipment which is not designed for lifting persons, but might in error be used for such a purpose, should be marked accordingly.

Regulation 8 concerns the organisation of lifting operations and is as follows:

(1) Every employer shall ensure that every lifting operation involving lifting equipment is
  (a) properly planned by a competent person;
  (b) appropriately supervised; and
  (c) carried out in a safe manner.
(2) In this regulation 'lifting operation' means an operation concerned with the lifting or lowering of a load.'

Regulation 9 requires the employer to carry out a thorough examination and inspection before the equipment is first used, unless it has not been used before, and there is an EC declaration of conformity with the Lifts Regulations. The regulations require further inspections to be carried out at specified times.

Regulation 10 provides for the person who makes the thorough inspection under Regulation 9 to notify the employer of any defect which in his opinion is or could become a danger to persons, sending a report to the enforcement agency if there is a risk of serious personal injury. Schedule 1 specifies the information which should be included in the report.

Regulation 11 requires the employer to keep copies of reports of inspections, and gives the time limits for which they should be held.

Temporary staff

The duty which is owed by the employer is owed not only to employees but also to temporary staff such as agency or bank staff who are called in to assist. All such employees are entitled to be included in the risk assessment process since, as has been seen, the assessment must take into account the individual characteristics of each employee. OTs who are unusually small in height or not as strong as the average might require special provisions in relation to manual handling.

OTs in independent practice

Independent OTs are not employees and as self-employed persons would be responsible for carrying out the assessments and taking the necessary precautions for themselves and any staff they employ. Where they work alongside employed OTs, they should ensure that the NHS trust takes into account hazards to their health and safety and that the agreement they have with the NHS trust reflects this duty (see Chapter 28).

Enforcement

What action can be taken if the employer ignores these regulations? The regulations are part of the health and safety provisions which form part of the criminal law. Infringement of the regulations can lead to prosecution by the Health and Safety Inspectorate. The Inspectorate has the power to issue enforcement or prohibition notices against any corporate body or individual. A health authority no longer enjoys the immunity from criminal sanctions that it once did as a crown authority and therefore these enforcement provisions are available against it. Similarly, an NHS trust is subject to the full force of the criminal law.

What remedies exist for compensation?

Breach of the regulations can be the basis of a civil claim for compensation unless the regulations provide to the contrary. Section 47 of HASAW, however, prevents breach of certain duties under the Act being used as the basis for a claim in the civil courts. Nevertheless, even where what is alleged is a breach of the basic duties, an OT who suffered harm as a result of the failure of the employer to take reasonable steps to safeguard her health and safety could sue in the civil courts on the basis of the employer's duty at common law (see later in this chapter).

The statutory duty to ensure the Act is implemented is paralleled by a duty at common law placed upon the employer to take reasonable steps to ensure the employee's health and safety. This duty is implied into all contracts of employment but it is preferable if the contract states clearly both the duty of the employer to take reasonable care of the employee's safety and also the employee's duty to co-operate with the employer in carrying out health and safety duties under the Act, the Regulations and at common law. It is, of course, in the long-term interests of the employer to prevent back injuries, thereby avoiding payment of substantial compensation to injured employees and also reducing the incidence of sickness and absenteeism.

Training

Training is essential to ensure that staff have the understanding required to carry out assessments and to advise on lifting and the appropriate equipment. Regular monitoring should take place to ensure that the training is effective and that policies for review are in place. There is also a duty on the employer to ensure that staff who are not expected to be regularly engaged in manual handling are aware of the risks involved.

Situation: how many to train?

A patient with complex needs requires specific manual handing support. The care agency has asked the occupational therapist to train each care staff in to how to handle this patient. This could require the OT to train 20 care staff over a few months period as the care staff change frequently. Is the OT legally required to train each individual carer or can cascaded training with effective documentation be legally adequate?

The legal responsibility upon the employer under the manual handling regulations is

so far as is reasonably practicable, avoid the need for his employees to undertake any manual handling operations at work which involve a risk of their being injured.

Where it is not possible to avoid such manual handling the employer must

> take appropriate steps to reduce the risk of injury to those employees arising out of their undertaking any such manual handling operations to the lowest level reasonably practicable.

This is the ultimate goal of the training. If the OT can be reasonably sure that by training significant care staff, others will be taught through them and thus the risks of injury will be reduced to the lowest level reasonably practicable, then cascading training would be a reasonable option. However if this is not a reasonable option, then all care staff must be individually taught. The obligation to arrange training is on the employer: in this scenario the care agency. It may be that other disciplines, such as physiotherapists, could be involved to lower the burden on the OT services.

Cases

There have been many cases involving claims for compensation for injuries caused by manual handling and the Court of Appeal has had the opportunity to lay down the basic principles which apply. In an early case[25] a social worker succeeded in a claim against the County Council where the failure of her employers to give her training in risk awareness was held to be a breach of the employer's duty to take reasonable care of the health and safety of the employee. Her lack of awareness of the dangers of manual handling meant that she sustained a lumber spine injury when she attempted with a neighbour to lift an older man who was halfway out of bed.

The implications of this decision are that even staff who are not expected to be involved in manual handling as part of their work must be trained in risk awareness in order to protect them if their work could involve reasonably foreseeable risks of injury from manual handling.

Court of Appeal decisions on manual handling

In the case of *Koonjul v Thameslink Healthcare Services*,[26] a care assistant hurt her back when attempting to move a bed. She failed in a claim based on alleged breach of Regulation 4 of the 1992 Regulations and her appeal to the Court of Appeal was dismissed. Lady Hale emphasised that there had to be an element of realism in making assessments under the Regulations.

The claimant failed in another decision of the Court of Appeal[27] which held that the employers were not in breach of the Directive or Regulations on manual handling. The facts of the case are given here.

Case: *King v Sussex Ambulance NHS Trust*

> King, an ambulance technician, suffered serious injuries carrying an older patient down the stairway of his home. He and his colleague had taken the patient down the stairway, which was narrow and steep, in a carry chair. He had been injured when forced for a brief moment to bear the full weight of the chair. He sued for compensation.

The judge found in favour of the ambulance technician, holding that the employers were in breach of Council Directive 90/269, Article 3(2) and the Manual Handling Regulations, and that the employers had acted negligently by discouraging employees in circumstances such as those in this particular case from calling the fire brigade to take patients from their homes. Sussex Ambulance NHS Trust appealed against the finding.

The Court of Appeal held that the NHS trust was not liable either under the Directive or under the Manual Handling Regulations. There was nothing to suggest that calling the fire brigade would have been appropriate in the case. The evidence showed that such an option was rarely used because it had to be carefully planned, took a long time and caused distress to the patient. There might be cases where calling the fire brigade would be appropriate, but that would depend on the seriousness of the problem, the urgency of the case and the actual or likely response of the patient or his/her carers and the fire brigade.

King had failed to show that more emphasis in training would have avoided his injuries. The ambulance service owed the same duty of care to its employees as did any other employer. However, the question of what was reasonable for it to do might have to be judged in the light of its duties to the public and the resources available to it when performing those duties. While the risks to King had not been negligible, the task that he had been carrying out was of considerable social utility.

Furthermore, Sussex Ambulance NHS Trust had limited resources so far as equipment was concerned. There was no evidence of any steps that the trust could have taken to prevent the risk and the only suggestion made was that it should have called on a third party to perform the task for it. Since calling the fire brigade was not appropriate or reasonably practicable for the purpose of the directive and the regulations, the Sussex Ambulance NHS Trust had not shown a lack of reasonable care. Accordingly, it had not acted negligently.

The King case was referred to in another manual handling case where there was a dispute between carers and East Sussex social services over the use of a hoist.[28] The facts of the East Sussex case are given.

Case: *East Sussex human rights and manual handling* (2003)

In February 2003 the High Court gave judgment on a case, where the claimants raised the issue of their human rights not to be hoisted. A and B were sisters born in 1976 and 1980 who suffered from profound physical and learning disabilities. They lived in the family home which had been specially adapted and equipped for them and were looked after on a full-time basis by their mother X and their stepfather Y. A dispute arose between the claimants and East Sussex County Council (ESCC), which provided community care services over the extent to which moving and lifting should be done manually. ESCC's policy on manual handling did not permit care staff to lift A or B manually. The claimants, supported by the Disability Rights Commission, argued that ESCC's manual handling policies, as applied to A and B, were unlawful and unjustifiable, on the basis that they improperly failed to take into account the needs of the disabled people involved. Its policy was subsequently amended to make it clear that ESCC did not operate a blanket no lifting policy. The claimants argued that the application of the policy to the specific circumstances of A and B's care and the draft protocols prepared by the independent handling adviser were unlawful.

The judge considered the effect of sections 2 and 3 of the Health and Safety at Work Act 1974, the Manual Handling Operations Regulations 1992 and the Management of Health and Safety at Work Regulations 1999; decided cases on manual handling and the implications of the European Convention for Human Rights and the Charter of Fundamental Rights of the European Union. He emphasised that one must guard against jumping too readily to the conclusion that manual handling is necessarily more dignified than the use of equipment. Hoisting is not inherently undignified, let alone inherently inhuman or degrading. He identified the principles that applied and stated that, ultimately, the employer must balance the impact of the assessment on both carer and the disabled person.

This balancing exercise is to be resolved in the context of Article 8 of the European Convention on Human Rights (see Appendix 1) by enquiring of each claimant whether the interference with his right to be respected is such as to be 'necessary in a democratic society'. Once the balance has been struck, if it comes down in favour of manual handling, then the employer must make the appropriate assessment and take all appropriate steps to minimise the risks that exist. The assessment must be properly documented and lead to clear protocols which cover all situations, including foreseeable emergencies and, in the case of patients such as A and B, events such as episodes of spasm and distress that might arise. The judge accepted that protocols developed by the employer cannot be too prescriptive. He emphasised that it was for ESCC to formulate its manual handling policy and to make the appropriate assessment in relation to A and B. Neither of those is a matter for the court. The making and drafting of the kind of assessments called for in a case such as this was outside the competence and expertise of the court. What the court could and should do was to assist ESCC by identifying the relevant legal principles.

The outcome of the case was that ESCC was required to complete with the assistance of the independent manual handling adviser the appropriate assessments and protocols. If these were not acceptable to the claimants, they could challenge them by way of judicial review.

Two other cases where the injured employees were successful in obtaining compensation are considered below.

Case: *Wiles v Bedfordshire CC*[29]

The County Court held that there was a breach of the Manual Handling Operations Regulations 1992 (Reg 4.1a) when W, a residential social worker, sustained an injury when taking a disabled girl, M, to the lavatory. W lifted the girl out of her wheelchair, propping her against the wall while she bent down to remove her underclothes, but the girl, whose upper limbs were prone to occasional involuntary spasms, threw out her hands and fell backwards on to W, who suffered a back injury.

W claimed that two persons should have carried out that activity. Following the incident, staff were instructed to use a hoist and two staff when taking M to the lavatory. The judge held that even though, at the precise time, W was not actually carrying out a manual handling operation, the whole task of taking M to the lavatory should be considered a manual handling operation. The employers were in breach of the regulations by failing to avoid the need for manual handling and for failing to carry out a proper assessment or taking steps to reduce the risk of injury.

Case: *O'Neil v DSG Retail Ltd*[30]

The Court of Appeal found in favour of an employee who had injured his back while carrying a microwave weighing between 15 and 20 kg. The Court of Appeal found that:

- The employers had failed to assess the specific risk in relation to the particular task to be performed by the employee and were therefore in breach of the Manual Handling Regulations (Reg. 4(1)(b)(ii)).
- The employers had failed to take appropriate steps to reduce the risk, by failing to give the training recognised as being necessary to increase awareness of the risk and reduce instinctive responses.
- It was reasonably foreseeable that an employee would twist while supporting a load.
- Failure to provide the appropriate training was therefore, on the balance of probabilities, a cause of the accident.

Jane Benten and Diane Ellis evaluated the practice of prescribing hoists in pre-discharge planning and concluded that as a result of devising a new proforma in an access home assessment a more uniform approach by OTs in discharge planning was achieved.[31]

Occupational therapists may be involved in manual handling litigation as a witness of fact or as an expert witness. For example see the following case.[32]

Case: *Mutuma v London Borough of Barnet*

An assistant day care worker with handicapped young people, Mr Mutuma, claimed compensation for back injuries sustained in the course of toileting a heavy patient using a specially designed hoist to lift him from his wheelchair. He claimed that the strain was caused by his fellow care worker, who suddenly let go of the patient's feet while Mr Mutuma was lifting the patient under his arms. This joint movement, according to Mr. Mutuma's case, was a necessary part of the lifting operation, designed to free the patient from the wheelchair and make the start of the hoist lift possible. The health authority denied liability on the basis that no manual handling was required and they also disputed whether there had been such an incident since it had not been reported. Crucial to the evidence was a document known as an MED4 which had been completed by an occupational therapist for this patient which contained specific instructions about the lifting and moving of the patient. Mr Mutuma said that he was following this MED4 when the accident occurred. Unfortunately this document had been mislaid. The occupational therapist who was responsible for laying down the manual handling procedures stated that she had a diary entry for August 23rd 1994: "Write up instructions re Stuart". She noted that this probably related to the patient in question, Stuart Edwards, but after all these years she could not be certain. The Court of Appeal allowed an adjournment so that inquiries could be made as to the whereabouts of the MED4.

Instructing others in lifting

OTs may be asked to instruct others such as carers, clients or other health or social services employees in the operations involving manual handling and compliance with the regulations. Before they instruct others they should be sure that they receive the necessary additional training to undertake the task of instruction, since failure to instruct competently could in itself give rise to an action in negligence if harm should occur as a result of negligent instructions.

Instructions not to instruct staff

Sometimes OTs are given instructions not to tell others how to lift, for example agency staff. It would be wise in this situation if the OTs pointed it out to management or the agency if the staff are not being trained and therefore the client, carer or other person is in danger.

Lifting extremely heavy persons

This is of considerable concern to occupational therapists. The National Institute for Health and Clinical Excellence defined morbid obesity as having a body mass index of more than 40 kg/m squared or between 35 and 40 k/m squared with comorbidities.[33] A review of methods of dealing with obese patients is provided by Graham Clews.[34] An article on support for bariatric employees includes the case study of a nurse who weighed 27 stone but was assessed as medically fit for practice by the occupational health consultant.[35] The legal issues arising are significant. Staff cannot cease to provide services for such persons, but the consequences in terms of costs and effort in minimising the risk of harm are considerable.

Publications by the BackCare (formerly the National Back Pain Association) including Safer Handling of People in the Community[36] are helpful in providing further guidance on manual handling. In the following case the court ordered arrangements to be made for a client to be moved from a wheelchair.

Case: *Wolstenholme*[37]

Lorraine Wolstenholme, a disabled woman of 50 in Milton Keynes, had slept in a wheelchair for 17 months after nurses stopped lifting her in case they were injured. A High Court judge ordered that arrangements for moving her should be made by 19 December 2003.

Reporting of Injuries, Diseases and Dangerous Occurrences Regulations 1995

The Regulations that were introduced in 1985 governing the reporting of injuries, diseases and dangerous occurrences have been replaced by new regulations which came into force on 1 April 1996. There is now one set of regulations (SI 1995/3163) in place of the four sets under the 1985 regulations. The list of reportable diseases has been updated, as has the list of dangerous occurrences. It will be legally possible for reports to be made by telephone. A pilot scheme was tested out in Scotland.[38] A new accident book (known as B1510) has been designed by the Department of Work and Pensions to take account of the Data Protection Act 1998 and the Human Rights Act 1998. Guidance on RIDDOR is provided by the Health and Safety Executive (HSE) and available from its website.[39]

Additional protection has been given by the Trade Union Reform and Employment Rights Act 1993, against dismissal or victimisation of employees (often known as whistleblowers) who report health and safety hazards and the Public Interest Disclosure Act 1998 is considered in Chapter 19 concerning employment law.

National Patient Safety Agency (NPSA)

Following the publication of *An Organisation with a Memory*,[40] the Department of Health published *Building a Safer NHS for Patients*[41] which set out details of a scheme for national reporting of adverse incidents, together with recommendations for an improved system for handling investigations and inquiries across the NHS. Subsequently the National Patient Safety Agency was set up with the aim that there would be a mandatory reporting system for logging all failures, mistakes, errors and near misses across the health services.[42] The National Patient Safety Agency published its first annual report in 2002 and indicated the ways in which it was establishing the service. Pilot schemes were set up. In February 2004 a National Reporting and Learning System was established by the NPSA using existing local risk management systems. Root analysis training was also being offered to NHS staff to pinpoint and tackle the root cause of patient. In its annual report for 2006/7 NPSA stated in the year ending in March 2007 1,406,416 patient safety incidents had been reported. It had initiated a project to evaluate and identify ways to improve reporting and learning. Following a successful pilot since May 2006 all reporting organisations had been able to access their incident data and compare their profile with similar NHS organisations. The first patient safety alert of the NPSA was issued on 23 July 2002 and was about preventing accidental overdose with intravenous potassium.[43] The alert notice refers to the possible risks from treatment with concentrated potassium and the need for additional safety precautions in the way potassium solutions are stored and prepared in hospital. Details of all the NPSA's alerts are available on its website.[44] An alert issued in March 2007 was concerned with safe practice with epidural injections and infusions.[45] The remit of the NPSA was extended in 2005 to include safety aspects of hospital design, cleanliness, and food. It was also given the task of ensuring research is carried out safely through its responsibility for the National Research

Ethics Service (NRES) (formerly the Central Office for Research Ethics Committees (COREC)). It is also responsible for the National Clinical Assessment Service (NCAS) which is concerned with the performance of individual doctors and dentists and has taken over from NICE (see chapters 10 and 17) responsibility for the three confidential enquiries: into maternal death and child health; patient outcome and death and Suicide and Homicide by persons with mental illness. In July 2007 the NPSA published a study which investigated the circumstances in a sample of deaths of patients admitted with acute illnesses. It stated that in 2005 1,804 serious incidents were reported as resulting in death and of these 576 were avoidable. It set out a series of recommendations including improvements in communication, training and the provision of appropriate equipment. The NPSA report came at the same time as new guidelines issued by NICE on how health professionals should manage sudden declines in patients' health. NICE and NPSA are collaborating on the production of technical patient safety solutions and have produced guidance on medicines reconciliation on admission of adults to hospital and ventilator-associated pneumonia in adults.

NPSA has introduced a twice yearly report on safety lapses known as the Organisation Patient Safety Incident Reports for each hospital in England and Wales. The NPSA published the first reports on 6 March 2009 on its website[46] which showed that there were 439,612 incidents reported by health trusts in England and Wales between April and September 2008. Of these 3,872 caused severe harm to patients and 1,915 incidents were linked to deaths. At present it cannot be assumed that an increase in the number of incidents indicates a worsening situation, since reporting levels may have been improved.[47]

The NPSA is also actively encouraging a Patient Safety First Campaign in England. Chief Executives of trusts and individuals can sign up to pledge their support by email.[48]

Implications for OT

The aim of ensuring that the NHS does not repeat the same errors is ambitious and difficult for one NHS trust to achieve, let alone the whole NHS. However, there are advantages in ensuring that within each occupational therapy department and throughout the OT services of the NHS, lessons are learnt from adverse events which occur. This requires an openness and honesty among staff to admit that mistakes have occurred, and the consultation paper *Making Amends*[49] suggested that in a new NHS Redress Scheme for giving compensation to patients following clinical negligence, if adverse events are reported, there should be an exemption from disciplinary or proceedings or disciplinary action by employers or professional regulatory bodies for those reporting adverse events, except where the healthcare professional has committed a criminal offence or it would not be safe for the professional to continue to treat patients. The NHS Redress Act is considered in Chapter 10. The final version of the Act did not include provisions relating to the reporting of adverse events.

NICE and NHS Employers Guidance

As part of its remit the National Institute for Health and Clinical Excellence has had the responsibility of producing public health guidance since 2005. It is producing guidance for employers to create a healthier workplace for the well-being of its staff. The Chief Executive of NICE explained this guidance in an article for the British Journal of Healthcare Management.[50] He stated that the guidance recommends that employers:

- Develop a plan to encourage employees to be physically active
- Encourage employees to walk or cycle etc. to travel part or all of the way to and from work
- Help employees to be physically active during the working day, for example by providing information about walking or cycling routes or putting up signs to encourage them to use the stairs.

NICE issued guidance for employers on how to support staff who want to stop smoking before the ban in July 2007.[51]

NHS Employers has also published guidance on a healthy workplace agenda[52] following the review by Carol Black on Working for a healthier tomorrow in March 2008 and the Government response Improving health and work; changing lives in November 2008. See Diana Kloss for the law relating to occupational health.[53]

The Occupiers' Liability Act 1957

This Act is enforceable in the civil courts where harm has occurred to a visitor, and places a duty of care upon the occupier (of whom there may be several) to take reasonable care of visitors. This duty of care is what is reasonable in the circumstances to ensure that the visitor will be safe for the purposes for which he is permitted to be on the premises.

Occupier

The occupier would be the person in control of the premises. This would normally be the NHS trust in respect of hospital property, and the ward sister would be acting as the agent of the occupier in respect of safety on her ward. There can, however, be several occupiers. For example, if painters employed by independent contractors come onto the premises they may also be in occupation of the premises and could be responsible for harm which occurs as a result of their lack of care.

Visitor

A visitor is a person on the premises with the express or implied consent of the occupier. In the context of hospitals the term would therefore include patients, staff, visitors, tradesmen and anyone else with a bona fide reason to be there who is not excluded by the occupier (see below).

The nature of the duty owed

The duty is set out in section 2(2) of the Act, and section 2(3) clarifies the duty further in relation to specific circumstances, as shown in Figure 11.11.

The OT and premises in the community

Where an OT is visiting private homes, the occupier may be the owner of the house who is also in occupation, or the occupier may be a tenant. If the OT is injured on the premises it will depend how the injury occurred as to who would be liable: thus if she is injured as the result of a frayed rug, the

Figure 11.11   Occupiers' Liability Act 1957 sections 2(1)–(4).

2(1)   An occupier of premises owes the same duty, the 'common duty of care', to all
          his visitors, except in so far as he is free to and does extend, restrict, modify or
          exclude his duty to any visitor or visitors by agreement or otherwise.

2(2)   The common duty of care is a duty to take such care, as in all the circumstances of
          the case is reasonable, to see that the visitor will be reasonably safe in using the
          premises for the purposes for which he is invited or permitted by the occupier to
          be there.

2(3)   The circumstances relevant for the present purpose include the degree of care, and
          of want of care, which would ordinarily be looked for in such a visitor, so that (for
          example) in proper cases: an occupier must be prepared for children to be less
          careful than adults.

2(4)(a)   In determining whether the occupier of premises has discharged the common duty
          of care to a visitor, regard is to be had to all these circumstances, so that (for
          example): where damage is caused to a visitor by a danger of which he had
          been warned by the occupier, the warning is not to be treated without more as
          absolving the occupier from liability, unless in all the circumstances it was enough
          to enable the visitor to be reasonably safe.

2(4)(b)   When damage is caused to a visitor due to the faulty execution of any work of
          construction, maintenance or repair by an independent contractor employed by
          the occupier, the occupier is not to be treated without more as answerable for the
          damage, if in all the circumstances he had acted reasonably in entrusting the work
          to an independent contractor and had taken such steps (if any) as he reasonably
          ought in order to satisfy himself that the contractor was competent and that the
          work had been properly done.

person in occupation whether tenant or owner would be liable; if she were injured as a result of a
structural defect then the owner or landlord would be liable depending on the nature of the tenancy
agreement.

The occupier has the right to ask any visitor to leave the premises. Should the visitor fail to leave,
she then becomes a trespasser and the occupier can use reasonable force to evict her. If, therefore,
an OT is asked by a client or carer to leave she should go. Should she be concerned for the well-being
of the client, she should ensure that social services are notified so that appropriate action can be
taken under the National Assistance Act 1948 or the Mental Health Act 1983. The College of
Occupational Therapists has updated its guidance on health and safety for home visits (September
2007). It covers the legal duties of employers, risk assessments, health and safety training and information and common hazards. It also provides a very useful home visiting check list for managers.

The Occupiers' Liability Act 1984

The 1957 Act does not cover the situation relating to trespassers. Until the 1984 Act was passed the
law relating to the nature of the duty owed to a trespasser was according to the common law (i.e.
the decisions of judges).

Under the 1984 Act, whether or not a duty is owed by the occupier to trespassers in relation to
risks on the premises depends on the factors set out in section 1(3) and shown in Figure 11.12.

Figure 11.12 Occupier's Liability Act 1984 sections 1(3) and (4).

1(3)(a) If the occupier is aware of the danger or has reasonable grounds to believe that it exists
   (b) If the occupier knows or has reasonable grounds to believe that the other is in the vicinity of the danger concerned or that he may come into the vicinity of the danger (in either case, whether the other has lawful authority for being in that vicinity or not)
   (c) The risk is one against which, in all the circumstances of the case, he may reasonably be expected to offer the other some protection.
1(4) The duty is to take such care as is reasonable in all the circumstances of the case to see that he (the trespasser) does not suffer injury on the premises by reason of the danger concerned.

In applying these factors to decide if a duty is owed to a trespasser, it would be rare for a duty to be owed to a mentally competent adult. It is, however, more likely that a duty will be owed to a child trespasser. Thus, for example, if a child on hospital premises is expressly told that he cannot go through a particular door or into another section of the hospital and he disobeys those instructions, then he becomes a trespasser for the purposes of the Occupiers' Liability Acts. Although not protected under the 1957 Act, it is likely that a duty to the child would then arise under the 1984 Act depending on the child's age and understanding.

The nature of the duty owed to trespassers

Once it is held that a duty of care is owed to a trespasser, the 1984 Act by section 1(4) defines the duty as: 'the duty … to take such care as is reasonable in all the circumstances of the case to see that he does not suffer injury on the premises by reason of the danger concerned.'

The duty can be discharged by giving warnings, but in the case of children this may have limited effect – it would depend on the age of the child.

Consumer Protection Act 1987

This enables a claim to be brought where harm has occurred as a result of a defect in a product. It is a form of strict liability in that negligence by the supplier or manufacturer does not have to be established. The claimant will, however, have to show that there was a defect. Further details are given in Chapter 15 on the law relating to equipment.

Control of Substances Hazardous to Health Regulations (COSHH) 2002

All health workers have responsibilities under the Regulations[54] relating to the control of substances hazardous to health. The OT who uses different substances in her work should be specifically alert to the need to ensure that the Regulations are implemented. New Regulations came into force in November 2002, replacing the 1999 Regulations. The HSE has set up a COSHH website to provide guidance for employers.[55]

Figure 11.13 Guidance on a COSHH assessment. Source: HSE (2003)[25]

(1) Work out what hazardous substances are used in your workplace and find out the risks to people's health from using these substances.
(2) Decide what precautions are needed before starting work with hazardous substances.
(3) Prevent people being exposed to hazardous substances, but where this is not reasonably practicable, control the exposure.
(4) Make sure control measures are used and maintained properly and that safety procedures are followed.
(5) If required, monitor exposure of employees to hazardous substances.
(6) Carry out health surveillance where your assessment has shown that this is necessary or where COSHH makes specific requirements.
(7) If required, prepare plans and procedures to deal with accidents, incidents and emergencies
(8) Make sure employees are properly informed, trained and supervised.

The eight steps to COSHH set out in the guide issued by the Health and Safety Executive[56] are shown in Figure 11.13.

There must be clarity over who has responsibility for carrying out the assessment, but the guide emphasises the importance of involving all employees in the task.

All potentially hazardous substances must be identified; these will include domestic materials such as bleach, toilet cleaner, window cleaner and polishes, and office materials such as correction fluids, as well as the medicinal products in the treatment room and the materials and substances used in occupational therapy. An assessment has to be made as to whether each substance could be inhaled, swallowed, absorbed or introduced through the skin, or injected into the body (as with needles). The effects of each route of entry or contact and the potential harm must then be identified. There must then be an identification of the persons who could be exposed and how. Once this assessment is complete, decisions must be made on the necessary measures to be taken to comply with the Regulations and who should undertake the different tasks. In certain cases, health surveillance is required if there is a reasonable likelihood that disease or ill-effect associated with exposure will occur in the workplace concerned.

OTs should be particularly vigilant about any substances used in their activities, such as paraffin or oils in art therapy and cleaning fluids, and ensure that a risk assessment is undertaken and its results implemented. Managers should ensure that employees are given information, instruction and training. Records should show what the results of the assessment are, what action has been taken and by whom, and regular monitoring and review of the situation. It was reported that a former trainee nurse, who had to give up her job after developing a potentially fatal allergy to latex, won a six-figure compensation payout. Tanya Dod who worked at Scarborough General Hospital was threatened with disciplinary action if she was caught using latex-free gloves.[57] The COSHH regulations have been relied upon in cases brought following MRSA infection (see below).

Corporate manslaughter and corporate homicide

As a consequence of the Corporate Manslaughter and Corporate Homicide Act 2007 it is possible for an organisation to which the Act applies to be prosecuted in the case of a death under both

Health and Safety Legislation and the 2007 Act. The jury can be instructed to find the accused organisation guilty of both offences. An organisation can be found guilty of an offence under the 2007 Act only if the way in which its activities are managed or organised by its senior management is a substantial element in the breach of duty of care owed by the organisation. Senior management means the persons who play significant roles in (i) the making of decisions about how the whole or a substantial part of its activities are to be managed or organised, or (ii) the actual managing or organising of the whole or a substantial part of those activities. The Act is further considered in Chapter 2.

Employers' Liability (Defective Equipment) Act 1969

Where:

- the employee suffers personal injury in the course of employment as a consequence of a defect in equipment, and
- the equipment is provided by the employer for the purposes of his business, and
- the defect is attributable wholly or partly to the fault of a third party,
- then the employee can recover compensation from the employer on the grounds that the injury is deemed to be also attributable to the employer.

The employer can raise any contributory negligence by the employee as a defence in the action and can recover a contribution or indemnity from the third party. The advantage of the Act is that it saves the employee from having to ascertain the identity of the third party and bring an action directly against them.

Employers' Liability (Compulsory Insurance) Act 1969

This requires all non-crown employers to be covered by an approved policy of insurance against liability for bodily injury or disease sustained by an employee and arising out of and in the course of employment. Despite the abolition of crown immunity, Schedule 8 of the NHS and Community Care Act 1990 preserves the immunity of health authorities and trusts from this Act, but local authorities are bound by it, as are independent hospitals and also independent practitioners who may be employers.

Common law duty implied in the contract of employment

Some of the terms in the contract of employment are implied by the law. These include the obligation of the employer to safeguard the health and safety of the employee by:

- employing competent staff
- setting up a safe system of work
- maintaining safe premises, equipment and plant.

The employee must obey the reasonable instructions of the employer and take reasonable care in carrying out the work. Thus, as has been seen in the discussion on manual handling above, the employee may have a claim for breach of contract by the employer if back injuries result from failure on the employer's part in not providing the appropriate training or equipment.

Failure by the employer to take reasonable care of the health, safety or welfare of the employee could result in the following actions by the employee:

- action for breach of contract of employment; and/or
- action for negligence, where the employee has suffered harm (the employee could also use as evidence any breach of specific health and safety regulations); and/or
- application to the employment tribunal claiming constructive dismissal (see Chapter 19) if it can be shown that the employer is in fundamental breach of the contract of employment.

Examples of cases brought in relation to the employer's duty of care at common law are the manual handling cases referred to earlier in this chapter and the stress cases discussed later in this chapter under 'stress and bullying'.

Special areas

Control of infection

A report by the National Audit Office (NAO) in 2000[58] raised major concerns about the level of hospital acquired infection (HAI). The Report suggested that HAI could be the main or a contributory cause in 20,000 or 4% of deaths a year in the UK and that there are at least about 100 000 cases of HAI with an estimated cost to the NHS of £1 billion. The NAO drew conclusions on the strategic management of HAI; surveillance and the extent and cost of HAI; and the effectiveness of prevention, detection and control measures. The Government has stated that the Commission for Health Improvement (subsequently the Commission for Health Audit and Inspection and now the Care Quality Commission, see Chapter 17) and the Audit Commission would conduct ward inspections and be given the right to seek information on HAI and to publish it.[59]

In the light of the acceleration of deaths resulting from failures to control cross-infection in the NHS, the DH published a strategy for tackling methicillin-resistant Staphylococcus aureus (MRSA) in November 2006. It was announced in June 2007 that the Healthcare Commission was to make unannounced spot checks on NHS trusts to cut rates of hospital-acquired infection.[60] The NHS trusts' performance would be measured against the DH hygiene code, which sets out 11 compulsory duties to prevent and cope with hospital superbugs. Sanctions for failure to comply with the Code could lead to a trust being placed under special measures. Further information on the DH strategy to reduce hospital acquired infections can be found on the DH website.[61]

The Healthcare Commission published in May 2008 the results of its annual survey on patient satisfaction and found that there was an increasing number of concerns about cleanliness. The new powers under the Corporate Manslaughter and Corporate Homicide Act may be used against NHS trusts which fail to control hospital acquired infections (see above and below and Chapter 2).

Homerton Hospital was issued with an improvement notice after a spot check by the Healthcare Commission which found dirty bedpans and commodes marked as ready for use. The Healthcare Commission said that the hospital had failed by July 2007 to implement changes to the hygiene procedures recommended.[62]

It was reported on 17 January 2007 that Leslie Ash an actress received a £5 million settlement after she caught MRSA at the Chelsea and Westminster Hospital. It caused her devastating disabilities and meant that she would never again be able to play active roles as an actress. The case was due to be heard at the High Court in April 2008 but the NHS Litigation Authority settled it out of court.

In May 2008 it was reported that Elizabeth Miller, a 71-year-old woman, had been given approval to bring a test case against the NHS for allegedly giving her MRSA. She contracted the superbug whilst recovering from a heart operation at the Glasgow Royal Infirmary. She is claiming £30,000 compensation from the Greater Glasgow NHS Trust because she can no longer play with her great-grandchildren because she is so ill. The defendants argued that she may have had MRSA before she was admitted. She is also arguing that there has been a breach of the COSHH regulations in her contracting the disease. In the case of *Kitty Cope v Bro Morgannwg NHS Trust* (2005) it was argued that there was a breach of COSHH regulations in an MRSA infection case which was settled out of court. In the case of *Ndri v Moorfields Eye Hospital* (2006) the judge ruled that COSHH did apply to MRSA infections.

In Winchester it was suggested that new rules on the use of intravenous fluids had cut the incidence of MRSA. The use of cannulae has to be authorised by a specialist and once in place tubes are flushed with a saline solution and inspected daily.[63]

A Risk and Regulatory Advisory Council is being set up to review regulations on health and safety. Its first project is to look at the Government initiatives in relation to MRSA to assess their effectiveness.[64] A DVD to combat the superbugs has been made available to all NHS Trusts in England and Wales by the NPSA[65]

Concerns also surround the increasing incidence of clostridium difficile. The Secretary of State, Alan Johnson, when appointed in 2007 was given £50 million to tackle MRSA and clostridium by doubling the size of the DH's infection improvement team who advise NHS trusts on developing plans to cut infections. In July 2007 the Healthcare Commission published a national study into healthcare-associated infection. In order to reduce the risk of infections the report recommended that trusts should develop a culture of safety, have a good system of corporate and clinical governance, review performance, manage risk and communicate with patients and the public. A report by the Healthcare Commission in October 2007 into Maidstone and Tunbridge Wells Trust revealed that up to 90 patients had died between 2004 and 2006 after being infected with clostridium difficile. The Minister of Health responded by announcing plans for a new super-regulator, the Care Quality Commission, to be established in April 2009, combining the Healthcare Commission, Mental Health Act Commission and the Commission for Social Care Inspection with powers to close NHS and private hospitals and residential care homes (see Chapter 17).

The day after the Care Quality Commission came into being on 1 April 2009 it issued a warning to 21 hospital trusts (including 4 foundation trusts) which had failed to meet standards on hygiene to meet strict conditions. Failure to comply could lead to warning notices, fines, prosecution and even closure. The chairwoman of CQC announced that the trusts' compliance would be monitored closely.[66]

Implications for Occupational Therapists

Like all NHS staff, occupational therapists have a significant role to play in maintaining high standards of cross-infection control and observing hospital policies on control of infection across the hospital and within their own departments. It is a duty placed on occupational therapists individually and upon their managers. Risk assessment and management of cross-infections should therefore be part of the basic philosophy of every department and ward, with a clearly identifiable person responsible for ensuring compliance. This would be required by statutory duties as well as the duties of the employer at common law and the occupier under the Occupiers' Liability Act (see earlier).

The possibility that compensation may be payable as a result of negligence leading to incidents of infection and the likelihood that the Corporate Manslaughter and Corporate Homicide Act could be used where deaths occur as a consequence of organisational failures to control infection should lead to higher standards being set and implemented. There could also be personal liability of an occupational therapist if she were to be negligent in allowing another person to be infected.

Criminal sanctions have been imposed on those spreading HIV. A man who infected his 2 lovers with HIV and exposed 13 others to the risk was jailed for 14 years. He was charged with exposing others to danger as well as having sex with under aged girls. A nurse died 8 years after contracting HIV when she accidentally jabbed her thumb when dealing with an HIV sufferer. She worked at the Maudsley Hospital. An inquest in February 2009 returned a verdict of accidental death.[67]

The COT/BAOT has provided a briefing for OTs on providing a safe service to people with infectious diseases.[68] This emphasises that the risk of infection can be minimised by:

- immunisation
- good hygiene practice
- safe sharps practice
- following infection control procedures.

Reference should also be made to the dangers of cross-infection from workers infected with hepatitis who are HIV positive or suffer from other infectious diseases. Advice from the NHS Executive on hepatitis B infected healthcare workers[69] adds to previous guidance[70] and recommends further testing of all hepatitis B infected healthcare workers who are e-antigen negative and who perform exposure-prone procedures or clinical duties in renal units; restriction of those who have a viral load which exceeds 1000 genome equivalents per ml from performing exposure prone procedures; and management of blood exposure incidents for both healthcare workers and patients.

Animals

Risk from animals in community care

An OT may be concerned with danger from dogs kept by clients and carers and needs to know her rights in this respect. Could she refuse to attend a client because there is an aggressive animal in the house? What are her rights if she is injured? If a client or carer has an animal which the owner does not have under control and as a consequence a visiting OT is injured, then she may be able to claim compensation under the Occupier's Liability Act 1957 above. She would need to establish that the owner as occupier of the premises failed to take reasonable care to ensure that she was safe. The fact that it was known that the animal could be aggressive would place upon the occupier a clear duty to protect visitors from it.

Where it is known that an aggressive animal is on the premises, then the owner can be warned that unless the animal is kept under control, the occupational therapy department cannot provide a service to the client in that home. This would, of course, be an extreme situation, but the employer has a duty to take reasonable care of its employees and cannot therefore force the employee to enter a dangerous situation or take unreasonable risks. Under the Dangerous Dogs Act 1991 persons are prohibited from having in their possession or custody dogs belonging to types bred for fighting and other specially dangerous dogs. The Act also makes further provision for securing that dogs are kept under proper control. Under the Dogs Act 1871 as amended by the Dangerous Dogs Act 1989 magistrates can give orders for a dog to be destroyed.

Therapeutic use of animals

One recent development in practice is the use of domestic animals to visit residential homes and other long-stay accommodation as part of the therapeutic care of the clients. The COT has prepared a statement in 1990[71] giving advice on the use of animals in therapy. It emphasised that the use of animals must be subject to the employing authority's approval and stated that 'under no circumstances should an animal be introduced into a work area'. The animal must also have been subject to appropriate veterinary checks to ensure there were no undue health risks. The COT warned that members were not covered by the British Association of Occupational Therapists' professional indemnity insurance for injury or damage caused by an animal which did not meet the conditions in the above stipulations. The charitable organisation Pets as Therapy[72] has prepared a handbook[73] which covers guidelines for pets as therapy visiting volunteers, an acknowledgement form which can be completed by the organisation which is being visited, policy and procedures for volunteers, confidentiality, complaints procedure and a vaccination policy. The COT produced a hot topic reference guide on animal assisted therapy in 2008.

Violence

Unfortunately there are more and more reports of attacks on health service employees, not just from strangers in the streets but also from carers and even clients. The rules relating to the terms of service of general practitioners were changed to enable them to arrange for the removal from their list of any patient who threatens violence to them. There have been reported cases of harm to OTs. Thus, in a case in 1983,[74] a voluntary patient at a mental hospital was charged with assault occasioning actual bodily harm to an OT employed at the hospital, and in 1993 an OT was killed by a mentally ill patient in the Edith Morgan Unit at Torbay. An inquiry[75] was set up following this death (see further Chapter 21). A survey by the Healthcare Commission in 2007 revealed that one in three NHS staff experienced violence or abuse in 2006.[76] The Public Accounts Committee found that overall only 5% of victims of violence claim compensation from the criminal injuries compensation authority (CICA) (See below) and that even when they do apply they are hampered by a complex application form and suffer delays in receiving their money because of bureaucracy.[77]

The employer has a duty to take reasonable care of the OT in relation to reasonably foreseeable violence. A risk assessment would therefore be required of this possibility and as a result any reasonable means to protect the employee should be adopted.

Is it possible to remove the risk altogether? If the answer to this is yes but, for example, only by stopping all home visits by OTs, this would not be 'reasonably practicable' in the term of the regulations.

What preventive action or protective measures can be taken? The answer to this might include the provision of two-way radios, personal alarms or, in very dangerous areas or on visits to clients who present a threat, OTs going in pairs or accompanied by another person. In the institutional setting protective measures may include more staffing, higher levels of supervision of difficult to manage patients and special security measures.

Review of the situation

A review should be undertaken to ascertain if the nature of the risk has changed (e.g. Is the district more violent than it was formerly assessed to be? Have the nature and condition of patients in a hospital ward deteriorated?) and the extent of the success of the measures taken to prevent harm to OTs. The question is raised whether any further measures are necessary. This type of analysis will not only relate to OTs but could be part of a wider assessment of all health professionals into which the OTs could have an input.

The COT and Department of Health guidance

Reference should be made to the guidance prepared by the COT.[78] This uses the definition of violence suggested by the Health and Safety Executive:

> Any incident in which an employee is abused, threatened or assaulted by a member of the public in circumstances arising out of the course of his or her employment.

The COT guidance deals with the issue of prevention, looking at assessment and problem identification and discussing various preventive strategies and monitoring. It also considers violence in the community. Other topics covered include reporting and recording incidents; counselling and support; compensation and legal assistance; and safety representatives.

A suggested pro forma for an incident report form is also given.

Monitoring of potentially violent situations is essential and the OT should play her full part to bring any concerns to the attention of the management and ensure that action is taken. The COT/BAOT has provided a briefing note no 51 on the Management of disturbed/violent behaviour (2005) which considers the precautions necessary in mental health settings and gives guidance on education and training, use of therapeutic occupations and risk assessment and risk management. That there is a need for occupational therapists to increase their awareness of the problems associated with aggression is the conclusion of an analysis of aggression shown by adults following brain injury.[79] The author recommends further training for OTs to increase awareness of how to use body language and communication skills effectively and how to increase awareness of potential environments and interventions where higher risk has been identified.

The Department of Health has introduced a zero tolerance policy on violence in the NHS and set up a web address[80] to provide information and advice. Guidance has been issued for managers in reducing violence to NHS staff. The Crime and Disorder Act 1998 establishes local Crime and Disorder Reduction Partnerships (CDRPs) led jointly by police and local authorities. They have a statutory responsibility to develop and implement a strategy to tackle crime and disorder in their area in consultation with health, education and the voluntary and independent sectors. The 1998 Act was amended by the Police Reform Act 2002 to extend responsibility for implementing the strategy to the fire and police authorities, and includes PCTs in the partnerships. In spite of the efforts, the National Audit Office[81] reported in March 2003 that reports of violence against NHS staff have risen by 13% over two years, costing the service at least £69 million annually. It estimated that about 40% of incidents were not being reported. In the light of this report, the Secretary of State for Health announced[82] that if the Department of Public Prosecutions failed to take action against those attacking health workers, then the victims could call on a new legal protection unit within the Department of Health to support private legal action against the attackers.

In April 2003 the NHS Security Management Service took over responsibility for all security management issues in the NHS including violence against staff. It published a strategy which set violence against NHS staff as a top priority to be dealt with, introduced a mandatory reporting system of violent incidents, and published a manual on tackling violence against staff. Whilst this initiative does not embrace local authority staff, there is no reason why managers within LAs could not make use of the guidance provided by the NHS Security Management Service. NHS Security Management Service is now incorporated in the NHS Counter Fraud and Security Management

Service Division of the NHS Business Services Authority and has developed a programme of work from the Zero Tolerance Campaign.[83] The NHS Security Management Service reported that there were 58,695 physical assaults on NHS staff in England in 2005–6.

An interesting analysis of the effect of violence on OT students is made by Alison Whitehead[84] who shows the importance of these findings for the education and training and support of OT students. Alison Blank has studied the literature relating to patient violence in community mental health[85] and draws the conclusion that there is an absence of information in OT literature about risk assessment and risk management of violence in community mental health, although there is much information on which they could draw.

Remedies following violent attacks

If a member of staff is injured as a result of violence the following actions could be taken:

- a public prosecution of the offender
- a private prosecution of the offender
- a civil action for compensation against the offender
- a civil action for compensation against the employer on the grounds that it has failed in its duty of care towards an employee as consequence of which the employee has been harmed
- a claim under the criminal injury compensation scheme (see below)
- social security benefits for injuries.

More than one of these courses of action could be taken.

The Court of Appeal held in 2006 that the NHS trust had failed in its duty of care to 6 nursing staff who were assaulted by a patient in Rampton Hospital. The Hospital had failed to carry out a risk assessment in accordance with the recommendations of the Tilt Report into Security in High Security Hospitals and as a consequence the staff were injured.[86]

In theory a health professional injured by a patient could sue the patient, but difficulties arise if the patient was suffering from a mental disorder. In such circumstances a preferable course of action would be for the injured employee to sue her employer if it can be established that there were failures in the risk assessment or the action taken to manage the risk of harm to the employee. In Wales the Welsh Assembly Government has launched the All Wales NHS Violence and Aggression Training Passport and Information Scheme and in Scotland the Scottish Executive is coordinating a Zero Tolerance Campaign. In September 2007 funding of £97 million was announced for further protection of NHS staff from violence. £29 million of this sum is to be used for safety alarms for lone workers and the remainder for training, additional local security management specialists, more prosecutions, a centralised reporting system to the NHS Security Management Service.[87]

Conclusion on violence

Unfortunately the possibility of violence at work is a reasonable foreseeability for the occupational therapist. The HSE in its guidance on workplace violence[88] notes that the main factors that can create a risk of violence are: impatience, frustration, anxiety, resentment and drink, drugs or inherent aggression/mental instability. Every employer has a responsibility to ensure that a risk assessment is undertaken and to take the appropriate action to protect health staff and others. Much guidance is now available from the Department of Health (and in particular the NHS Counterfraud and Security Management Service in England and the All Wales NHS Violence and Aggression Training Passport and Information Scheme) and from the Health and Safety Executive websites.

Domestic violence

Occupational therapists may become aware especially in their community work, of domestic violence taking place. They should remember that such aggression is a criminal offence and under the Domestic Violence Crime and Victims Act 2004 more powers are available against the aggressor. Advice should be taken from senior management on the reporting of such incidents which would be a justifiable exception to the duty of confidentiality on the grounds of public safety. The literature on occupational therapy with women and children who are survivors of domestic violence is reviewed by Anthea Cage.[89] She notes that there is a gap in the profession's knowledge and skills in identifying and working with victims of violence.

Stress and bullying

Concern with stress at work is now recognised as part of the employer's duty in taking reasonable care of the health and safety of the employee. In a reported case[90] in 1994 a social work manager obtained compensation when his employer failed to provide the necessary support in a stressful work situation after he returned to work following an earlier absence due to stress. The employer was not liable for the initial absence, but that put it on notice that the employee was vulnerable and its failure to provide the assistance it was acknowledged he needed was a breach of its duty to provide reasonable care for his health and safety as required under the contract of employment. The Court of Appeal[91] has emphasised that when a court decided whether or not the claimant was entitled to compensation for mental illness caused by stress at work, the threshold question was whether the kind of harm to the particular employee was reasonably foreseeable and not whether psychiatric injury was foreseeable in a person of ordinary fortitude. The House of Lords allowed one appeal: an employer had to take steps to support an employee who could not cope.

In a subsequent case it was held that the mere fact that the employers had provided counselling services did not relieve them of the duty to take reasonable care of an employee who was being subjected to considerable stress because of overwork and a lack of clear management controls.[92] The Court of Appeal dismissed the employer's appeal against the finding of a breach of the duty of care and the award of £134,000.

The Health and Safety Executive issued its first enforcement notice for failure to protect staff from stress in August 2003.[93] Failure to observe the enforcement notice could lead to prosecution. The notice was issued against the West Dorset Hospitals NHS Trust which was given six months to assess stress levels among its 1100 staff and introduce a new programme to reduce it. Stress reduction is one of eight key targets set by the HSE which has set up a stress website[94] covering the reasons why stress must be tackled, management standards, advice for individuals and good practice. It has also provided a guide on improving efficiency which shows how tackling stress at work can improve an organisation's efficiency.

Reference should also be made to Chapter 10 on negligence, Chapter 15 on equipment issues and Chapter 16 on transport issues.

Sexual harassment

It is essential that OTs are sensitive to the dangers of sexual harassment and make every effort to avoid potentially difficult situations. On the one hand they must be aware of the sex discrimination laws (see Chapter 19) and must ensure that they do not discriminate either directly or indirectly.

On the other hand they must ensure that they are chaperoned in any situation which could lead to the client bringing accusations of harassment by the OT or where the OT is herself at risk. The COT identified in 1995 the circumstances where a chaperon is recommended[95] in the interests of both the client and the OT. Guidance issued by the Council for Healthcare Regulatory Excellence published in January 2008 on sexual boundaries is discussed in Chapter 4.

The Protection from Harassment Act 1997

The Protection from Harassment Act 1997 can also provide some protection in the workplace if an individual considers that they are subject to unreasonable unwanted attention.

The Act creates the following:

- A criminal offence of harassment (section 1) which is defined as a person pursuing a course of conduct which amounts to harassment of another and which he knows or ought to know amounts to harassment of the other (the reasonable person test (see glossary) is applied).
- A civil wrong whereby a person who fears an actual or future breach of section 1 may claim compensation including damages for anxiety and financial loss.
- The right to claim an injunction (see glossary) to restrain the defendant from pursuing any conduct which amounts to harassment.
- The right to apply for a warrant for the arrest of the defendant if the injunction has not been obeyed.
- An offence of putting people in fear of violence, where a person on at least two occasions causes by his conduct another person to fear that violence will be used against them.
- Restraining orders made by the court for the purpose of protecting the victim of the offence or any other person from further conduct amounting to harassment or to fear violence.

Certain defences are permitted in the Act including that an individual is preventing or detecting crime.

Bullying at work

The Healthcare Commission, following a survey, estimated in February 2008 that one in 12 NHS staff are bullied by their managers. Only 2 out of 5 staff felt that their NHS Trust was taking effective action to deal with bullying. NHS Employers has issued guidance on how trusts can combat workplace bullying.

In June 1996 Unison negotiated for Janet Ballantyne an out-of-court settlement of £66 000 as compensation for the stress that she had suffered as a residential social worker. Bullying issues were central to her stress and compensation was paid for the anxiety, depression and panic attacks which were caused by the style of her abusive manager.[96]

£100 000 was accepted in an out-of-court settlement by a teacher who alleged that he had been bullied by the head teacher and other staff, when he was teaching in a school in Pembrokeshire.[97] Dyfed County Council denied negligence. He suffered a minor breakdown in October 1996 and was returned to the same school although he had asked for a transfer. He claimed that he was isolated, ignored and subjected to a series of practical jokes. He then suffered a second nervous breakdown. It was claimed that a support plan worked out for him by the Council had not been properly implemented. The lessons for managers from this case are obvious.

A review on the literature on bullying at work from the Health and Safety Laboratory is available from the HSE website.[98] The aim of the project is to enable the HSE to develop guidance for organisations on primary interventions in relation to bullying. The Chartered Management Institute published a report on bullying at work in 2008[99] which showed that 70% of those managers polled by the CMI had witnessed bullying in the past three years and 42% had been bullied themselves. Root causes appeared to be lack of management skills, personality clashes and authoritarian management styles.

The British Association of Occupational Therapists together with Unison published in October 2006 a guide for occupational therapy staff on bullying at work. It defines what is meant by workplace bullying and harassment, analyses the effects of bullying, sets out the law and explains how a successful policy could be developed. It also considers bullying by clients and the public.

Criminal injuries compensation authority (CICA)

A scheme to compensate those who have suffered personal injuries as the result of criminal action has been in existence since 1964. A new scheme for compensation following injuries or death as a result of a crime was established on 1 April 1996 under the Criminal Injuries Compensation Act 1995, based on a statutory scale of awards known as the 'tariff'. Details of the current scheme[100] is available from the Criminal Injury Compensation Authority (CICA) headquarters in Glasgow[101] or from the CICA website.[102] Claims are processed by the CICA and claims officers and adjudicators on a panel determine whether a claim can be met. Evidence is obtained from applicants, the police medical bodies and others such as witnesses to the incident. The CICA determines whether payments are to be made to victims of criminal acts. Those eligible (and these include the victims of crime as well as the dependents of homicide victims) must have reported the crime to the police as soon as possible. The application should be made within two years of the incident, but exceptions can be made to both these requirements. Payments are made against a tariff system up to a maximum of £500,000 (see Paragraph 24 of the scheme) and include the following items:

- medical expenses
- mental health expenses
- lost wages for disabled victims (but not for the first 28 full weeks of lost earnings or earning capacity)
- lost support for dependants of homicide victims
- funerals
- travel
- rehabilitation for disabled victims
- pain and suffering
- bereavement
- loss of parental services.

Loss of earnings and special expenses (damage to property and equipment used as physical aids), NHS prescription, opticians' and dentists' charges, special equipment, adaptations to home and disability aids, cost of care relating to bodily functions and preparation of food and supervision are also payable.

Staff health

The standard of the health of health service staff has been a concern for some time of many health and safety bodies and the Department of Health. In March 2010 the Department of Health published the report of a working group on the health of health professions called *Invisible patients*, The report focuses on the health issues facing regulated health professionals and identifies priorities for addressing them. It looks at how ill health may affect their professional practice and the difficulties they face in seeking help. Its recommendations include the development of occupational health services, and greater involvement of the health professional regulatory bodies and education services in promoting higher standards. The report can be downloaded from the DH website.

Conclusions

A risk management strategy is at the heart of any policy relating to health and safety, not just for employees but also for the clients and general public. Regular monitoring of the implementation of a risk management policy should ensure that harm is avoided and that a quality service is maintained for the public. This should be accompanied by clear, comprehensive documentation.

 Questions and exercises

1   Undertake a risk assessment of your department.
2   Show the differences between the implementation of HASAW by the health and safety inspectorate and a case brought by an employee for compensation because of breach of the duty to care for the health and safety of an employee by the employer.
3   An OT reports that a house she visits is in a dangerous condition. What action should her manager take?
4   Examine the systems for reporting untoward incidents in your department. To what extent are they effective in ensuring accountability and improvements in the quality of the service?
5   How are the risks of violence from patients and the general public managed in your department?

References

1   *R v Porter* The Times Law Report 9 July 2008.
2   *R v Chargot and others* The Times Law Report 16 December 2008.
3   Management of Health and Safety at Work Regulations 1999 Statutory Instrument 1999/3242; Health and Safety Commission (2000) Approved Code of Practice and guidance (ACOP).
4   *Allison v London Underground Ltd* The Times Law Report 29 February 2008.
5   Management of Health and Safety at Work Regulations 1999 SI No 3242.
6   Provisions and Use of Work Equipment Regulations 1998 SI No 2306.
7   *Smith (Jean) v Northamptonshire County Council* The Times Law Report 24 March 2008.
8   *Smith (Jean) v Northamptonshire County Council* The Times Law Report 21 May 2009.
9   *Spencer-Franks v Kellog Brown and Root Ltd and Another* The Times Law Report 3 July 2008 HL.
10   Provision and Use of Work Equipment Regulations SI 1998/2306.
11   *Baker and others v Quantum Clothing and others* The Times Law Report 18 June 2009 CA.
12   *Craner v Dorset County Council* The Times Law Report 27 February 2009.
13   College of Occupational Therapists (2006) Risk Management College of Occupational Therapists Guidance 1. COT, London.

14   Clarke, C. (2000) Risk management: a user guide. *British Journal of Occupational Therapy*, **63**(11), 529–31.

15   Hignett, S. (2001) Manual handling risk assessments in occupational therapy. *British Journal of Occupational Therapy*, **64**(2), 81–6.

16   Health and Safety Executive (1992) *Manual Handling: Guidance on Regulations*. HMSO, London.

17   Health and Safety Commission (1992) Guidance on Manual Handling of Loads in the Health Services. HMSO, London.

18   Health and Safety Executive (2007) *Getting to Grips with Manual Handling*. HSE, London.

19   College of Occupational Therapists (2006) *Manual Handling*. COT, London.

20   Mandelstam, M. (2001) Safe use of disability equipment and manual handling: Legal aspects. *British Journal of Occupational Therapy Part 1 Disability Equipment*, **64**(1), 9–16; *Part 2 Manual Handling* **64**(2), 73–80.

21   Backcare (1999) Safer Handling of People in the Community National Back Pain Association.

22   Smith, J. (ed) (2005) *A Guide to the Handling of People*, 5th edn. Backcare, Teddington.

23   Statutory Instrument (Health and Safety (Miscellaneous Amendments) Regulations 2002, SI 2002/2174.

24   *Egan v Central Manchester and Manchester Children's University Hospitals NHS Trust* The Times Law Report 3 February 2009.

25   *Colclough v Staffordshire County Council*, 30 June 1994, Current Law No. 208, October 1994.

26   *Koonjul v Thameslink Healthcare Services* [2000] PIQR P 123.

27   *King v Sussex Ambulance NHS Trust* [2002] EWCA 953; Current Law No. 408, August 2002.

28   *R (on the application of A, B, X and Y) v East Sussex County Council (Disability Rights Commission an interested party)* [2003] EWHC 167 (Case No. CO/4843/2001); 10 February 2003, QBD.

29   *Wiles v Bedfordshire CC*, Current Law No. 365, June 2001.

30   *O'Neil v DSG Retail Ltd*, The Times, 9 September; Current Law No. 209, October 2002.

31   Benten Jane and Ellis Diane (2008) Implications of hoist provisions when planning discharge home from an acute hospital. *British Journal of Occupational Therapy*, **71**(5), 209–14.

32   *Mutuma v London Borough Of Barnet* [2002] EWCA Civ 308.

33   National Institute for Health and Clinical Excellence (2002) Guidance on surgery for morbid obesity.

34   Graham Clews (2008) Under Pressure. *Frontline* **14**(2), 12–14.

35   Jane Charlton and Julian M Pearce (2007) Supporting bariatric employees. *The Column* **19**(1), 12–16.

36   BackCare (1999) *Safer Handling of People in the Community*. BackCare, Teddington.

37   News item, *The Times*, 19 November 2003.

38   Enquiries can be made to: Health and Safety Executive Information Centre, Sheffield, Tel. 0114 2892345, Fax 0114 2892333.

39   www.hse.gov.uk/riddor/

40   Department of Health. *An Organisation with a Memory*: report of an expert group chaired by Professor Liam Donaldson Chief Medical Officer, Department of Health. Copies are available from the Stationery Office, PO Box 29, Norwich NR3 1GN or from the Department of Health website www.doh.gov.uk

41   Department of Health (2001) Building a Safer NHS for Patients.

42   Department of Health (2001) Press release *National patient safety agency to be launched*. National Patient Safety Agency (Established and Constitution) Order 2001, SI 2001/1743; National Patient Safety Agency (Establishment and Constitution) (Amendment) Order 2003, SI 2003/1007.

43   National Patient Safety Agency, Patient Safety Alert PSA 01, London, NPSA, 2002.

44   www.npsa.nhs.uk

45   National Patient Safety Agency Patient Safety alert No 21: Safer Practice with epidural injections and infusions March 2007.

46   www.npsa.nhs.uk

47   Lister Sam Hospitals can make you sick, but which are the worst? Report cards will tell all. The Times 7 March 2009.

48   patientsafetyfirst@npsa.nhs.uk

49   Department of Health (2003) *Making Amends*. A consultation paper setting out proposals for reforming the approach to clinical negligence in the NHS.

50 Andrew Dillon (2008) NICE guidance for healthy workplaces. *British Journal of Healthcare Management*, **14**(6), 249.

51 www.nice.org.uk/phi005

52 NHS Employers (2008) The Healthy Workplace Agenda Briefing note No 56.

53 Kloss Diana Occupational Health Law (2005) Blackwells Oxford.

54 Control of Substances Hazardous to Health (COSHH) Regulations 2002, SI 2002/2677.

55 www.coshh-essentials.org.uk

56 Health and Safety Executive (2003) Preventing or controlling exposure to hazardous substances at work: www.hse.gov.uk/hthdir/noframes/coshh/coshh9a.htm

57 News item, The Times 14 March 2008.

58 National Audit Office (2000) The Management and Control of Hospital Acquired Infection in Acute NHS Trusts in England. Stationery Office, London.

59 DoH Press notice 12 June 2000; Jill Sherman, Infections caught in hospital to be exposed. *The Times*, 13 June 2000.

60 David Rose. Hit squads to stamp out hospital superbugs. The Times 4 June 2007 page 18.

61 www.dh.gov.uk/en/Policyandguidance/Healthandsocialcare

62 News item Hospital reprimanded over hygiene. The Times 31 December 2008.

63 News item The Times 9 May 2008.

64 Rosemary Bennett Risk assessment watchdog set up to halt march of the nanny state. The Times 16 January 2008.

65 www.npsa.nhs.uk/clearnyourhands/the-campaign/training-video/

66 Lister Sam New 'Super-regulator' orders 21 hospital trusts to clean up 3 April 2009.

67 News item the Metro 12 February 2009.

68 COT/BAOT (2003 revised 2005) Briefing: Providing a Safe Service to People with Infectious Diseases. COT, London.

69 NHS Executive (2000) *Hepatitis B Infected Health Care Workers* HSC 2000/020 DoH, London.

70 HSG (93)40 Protecting health care workers and patients from hepatitis B, and its addendum EL(96)77.

71 College of Occupational Therapists (1990) *Statement on Animals in Occupational Therapy Practice*, SPP 130. COT, London.

72 reception@petsastherapy.org

73 Pets as Therapy. *Visiting Dogs and Cats*. Handbook; www.petsastherapy.com

74 *R v Lincolnshire (Kesteven) Justices, ex parte Connor* [1983] 1 All ER 901, QBD.

75 Blom-Cooper, L., Hally, H. & Murphy, E. (1996) *The Falling Shadow – One patient's mental health care 1978–1993*: Report of an Inquiry into the death of an occupational therapist at Edith Morgan Unit, Torbay 1993. Duckworth, London.

76 Healthcare Commission (2007) Annual NHS Staff survey; www.healthcarecommission.org.uk

77 Public Accounts Committee Compensating Victims of Violent Crime 2008.

78 College of Occupational Therapists (1995) *Violence at Work* (Position Statement). COT, London.

79 Beaulieu Karen (2007) Occupational Therapists' perceptions and management of aggression related to adults with a brain injury. *British Journal of Occupational Therapy*, **70**(4), 161–70.

80 www.nhs.uk/zerotolerance/

81 National Audit Office (2003) A Safer Place to Work: Protecting NHS Hospital and Ambulance Staff from Violence and Aggression. www.nao.gov.uk/publications/nao_reports/02-3/0203527es.pdf

82 Sam Lister, Ministers to fund action on abusive patients, *The Times*, 15 April 2003.

83 www.cfsms.nhs.uk/ Free phone line 0800 028 40 60.

84 Whitehead, A. (2003) The legacy of violent attack: an exploratory study of occupational therapy students' experiences of violent attack. *British Journal of Occupational Therapy*, **66**(3), 94–100.

85 Blank, A. (2001) Patient violence in community mental health: A review of the literature. *British Journal of Occupational Therapy*, **64**(12), 584–9.

86 *Bucks and others v Nottinghamshire Healthcare NHS Trust* [2006] EWCA Civ 1576.

87 Department of Health press release 25 September 2007.

88   www.hse.gov.uk/healthservices/violence/index.htm
89   Cage Anthea (2007) Occupational Therapy with women and children survivors of domestic violence: are we fulfilling our activist heritage? A review of the literature. *British Journal of Occupational Therapy*, **70**(5), 192–8.
90   *Walker v Northumberland County Council* (QBD) Times Law Report, 24 November 1994; [1995] 1 All ER 737.
91   *Sutherland v Hatton: Somerset CC v Barber; Sandwell MBC v Jones; Baker Refractories Ltd v Bishop* [2002] EWCA Civ 76; The Times, 12 February 2002, CA. *Barber v Somerset CC*, The Times, 5 April 2004, HL.
92   *Daw v Intel Corp (UK) Ltd* [2007] EWCA Civ 70; [2007] 2 All ER 126, (2007) 104(8) L.S.G 36.
93   Simon de Bruxelles, Oliver Wright and Helen Rumbelow, Bosses will be fined for workers' stress, *The Times*, 5 August 2003, p. 1.
94   www.hse.gov.uk/stress/imdex.htm
95   College of Occupational Therapists (1995) Gender Issues Relating to Personal Care Tasks in the Practice of Occupational Therapy (Position Statement). COT, London.
96   Chartered Society of Physiotherapy Industrial Relations Department (1997) Health and Safety Briefing Pack No. 5 (July 1997) Bullying At Work. CSP, London.
97   Victoria Fletcher 'Teacher "bullied by staff" wins £100 000' *The Times*, 17 July 1998.
98   Johanna Beswick et al Bullying at work: a review of the literature WPS/06/04 Health and Safety Laboratory 2006.
99   Chartered Management Institute (2008) Bullying at Work: the Experience of Managers CMI.
100   Criminal Injuries Compensation Scheme 2008 Home Office.
101   Criminal Injuries Compensation Authority, Tay House, 300 Bath Street, Glasgow G2 4JR; Tel 0800 358 3601.
102   www.cica.gov.uk

12 Record Keeping

Record keeping is considered in this section because the standard of record keeping is most likely to come to the fore when litigation commences, a prosecution is initiated or a complaint is made. However, it should not be ignored that the principal purpose of record keeping is to ensure the quality of care provided for the patient, to facilitate communication between professionals, and maintain a record of the diagnosis, treatment and future plans for the patient. A good standard for documentation would be that if any health professional were to be called away in an emergency, his or her colleagues would be able to provide continuity of care on the basis of the full comprehensive clear records of the absent occupational therapist (OT). The following topics are covered in this chapter:

- Principles of record keeping and standards of practice
- Guidelines on actual recording
- Changing records
- Documentation and referrals
- Storage of records and length of time they should be kept

- Destruction of records
- Ownership and control of records
- Unified systems of record keeping
- Electronic health records
- Legal status and evidential value of records
- Client held records
- Audit and standard setting

Reference should also be made to Chapter 13 on statements, reports and giving evidence in court, Chapter 8 on confidentiality and data protection, and Chapter 9 on access to records.

Legal Aspects of Occupational Therapy, Third Edition By Bridgit Dimond
© 2010 Bridgit Dimond

Principles of record keeping and standards of practice

Standard 10 of the HPC Standards of conduct, performance and ethics[1] requires the registrant to keep accurate patient, client and user records and explains that:

> making and keeping records is an essential part of care and you must keep records for everyone you treat or who asks for professional advice or services. All records must be complete and legible, and you should write, sign and date all entries.

Failure to comply with the standards set by the HPC could lead to a fitness to practice hearing and being struck off the register and are discussed in Chapter 4 where several cases show examples of unsatisfactory record keeping as ground for unfitness to practice.

In 2006 the COT issued guidance on record keeping[2] which covers the topics shown in Figure 12.1. It also issued a briefing note[3] on issues of responsibility. This covered the purpose of records; signing and countersigning OT entries in health and social care records; ensuring accuracy in electronic care records and records held by service-users and duplication. Subsequently in 2007 the COT has published Professional Standards for OT practice which include a general statement on record keeping.[4]

Figure 12.1   Record keeping COT (2006).

1 Introduction
1.1   What constitutes a care record?
1.2   The purpose of care records
1.3   The legal status of records and responsibility for them
2 The quality of care records
2.1   Inclusion
2.2   The use of 'Violent' warning markers
2.3   The use of acronyms and abbreviations
2.4   Signing and countersigning record entries
2.5   Timing and dating record entries
2.6   Timely record keeping
2.7   The Climbié Inquiry recommendations
3 The format of care records
3.1   Specific or shared care records
3.2   Electronic care records
3.3   Integrated children's systems
3.4   Care records held by service users
4 The handling and management of care records
4.1   The Caldicott Review recommendations
4.2   Confidentiality and consent
      4.2.1   The Data Protection Act 1998
      4.2.2   The Human Rights Act 1998
4.3   Access to care records
4.4   Social care information governance
4.5   Information governance toolkits
4.6   Transferring information to another professional or agency
4.7   Storage of paper records
4.8   Retention of records
      4.8.1   Retention of diaries

Record keeping – as either an occupational therapy record or part of a multi-disciplinary record – is an essential and integral part of care. The purpose of the records is to give a comprehensive, accurate and justifiable account of the care, treatment and support provided or planned for a service user. The information also supports the use of audit, evidence-based clinical practice and improvements in clinical effectiveness through research.

Three record keeping standards are provided. The statements are as follows.

(1) A record should be kept of all occupational therapy activity and intervention made with, or on behalf of, the service user person.
(2) OT records should be well-organised, well-managed and clear, to ensure that they are accessible to those who may need to refer to them.
(3) Occupational therapy staff should be aware of, and abide by, legal requirements for the confidentiality, storage and disposal of records, and a service user's right to access their own records. They should also be guided by local policy on these matters.

It should be clear from Chapters 10, 11 and 13 that the documentation can play a significant part in any court hearing and it is essential therefore that clear principles on content, style, clarity, comprehensiveness and accuracy should be followed. Many civil cases are contested several years after the events to which they relate and the records are therefore extremely important. The criteria set by the COT in relation to professional records are shown in Figure 12.2. Reference can also be made to the principles set out in the Department of Health NHS Code of Practice on Confidentiality 2003 DH London which superseded the NHS Training Directorate booklet.[5] The Department of Health statement on record keeping principles is set out in Figure 12.3. A helpful guide albeit American on records is by Ginge Kettenbach.[6]

Obvious defects which can be picked up in any internal audit (see later in the chapter) include illegible handwriting, too little or too much information where basic facts are missing, and failure to write up the records within 24 hours of the contact/intervention. Whilst it is not realistic to ban

Figure 12.2   Criteria set by COT.

(1)   Each client has a record.
(2)   The information contained in the record is objective, accurate and factual.
(3)   The record is systematically organised and complete.
(4)   Each entry is contemporaneous, i.e. recorded within one working day of the contact or intervention.
(5)   The record is legible and without slang, abbreviations or unexplained acronyms.
(6)   Any amendment to the record is made in such a way that the original text can still be read and the amendment has been signed and dated by the OT.
(7)   Each entry is signed and dated by the responsible occupational therapy staff member.
(8)   Records made by a student are countersigned and dated by a state registered OT.
(9)   Records made by support staff are countersigned and dated by the supervising OT, if required by the employer's policy.
(10)   OT staff are familiar with and follow the employing organisation's policies on record keeping. Where local policies differ from professional guidelines, the employer is responsible for any consequences arising from the quality of the OT's record keeping, provided the OT has followed local policies.
(11)   Where electronic records are used, OT staff are aware of new developments and guidance issued on the use of electronic systems.

Figure 12.3   Principles to follow in record keeping.

(1)   Records should be made as soon as possible after the events which are recorded.
(2)   They should be accurate, comprehensive and clear.
(3)   They should be written legibly and be jargon-free.
(4)   They should avoid opinion and record the facts of what is observed.
(5)   They should not include abbreviations (unless these have been identified).
(6)   They should not be altered, unless the changes are made so that the original entry is clearly crossed out, but still readable.
(7)   Any change should be dated and signed.
(8)   They should be dated, timed and signed by the maker.

---

abbreviations entirely, because their use can be time saving, it is essential that a procedure should be in place to ensure that there are no ambiguities over the meaning. It is therefore suggested that there should be an agreed list of permissible abbreviations, which should be attached to the patients' records. To enforce the use of the approved list, it should be a disciplinary offence to use an abbreviation which is not on the approved list, or to use an abbreviation on the list for another meaning. All that has been said about abbreviations also applies to the use of symbols and signs and other hieroglyphics. Reference should also be made to the NHS Code of Practice on record keeping standards which replaces earlier publications from the NHS Training Authority.[7]

It is preferable if records document the facts of a situation, or where an opinion, such as a diagnosis is required, that the opinion is supported by the facts on which it is based. Clearly no derogatory personal opinions of the patient should be recorded. (It is also worth noting the dangers of failing to hang up after leaving a phone message on an answer phone. This occurred when a hospital left a message for a patient rearranging an appointment, but the machine also recorded the slanderous statements subsequently made by the operator about the patient.[8])

Professional opinions

Records should contain the facts of what took place between patient and professional, the assessment, the diagnosis, treatment and care and outcome, together with details of what the patient has stated, the fact that consent was given and the information given to the patient about the risks of the recommended treatment. Sometimes however it is necessary to record the opinion of the professional. A Data Protection Good Practice Note has been provided by the Information Commissioner on how the DPA applies to professional opinion.[9] The ICO suggests the following:

When an opinion is recorded it is good practice to do the following:

- Make it clear that it is an opinion, showing who gave the opinion and when
- If possible, provide contact details
- Structure the record so that if someone objects to its accuracy, their view or challenge can be included in such a way that it is given proper weight
- Have a records policy that lays down the criteria that should be considered for continuing to keep the information or, where appropriate, specific retention periods for certain categories of information.

Changing records

Records should not be altered. If, however, the writer discovers that the wrong information was recorded, it would be possible to put a line through that information, sign and date this and then write the correct information. Any attempt to cover what was previously written by whiting it out or heavy blocking out is unacceptable practice and will arouse suspicions. What was erroneously recorded should still be legible. It was reported in *The Times* newspaper[10] that a casualty nurse who told the parents of a sick baby that he probably had a sniffle and they should take him to the family doctor, altered the notes when the baby died one hour later. She changed the words 'extremely pale' to 'quite pale' and added a pulse reading, although she had not taken his pulse. Even though an independent inquiry found that her actions probably had no bearing on the child's outcome, she faced internal disciplinary proceedings at which she was dismissed, and such circumstances could also lead to professional conduct proceedings with the possibility of being struck off the register of the UKCC (now replaced by the NMC).

An OT should not give into pressure from a patient to alter records, as the following case illustrates. In July 1998 a GP who allowed a patient to destroy part of her records was found guilty of serious professional misconduct by the GMC.[11] He had allowed the patient, who was involved in an acrimonious property dispute with her children, to remove a letter in which she was described as 'bad tempered' and another document which referred to her drinking.

Under the Data Protection Act 1998, a patient who considers that the records are inaccurate can make a formal request for them to be changed, but the health professional has a discretion over whether to accept the alteration and can refuse, simply recording the patient's objection in the margin.

Consequences of failure to maintain good record keeping standards

Record keeping failures are one of the most common reasons for professional conduct disciplinary measures. For example in August 2009 a panel of the HPC Conduct and Competence Committee heard oral evidence from five witnesses who had worked with Kerry Campbell, a senior OT in Surrey. The panel found that she had failed to maintain adequate records of assessments of patients, provided inappropriate treatment to patients and wrote up case notes retrospectively. They also found that she falsely wrote up case notes and incorrectly closed cases that required further assessment. The panel chair stated that "The facts proved are breaches of core competencies and thus the panel finds that in not discharging her duties she knew what was required of her and deliberately chose not to do so." She was struck off the Register.

In June 2009 an OT Mr Gary Byrom was struck off the HPC Register after a HPC Conduct and Competence Committee found that his record keeping was incomplete and not of the standard required of an experienced OT. The Panel heard that Mr Byrom had been given numerous opportunities to complete his record keeping and despite being given time and resources, failed to do so. HPC Panel Chair, Mr Martin Ryder, commented:

> The Registrant's misconduct constituted breaches of standards 1 and 10 of the HPC Standards of Conduct, performance and ethics in operation at the time. These provide that the registrant must always keep high standards of conduct, act in the best interest of patients, clients and users and keep accurate patient, client and user records. The Registrant's failure to keep and maintain proper records, placed clients at risk and it is necessary to make a striking off order to protect adequately the public and in the wider public interest.

The Panel decided to strike Mr Byrom from the Register with immediate effect. The details of the allegations were that:

1. He failed to carry out instructions with regard to basic record keeping, in that:
    (a) No diary records were found in 39 of his 56 cases.
    (b) No written records were found for his entire case load.
    (c) 14 files were found in the filing cabinet which were not open to him.
2. The matters set out in paragraph 1, a, b and c was seen to constitute misconduct and/or lack of competence.
3. By reason of that misconduct and/or lack of competence, his fitness to practise was impaired.

In addition to fitness to practise hearings before the HPC Conduct and Competence Committee, failures to maintain good record keeping standards can also be followed by disciplinary proceedings held by the employer and could lead to dismissal.

Documentation and referrals

In its Standards document[12] the COT sets a standard for documentation for referrals. Its referral standard statement 2 requires occupational therapists to respond to referrals within a stated time frame, based on local need, resources and policy. For monitoring, the OT is asked if her service has:

● a clearly documented policy stating a time frame for responding to referrals
● a clearly documented system for prioritising referrals that recognises levels and degrees of need and optimises the use of resources.

The Standards document advises that occupational therapists should have and abide by clearly documented procedures and criteria for referral to their service. On receipt of a referral the OT should record the source and date of the referral and the services requested.

In addition, documentation relating to priorities and waiting lists should be recorded and the relevant management agencies notified at regular intervals. This should include information on waiting lists and unallocated or uncompleted work.

Reference should also be made to the publications of the Department of Health on standards for record keeping,[13] and the NMC *Guidelines for Records and Record Keeping*[14] are of value to all health professionals (see Figure 12.4).

Use of emails

Correspondence between professionals and with patients is increasingly through the use of emails. This can give rise to some legal queries such as how is confidentiality protected? What record should be kept of any such correspondence? What information, if any, should not be sent by email? At present there are no national guidelines for the use of email with patients and it is advisable for each NHS organisation or professional group to develop their own protocols.

The Department of Health's NHS Code of Practice on Records Management[15] suggests the use of Contact for email within the NHS. "Contact" is a secure national email and directory service provided free of charge for NHS staff and developed specifically to meet the BMA requirements for clinical email between NHS organisations. The DH guidance suggests that Contact can be used to replace paper communications for the following:

Figure 12.4   Record keeping best practice.

Patient records should:
Be factual, consistent and accurate
- be written as soon as possible after an event has occurred, providing current information on the care and condition of the patient;
- be written clearly, legibly and in such a manner that they cannot be erased;
- be written in such a manner that any alterations or additions are dated, timed and signed in such a way that the original entry can still be read clearly;
- be accurately dated, timed and signed or otherwise identified, with the name of the author being printed alongside the first entry;
- be readable on any photocopies;
- be written, wherever applicable, with the involvement of the patient or carer;
- be clear, unambiguous, (preferably concise) and written in terms that the patient can understand. Abbreviations, if used, should follow common conventions;
- be consecutive;
- (for electronic records) use standard coding techniques and protocols;
- be written so as to be compliant with the Race Relations Act and the Disability Discrimination Act.

Be relevant and useful
- identify problems that have arisen and the action taken to rectify them;
- provide evidence of the care planned, the decisions made, the care delivered and the information shared;
- provide evidence of actions agreed with the patient (including consent to treatment and/ or consent to disclose information).

And include
- medical observations: examinations, tests, diagnoses, prognoses, prescriptions and other treatments;
- relevant disclosures by the patient – pertinent to understanding cause or effecting cure/ treatment;
- facts presented to the patient;
- correspondence from the patient or other parties.

Patient records should not include
- unnecessary abbreviations or jargon;
- meaningless phrases, irrelevant speculation or offensive subjective statements;
- Irrelevant personal opinions regarding the patient.

- patient referrals from GP to hospital
- hospital to hospital – or internal hospital referrals
- discharge letters
- clinical enquiries
- research links and
- clinical team communications.

The NHS Code of Practice recommends that local procedures need to be in place at the sending and receiving ends of communication. Clinical information should be clearly marked and properly addressed. It should be stored securely and added to patients' records when appropriate. Contact tracks what is received, by whom and when it is read. ContactPoint has a database of 11 million children in England.

Storage of records and length of time they should be kept

Records should be kept so that they are easily accessible to those who require to access them but at the same time with efficient controls to prevent unauthorised access and disclosure. The Audit Commission, in its report on hospital records,[16] considered that patients were being put at risk because their medical records are kept in a mess and sometimes lost. Failure to find records led to consultations being cancelled and to operations being postponed. It recommended that each hospital set up one main records library with good security.

Where litigation is being contemplated, reference should be made to the time limits within which action can be brought, as discussed in Chapter 10. In such circumstances, where there is a possibility of litigation, it would be extremely unwise to destroy any records. Records could be destroyed according to the advice given by the Department of Health in its NHS Code of Practice on Records Management.[17] Clearly this guidance would be subject to checking through the material to ensure that records which are likely to be the subject of litigation or complaints are kept for longer. Where the records are so old as to amount to historical documents, the Public Records Act 1958 comes into play and legal advice should be taken on their destruction.

The Information Security Management

A Code of Practice on Information Security Management has been prepared by the DH[18] and is available on its website. This Code of Practice is a guide to the methods and required standards of practice in the management of information security for those who work or under contract to, or in business partnership with NHS organisations in England. It is based on current legal requirements, relevant standards and professional best practice. The Code of Practice replaces the manual published in 1996.

Destruction of records

When records are destroyed, given their confidential nature this should be done by the health professional, department or organisation concerned, or else a firm offering secure disposal should be used.

Ownership and control of records

NHS records are owned by the Secretary of State and responsibility is delegated to the statutory health authorities. This also applies to the NHS records kept by general practitioners as part of their terms of service. Primary care trusts are responsible for arranging the transfer of the records to a new GP where a patient has indicated his or her wish to transfer, and for collecting the records from the GP when a patient has died.

The ultimate decision on disclosure to others rests with the chief executive officer of the NHS trust or primary care trust. Thus statutes such as the Data Protection Act 1998 give to the holder of the records the right to decide whether the exceptions apply or whether access should be permitted. The holder should, however, consult the health professional who cared for the patient (see Chapter 9).

Records relating to independent practice are owned by the health professional who made them. It can be agreed between the independent practitioner and the patient, before assessment and treatment commences, what access is to be arranged and whether there should be patient-held records. The patient receiving independent care has the same statutory rights of access under Data Protection Act provisions as the NHS patient (see Chapter 9).

Unified systems of record keeping

The development of a unified system of record keeping has now been achieved by many NHS trusts and community units. The aim is that all members of the multi-disciplinary team keep their patient records in the same patient folder to ensure that maximum co-operation and multi-disciplinary planning in the care of the patient takes place. Some OTs may fear loss of control over their records as a result of this development. They may also be tempted to provide an additional set of records in case the main set goes missing. The danger of this cautionary practice is that neither set may be complete or it may be assumed that there is only one set and the fact that there are other records is not known. The introduction of electronic records (see below) is likely to remove most of these problems.

At present there is also a problem if the records kept by one discipline apparently contradict the records kept by another. Should this be the situation, the OT should not amend her records unless she knows them to be wrong. If this is the case, any changes should be made so that the original writing is retained (see above). Any changes should be signed and dated.

Health and social services records

Difficulties have arisen over attempts to set up a unified record system which covers both health and social services records, since different statutory instruments apply to the two in relation to access (see Chapter 9). Such differences are not insurmountable but any joint sharing of records should ensure adequate controls over storage, access, confidentiality and standards.

Electronic health records

On 4 February 2001 the Department of Health issued a press release saying that by March 2005 every person in the country will have their own electronic health record (EHR).[19] The electronic health record is defined by the Department of Health as holding summarised key data about patients, such as name, address, NHS number, registered GP and contact details, previous treatments, ongoing conditions, current medication, allergies and the date of any next appointments. It was intended that it would be securely protected, created with patient consent, and with individual changes made only by authorised staff. The timetable for the EHR envisaged that 5 million people would have their own lifelong EHR by 2003, rising to around 25 million by 2004 and then everyone by March 2005. In addition, an electronic patient record (EPR) was to be created at a later date, which would provide full information about the patient's health admissions and consultation. Whilst this timetable has now been amended, significant developments are taking place within the NHS. The National Programme for Information Technology is overseeing the implementation of an electronic integrated care records service, an electronic booking system, electronic transmission of prescriptions and an underpinning IT infrastructure. A National Clinical Advisory Board and a Public Advisory Board advise on strategy and implementation. Further details can be obtained from the Department of Health website.[20] The COT has provided a briefing note on Electronic Care Records (ECRs).[21]

There are two parts to the NHS care records service:

1. Services that are common to all users nationally are the responsibility of the national application service provider (NASP).
2. Services delivered at a more local level will be the responsibility of five local service providers (LSPs). Together, they are to ensure the integration of existing local systems and implement the new systems, if necessary.

The NASP and the LSPs will make IT work across the NHS to support the creation of the NHS care records service. Further information is available on the dedicated website.[22]

The Department of Health pledged guarantees in May 2005 relating to patients' control over access to their health records.[23]

Electronic Social Care Record (ESCR)

The ESCR brings together all relevant information for a social care user in one place. It holds three types of information:

- structured information, which typically includes:
  - national forms, such as those used for recording children's information, local forms and forms completed by service users, such as self-referral or financial assessment forms.
- unstructured information, which covers all other recording including:
  - letters
  - emails
  - records of phone calls
  - meetings notes and
  - video clips
- coded data which is mainly for management and statistical reports.

Guidance has been issued by the DH and is available on its website.

NHS Care Record Guarantee

The NHS Care Record Guarantee sets out the rules that will govern information held in the NHS Care Records Service. This is an important part of the public information campaign about NHS Care Records. The NHS Care Record Guarantee is regularly reviewed by the National Information Governance Board.[24] It was developed by the Care Record Development Board (CRDB). The Guarantee covers people's access to their own records, controls on others' access, how access will be monitored and policed, options people have to further limit access, access in an emergency, and what happens when someone cannot make decisions for themselves. The Care Record Guarantee was first published in 2005 and revised in 2006 and 2007. The 2007 version of the Care Record Guarantee has emphasised and strengthened the clear commitment to the confidentiality and security of patient's information.

There were several minor changes including the introduction of standardised terms to reduce ambiguity and improve clarity. The implementation of the 2005 Mental Capacity Act was referred to, and there were several new sections regarding;

- the Summary Care Record - introducing the summary care record and indicating that patients have the choice to not have one at all;

- information for parents and young people - emphasising the importance of parents and health-care professionals in supporting and encouraging children to make decisions for themselves;
- an extra section that clearly outlines the processes involved in keeping patient electronic records secure and confidential; and
- a 'how to complain section', which directs patients to their local PALs office if they feel the commitments of the Care Record Guarantee are not being upheld.

The need to evolve consistent terminology to support electronic health and social care records is considered by Mary Brewin.[25] She welcomes the advantages of electronic health records but highlights the work that OTs must do to prepare for their introduction.

Whilst the computer will avoid problems of illegibility, considerable care will still have to be taken. In August 1998 it was reported[26] that a student suffering from meningitis may have died as a result of her name being wrongly spelt on a computer. The omission of the letter 'p' in her surname Simpkin meant that her records could not be accessed and an inquiry found that she might have lived if vital results of blood tests, entered into the computerised records under the wrong name, had been seen by staff.

The advantages of computerised records covering the whole of the NHS cannot be exaggerated, but care will be required to ensure security over access and to ensure that they are correctly kept.

It will be apparent from Chapter 10 in relation to accountability, and the discussion on the extended times within which an action can be brought, that it is mainly documentation rather than unaided memory that is relied on in any court hearing. There is considerable value in staff who have been involved in litigation, disciplinary proceedings and other hearings sharing the lessons they have learnt with their colleagues and illustrating the significant role which documentation played in their giving evidence. This topic is further discussed in Chapter 13.

The Department of Health, the General Medical Council and the Office of the Information Commissioner issued joint guidance on the use of IT equipment and access to patient data on 25th April 2007. It can be down loaded from the relevant websites. The joint statement was made to ensure that all those who have access to patient information in the course of their work are clear about what is expected of them. The DH strongly supported the call of the ICO for stronger penalties to apply where individuals obtain information unlawfully, and for the law to be changed to provide the possibility of a custodial sentence for those found guilty. In the case of the new NHS IM&T systems, authorised individuals will have to sign a statement to indicate their understanding and agreement to adhere to the standards set out in the joint guidance.

The Information Commissioner published his views on NHS electronic care records in January 2007 in response to the concerns of those made to the ICO that their health records would be available to everyone across the NHS. The ICO had been informed by NHS Connecting for Health that every one, in the initial trial areas, whose Summary Care Record (current medication, known allergies and adverse reactions) are to be loaded onto the NHS Care Record Service will be contacted and given information about their options. Once the information is uploaded, patients can choose to remove some or even all of the information initially loaded or keep the uploaded information but make the Summary Care Record invisible. The ICO also referred to the range of access controls to be introduced by the NHS as the new systems develop. All access to the Summary Care Record will be logged and unusual access will be investigated by a member of staff in every NHS trust (known as the Caldicott Guardian – see Chapter 8). NHS Connecting for Health had also informed the ICO that health information uploaded onto the NHS Care Records Service will not be accessible to any other organisations beyond the NHS without the patient's explicit consent, except where this is allowed or required by law. The ICO stated that the NHS must continue to comply with the Data

Protection Act 1998 and this is vital to guarantee that public confidence is maintained. The ICO would monitor the implementation and operation of the NHS Care Records Service to ensure patients are provided with adequate information and choices and that their health data is maintained in a safe and secure way.

A National Audit Office progress report published on 15 May 2008[27] on the national programme for electronic medical records stated that the Care Records Service is unlikely to be in place before 2014–5 at the earliest, because of serious delays in installing new software; the estimated total cost of the programme is broadly unchanged; some benefits from the programme are starting to emerge such as financial savings; trusts have experienced some technical problems in using the new care records system. The NAO made several recommendations including the fact that the DH and NHS should give priority to data protection, monitor levels of public confidence and review how the levels are being influenced by its communications about the protections in place to secure and manage access to care records. Separate recommendations are given for NHS trusts and for the DH and strategic health authorities.

The Public Accounts Committee warned in January 2009 that the upgrading of the NHS computer system which would provide electronic records for patients was running at least 4 years behind schedule. BT was seeking to renegotiate a contract worth £1 billion to provide medical records systems for all NHS hospitals in London.

As delays and concerns about confidentiality continue to frustrate the NHS electronic record system some patients are turning to smart cards which they keep and which provide sensitive details of their medical condition. A Health eCard is available for £40 with about 21 surgeries mainly in London and the South East using it.[28]

Legal status and evidential value of records

When does a record become a legal record? This question is often asked and the answer is that any record and any information, however recorded, can be ordered to be produced in a court of law if it is relevant to an issue which arises in the court proceedings and if it is not privileged from disclosure. (Reference should be made to Chapter 8 on confidentiality for the powers and limitations of the court in requiring the production of witnesses and documents.)

It does not follow that what is contained in any record is necessarily accurate or true. It is possible for a completely fictitious account to be recorded. If, for example, the nurse referred to above had not immediately written up her notes so that rather than adding to the record she had put down a totally fictitious pulse rate and written 'quite pale' in the first instance, the deception would possibly not have been discovered and the false record would have been taken at its face value on an initial enquiry into the baby's death. Therefore, in determining the weight to be attached to records and assessing their evidential value, the judge in any court hearing listens to the makers of such records being cross-examined and, in the light of that oral evidence, decides how much value can be placed on the written records.

Client-held records

Many different professionals are increasingly allowing clients to hold their own records. There are considerable advantages in occupational therapy practice if clients are encouraged to keep their own records and become responsible and involved in their progress. There are some fears associated with the patient acting as custodian of the records. Fears, however, that records could be lost if the health professional ceases to be in control of the records are generally unfounded. The evidence from ante-natal care with mothers holding their own records seems to indicate that records are less likely to go missing. Nevertheless, such fears could lead to the setting up of a second system of record keeping at a central point. The danger of a dual system is that neither set might be complete and there might not be consistency in what was recorded in each place.

There is also a fear that if records in the custody of the client go missing and litigation is commenced, then the professionals will be at a disadvantage in defending themselves. The burden is, however, on the claimant to establish negligence and this may be difficult to do if the documentation is missing and it is the claimant who is responsible for that loss.

Audit and standard setting

To maintain consistently high standards in record keeping across an OT department is difficult. Standards of record keeping should be audited periodically to highlight aspects not being attained and to enable improvements to be made if necessary. The service monitoring forms which accompany the record keeping standard statements in the COT Professional Standards for OT practice[29] can be used to audit OT records. Local audit within a department or across the trust can be supported by outside bodies such as the King's Fund. In addition, the Clinical Negligence Scheme for Trusts (CNST) identified hospital records as one of its core standards. Standard 6 requires that 'a comprehensive system for the completion, use, storage and retrieval of health records is in place. Record keeping standards are monitored through the clinical audit process.' Inspections by the CNST of member trusts can assist in maintaining high standards. The NHS LA standards for 2009–2010 on risk management for acute units, primary care trusts and independent sector providers of healthcare can be found on the NHSLA website.[30] Inspections by the Care Quality Commission (which replaced the Healthcare Commission in April 2009) should also support good record keeping practice.

Conclusions

Records are kept as part of the professional duty of care owed to the patient. Sound professional practice therefore requires standards to be identified and regularly monitored. If these standards are maintained, then in the event of a complaint, litigation, an inquiry or other investigation, they are likely to provide good evidence of the events and interventions which took place.

   Questions and exercises

1   With some colleagues, carry out an audit of the standards of record keeping among yourselves. Imagine that you were having to answer questions on the records in ten years' time.
2   What abbreviations do you consider could be usefully used in record keeping by OTs? What steps would you take to ensure that there was no confusion arising from their use?
3   Consider ways in which the keeping of occupational therapy records could be made more efficient.

References

1   Health Professions Council (2004 reprinted 2007) *Standards of conduct, performance and ethics*. HPC, London.
2   College of Occupational Therapy (2006) Record Keeping Guidance No 2.
3   College of Occupational Therapy (2006) Record keeping – Issues of Responsibility Briefing note 43. COT, London.
4   College of Occupational Therapists (2007) *Professional Standards for Occupational Therapy Practice*. COT, London.
5   NHS Training Directorate (1994) Just for the Record: A guide to record keeping for health care professionals. NHS Training Directorate, Bristol.
6   Kettenbach Ginge (2003) *Writing SOAP Notes*, 3rd edn. F.A Davis Company, Philadelphia.
7   Department of Health Records Management NHS Code of Practice April 2006.
8   Jack Malvern Patient bruised by hospital's blunt message The Times 15 May 2008 page 23.
9   Information Commissioner's Office (2006) Data Protection Good Practice Note How Does the Data Protection Act apply to professional opinions? ICO, London.
10 Paul Wilkinson, Notes on dead baby altered by nurse, *The Times*, 7 November 1995.
11 Peter Forster GP allowed patient to tamper with records. *The Times*, 7 July 1998.
12 College of Occupational Therapists (2003 revised 2007) *Professional Standards for Occupational Therapy Practice*. COT, London.
13 www.dh.gov.uk
14 UKCC (1998) *Guidelines for Records and Record Keeping*. UKCC, London; now reprinted by NMC 2008.
15 Department of Health Records Management NHS Code of Practice April 2006.
16 Audit Commission (1995) Setting the Records Straight: A Study of Hospital Medical Records. HMSO, London.
17 Department of Health Records Management NHS Code of Practice April 2006.
18 Department of Health (2007) Information Security Management: NHS Code of Practice.
19 Department of Health, 4 February 2001, *Patients to gain access to new at-a-glance Electronic Health Records*.
20 www.doh.gov.uk
21 College of Occupational Therapists (2007) Electronic Care Records- Involving OTs in design and implementation Briefing note no 95. COT, London.
22 www.nhscarerecords.nhs.uk
23 Department of Health Clear rules set for patients' electronic records May 2005.
24 www.nigb.nhs.uk
25 Brewin, M. (2002) Moving on: evolving consistent terminology to support electronic health and social care records. *British Journal of Occupational Therapy*, **65**(11), 522–4.
26 Helen Johnstone, Spelling mistake may have cost student her life. *The Times*, 28 August 1998.
27 National Audit Office (2008) The National Programme for IT in the NHS – progress since 2006 HC 484-1 Session 2007–8. Stationery Office, London.
28 Rose David Patients avoid NHS database blunders by keeping cards close to their chest The Times 26 December 2008.
29 College of Occupational Therapists (2007) *Professional Standards for Occupational Therapy Practice*. COT, London.
30 www.nhsla.com

13 Statements, Reports and Giving Evidence in Court

The increase in the number of cases in which patients are seeking compensation for harm has led to a greater possibility that the occupational therapist (OT) may be involved in giving evidence in court. In addition many OTs (especially those in independent practice) are developing their role in giving expert evidence. This chapter covers both aspects and also looks at the preparation of statements and reports and at some of the rules of evidence and the terminology which are likely to be encountered in court. The following topics are covered:

- Civil Procedure Rules introduced in April 1999
- Case Management in civil proceedings
- Statement making
- Report writing
- The OT in court or tribunal
- Witness of fact
- Expert witness
- Clinical negligence pre-action protocol
- Litigation in the NHS

Civil Procedure Rules introduced in April 1999

Failures in the old system of civil procedure were notorious and Lord Woolf was invited to examine the deficiencies and make recommendations for reform. In his report *Access to Justice* Lord Woolf noted the many hindrances to justice. In June 1995 he issued an interim report on access to justice.[1] This reported on recommendations to change our system of obtaining compensation for personal injuries. It was followed in January 1996 by a consultation document[2] with papers covering the following issues: 1. Fast track; 2. Housing; 3. Multi-party actions; 4. Medical negligence; 5. Expert evidence; 6. Costs.

Legal Aspects of Occupational Therapy, Third Edition By Bridgit Dimond
© 2010 Bridgit Dimond

The consultation paper on medical negligence cases considered that there should be considerable benefits from Lord Woolf's proposed reforms.[3] His specific proposals on medical negligence included:

- training of health professionals in negligence claims
- GMC and other regulatory bodies to consider the need to clarify the professional conduct responsibilities in relation to negligence actions
- improvement of record systems to trace former staff
- use of alternative dispute mechanisms
- a separate medical negligence list for the High Court and County Courts
- specially designated court centres outside London for handling medical negligence cases
- methods to reduce delays by improving arrangements for listing of cases
- investigation of improved training for judges in medical negligence
- standard tables to be used where possible to determine quantum
- practice guide on the new case management
- pilot study to consider medical negligence claims below £10 000.

Lord Woolf's final report was published in July 1996[4] and led to the implementation of a new procedure for civil claims in April 1999. The general rules form the core of a single, simpler procedural code which applies to civil litigation in the High Court and county courts.

Features of the new scheme include:

- A new system of case management, with the courts rather than the parties taking the main responsibility for the progress of cases.
- Defended cases are allocated for the purpose of case management by the courts to one of three tracks:
  - Small claims (up to £5000). This provides a procedure for straightforward claims which do not exceed £5000, without the need for substantial prehearing preparation and the formalities of a traditional trial, and where costs are kept low.
  - A new fast track with limited procedures and reduced costs (up to £10 000). Factors deciding whether a case is allocated to the fast track include: the limits likely to be placed on disclosure; the extent to which expert evidence may be necessary and whether the trial will last longer than a day. However, certain exceptions to the fast track were recommended and these included medical negligence cases.
  - A new multi-track (for more complex cases over £10 000).

The court allocates each case to one of these three tracks on the basis of information provided by the claimant on the statement of case. If it does not have enough information to allocate the claim then it will make an order requiring one or more parties to provide further information within 14 days.

Case management (see below) directions are given at the allocation stage or at the listing stage.

Case management in civil proceedings

The overriding principle enshrined in the new Civil Procedure Rules[5] (see Figure 13.1) is that all cases should be dealt with justly. The court must seek to give effect to this overriding principle when it exercises any powers under the rules and when it interprets any rule. The parties also have a duty to help the court to further this overriding objective. The court in furthering this principle of dealing with cases justly must actively manage the cases. Active management includes:

Figure 13.1   Overriding objective in civil proceedings.

The Civil Procedure Rules are a new procedural code with the overriding objective of enabling the court to deal with cases justly. Dealing with a case justly includes, so far as is practicable:

(1)   Ensuring that the parties are on an equal footing
(2)   Saving expense
(3)   Dealing with the case in ways which are proportionate:
    (a)   to the amount of money involved
    (b)   to the importance of the case
    (c)   to the complexity of the issues
    (d)   to the financial position of each party
(4)   Ensuring that it is dealt with expeditiously and fairly
(5)   Allotting to it an appropriate share of the court's resources, while taking into account the need to allot resources to other cases

- encouraging the parties to co-operate with each other in the conduct of the proceedings
- identifying the issues at an early stage
- deciding promptly which issues need full investigation and trial and accordingly disposing summarily of the others
- deciding the order in which the issues are to be resolved
- encouraging the parties to use an alternative dispute resolution procedure if the court considers that appropriate, and facilitating the use of such procedure
- helping the parties to settle the whole or part of the case
- fixing timetables or otherwise controlling the progress of the case
- considering whether the likely benefits of taking a particular step justify the cost of taking it
- dealing with as many aspects of the case as it can on the same occasion
- dealing with the case without the parties needing to attend court
- making use of technology
- giving directions to ensure that the trial of a case proceeds quickly and efficiently.

Statement making

Witnesses can refer to any contemporaneous records and statements in giving evidence and since it takes many years for some court hearings to take place, it is therefore vital that comprehensive clear records have been kept and statements made at the time of the incident. Before preparing a statement a health professional should have advice from a senior colleague and if possible a lawyer. (Many NHS trusts and primary care trusts and all local authorities have lawyers who would be able to provide advice and assistance on drawing up a statement.) The elements shown in Figure 13.2 should be contained in a statement.

The statement writer should ensure that the statement is:

- accurate
- factual
- concise
- relevant

Figure 13.2 Elements to include in a statement.

(1) Date and time of the incident
(2) Full name of maker, position, grade and location
(3) Full names of any persons involved, e.g. patient, visitor, other staff
(4) Date and time the statement was made
(5) A full and detailed description of the events which occurred
(6) Signature
(7) Any supporting statement or document attached

- clear
- legible (it will usually be typed)
- signed.

The statement maker should read it through, checking on its overall impact and whether all the relevant facts are included. A copy should be kept. Advice should be sought on its clarity and comprehensiveness and it should not be signed unless the maker is completely satisfied that it records an accurate, clear account of what took place. Many years later the statement could be used in evidence in court and it is an easy point for cross-examination (see later) if the witness contradicts in court what she put in her statement.

Report writing

Report writing to the OT will have a very different meaning from report writing to an expert witness. Both areas will be covered in this section.

Reporting on clients

The OT would be required to follow the accepted standards of report writing. The COT has, as part of its material on the occupational therapist and the court,[6] provided advice on report writing with a useful checklist for the format of any report.

Principles to be followed in report writing

- Identify the purpose of the report (likely readership and the kind of language which can be used) and therefore the appropriate style to be used.
- Identify the main areas to be included.
- Decide the order to be followed: sometimes chronological order is appropriate, at other times subject order may be preferable.
- Identify the different kinds of information used in the report and state the source of the material (e.g. hearsay evidence; factual evidence observed or heard by the author of the report; evidence of opinion of another person; statements by others and similar fact evidence).
- Sign and date the statement but only after reading it through and being 100% satisfied with it.

Good report writing

For most purposes the style likely to be of greatest use is one of simplicity, with short sentences, clear paragraphing and sub-paragraphing, and avoidance of jargon and meaningless clichés. The report should begin with the statement as to its purpose, the person(s) to whom it is addressed, and the name and status of the writer. Other documents which are relevant should be carefully referenced. A conclusion should be reached at the end of the report which is substantiated by the contents of the report.

An analysis of possible conflicts for OTs who write reports for personal injury litigation with the COT Code of Ethics and Professional Conduct is made by Mary Sterry[7] in an article which contains useful advice for OTs in report writing.

Common mistakes in report writing

The following are some of the common mistakes found in report writing:

- lack of clarity
- too complex a style for the reader
- use of inappropriate jargon
- use of misleading abbreviations
- failure to follow a logical order
- inconsistency
- ambiguities
- inaccuracies
- lack of dates within the report
- wrong names included
- confusing account
- mix of evidence and sources
- opinion without facts
- failure to cite facts to support statements
- failure to give conclusions
- failure to base conclusions on the evidence
- lack of signature and/or date
- failure to ask someone else to read it through.

Reports by expert witnesses

Expert witnesses will normally be asked, by a solicitor representing one of the parties to the case, to prepare a report. This report is vital since, if it is unfavourable to the party seeking it, the outcome may be that the case is settled or even withdrawn. The effect of the Woolf recommendations on the role of the expert witness is considered below. Appendix 2 of the Medical Legal Forum's standards for expert witnesses provides extremely helpful advice and check lists for report writing.[8]

Reports and privilege

At present where an expert has prepared a report for a solicitor in anticipation or in the course of litigation, that report and any correspondence connected with it are protected by legal professional privilege and it cannot be ordered to be disclosed in court or the expert compelled to appear by the other side (see Chapter 8 on legal professional privilege). However, once the report is disclosed to the court it loses its professional privilege although this continues to attach to any correspondence between the parties which has not been disclosed. For example an expert may prepare a report on request but in the covering letter advise the solicitor that his client is likely to lose the case. Even if the solicitors do decide to disclose the report, the letter remains privileged. Under Rule 35(13) a party who fails to disclose an expert's report may not use the report at the trial or call the expert to give evidence orally, unless the court gives permission.

Some of the requirements on the form and content of an expert's report set out in Rule 33.3 of the Civil Procedure Rules[9] are as follows:

(1) An expert's report must:
    (a)   give details of the experts qualifications, relevant experience and accreditation;
    (b)   give details of any literature or other information which the expert has relied on in making the report;
    (c)   contain a statement setting out the substance of all facts given to the expert which are material to the opinions expressed in the report or upon which those opinions are based;
    (d)   make clear which of the facts stated in the report are within the expert's own knowledge;
    (e)   say who carried out any examination, measurement, test or experiment which the expert has used for the report and:
        (i)   give the qualifications, relevant experience and accreditation of that person,
        (ii)   say whether or not the examination, measurement, test or experiment was carried out under the expert's supervision, and
        (iii) summarise the findings on which the expert relies;
    (f)   where there is a range of opinion on the matters dealt with in the Report:
        (i)   summarise the range of opinion, and
        (ii)   give reasons for his own opinion;
    (g)   if the expert is not able to give his opinion without qualification, state the qualification;
    (h)   contain a summary of the conclusions reached;
    (i)   contain a statement that the expert understands his duty to the court, and has complied and will continue to comply with that duty; and
    (j)   contain the same declaration of truth as a witness statement.
This declaration of truth includes a statement as to whether he can or cannot give an opinion without qualification. The expert must also make a statement that he understands his duty is to the court and he has complied and will continue to comply with that duty.

The OT in court or tribunal

Giving assistance to the court

The College of Occupational Therapists (COT) has provided a step-by-step guide covering the basic information which an OT would require if she is asked to appear in court[10] It provides practical advice for an OT who is called as a witness of fact and has to provide statements and reports. It also covers the roles of the defendant and claimant, and going to court. In addition, it provides memory techniques and guidance to some of the common legal terms (see glossary of this book). Sections also cover Scotland and Northern Ireland. The COT has also published a briefing note on giving evidence in court in relation to the scope of professional practice.[11] In 2009 the COT Medical Legal Forum published guidance setting standards for expert witnesses which is considered below.[12] The skills of OTs in assessment mean that their evidence is relevant in a wide variety of court and tribunal hearings, as expert witnesses as well as witnesses of fact. An OT may be required to give evidence about a client's disability in relation to a client injured in a road accident where the amount of compensation is in dispute, where there is a dispute over the provision of services by the statutory authorities, or about any of the different client groups considered in Chapters 20–24 of this book. Other frequent occasions for an OT to give evidence are in applications relating to special educational needs, which are discussed in Chapter 23.

There are many examples of OTs being congratulated by the judge on their giving evidence, their report or the information they have provided to the court. Their assessments must of course be related to the evidence given to the court and in one case the Court of Appeal disallowed a sum for counseling. In this case[13] the claimant, Mrs Wells was severely injured in a road accident for which her husband had accepted liability. An occupational therapist had given evidence on behalf of the claimant that, although she had a limited intellectual function, she had some awareness of her condition and that could benefit from counselling. The Court of Appeal stated that in its view, the Judge should not have acted on that suggestion. The other evidence, including the video-film, demonstrated its invalidity. Mrs Wells has far too low a level of brain function to benefit from counselling as distinct from, and in addition to, the constant stimulus which her attentive family, the permanent company of her carers and her weekly physiotherapy and occupational therapy will give her. "Accordingly, we disallow the award for counselling in its entirety."

In another case[14] where defendants in a road traffic accident appealed against the award for personal injuries, the Court of Appeal was not prepared to allow the appeal:

> The claimant's representative stated that defendant had never suggested any job which Mr Pinnington might be capable of undertaking. During the evidence no realistic suggestions had been put to him or had been established on the evidence. At the time of his accident he was working as a craftsman with his hands. He has severe injuries to his right hip and knee and stiffness of his back and neck which limit his mobility, although of course they may be improved by surgery in the future. The modest computer skills he has acquired out of necessity are not a basis for employment. Reading is difficult because of his eye injury and a great deal of time is taken up in coping with the effect of his disabilities. In these circumstances the judge's acceptance of the evidence of an occupational therapist who had conducted three detailed assessments of Mr Pinnington could not reasonably be challenged on appeal.

Evidence in chief

Where a witness gives evidence and is questioned by the lawyer for the side who called her, this is known as evidence in chief. The witness cannot be asked leading questions when examined in chief, and the lawyer will take the witness through the statement that she has made.

Cross-examination

Cross-examination is the term applied to the opportunity for one side, A, (usually through lawyers) to question the witnesses called by the other side, B (and vice versa). There are two distinct objectives in cross-examination. The one is to discredit the witness or show that his or her evidence is irrelevant to the point being established. The other is to use this witness to strengthen the case of one's own side.

In pursuing the first aim, the cross-examiner will attempt to:

- undermine confidence of the witness
- show up inconsistencies and/or ambiguities in the evidence

- show how the evidence being given is contradicted by other witnesses
- show how the witness is unreliable and/or unintelligent.

In pursuing the second aim, the cross-examiner will attempt to ensure that the witness (for side A):

- gives evidence helpful to side B
- praises side B
- corroborates evidence being given by side B.

Attempts may also be made to use the witness to testify on professional/expert matters and express opinions useful to the other side.

Preparation and an unshakeable conviction in the accuracy of your evidence is essential for cross-examination.

Re-examination

After cross-examination, the side which has called the witness can re-examine the witness on any issues which have been raised in the cross-examination, in order to repair any damage created by the cross-examination.

Procedure

The stages which are followed in criminal courts and civil courts are shown in Chapter 2 on the legal system. Lord Woolf reviewed the system for obtaining compensation in civil litigation, and the recommendations contained in his paper were implemented in April 1999 and are considered at the beginning of this chapter. The implications for the use of expert witnesses are considered below.

Rules of evidence

This is a complex area and the rules depend on the nature of the court hearing. For example, hearsay evidence (where a witness gives evidence about what was reported to him/her by an eye witness and of which he or she does not have direct evidence) may be acceptable in some hearings, e.g. social security tribunals, but not acceptable in civil or criminal hearings except in very specific circumstances.

Some of the issues which are covered by the rules include:

- rules on relevance, admissibility and hearsay
- weight of evidence
- burden of proof
- degrees (standard) of proof
- presumptions
- judicial notice
- competence of witness
- compellability of witness
- corroboration
- doctrine of privilege (see Chapter 8).

It is not possible in a work of this kind to give full details of the significance of the rules of evidence on the above topics and reference must be made to one of the specialist books listed for further reading.

Witness of fact

Anyone who can give evidence on a matter relevant to an issue before the court can be summoned to appear. The only grounds for refusing to attend and give evidence are if the evidence is protected by legal professional privilege against disclosure in court, or if, on grounds of national security or other public interest, a minister of state has signed a public interest immunity certificate that the information should not be disclosed. (Legal professional privilege and public interest immunity are considered in Chapter 8 on confidentiality.)

As a witness of fact the OT may be required to give direct evidence over a matter with which she has been involved. She should ensure that she keeps to the facts and does not offer an opinion. In some cases she may be asked to pronounce upon the prognosis of the client; she should not magnify the extent of the disability and the poor prognosis in order to obtain more compensation for the client. The practitioner has to ensure that her professional standards are maintained and that she tells the court honestly the nature of the prognosis as she sees it. She may need guidance and training in how to withstand cross-examination. It is vital that she does not express views outside her competence. Thus, whichever party calls her as witness, she should not alter the facts or emphasis to support that party but should give her evidence according to professional standards of integrity.

Evidence from witnesses of fact could also be given at criminal court hearings. Thus, in a case where a consultant psychiatrist was charged with indecent assaults on four women, two OTs were among the witnesses who gave character evidence called in his support.[15] His convictions were quashed by the Court of Appeal.

Key points for witness of fact

Preparation

- Ensure that the records are available.
- Identify with stickers significant entries, but do not mark or staple or pin anything to the records.
- Read the records through so that you are familiar with them.
- Try to obtain assistance from a lawyer or senior manager in preparation for the court hearing, so that you are prepared for giving evidence in chief and answering questions under cross-examination.
- Try to visit the court in advance to familiarise yourself with its location, car parking, toilet facilities, etc.

At the court before the hearing

- Be prepared for a long wait and take work to do or something to occupy yourself with.
- Dress appropriately and comfortably but not too casually.
- Try to relax.

Giving evidence

- Keep calm.
- Give answers clearly and without exaggeration.
- Tell the truth.
- Do not feel that you are there to represent only one side.
- Answer questions honestly even though it might put the side cross-examining you in a good light.
- Take time over your answers.
- Do not make up replies if you are unable to answer the question raised.
- Do not answer back or allow yourself to be flustered during the cross-examination.
- If you do not understand any legal jargon which is used, ask for an explanation.
- Keep to the facts and do not express an opinion.
- Ask for time to refer to the records if necessary.

Expert witness

An expert witness is invited to give evidence of opinion on any issue which is subject to dispute. It might be on what would be the appropriate standards of care which would have been expected according to the Bolam test (see Chapter 10). It may be for an opinion on the prognosis of the patient where the amount of compensation is disputed.

Impartiality and professional integrity

Under Part 35 of the new Civil Procedure Rules introduced in April 1999 following the Woolf Report, new rules apply to expert witnesses:

- Expert evidence must be restricted to that which is reasonably required to resolve the proceedings.
- It is the duty of an expert to help the court on matters which his expertise covers.
- This duty overrides any obligation to the person from whom he has received instructions or by whom he is paid.
- No party may call an expert or put in evidence an expert's report without the court's permission.
- The court has power to limit the amount of the expert's fees and expenses that the party who wishes to rely on the expert may recover from any other party.
- Expert evidence is to be given in a written report unless the court directs otherwise.
- The expert can ask the court for directions.
- A party who fails to disclose an expert's report may not use the report at the trial or call the expert to give evidence orally unless the court gives permission.

A Practice Direction[16] has given further instructions about expert evidence and has emphasised:

- Expert evidence should be the independent product of the expert uninfluenced by the pressures of litigation.
- An expert should assist the court by providing objective, unbiased opinion on matters within his expertise, and should not assume the role of an advocate.

Figure 13.3   Civil Procedure Rules on Experts and Assessors Rule 35.

- Interpretation
- Expert's overriding duty to court
- Court's power to restrict expert evidence
- General requirement for expert to give written report
- Written questions to expert
- Court's power to direct that evidence is to be given by a single joint expert
- Instructions to single joint expert
- Power of court to direct a party to provide information
- Contents of report
- Use by one party of expert's report disclosed by another
- Discussions between experts
- Consequences of failure to disclose expert's report
- Expert's right to ask court for directions
- Assessors

- An expert should consider all material facts, including those which might detract from his opinion.
- An expert should make it clear:
  - when a question or issue falls outside his expertise
  - when he is not able to reach a definite opinion, for example because he has insufficient information.
- If, after producing a report, an expert changes his view on any material matter, such change of view should be communicated to all parties without delay, and when appropriate to the court.

The Civil Procedure Rule 35, which can be accessed on the Ministry of Justice website,[17] sets out the rules relating to experts and assessors. It states that there is a duty to restrict expert evidence to that which is reasonably required to resolve the proceedings (Rule 35(1) and covers the topics shown in Figure 13.3. The overriding duty of the expert to the court is discussed below. The Civil Justice Council prepared a protocol for the instruction of experts to give evidence in civil claims in June 2005.[18] It is available on the Ministry of Justice website.[19]

It follows from these rules that an expert witness should not change her views according to the side which calls her. One useful rule for the practitioner to follow is to give an honest reasoned opinion whichever side calls her. She must not be partisan, nor should she on the one hand exaggerate or on the other belittle the amount of compensation. If she always gives an honest and professional view she will be respected by the solicitors who will know that they can trust her to withstand cross-examination as an expert witness and will know her to be reliable. She will not see the court battle as personally involving her and thus, whichever side wins, she will be able to feel that she has given an honest report to the court. In many cases judges have commented on the excellent evidence given by OTs and these cases show that a carefully prepared report, well substantiated, can reduce the length of a court hearing and enable many matters to be agreed by the parties, thus saving court time. Extremely helpful guidance is given by the COT's Medical Legal Forum which has set standards for the OT in giving expert evidence. There are also useful appendices setting out background training and information; guidelines for preparing an expert report and business aspects for those OTs who are independent practitioners (see Chapter 28).

Joint expert

The court has the power under the CPR to require a single expert to be appointed but there may be good reasons to accede to a party's request for another expert. For example in the case of *Daniels v Walker*[20] an injury was suffered by the claimant some ten years previously when he was six or seven and had been struck by a car. His injuries were very serious. There was a very substantial report by a jointly instructed occupational therapist, about which the defendant's solicitors were unhappy. However, the claimant's solicitors refused to make their client and his family available to be interviewed by an expert nominated by the defendant's solicitors. The defendant applied to the judge, who refused him permission to call any further expert evidence on the point, but allowed him to put written questions to the expert. The defendant appealed to the Court of Appeal, which allowed his appeal. Giving the leading judgment, the Lord Chief Justice, Lord Woolf, neatly encapsulated the point in the following two paragraphs:

> Where a party sensibly agrees to a joint report and the report is obtained as a result of joint instructions in the manner which I have indicated, the fact that a party has agreed to adopt that course does not prevent that party being allowed facilities to obtain a report from another expert, or, if appropriate, to rely on the evidence of another expert.
>
>   In a substantial case such as this, the correct approach is to regard the instruction of an expert jointly as the first step in obtaining expert evidence on a particular issue. It is to be hoped that in the majority of cases it will not only be the first step but the last step. If, having obtained a joint expert's report, a party, for reasons which are not fanciful, wishes to obtain further information before making a decision as to whether or not there is a particular part (or indeed the whole) of the expert's report which he or she may wish to challenge, then they should, subject to the discretion of the court, be permitted to obtain that evidence.

This ruling was cited with approval in a case[21] involving alleged non-accidental injury of a child where the parents challenged the fact that the court had relied upon the evidence of only one paediatric neuro-radiologist.

Client pressures

Some OTs find that clients place considerable pressure on them to make assessments in their favour, since a considerable sum of compensation may be dependent on the outcome, but this pressure must be resisted.

Situation: court assessment

> An OT was asked to assess a client for the purposes of quantifying the compensation payable in a road traffic case. The OT formed the view that the client was exaggerating his symptoms and that he in fact had far greater movement than he was admitting to. She noticed in particular that he was able to bend down and pick up his tea cup and saucer from the floor as they spoke. She included this fact in her report and received an extremely abusive reply from the client contradicting her.

In such a situation the OT has a professional responsibility to undertake an honest and thorough assessment and should not omit aspects of her findings even though these might be unwelcome to the client. It might help if she points out at the time some of those features she observes which the client might later disagree with.

Conflicting expert evidence

What is the situation if there is a clash between the evidence given by expert witnesses, who both purport to speak on behalf of a body of competent professional opinion? This was the situation which arose in the Maynard case,[22] mentioned in Chapter 10. The House of Lords held that where both sides were supported by equally competent professional opinion, then the claimant had not established the case.

Points to remember

The expert witness:

- does not take sides
- outlines her professional credentials (status, experience, appointments and academic qualifications)
- gives a professional, not personal, opinion
- understands on what issues and topics he or she has expertise
- provides a logical report (see above)
- always supports opinion with fact
- avoids confusing technical language and jargon
- avoids being verbose
- gives concrete understandable examples and uses everyday analogies
- keeps facts and opinions relevant to the issues before the court
- ensures that she understands the purposes of the proceedings
- dates and signs the report
- finds out where the court is and turns up
- makes sure that the case has not been adjourned before travelling
- does not stand on her dignity
- is acquainted with court procedure and the role of the judge, jury and counsel
- knows how to address the judge and others
- dresses appropriately
- does not get emotional and forget what to say
- knows the report and the facts contained in it
- does not deviate from the report or introduce new material
- believes what she has written and what she is saying
- is dispassionate about the outcome
- does not take an adversarial stance
- prepares for cross-examination
- remains calm under cross-examination
- does not exaggerate
- keeps to the facts
- does not try to hasten the case along
- does not try to be humorous.

Mediation

One of the results of the Woolf Reforms in civil justice is that the parties are encouraged to resolve the dispute before going to court, using mediation or other forms of resolution such as alternative dispute resolution. Often such processes can be linked with the complaints procedure (see Chapter 14) to avoid litigation. In mediation an independent mediator attempts to assist the parties to bring about an agreement to resolve the dispute. Unlike arbitration, the parties are under no compulsion to accept any ruling by the independent person. The annual report for 2000 of the NHS Litigation Authority points out the low uptake of mediation:

> Virtually everyone engaged in civil litigation pays lip service to the benefits of mediation, but in practice it is proving extremely difficult to persuade the parties to put their words into practice.

Clinical negligence pre-action protocol

As a consequence of the Woolf Reforms and the work of the Clinical Disputes Forum (a multi-disciplinary group formed in 1997 as a result of the Woolf recommendations) a clinical negligence pre-action protocol was drawn up which is now part of the Practice Directions which are part of the Civil Procedure Rules. This protocol requires parties to follow specific steps at the beginning of an action and they are penalised if they fail. Times are set for the response to requests for records etc.

Claim form is issued

The issuing of the claim form marks the beginning of the case. There are important time limits (see Chapter 10) within which the claim form (originally known as a writ) is issued. The claim form indicates that action is now being commenced. The claim form usually names the NHS trust as the defendant but it is possible for an individual employee to be named as a party and more than one defendant can be named.

Service of the claim form

The claim form must be sent to the defendant within four months of its issue. (In the past there was a requirement for personal service, i.e. the claim form had to be handed to the defendant personally. Now, however, the claim form is sent to a known address.) The defendant must then respond by filing a defence or an admission, or an acknowledgement of service. If the defendant fails to respond then the claimant may be able to obtain judgment in default.

The drafting of the documents or statements of case (once known as pleadings) is arranged by the respective parties' solicitors who often instruct counsel (i.e. barristers). A litigant may, however, represent himself. Strict time limits are laid down for the service and response to the documents. Under the Woolf reforms the documents exchanged between the parties should be simpler and be verified by the parties. If there are uncertainties, the court can require the parties to clarify any matter in dispute.

Pre-trial review

Eventually there will be an assessment of the situation by the parties, together with a registrar or judge, account taken of the number of witnesses to attend, exchange of any experts' medical reports and, finally, the case will be set down for hearing.

Payment into court

Rules about offers to settle and payments into court are set out in Parts 36 and 37 of the Civil Procedure Rules. In some cases where there is dispute over the amount of compensation but liability is accepted, the defendant will probably be advised to pay a sum in settlement of the case into court. If the claimant accepts this payment in, the defendant will be liable for the claimant's costs up to that point. The court will be notified that there has been a settlement of the case. A payment in may also be made where the defendant does not accept liability but is not confident of winning the case, and rather than risk losing and having to pay the costs of both sides, he offers a sum in full and final settlement.

If the claimant decides that the payment in is not acceptable, the case will continue. In these circumstances the judge is not told that there has been a payment in. He will not therefore be influenced by that in determining the case and deciding what compensation to award. If he awards less than the payment in or if he decides there is no liability by the defendant, then the claimant will have to pay both the defendant's costs from the time of the payment in as well as his own, since, of course, had the claimant accepted that sum deemed reasonable in comparison with the judge's award, there would have been no time-consuming and costly court hearing. These costs may well exceed the amount of the award. The judge has a discretion over whether to award the defendant the costs in these circumstances.

No win – no fees

Legal aid is being phased out from personal injury litigation. The Government has approved the system of conditional fees being introduced into this country. The claimant is able to negotiate, with a solicitor, payment on a 'no win – no fees' basis, i.e. if the claimant loses, his or her solicitor does not charge any fees. Costs of the successful defendant would still be owing, and insurance protection is taken out to meet these and other costs not covered by the agreement with the solicitor. Recent statutory changes enable a successful party to claim from the unsuccessful the enhanced fees agreed with lawyers under the conditional fee agreement.

The future

Ten years have now passed since the implementation of the Woolf Reforms in Civil Procedure and there are criticisms that there has been over management by judges and that the number of cases being brought to court has drastically reduced because of the burdensome pre-action protocols which require cases to be virtually ready for trail before proceedings can be issued.[23] In addition it is feared that the results of the no-win no-fee system has greatly reduced public funding of civil litigation and increased disproportionately the fees paid to lawyers. A consultation paper was published by the Law Society of England and Wales in April 2009 which invited views on a wide range of issues linked to the funding of litigation.

Conclusion

There are considerable fears about giving evidence in court and it is vital that any witness, whether expert or witness of fact, should be properly prepared for the occasion. Even though they are not on trial themselves, their professional standing and integrity is being put to the test and it is therefore essential that they follow the highest standard of professional practice. Developments in compensation schemes within the NHS and the NHS Redress Scheme are considered in Chapter 10. Criticism has been made of the Woolf Reforms and also of the No Win- No fee system of payment. A policy paper prepared by the Bar Council of England and Wales published on 23 April 2009 recommends a self-funding scheme that would pay lawyers at ordinary rates, with a successful claimant putting a slice of his damages into the fund to pay for future cases. It would sit alongside the legal aid scheme. Lord Justice Jackson is undertaking a review of the costs of litigation.

 Questions and exercises

1   You have been asked to appear as a witness in a case. Draw up a list of your fears and try to work out ways in which these fears could be resolved. Refer to the COT guidance on the OT and the court.
2   Try to attend a court hearing and analyse the way in which it operates, the procedure followed and the actions of judge, jury (if present), barristers, solicitors, court clerk, court usher, witness, and any other person taking part in the court proceedings.
3   Prepare a protocol for the preparation of a report as an expert witness.

References

1   Lord Woolf (1995) *Interim Report on Access to Justice Inquiry*. Lord Chancellor's Office.
2   Para. 13, Medical negligence in the new system, from *Final Report on Access to Justice*, July 1996. HMSO, London.
3   Lord Woolf (1996) *Access to Civil Justice Inquiry*. Consultation paper. Lord Chancellor's Office.
4   Lord Woolf (1996) *Final Report Access to Justice*. HMSO, London.
5   Grainger, I. & Fealy, M. (1999) *Introduction to the new Civil Procedure Rules*. Cavendish Publications Ltd, London.
6   Bond Solon Training (2006) *The Occupational Therapist and the Court: A step by step guide for occupational therapists and their staff*. COT, London.
7   Sterry, M. (1998) Personal injury litigation and the College of Occupational Therapists' Code of Ethics and Professional Conduct. *British Journal of Occupational Therapy*, **61**(6), 263–6.
8   College of Occupational Therapist (2009) *Medical Legal Forum Standards for practice for expert witnesses*. COT, London.
9   Civil Procedure Rules Stationery Office 2001, also available on the Lord Chancellor's website: www.opengov/lcd.org
10 Bond Solon Training (2006) *The Occupational Therapist and the Court: A step by step guide for occupational therapists and their staff*. COT, London.
11 College of Occupational Therapists (2007) *Occupational Therapists – Giving evidence in court and scope of practice*. Briefing note no 87. COT, London.
12 College of Occupational Therapist (2009) *Medical Legal Forum Standards for practice for expert witnesses*. COT, London.
13 *Wells v Wells* [1996] EWCA Civ 784, [1997] 1 WLR 652.
14 *Pinnington v Crossleigh Construction* [2003] EWCA Civ 1684.
15 *R v Ananthanarayanan* [1994] 2 All ER 847, CA.
16 www.justice.gov.uk/civil/procrules_fin/contents/parts/part35/practicedirection

17   www.justice.gov.uk/civil/procrules_fin/contents/parts/part35
18   Council of Justice (2005) *Protocol for the Instruction of Experts to give Evidence in Civil Claims.* Ministry of Justice, London.
19   www.justice.gov.uk
20   *Daniels v Walker* [2000] 1 WLR 1382.
21   *GW & Anor v Oldham Metropolitan Borough Council & Anor* [2005] EWCA Civ 1247.
22   *Maynard v West Midlands Regional Health Authority* [1985] 1 All ER 635.
23   West Lawrence Have the Woolf reforms worked? The Times 9 April 2009.

14 Handling Complaints

It is a statutory requirement that every healthcare and social service organisation has an efficient procedure for handling complaints. Handling complaints should not be seen as a negative exercise since feedback through the complaints machinery can become an effective method of quality assurance and improving standards. The following topics are covered in this chapter:

- Background to present complaints procedures
- The 2004 complaints procedure
- NHS and Social Services Complaints – a unified procedure
- Patient representative organisations
- Complaints and the private sector
- Other quality assurance methods
- Future developments

Background to present complaints procedures

A statutory duty was established under the Hospital Complaints Procedure Act 1985 for each health authority to set up a complaints procedure. This was evaluated in by the Wilson Committee in 1994[1] which saw the system for dealing with complaints relating to health services to be confusing, bureaucratic, slow and inefficient. The report reviewed the current situation and set objectives for any effective complaints system. The principles it identified are set out in Figure 14.1.

A new complaints procedure came into effect on 1 April 1996 implementing the majority of recommendations contained in the Wilson Report. It established three levels of complaints handling: local level; Independent review and the Health Service Ombudsman. This complaints procedure was itself reviewed in 2003 when the Department of Health published the results of an investigation

Legal Aspects of Occupational Therapy, Third Edition By Bridgit Dimond
© 2010 Bridgit Dimond

Figure 14.1   Principles of an effective complaints system.

(1)   Responsiveness
(2)   Quality enhancement
(3)   Cost-effectiveness
(4)   Accessibility
(5)   Impartiality

(6)   Simplicity
(7)   Speed
(8)   Confidentiality
(9)   Accountability

into the effectiveness of the complaints procedure established following the Wilson Report. The Department of Health publication, 'NHS Complaints Reform: making things right'[2] noted the following criticisms of the 1996 complaints procedure:

- It is unclear how, and difficult, to pursue complaints and concerns.
- There is often delay in responding when concerns arise.
- Too often there is a negative attitude to concerns expressed.
- Complaints seem not to get a fair hearing.
- Patients do not get the support they need when they want to complain.
- The independent review stage does not have the credibility it needs.
- The process does not provide the redress the patients want.
- There does not seem to be any systematic processes for using feedback from complaints to drive improvements in services.

The aims of the 2003 reforms to the complaints procedure were to establish clear national standards and accountabilities, devolution to clinicians and managers backed up by independent scrutiny, flexibility and ensure that patients can choose how they wish to pursue their concerns and have the support they need to help them do so.

The Department of Health recommended that there should be:

- Increasing support and information for people who make complaints through local patient advice and liaison services and independent complaints and advice services (see below).
- Patient feedback and customer care and training for NHS staff, including board members, to improve the way people are dealt with to help resolve complaints quickly.
- Subject to legislation, placing responsibility for independent complaints review with the Commission for Healthcare Audit and Inspection (CHAI), known as the Healthcare Commission.

The complaints procedure of 2004 (revisions in 2006 and 2009)

The new complaints procedure envisaged the similar three stages to the procedure following the Wilson report: local intermediate and Health Service Ombudsman, but the intermediate stage was made more independent by its being placed upon the Healthcare Commission. Regulations were brought into force on 30 July 2004[3] on a new complaints system and amended in 2006.[4] Guidance is provided by the DH on both sets of regulations and is available on its website. From the 1 April 2009 the independent stage of complaints investigation which was carried out by the Healthcare Commission (which was abolished and replaced by the Care Quality Commission) was taken over by the Health Service Ombudsman thus turning the 3 stage complaints procedure into a two stage complaints procedure.

The regulations cover:

- nature and scope of arrangements for the handling and consideration of complaints
- handling and consideration of complaints by NHS bodies
- handling and consideration of complaints by the Healthcare Commission (this stage was subsequently abolished in April 2009 and complainants who are dissatisfied can apply to the health service Ombudsman for further investigation)
- publicity, monitoring and annual reports.

The regulations require each NHS body and each primary care trust to make arrangements for the handling of complaints in accordance with the regulations:

> The arrangements must be accessible and such as to ensure that the complaints are dealt with speedily and efficiently, and that complainants are treated courteously and sympathetically and as far as possible involved in decisions about how their complaints are handled and considered.

The arrangements must be in writing with a copy given free of charge to any person who requests a copy.

Amendments were made to the Regulations in 2006[5] to facilitate the transfer of complaints which relate to social services, extending the persons who can be appointed as complaints managers (the complaints manager does not have to be an employee of the NHS body and can be appointed for more than one NHS body), changing the time limit for response to a complaint and broadening the remit of the Healthcare Commission in relation to complaints about NHS Foundation Trusts. (This second stage of the complaints procedure was abolished in April 2009 – and complainants can now apply to the health service Ombudsman)

A primary care provider (and this includes pharmacists, ophthalmic opticians, dentists, GPs and primary care trusts) must ensure that a complaints procedure is in place. A complex complaint is one that relates to several different NHS bodies or local authority or primary care providers or is already subject to a concurrent investigation. If the NHS trust or primary care trust arranges for the provision of services through an independent provider, they are required to ensure that the independent provider has arrangements in place for the handling of complaints in accordance with the regulations.

Excluded from the complaints regulations are:

- complaints made by an NHS body that relate to the exercise of its functions by another NHS body
- complaints by a primary care provider that relate either to the exercise of its functions by an NHS body or to the contract or arrangements under which it provides primary care services
- complaints made by an employee of an NHS body or primary care provider about any matter relating to his contract of employment
- complaints made by an independent provider about any matter relating to arrangements made by an NHS body with that independent provider
- complaints which relate to the provision of primary medical services in accordance with arrangements made by a PCT with a Strategic Health Authority under S.28C of the 1977 Act or under a transitional agreement
- complaints that are being or have been investigated by the Health Service Ombudsman
- complaints arising out of an NHS body's alleged failure to comply with a data subject request under the Data Protection Act 1998 or a request for information under the Freedom of Information Act 2000
- a complaint about which the complainant has stated in writing that he intends to take legal proceedings

- a complaint about which an NHS body is taking or is proposing to take disciplinary proceedings in relation to the substance of the complaint against a person who is the subject of the complaint
- a complaint the subject matter of which has already been investigated under these Regulations
- a complaint relating to a scheme under the Superannuation Act 1972.

The regulations require a complaints manager to be appointed by each NHS body. This may include a person who is not an employee of the NHS body and a person who is appointed as a complaints manager for more than one NHS body.

A complaint can be made by a patient, or any person who is affected by or likely to be affected by the action, omission or decision of the NHS body which is the subject of the complaint. A complaint may also be made by the representative of a person who has died, is a child or is unable by reason of physical or mental incapacity to make the complaint himself or has asked the representative to act on his behalf.

Time limits for making a complaint are six months from the date on which the matter which is the subject of the complaint occurred or first came to the notice of the complainant, but the complaints manager can investigate complaints outside these time limits if he is of the opinion that having regard to all the circumstances, the complainant had good reasons for not making the complaint within that period and it is still possible to investigate the complaint effectively and efficiently.

The College of Occupational Therapists has provided a briefing note on complaints and the OT.[6]

Procedure

The complaints manager must send to the complainant a written acknowledgement of the complaint within two working days of the date on which the complaint was made, together with details of the right to assistance from independent advocacy services.

Where the complaint was made orally, the acknowledgement must be accompanied by the written record with an invitation to the complainant to sign and return it.

The complaints manager must send a copy of the complaint and his acknowledgement to any person identified as the subject of the complaint.

Investigation

The complaints manager must investigate the complaint to the extent necessary and in the manner which appears to him most appropriate to resolve it speedily and efficiently. Where the manager thinks it would be appropriate to do so he can, with the agreement of the complainant, make arrangements for conciliation, mediation or other assistance for the purpose of resolving the complaint. The NHS body must ensure that appropriate conciliation or mediation services are available. He must take such steps as are reasonably practicable to keep the complainant informed about the progress of his investigation.

Response

The complaints manager must prepare a written response to the complaint which:

- summarises the nature and substance of the complaint
- describes the investigation under regulation 12 and
- summarises its conclusions.

The letter must be signed by the chief executive of the NHS body except in cases where for good reason the chief executive is not himself able to sign it, in which case it may be signed by a person acting on his behalf.

The letter must be sent to the complainant within 25 days (amended from 20 by the 2006 Regulations) beginning with the date on which the complaint was made unless the complainant agrees to a longer period in which case the response may be sent within that longer period.

The letter must notify the complainant of his right to refer the complaint to the Health Service Ombudsman

Copies of the response must be sent to any person who was the subject of the complaint and any other person to whom the complaint has been sent under the regulations.

Handling and considerations of complaints by the Health Service Ombudsman

Part III of the regulations enable a complainant:

- who is not satisfied with the results of an investigation (except where the complaint relates to an NHS Bursary scheme)
- where the investigation has not been completed within six months of the date on which the complaint was made or
- where the complaints manager has decided not to investigate because it was out of time

to request a consideration of the complaint by the Health Service Ombudsman within 6 months of the response being made. (Increased from 2 months by the 2006 Regulations).

The Health Service Ombudsman is then required to assess the nature and substance of the complaint and decide how it should be handled having regard to the views of the complainant, the views of the body complained about, the views of the Independent Regulator (where the complaint relates to a Foundation Trust) any investigation of the complaint and action taken as a result and any other relevant circumstances. The Health Service Ombudsman must notify the complainant as to whether it has decided to:

- take no further action
- make recommendation to the body which is the subject of the complaint as to what action might be taken to resolve it
- investigate the complaint further, whether by establishing a panel to consider it or otherwise
- consider the subject matter of the complaint as part of or in conjunction with any other investigation or review
- refer the complaint to a health regulatory body

Where the Health Service Ombudsman proposes to investigate the complaint it must within ten working days of the date on which it sent the notification, send the complainant and any other person to whom the notice was sent its proposed terms of reference for its investigation.

The Regulations cover the investigation by the Health Service Ombudsman, including the use of an independent panel to hear and consider complaints and its powers to request the production of such information and documents as it considers necessary to enable a complaint to be considered properly. Members and employees of an NHS body and any person who is or was a healthcare professional or employee of a healthcare professional are excluded from being a member of a panel. Detailed procedural rules are laid down for the panels. The report of the Health Service Ombudsman's investigation must include the specified information and be completed as soon as reasonably practicable. The report must be sent to the complainant with a letter explaining to him his right to take his complaint to the NHS body that was the subject of the complaint (and, in the case of a complaint involving a primary care provider, to the PCT), to any relevant strategic health authority and to the Independent Regulator for complaints about an NHS foundation trust, where he so requests. The Independent Regulator may make an individual request for a report or make a standing request that identifies a type of complaint for which he wishes to receive a report.

Part IV of the regulations requires each NHS body and the Health Service Ombudsman to ensure that there is effective publicity for its complaints arrangements. For monitoring purposes, each NHS body must prepared a quarterly report specifying the number of complaints received, the subject matter of the complaints, summarise how they were handled including the outcome and identify any complaints where the recommendations of the Health Service Ombudsman were not acted upon, giving the reasons. An annual report must be prepared on the handling and consideration of complaints and be sent to specified bodies including, the Health Service Ombudsman, the strategic health authority and PCT, as appropriate.

Criticisms by the Healthcare Commission and Patients Association

In October 2007 the Healthcare Commission (since April 2009 the Care Quality Commission) published its first audit on how the NHS trusts handled complaints which is available on the CQC website.[7] It found considerable variation in how complaints were handled across the country. Its report highlighted the issues shown in Figure 14.2. (The Healthcare Commission was absorbed within the Care Quality Commission in April 2009.) The Healthcare Commission was required to liaise with the Health Service Ombudsman on the transitional arrangements for complaints being passed from the former to the latter.

In September 2008 the Patients Association described the NHS complaints system as cumbersome, variable and as taking too long. Of the 500 patients polled, 69% said that they had wanted to complain about the healthcare they had received in the past 5 years. 29% of those who complained described the process as totally pointless, 20.5% as pointless and 19% as slightly pointless. More than 80% believed that there was not a culture of openness in the NHS when errors occurred and staff were not encouraged to report mistakes. The DH responded to the report by saying that it would be reforming the system so that patients' concerns were taken seriously. The Patients Association called for NHS trust boards to be publicly accountable for an open, transparent and

Figure 14.2 Criticisms by the Healthcare Commission on the 2004 complaints system.

- More needs to be done to make the complaints systems open and accessible, especially for those with learning disabilities and from ethnic communities;
- People who complain should be confident that their care will not suffer;
- Trusts should use complaints data to inform decision making
- Whilst there is no one-size-fits-all approach to investigating complaints, a common approach would improve risk management of complaints and manage the expectations of complainants
- There are no nationally available standard tools and resources such as case studies, checklists and training aids for staff.

timely resolution of complaints.[8] Following the Healthcare Commission Report into the deaths and A&E failures at Mid Staffordshire NHS Foundation Trust in March 2009 (available on the website of the Care Quality Commission), the Department of Health announced that all hospitals in England would have to publish the number and details of complaints that they receive and they would be published on the NHS website.[9]

NHS and Social Services Complaints: a single comprehensive procedure

Regulations relating to Social Services Complaints[10] came into force on 1st September 2006 They impose time-limits on making complaints, new timescales for handling stages of the process and provide greater independence at the final review panel stage. They can be downloaded from the Office of Public Sector Information[11] The NHS Complaints regulations were amended[12] following the White Paper commitment to develop a single comprehensive complaints procedure across health and social care by 2009. The amendments are intended to make the system more responsive and give better links with the arrangements for responding to social care complaints. Those people who fund their own care can voice their complaints about residential care to the Local Government Ombudsman. The Chief Executive of Counsel and Care echoed complaints about the current procedures being bureaucratic and unwieldly in a letter to the Times.[13] Stephen Burke stated that at present the length of time it currrently takes to negotiate the system and the amount of paperwork and effort involved actively discourages many older people and their families from raising a complaint.

The Department of Health issued a letter on 25 November 2008 to NHS Chief Executives and to LA Adult Social Services Directors setting out the key features of the single complaints system which was from 1 April 2009 to cover all health and adult social care services in England. These included:

- NHS and social care organisations being encouraged to ask people about their experiences of care and to use this information to help improve standards.
- A greater emphasis upon the quick resolution of straight-forward cases by managers and commissioners, as well as greater use of options such as mediation to resolve complex cases locally.
- Complainants and NHS and social care organisations being able to agree upon an individual timescale and approach to resolving a case.
- Complainants being able to complain directly to the PCT or local authority Adult Social Services commissioner rather than to the provider of the service.
- An end to the role of the Healthcare Commission as the first point of appeal for NHS cases that cannot be resolved locally.
- A complainant who is unhappy with the way their case has been handled still being able to ask the Health Service Ombudsman or the Local Government Ombudsman to review their case.

National Audit Office Report

The National Audit Office on 10 October 2008[14] published a report of the complaints system for the NHS and social care sector which was highly critical of existing procedures. Amongst the many issues which the DH was required to address were:

- The infrastructures for the two complaints systems have different legislative frameworks, accountability arrangements, numbers of stages and approaches to independent review.

- Potential demand is understated by the current volume of complaints in health and social care.
- The removal of the Healthcare Commission's independent review stage requires NHS trusts to improve the capability and capacity of their complaints handling functions.
- There are variations in approach to the investigation of social care complaints locally, with a mix of internal and external investigators and a lack of standards for investigations or investigators.
- There is currently limited dissemination of lessons on how services have been improved as a result of learning from complaints.
- It should be a requirement for registration with the CQC that providers show evidence of consistently acting on complaints.
- Networks of complaints managers can provide valuable support in improving complaints handling.
- Key features of effective local complaints handling include:
  - There is a need to establish an open and constructive complaints handling culture with commitment and leadership from senior management.
  - Complaints managers should be equipped with the requisite skills and training based on standards and guidelines agreed by VIAN (Voice for improvement action network).
  - All front-line staff should be provided with the skills and confidence to respond to concerns and complaints in an open and constructive manner, including training in customer service and complaints handling.
  - Clarity to service users should be provided about how to make a complaint and how, in general, their complaint will be handled.
  - There should be a tracking system which records how the complaints have been handled.
  - A comprehensive approach should be developed to getting feedback from the complainant.
  - The implementation of recommendations, service changes and improvements arising from complaints should be publicised.

Commission for Patient and Public Involvement in Health (CPPIH)

In accordance with the strategy set out in the NHS Plan,[15] the Commission for Patient and Public Involvement in Health (CPIHH) was established under section 20 of the NHS Reform and Health Care Professions Act 2002 in January 2003. Its functions, set out in section 20(2) of the 2002 Act, included advising the Secretary of State about arrangements for public involvement in and consultation about matters relating to the health service in England and the provision of independent advocacy services. It was abolished in 2008 when the Local Government and Public Involvement in Health Act 2007 set up Local Involvement Networks, came into force (see below).

Independent complaints and advice services (ICAS)

Under section 12 of the Health and Social Care Act 2001, the Secretary of State has a responsibility to provide independent advocacy services to assist patients in making complaints against the NHS. The independent complaints advisory services[16] were available nationally from September 2003. A consultation paper, 'Involving Patients and the Public in Healthcare'[17] was issued by the Department of Health in September 2001 for consultation on proposals for greater public representation to replace the community health councils (CHCs).

ICAS focus on helping individuals to pursue complaints about NHS services. They aim to ensure complainants have access to the support they need to articulate their concerns and navigate the complaints system, maximising the chances of their complaint being resolved more quickly and effectively. ICAS work alongside the trust-based patients' forums and patient advocacy and liaison services. Information about ICAS and the current range of pilot services is available on the Department of Health website.[18] It was announced in January 2006 that following a rigorous exercise, the DH awarded contracts to three organisations to deliver a new and improved Independent Complaints Advocacy Service from 1 April 2006. Community Health Councils were abolished in 2003 in England but retained in Wales.

Patient advice and liaison services (PALS)

A significant proposal in the NHS Plan[19] (see Chapter 17) was the patient advocacy and liaison services (PALS). The Plan envisaged that by 2002 PALS will be established in every major hospital with an annual national budget of around £10 million. All NHS trusts were required to establish a PALS service by April 2002. Their core functions were:

- to provide on the spot help and speed resolution of problems
- to act as a gateway to independent advice and advocacy services
- to provide accurate information about the trust's services and other related services
- as a key course of feedback to the trust, to act as a catalyst for change and improvement
- to support staff in developing a responsive, listening culture.

Patients' forums

Under section 15 of the NHS Reform and Health Care Professions Act, the Secretary of State had a duty to set up in every trust and primary care trust a body which was to be known as a patients' forum. The members of each patients' forum were appointed by the Commission for Patient and Public Involvement in Health. Statutory functions[20] were laid down in section 15(3) of the 2002 NHS Reform and Health Care Professions Act. In 2006 the DH published its report A Stronger Local Voice which announced that Patient Forums in England were to be abolished and replaced by local authority run Local Involvement Networks (LINKS) under the Local Government and Public Involvement in Health Act 2007.

Local Involvement Networks

Part 14 of the Local Government and Public Involvement in Health Act 2007 established local involvement networks for health and social services. Under section 221 each local authority is required to make contractual arrangements for the purpose of ensuring that there are means by which specified activities can be carried on in the area. The activities specified include:

- promoting and supporting the involvement of people in the commissioning, provision and scrutiny of local care services
- enabling people to monitor for the purposes of their consideration of specified matters (standard of provision of local care services, how they could be improved and whether and how they ought to be improved) and to review for those purposes the commissioning and provision of local care services

- obtaining the views of people about their needs for, and their experience of local care services and
- making these views known and making reports on recommendations about how local care services could or ought to be improved, to persons responsible for commissioning, providing, managing or scrutinising local care services.

Local care services means services provided as part of the health services and services provided as part of the social services of a local authority. The local involvement network (LINK) which results from these arrangements cannot include a local authority or health services organisation. The service providers must allow entry by local involvement networks. The local involvement network must provide an annual report which contains matters to be specified by the Secretary of State and sent to the local authority and NHS organisations in the area.

Regulations on local involvement networks came into force on 1 April 2008.[21] As a consequence of this, the patient forums and the Commission for Public and Patient Involvement in Health were abolished. The Audit Commission and the Healthcare Commission reported in June 2008 that the reforms costing £1 billion to make the NHS more efficient and patient-friendly have failed to have much impact. They stated that services have improved as a result of central targets and extra money but the marketisation initiative has yet to contribute much.

Consultation with patients

Section 11 of the Health and Social Care Act 2001 (now section 242 of the National Health Service Act 2006) places a duty on NHS trusts, Primary Care Trusts and Strategic Health Authorities to make arrangements to involve and consult patients and the public in service planning and operation and in the development of proposals for changes. An action seeking judicial review of a decision to close twin inpatient wards without consultation in breach of section 11 succeeded, the trust's defence of it being a decision taken in an emergency situation was not accepted.[22]

Complaints and the private sector

Individual hospitals and private practitioners can set up their own complaints procedures. There would be advantages, however, in their following the same principles as those accepted for the public sector. There would in particular be benefit to them in ensuring that at some stage in the procedure the complainant would be able to secure the assistance of an independent person or review panel. It may be that those working in independent practice could provide a panel from which independent persons could be chosen to investigate or mediate a complaint. Under the 2004 complaints procedure if an independent occupational therapist were to contract with an NHS organisation for the provision of services, it would be a requirement that the occupational therapist has in place a complaints procedure.

Concern was expressed that elderly people who paid for their care (and they make up almost half of the 440,000 care home residents in the UK) did not have recourse to any body to whom they could make their complaints since CSCI did not have the jurisdiction. It has been suggested by the Department of Health that they should make their complaints about social care to the Local Government Ombudsman. The current review of the complaints system should take into account the complaints of those who fund their own care. The Health Act 2009 includes provision for the Commission for Local Administration in England to have powers to investigate complaints about privately arranged or funded adult social care. Schedule 5 to the Act 2009 sets out the detailed provisions.

Complaints and litigation

Case: *R v Canterbury and Thanet DHA and another, ex parte F and W*[23]

Complaints were made under the previous hospital complaints procedure by eight families that a doctor employed by the first defendants and seconded to the second defendants diagnosed sexual abuse when it should not have been so diagnosed and delayed in telling the parents of the diagnosis. A legal aid certificate was obtained by one of the complainants. The doctor withdrew her co-operation in view of the possibility of legal proceedings. The defendants subsequently considered that an inquiry was inappropriate. The complainants applied for judicial review contending *inter alia* that there was a duty to review their complaints.

The court held that the complaints procedure was not appropriate where litigation was likely because:

- the purpose of the inquiry was either to obtain a second opinion and a change of diagnosis or to enable the health authority to change its procedures in the light of matters brought to its attention during the investigation; and
- the procedure depends on the co-operation of the doctor concerned which obviously would not be forthcoming if legal proceedings were likely.

Complaints and the Occupational Therapist

Reports on the investigation of complaints have frequently shown that whatever the substance of the original complaint, the way in which it has been handled gives grounds for complaint. It is essential that all OTs are familiar with the complaints procedure, that they know how an informal complaint should be dealt with, how the complainant should be advised and take every step to prevent the handling of the complaint becoming itself a ground for complaint. It is a challenge for OTs to use complaints constructively to ensure that the quality of services is improved.

Individuals who have complaints about the services provided in the NHS do not have any contractual right to bring an action before the court for breach of contract. If harm has been suffered as a result of a failure or omission, they may have a successful claim in the law of negligence (see Chapter 10) or if a service has not been provided they may in exceptional circumstances be able to bring a case of breach of statutory duty for failure to provide that service (see Chapter 6) or seek judicial review of administrative failures. They may now, depending on the nature of the complaint be able to argue a violation of one of the principles set out in the NHS Charter (see appendix 2 and Chapter 6). The NHS Constitution recognises the following rights of patients:

Complaint and redress:

You have the right to have any complaint you make about NHS services dealt with efficiently and to have it properly investigated.

You have the right to know the outcome of any investigation into your complaint.

You have the right to take your complaint to the independent Health Service Ombudsman, if you are not satisfied with the way your complaint has been dealt with by the NHS.

You have the right to make a claim for judicial review if you think you have been directly affected by an unlawful act or decision of an NHS body.

You have the right to compensation where you have been harmed by negligent treatment.

Other quality assurance methods

There are, however, many other mechanisms to ensure the maintenance of high standards of health-care although these cannot be directly implemented by the patient. The White Paper put forward a strategy for improving quality assurance and its mechanisms which included the establishment of a National Institute for Health and Clinical Effectiveness (NICE), a Commission for Health Improvement which was replaced by the Commission for Health Audit and Inspection (CHAI) (known as the Healthcare Commission) and which was subsequently absorbed into the Care Quality Commission, and National Service Frameworks for national standards. The statutory duty to ensure quality of services was the foundation for the establishment of Clinical Governance whereby chief executives and Trust Boards are held accountable for the clinical performance of their organisations. These initiatives are further considered in Chapter 17.

Conclusions

Radical changes have been made to the scheme for handling complaints and for obtaining compensation in respect of clinical negligence. Yet the complaints scheme established in 2004 has met with considerable criticisms. It remains to be seen if revisions can be made to ensure that the principles set out in Figure 14.1 can be met.

The Health Service Ombudsman has since 1 April 2009 taken over the second stage of independent review of a complaint. It can provide reports on the effectiveness of the local procedures in resolving complaints and can also indicate how the lessons learnt from complaints have led to improvements in overall quality standards. If league tables are published relating to the level of complaints, care must be taken on how they are used. It is dangerous to assume that an absence of complaints is indicative of a satisfactory service or, conversely, that many complaints show that an organisation is worse than one with fewer complaints. There are many reasons why people do not complain even when there is a perceived reason to complain and it could be that the organisation with no complaints is so appalling that patients consider that complaining would be a waste of time. Any league tables should, however, highlight the speed and efficiency with which complaints are handled.

It is in the interests of all health professionals to ensure that any complaints by parents and children relating to the provision of health and social services are resolved informally, as speedily as possible, without requiring the complainant to make use of the formal procedure.

OTs should have the confidence to realise that complaints can be a useful way of monitoring and improving the services to clients and that it takes courage to make a complaint, especially where the client suffers from a chronic condition. Constructive advances can be made if clients are prepared to discuss with health professionals ways in which the services could be improved. Every complaint should be dealt with objectively and no assumptions made about the genuineness of the complaint or grounds for it until it has been effectively and thoroughly investigated.

Questions and exercises

1   Obtain a copy of the report prepared in October 2007 by the Healthcare Commission on complaints and the National Audit Report of 2008 on complaints handling and see if there are any lessons for your particular OT services.
2   A client tells you that he is not happy with the care provided by another health professional. What action do you take and what advice do you give?
3   In what way could the handling of informal complaints be improved?

References

1   DoH (1994) *Being Heard. The Report of a review committee on NHS complaints procedures.* Department of Health, London. (The Wilson Report).
2   Department of Health, NHS Complaints Reform: making things right, DH, London, 2003.
3   The National Health Service (Complaints) Regulations 2004 SI 1768.
4   The National Health Service (Complaints) Amendment Regulations 2006/2084.
5   The National Health Service (Complaints) Amendment Regulations 2006/2084.
6   College of Occupational Therapists (2007) Complaints against the occupational therapist Briefing note no 80. COT, London.
7   www.cqc.org.uk/
8   Rose David 'Pointless' NHS complaints system to become less rigid The Times 22 September 2008.
9   Rose David Hospitals will be forced to publish complaints details The Times1 May 2009.
10 The Local Authority Social Services Complaints (England) Regulations 2006 SI 2006/1681.
11 www.opsi.gov.uk
12 The National Health Service (Complaints) Amendment Regulations 2006 No 2084.
13 Burke Stephen Letter to the Editor The Times 11 October 2008.
14 National Audit Office (2008) Feeding Back Learning from complaints handling in health and social care Report by the comptroller and auditor General HC 853 Session 2007–2008.
15 DH, NHS Plan Cm 4818, 1 July 2000 (Chapter 10).
16 Information on ICAS is available from the DH website www.dh.gov.uk/complaints/
17 Department of Health, Involving Patients and the Public in Healthcare, DH, London, September 2001.
18 www.dh.gov.uk/complaints/advocacyservice.htm
19 Department of Health, The NHS Plan: a plan for investment, a plan for reform, Cm 4818-1, DH, London, 2000; www.nhs.uk/nhsplan/contentspdf.htm
20 Section 15(3) NHS Reform and Health Care Professions Act 2002.
21 The Local Involvement Networks Regulations SI 2008/528.
22 *R (On the application of Morris) v Trafford Healthcare NHS Trust* [2006] EWHC 2334.
23 *R v Canterbury and Thanet District Health Authority and South East Thames Regional Health Authority, ex parte F and W (QBD)* [1994] 5 Med LR 132.

15 Equipment and Medicinal Products

Occupational therapists (OTs) spend much of their time in assessment for and provision, installation and maintenance of equipment. The law relating to this is therefore of importance to their practice. Liability in relation to the transport of equipment is considered in Chapter 16. See also Chapter 18 and the direct payment scheme for community care services including equipment. The following topics are considered in this chapter:

- Community Equipment Services
- Supply of equipment and determination of priorities
- Refusing to supply equipment
- Choice of equipment
- Wheelchairs
- Referral by non-occupational therapists
- Disputes with clients
- Reissue of equipment
- Manufacturing equipment for specific needs
- Adaptations to equipment by the OT

- Common law rights against a supplier
- The Consumer Protection Act 1987
- Medical Devices Regulations
- Adverse incident reporting procedures
- Installation options
- Maintenance
- Exemption from liability
- Use of equipment by a non-client
- Failure by the client to follow instructions
- Insurance cover
- Medicinal products

The legal issues relating to the safe use of disability equipment and manual handling are considered in a two-part article by Michael Mandelstam[1] and also in a book by the same author.[2] The COT in 2008 published a position statement on community equipment[3] setting out the role of OTs and the COT and declaring that:

Everyone in England, regardless of whether they pay for themselves or are supported by the state, has the right to information, advice and assistance to help them select the most appropriate equipment.

The COT has also published in 2008 guidance on how equipment can make your life easier.

Legal Aspects of Occupational Therapy, Third Edition By Bridgit Dimond
© 2010 Bridgit Dimond

Community equipment services

In the past there has been confusion over which of the statutory authorities had the responsibility of providing equipment, and funding problems led to disputes. A report by the Audit Commission in 2000[4] drew attention to the deficiencies in community equipment services. A revisit two years later by the Audit Commission found that some services still remained in a parlous state and that although £220 million in additional funding was made available, little had actually reached frontline equipment services.[5] Current planning within the NHS and social services is based on greater co-operation and co-ordination in the provision of community equipment services. Guidance issued in 2001[6] sets out the action which should be taken to improve provision of community equipment by the development of integrated local authority and NHS equipment services. A lead senior officer in each organisation and a single lead officer to head the planning work had to be appointed by the end of July 2001. Additional guidance was provided in March 2001.[7] The strategy for an integrated community equipment service was envisaged in the intermediate care guidance.[8] The guidance is discussed in Chapter 24. The National Service Framework for older people (see Chapter 24) Standard 2 required that single integrated community equipment services were in place by April 2004. The new resources for community equipment in the access and systems capacity grant must be invested in a pooled budget in accordance with the grant conditions.[9] Any services which form part of a package of intermediate care (see Chapter 18) must be provided free of charge for six weeks (the time limit can be extended in exceptional circumstances). Any item of community equipment which a person (or their carer) is assessed as needing as a community care service, and for which the individual (or their carer) is eligible, is required to be provided free of charge.[10] All minor adaptations costing £1000 or less (which includes the cost of buying and fitting the adaptation) are required to be provided free of charge. Councils retain the discretion to make a charge in relation to minor adaptations that exceed £1000 to provide. The COT published guidance on the changes to the LA charging regime for community equipment in 2003 which was revised in 2007.[11]

The Prime Minister launched the transforming community equipment and wheelchair services (TCEWS) programme in June 2006. The aim of the programme was to develop a new model for community equipment and wheelchair services in England and to look at how to make the best use of the strengths of the third and private sector. The model is not mandatory but it effectively demonstrates a way to deliver a personalised service, for both self funders and those supported by the state. Further information can be obtained from the DH website.[12] (See also Chapter 18 for a discussion on the social care reform agenda and the care services efficiency delivery programme.)[13] Integrated Community Equipment Services (ICES) Team supports and encourages the development of modern, integrated community equipment services in England.[14]

Supply of equipment and determination of priorities

Given the limitation on resources it is inevitable that there is a waiting list for equipment for home use. Even if the equipment is available there might still be a delay in arranging installation. This is a major concern to those who have recommended equipment since there may be liability if harm should occur while the client is waiting for the delivery and/or installation. The determination of priorities is part of the duty of care owed by the community professional to the client. If a community professional fails to assess the urgency of a client's need for equipment and harm befalls the client, then there is likely to be an investigation as to the priority which had been attached to that client's needs in comparison with the needs of others. In the case of *Deacon v McVicar*[15] the judge ordered the disclosure of the records of the other patients on the ward at the same time as those of the claimant patient, in order to assess whether sufficient regard had been made to the needs of the claimant patient in comparison with the needs of the other patients on the ward at the same time. This is an unusual step but it indicates that the determination of priorities is a legal duty and can be evidenced from the records if they are properly kept.

Priority setting has become even more important since the introduction of a legal duty under the NHS and Community Care Act 1990 for social services to assess patients, in conjunction with health service professionals and others, for community care. It is clear that a thorough assessment will reveal needs not all of which can be met immediately. The House of Lords[16] has accepted the principle that both the duty to assess for care and the duty to provide care under the Chronic Sick and Disabled Persons Act 1970 are influenced by the resources available and this is further discussed in Chapter 20.

Determining priorities must take into account both the care and facilities available and also the priority between different patients. It is essential that the different professional groups working in the community have a major input into the determination of priorities and all levels of decision making (see Chapter 10 on the accountability aspects of this). Caroline Wright and Elizabeth Ritson[17] carried out an investigation into prioritising in a London Borough and concluded that the study highlighted the importance of receiving accurate information at the point of referral, and the necessity of discussing needs and priorities with service users before deciding how quickly a client should be seen by the service. The study also demonstrated how the priorities of service users may differ from those of the service provider. The study led to a need for change within the priority system and the way that referrals were processed by the department. It also led to further discussions about the importance of bathing and furthered the debate on essential activities versus those that enhance quality of life. Often there are significant waiting times for assessments by social services OTs for clients with learning disabilities/dementia or other conditions to determine whether they can remain in their own homes and what equipment is required. Setting priorities is essential.

Costly equipment

An example of the range of sophisticated equipment now available and for which there may be inadequate funding is the facility known as Snoezelen, for those with learning or other disabilities. Such a facility requires not simply the tubes, other equipment and mattresses, but also the accommodation. It is important that the value and effectiveness of such equipment is researched to justify any priority given to its purchase.[18] A more recent evaluation of Snoezelen in dementia is provided by Erik van Diepen and colleagues.[19] They conclude that the effects of Snoezelen on agitated behaviour in patients with dementia were encouraging.

Even more costly than Snoezelen is the equipment for tetraplegic patients, including computers and environmental control units (ECUs). Curtin[20] points out that objective assessments and demonstrations are essential if patients with a tetraplegic spinal cord injury are to achieve the maximum benefit of technical equipment such as computers and ECUs. Similar considerations apply to the use of powered wheelchairs.[21] In Curtin's study a research OT was able to work with OTs at the National Spinal Injuries Centre to evaluate those powered chairs available in the UK, to establish an effective and objective assessment procedure, and to implement a training programme so that OTs remain aware of new developments.

Refusing to supply equipment

It may be that the decision following a request for equipment is that none should be provided. This decision is also part of the duty of care and the professional who makes that determination should be able to justify it. It is therefore essential that comprehensive records are kept in case the decision is questioned at a much later date. Each such decision involves the use of professional discretion which can rarely be supplanted by written procedures and policies. An occupational therapist exercising her professional judgement that equipment is not required according to the clinical criteria of the patient's condition cannot be forced to provide the equipment (see Chapter 6 and the case of *Burke v GMC*).

Where equipment is supplied by the NHS charges cannot be levied and maintenance must be carried out by the NHS. Where NHS budgets are tight and the OT is aware that a patient receiving continuing healthcare is being refused vitally required equipment, she would have a duty to put in writing to her managers the situation, so that a decision on priorities can be properly made.

Another aspect of the decision over whether OT services should be provided is the following situation.

Situation: Failure to collect prescribed equipment

An OT becomes aware that a patient has no intention of collecting prescribed equipment (e.g. a 4 wheeled walker for mobility practice). Would she be legally entitled to cease further therapy if the equipment is essential to it?

The OT has a duty of care to the patient. She also has a duty to ensure that she uses resources reasonably. If she is aware that failures on the patient's part (e.g. failing to collect equipment, failing to carry out instructions) reduce the value of her services to the patient, then she has to decide whether the provision of her services is of benefit to the patient. Clearly there needs to be good communication with the patient to explain the position and excellent documentation of the information given and the action taken. In the end she would have to satisfy the Bolam Test of what the OT following reasonable professional practice would do (see Chapter 10). In such situations it would be helpful to discuss the situation with a manager or colleague.

Choice of equipment

The community professional has to make a determination of the nature of the equipment required by the client, choice of supplier and any other features in relation to the individual circumstances and physical and mental capabilities of the client. The individual circumstances will also require consideration of the carers and their capacities. Alternatives other than the provision of equipment are also important. For example, it may be that there is a danger in clients making use of the equipment on their own and additional visits by community staff are advisable instead. Or it may be unsafe for a client to attempt to bath on her own and the provision of equipment for her to do so might endanger her safety.

The decision of which manufacturer out of a bewildering range of products, many of which are newly on the market, requires the OT to keep constantly up to date with new items or designs and requires constant training and contact with manufacturers and suppliers. The most frequent articles to be found in professional journals for OTs are those relating to equipment.

Failures by the OT, in selecting equipment which no reasonable therapist would have selected for a specific client, could lead to liability if harm is incurred. The Bolam test would be applied to determine the standard of care which the OT should have followed (see Chapter 10). In addition, the OT must be aware of the cost implications of the equipment she is recommending and have access to a value for money audit which is kept up to date. Disability Living Centres and Equipment Assessment Centres can provide guidance. For example, the Disability Equipment Assessment Centre at Southampton, a Department of Health funded programme, provides such a service of equipment evaluation.[22] Helen Pain at that DEAC has written with others a guide on choosing disability equipment.[23] All OTs should recognise their duty to give feedback to such centres and to manufacturers and suppliers, to ensure that any potential dangers, hazards or weaknesses in equipment are identified and the appropriate action taken. Paying top prices will not necessarily fund the most appropriate equipment as an evaluation of chairs for people with arthritis and low back pain showed.[24]

In the choice of equipment it is important that the OT has access to feedback from monitoring reviews. For example, Chamberlain and colleagues[25] looked at the long-term usefulness of equipment and adaptations provided by social services OTs. They found that 83% of the equipment was still being used 18 months to 2 years after issue and 69% on a daily basis. They also noted that people rated the equipment more useful if they were able to use it alone. As a consequence of the study they recommended that there should be a review of systems to ensure that service users and carers are competent in using the equipment issued to them and are aware of how to contact the service if reassessment, repair or return of the equipment is needed.

Janet Heaton and Claire Bamford[26] provide a useful analysis of the key information required to assess the outcomes of equipment and adaptations and provide useful tables of existing measures of functional and health status.

Situation

An OT recommends that a disabled person should have a shower installed. Unfortunately when the client turns it on scalding water rushes out and because of his incapacity he cannot switch it off quickly and is therefore severely injured. Who is liable for his injury?

The OT would have a duty to ensure that any shower she recommended was suitable to meet the specific disability needs. A person with learning disabilities would therefore have a shower where the temperature was controlled. A person with physical disabilities, who was unable to manage certain types of controls, should have that taken into account in selecting the equipment. If, however, the shower was of faulty manufacture, then the makers or suppliers would be liable under the Consumer Protection Act 1987 discussed below.

The choice of equipment for people with restricted growth is considered by Jill Jepson.[27]

Wheelchairs

One area where constant training is required is in the selection of wheelchairs. An article by Silcox[28] starts with a quote from the McColl report:[29]

The number of people in unsuitable wheelchairs indicates that standards of wheelchair assessment, prescription and advice are inadequate.

Many accidents occur with wheelchairs and clearly the OT owes a duty of care to the client to ensure that her advice and prescription for the appropriate wheelchair is in accordance with the standards of the reasonable practitioner. Silcox points out:

> It would seem to be important to get uniformity into this area of therapist training, if therapists are to say that they offer an informed, caring and professional service to their disabled customers.

The need for alternative controls for wheelchairs may also require investigation[30] as well as the use of stump boards.[31]

The need to ensure that other professional staff, such as general practitioners, are also trained in the appropriate prescribing of wheelchairs has been demonstrated.[32] Research by White into referrals for wheelchairs[33] showed a fragmented service where the referrals for wheelchairs were being increasingly devolved to OTs, many of whom were part-time. The need to provide training was clear and also there was a need to provide training for doctors and other personnel who make referrals, to reduce the number of inappropriate referrals. She suggests also that there should be a national policy specific to wheelchair provision to ensure a fair system for all wheelchair users. The needs of short-term users with specialist needs should be recognised. There is also a need for funding to ensure that specialist assessment can take place and for the development of a database.

In February 1996 John Bowis, a junior health minister, announced[34] that severely disabled persons were to be offered powered wheelchairs (electrically powered indoor/outdoor wheelchairs (EPIOC)) on the National Health Service under a £50 million scheme. The need for training by OTs in the selection and use of such equipment was emphasised. The funding was for four years only. The scheme for EPIOCs was reviewed by the Department of Health in 2000.[35] In October 2003 a programme was introduced to develop mobility and functional maps to be completed by consumers when they choose wheelchairs. Rosemary Evans[36] studied users' views on the effect of EPIOC on occupation. She found that participants had increased opportunity to be independent and to have control over their occupations as a result of EPIOC use, and that it may also have had a positive effect on health. She suggested that further research with a larger sample might justify continued provision.

White's research raises numerous issues which apply across the whole field of the prescription and supply of equipment. There are considerable advantages in more central direction in the guidance from Government departments. Elizabeth White followed up her earlier investigations with research into the effectiveness in the post-devolution wheelchair service.[37]

The NHS Wheelchair Service

The NHS Wheelchair services are run by strategic health authorities which are responsible for allocating funds to the Wheelchair Service and PCTs who provide the service. This may include contracting out the running of the service to an outside company. Eligibility criteria, the timescales of provision and the types of chair offered vary between different areas. Four types of powered wheelchair are offered because a user cannot propel or use a manual wheelchair: electric indoor chair (user-controlled); electric outdoor chair (attendant-controlled); electrically powered indoor/outdoor chair (user-controlled) and dual purpose chair – user-controlled indoors, attendant-controlled outdoors. Further information on the service, referrals, assessments, maintenance and repairs can be obtained from the direct government website.[38] Information on the voucher schemes for hiring or buying a wheelchair is available from the same site, which considers other options for obtaining a wheelchair. A new wheelchair service for Wales was announced in 2002 and information on it provided by the CSP Wales.[39] The National Wheelchair Managers Forum published standards for wheelchair services in 2004.[40]

Safety of wheelchairs

Many warnings have been issued by the MHRA (see below) in relation to wheelchairs – some have been noted above. A MHRA warning issued in 2005[41] noted that an incorrectly fitted or adjusted posture belt attached to a wheelchair can lead to death or serious injury to a wheelchair user. Were an occupational therapist to act in ignorance of these warning notices and harm were to be caused to a client or other person, there would be a prima facie case of negligence. If death occurred there could be criminal prosecution for manslaughter. There would also be disciplinary action by an employer and possibly fitness to practice proceedings before the Health Professions Council. The MHRA issued guidelines on wheelchair stability in 2004[42] which were followed by discussions with manufacturers to produce a simplified set of guidelines. These are available from the MHRA website.[43] The Muscular Dystrophy Campaign published guidelines on best practice in providing wheelchairs and special seating for those with muscular dystrophy in 2006.[44] It can be downloaded free from the website[45]

Care Services Efficiency Delivery

In June 2006 the then Prime Minister announced the launch of a Transforming Community Equipment and Wheelchair Services Programme as part of the Care Services Efficiency Delivery (CSED) Programme (see above and Chapter 18). The new system changed the way that equipment is provided with accredited retailers exchanging equipment for a prescription. The aim is to give state supported users the choice that they have not previously enjoyed. They also have the option of topping up existing prescriptions to a different product within the same functional range to suit the user's lifestyle or preference. Further information can be obtained from the CSED website[46] and from the DH community equipment services' site.[47] The Wheelchair services programme has, at the time of writing not been established and further evidence is being collated. Details of the objectives and content of the programme can be found on the CSED website. The retail equipment prescription scheme can lead to legal issues as the following situation illustrates:

Situation: Too costly

A patient, with multiple sclerosis, requires a profiling bed which would enable her to transfer from the bed without the support of her husband who has back problems and would also prevent painful spasms at night. The equipment service will provide a single profiling bed for her, but not for the husband. They are willing to pay towards a double bed with profiling on one side, but the equipment service say that this is not an option and they would have to pay the full cost. What are the legal implications?

If the equipment service is able to provide a single profiling bed, then there would appear to be no reason in law, why the cost of this could not be used as a contribution to the double bed with the couple paying the remainder. The bed would probably have to be made to order and therefore the cost to the couple quite high.

Donations of used items

Situation: a dubious gift

> Mary White, an occupational therapist, is offered a wheelchair which belonged to an MS sufferer who had recently died. The family had bought it for the patient and it was almost new. Mary was grateful to receive it, since she knew of a client, Angela Jones, who was anxious to have a wheelchair as soon as possible. She arranged for it to be collected and delivered to Angela. Only a few days later, she learnt to her horror that one of the wheels on the chair had broken and Angela had suffered serious injuries from falling from the chair. Mary is concerned that she may be liable. What is the law?

In the above situation Mary has a duty of care to Angela. The question would be asked: what would be the reasonable standard of an OT in arranging for the issue of a wheelchair whatever its provenance? Clearly Mary should have arranged for the chair to be checked thoroughly before it was issued to Angela. As well as having a potential action in the law of negligence against Mary's employers, Angela may also have remedies under the Consumer Protection Act 1987 against the supplier of the equipment, which would be Mary's employers (see later in the chapter).

Referral by non-occupational therapists

What if the referral by a non-OT is defective? What is the situation in law if non-OTs, e.g. doctors, nurses or non-professionals, do the prescribing of equipment and they do it wrongly? If the OT is aware that people who do not have the training are making the prescriptions for equipment, and that the clients could suffer harm, she should take up this issue with management and, on the lines of the policy recommended by White above, ensure that either the appropriate training was given to such referrers or that all such requests came via the occupational therapy or physiotherapy department. If she is aware that a client has been given the wrong or unsuitable equipment for his or her needs and she fails to take the appropriate action, she may be liable should harm occur to the client as a result.

Disputes with clients

Because the provision of equipment by social services can be means tested, there is a danger that a client could opt for a cheaper solution to a problem than the OT would advise.

Situation

> A client is not prepared to fund the necessary access to the house and wants a cheaper ramp provided. In the opinion of the OT such a ramp would be dangerous because of an unacceptable slope. The OT makes it absolutely clear that such a ramp would be completely contrary to her professional judgment, but the client ignores the advice and arranges for its installation. The client subsequently suffers personal injury when the wheelchair comes off the ramp. Is the OT liable?

The answer should be no, but the OT would have to show that she strongly warned against the installation and her documentation would be extremely important. Clearly, if the installation was effected through social services there would be some liability, since the department should not arrange the installation of fittings which could be dangerous. However, it is difficult to prevent people doing adaptations in their own homes, unless planning permission would be required. Should anyone on the premises be harmed by the installation, the occupier could, of course, be responsible (see Chapter 11 on health and safety and the case of *Smith (Jean) v Northamptonshire County Council*[48]).

Reissue of equipment

If the OT is responsible for reissuing equipment which has been collected from the homes of clients who have ceased to use it, then care should be taken to ensure that it is safe, clean and, where appropriate, serviced.

Situation

An OT reissues toilet seats and frames which have been collected from the house of a client who has died. Unfortunately, she had assumed that the equipment had been cleaned and checked for faults prior to reissue, but this was not the case. Where does she stand if following reissue it is discovered that the frame has not been properly decontaminated and as a result a client is infected?

The OT's liability will depend on the reasonableness of her assumption that the equipment had been properly cleaned and maintained. However, once fault is established the client should be able to obtain compensation because the employer of the OT should have ensured that there was a proper system established before the equipment was reissued.

Situation

An OT retains a returned wheelchair and then loans it to another patient. Where does the OT stand if the brakes on the wheelchair fail and the second patient is harmed?

It may be entirely appropriate for returned equipment to be used elsewhere, but where equipment has been specifically made for one client it is preferable that any new client has a personal fitting carried out by properly qualified persons, rather than the OT becoming responsible for the reissuing. However, if it is entirely reasonable for the OT to reissue equipment, then there must be an established procedure, which is complied with, for the equipment to be checked by a qualified person and for any cleaning to be undertaken, and appropriate records must be kept.

The issue of equipment by OTs to schools for disabled children can also give rise to legal concerns as to responsibility when things go wrong. For example if an OT were to issue seating splints for a child and the carer of the child in the school did not have the appropriate manual handling training and the child is harmed, would the OT be held liable? The answer is that the OT has in law a duty to take all reasonable care to ensure that reasonably foreseeable harm is prevented. She should when issuing the equipment take reasonable care to ensure that those who are caring for the child are familiar with the equipment and have had the appropriate training. If she is aware of deficiencies in that respect, she would have a responsibility to point out the dangers to those in charge of the school's health and safety. Advice on safety in relation to medical devices can be obtained from the Medicines and Healthcare Products Regulatory Agency (MHRA) (see below).

Manufacturing equipment for specific needs

It may happen that an OT and technician create equipment specifically for an individual client's needs and supply this to the client. If harm were to befall the client as a result of the use of this equipment, the OT and technician and their employer may be liable. If an action is brought under the rules of negligence (see Chapter 10), then fault, i.e. a failure to follow the reasonable standard of care, would have to be shown. However, it is possible that an action could be brought against them as the manufacturer or supplier under the provisions of the Consumer Protection Act 1987. Under this Act fault does not have to be proved, merely that there is a defect in the product which has caused the harm (see below). The existence of the defect would be judged against what was known at the time.

Adaptations to equipment by the OT

Where an OT makes adaptations to equipment to fit it for a specific patient, both she or her employer could be liable if harm befalls the client.

Situation

> An OT adapts a wheelchair in order to facilitate the discharge of a patient from hospital, but her adaptation is not checked over by the wheelchair suppliers. The client is injured as a result of this adaptation proving defective.

If in making this adaptation and in failing to get it checked by the appropriate specialist the OT was failing to follow the reasonable standard of care, then the client is likely to succeed in any claim for negligence against the OT or her employer. In addition, in making the adaptation she becomes the supplier of the goods, for the purposes of the Consumer Protection Act 1987 (see below), and the original manufacturer could deny liability on the basis that the product has been changed.

Pick and mix

The OT may also use parts of one company's equipment for use with another company's product. For example, the hoist sling from one hoist could be used on a hoist made by a different firm. If this cross-matching of equipment were to lead to harm, there could be liability if it could be established that the accident happened as a result of the misuse/adaptation. It would have to be proved, however, that it was unreasonable for the OT to use the equipment in this way and that she would not be supported by a responsible body of professional opinion in that use (the Bolam test).

Common law rights against a supplier

Common law action in negligence

The law of negligence enables an action to be brought against the manufacturer of a defective product if harm has been caused to a consumer or third person. This principle was established in the leading case of *Donoghue v Stevenson*.[49] This form of action is discussed in detail in Chapter 10 on negligence. It should be noted that in order to succeed the plaintiff must establish:

- that there was a duty of care
- that there has been a breach of this duty of care and
- that as a reasonably foreseeable result of that breach of duty
- harm has been caused.

Contractual action against supplier

The supplier is under a contractual duty to provide goods in accordance with the contract terms. In addition, where the purchaser is an independent individual, he or she can rely on the legal rights under the sale and supply of goods and services legislation, which give additional protection over and above that contained in the contract documents by implying certain terms into the contract. Where the purchaser is a large consortium or organisation in its own right, the fact that it could threaten to remove the contract to other suppliers may assist in the performance of the contractual terms without any recourse to legal action.

The Consumer Protection Act 1987

Part 1 of the Act covers product liability and Part II of the Act covers consumer safety. The sections under Part 1 on Product liability are shown in Figure 15.1. The provisions of this Act are discussed in this chapter but reference should be made to other legal rights of action in Chapter 11 on health and safety.

Basis of the Act

The Consumer Protection Act 1987 enables a claim to be brought where harm has occurred as a result of a defect in a product. It was enacted as a result of the European Community Directive No. 85/374/EEC. It is a form of strict liability in that negligence by the supplier or manufacturer does

Figure 15.1   Product liability under the Consumer Protection Act 1987.

section 1   Purpose and construction of Part I
section 2   Liability for defective products
section 3   Meaning of defect
section 4   Defences
section 5   Damage giving rise to liability
section 6   Application of certain enactments
section 7   Prohibition on exclusions from liability
section 8   Power to modify Part I
section 9   Applications of Part I to the Crown

not have to be established. The claimant will, however, have to show that there was a defect. The supplier can rely on a defence colloquially known as 'state of the art', i.e. that the state of scientific and technical knowledge at the time the goods were supplied was not such that the producer should have discovered the defect (see below).

A product is defined as meaning any goods or electricity and includes a product which is comprised in another product, whether by virtue of being a component part or raw material or otherwise.

Who is liable under the Consumer Protection Act?

The producer

Section 2(1) states that 'where any damage is caused wholly or partly by a defect in a product, every person to whom section (2) below applies shall be liable for the damage'.

Section 2(2) includes the following as being liable: the producer of the product; any person who, by putting his name on the product or using a trade mark or other distinguishing mark, has held himself out to be the producer of the product; and any person who has imported the product into the EC in the course of business.

The supplier

In addition to producers or original importers as set out under section 2(2), section 2(3) provides that any person who has supplied the product to the person who suffered the damage or to any other person shall be liable for the damage, if:

- the person who suffered the damage requests the supplier to identify the producers (as set out above)
- that request is made within a reasonable period after the damage occurs and when it is not reasonably practicable for the person making the request to identify the producers, and
- the supplier fails, within a reasonable period after receiving the request, either to comply with the request or to identify the person who supplied the product to him.

This provision makes it is essential for the OT to keep records of the manufacturer/supplier of any goods (including both equipment and drugs) which she provides for the client. In the absence of her being able to cite the name and address of the manufacturer or the company that supplied the goods to her, she may become the supplier of the goods for the purposes of the Act and therefore have to defend an action alleging that there was a defect in the goods which caused harm. Harm includes both personal injury or death and loss or damage to property.

Where a social services authority or health service body supplies equipment for use in the community, that body can become the supplier for the purposes of the Consumer Protection Act. If harm results from a defect in the equipment, the appropriate supplier must provide the client with the name and address of the firm from which the equipment was obtained, otherwise it will itself become liable for the defects. Records of the source of equipment are therefore essential in order that the client can be given this information.

Some OTs may hesitate to tighten a bolt or replace a nut for fear that they may be deemed to have become the supplier of the equipment in so doing. Common sense is required in such situations. The instructions of the manufacturer on the maintenance of the equipment must be followed.

What is meant by a defect?

This is defined in the Act as set out in Figure 15.2.

Defences

Certain defences are available under section 4 and are shown in Figure 15.3.

Figure 15.2   Definition of defect: Consumer Protection Act 1987 – section 3.

(1)   Subject to the following provisions of this section, there is a defect in a product for the purposes of [Part 1 of the Act] if the safety of the product is not such as persons generally are entitled to expect; and for those purposes 'safety', in relation to a product, shall include safety with respect to products comprised in that product and safety in the context of risks of damage to property, as well as in the context of risks of death or personal injury.

(2)   In determining … what persons generally are entitled to expect in relation to a product all the circumstances shall be taken into account, including—

　(a)   the manner in which, and purposes for which, the product has been marketed, its get-up, the use of any mark in relation to the product and any instructions for, or warnings with respect to, doing or refraining from doing anything with or in relation to the product;

　(b)   what might reasonably be expected to be done with or in relation to the product; and

　(c)   the time when the product was supplied by its producer to another.

Figure 15.3   Defences under the Consumer Protection Act 1987 – section 4(1).

(a)   that the defect is attributable to compliance with any requirement imposed by or under any enactment or with any Community obligation; or

(b)   that the person proceeded against did not at any time supply the product to another; or

(c)   that the following conditions are satisfied, that is to say—

　(i)   that the only supply of the product to another by the person proceeded against was otherwise than in the course of a business of that person's; and

　(ii)   that section 2(2) [that the person is the producer or importer] above does not apply to that person or applies to him by virtue only of things done otherwise than with a view to profit; or

(d)   that the defect did not exist in the product at the relevant time; or

(e)   that the state of scientific and technical knowledge at the relevant time was not such that a producer of products of the same description as the product in question might be expected to have discovered the defect if it had existed in his products while they were under his control [the 'state of the art' defence]; or

(f)   that the defect—

　(i)   constituted a defect in a product ('the subsequent product') in which the product in question had been comprised; and

　(ii)   was wholly attributable to the design of the subsequent product or to compliance by the producer of the product in question with instructions given by the producer of the subsequent product.

What damage must the plaintiff establish?

Compensation is payable for death, personal injury or any loss of or damage to any property (including land) (section 5(1)). The loss or damage shall be regarded as having occurred at the earliest time at which a person with an interest in the property had knowledge of the material facts about the loss or damage (section 5(5)). Knowledge is further defined in subsections 5(6) and (7).

There have been few examples of actions being brought under the Consumer Protection Act 1987 in healthcare cases and only a handful of cases have been reported. One, reported in March 1993,[50] led to Simon Garratt being awarded £1400 against the manufacturers of a pair of surgical scissors which broke during an operation on his knee, with the blade being left embedded. A second operation was required to remove it. Had he relied on the law of negligence to obtain compensation he would have had to show that the manufacturers were in breach of the duty of care which they owed to him. Under the Consumer Protection Act 1987 he only had to show the harm, the defect and the fact that it was produced by the defendant. In another case,[51] patients who had contracted hepatitis C from blood and blood products used in blood transfusions were able to succeed in a claim brought under the Consumer Protection Act 1987. This decision may well lead to greater use of the Consumer Protection Act 1987 where personal injuries are caused as a result of defective products, since negligence does not have to be established under the Consumer Protection Act 1987, only that there was a defect in the product which has caused the harm.

In one of the few cases[52] involving hospital treatment, a claimant brought an action against manufacturers of an artificial hip which sheared in two beneath the femoral head close to the radial base of the spigot region of the stern. A further operation was required which lead to less movement and mobility. At the trial it was agreed that the prosthesis fractured as a result of fatigue failure initiating from a defect in the titanium alloy from which it was made. The defendants argued that there was no defect in the product when it left them, and that the defect occurred at the time of implantation. The trial judge found in favour of the defendants. The claimant's appeal failed.

The meaning of "defect" in the CPA was considered by the Court of Appeal in a case brought against Tesco Stores.[53] In this case the trial judge had found Tesco and the manufacturer of the bottle to be in breach of the CPA in that the fitting on a bottle of dishwasher powder was not child proof. The mother had left her child of 13 months whilst she went to answer the phone and found the child sitting in the kitchen with the powder on his lips and his head right back. The mother was not found to be negligent. The Court of Appeal unanimously held that the definition of defect in the Act as "if the safety of the produce is not such as persons generally are entitled to expect" could not be interpreted to imply that every producer of a product warrants that the product fulfils its design standards. The public would expect that the bottle was more difficult to open than an ordinary screw top, though not so difficult as if the British Standard had been met. A requirement to meet British Standards could not be read into the CPA. There was therefore no breach of the CPA. In contrast in another case[54] brought under the CPA and the common law of negligence the Court of Appeal unanimously dismissed an appeal against an award of damages of almost £40,000 to a boy who at 12 years old was injured in the eye by the buckle on elastic straps attached to Cosytoes, a fleece lined sleeping bag, which he was helping his mother attach to a pushchair. He lost the central vision of his left eye. The Court of Appeal held that there was a defect in the product because of the risk of the elasticated strap springing back into the eye. The defendants' argument that at the time the scientific and technical knowledge of the defect was not available at that time did not succeed. The safety of the product was not such as persons generally are entitled to expect. There was however no finding of negligence at common law.

In a claim for damages in relation to a defect in vaccination, the Court of Appeal unanimously dismissed an appeal against the trial judge's permitting the substitution of SmithKline Beecham in place of Merck as defendant even after the expiry of ten years referred to in section 11A(3) of the Limitation Act 1980.[55]

Injuries to employees by equipment

Employees who are harmed as a result of defects in equipment can use the provisions of the Employer's Liability (Defective Equipment) Act 1969 (see Chapter 11). Patients or clients would not be able to make use of the provisions of this statute.

Responsibility for equipment

It is essential when equipment is first supplied that the responsibility for it and the rights of action, if any defect be discovered, should be clearly defined. This is discussed below.

Situation

A local authority decided on grounds of cost savings and efficiency to purchase a shower which could be reused in another house. Unfortunately the shower broke when being used by a client, who was consequently injured. Who is liable for the injuries?

In the situation above possible defendants include:

- The local authority if its employees failed to purchase safe equipment or if its employees fitted the equipment negligently (see later for installation).
- The suppliers or manufacturers if there was a defect in the shower. They could be liable under the Consumer Protection Act 1987. However, if it were shown that the reuse of the shower and its new installation was not carried out by the firm, they may not be responsible.
- Any person who negligently fitted or refitted the shower (see later).

The causes of the shower collapsing would have to be investigated in order to establish responsibility.

Assistive devices or assistive technology (wheelchairs, lifts, special electric beds, postural aid, non-oral communication devices, writing aids and safety equipment used in bathrooms) can be of considerable help in promoting independence for people with disabilities, but they are also extremely costly. The possibility of recycling such equipment on a national or even international basis is explored by Claude Vincent.[56] He discussed a policy for recycling adopted in the Canadian Province of Quebec and showed how 99 factors were important for any strategy for recycling, covering technocratic, professional, market and political elements. The role of the OT in a recycling strategy is also considered. In this country any recycling policy would have to take note of the Medical Devices Regulations.

Medicines and Healthcare Products Regulatory Agency (MHRA) and Medical Devices

The Medical Devices Agency (MDA) was established in September 1994 as an executive arm of the Department of Health, to promote the safe and effective use of devices. (Since 2003 its role has been taken over by the Medicines and Healthcare Products Regulatory Agency (MHRA) (see below) In particular its role is to ensure that whenever a medical device is used, it is:

- suitable for its intended purpose
- properly understood by the professional user
- maintained in a safe and reliable condition.

Its primary responsibility is to ensure that medical devices achieve the potential to help healthcare professionals give patients and other users the standard of care they have a right to expect. In fulfilling this role it has six main functions which include investigating adverse incidents, providing advice and guidance, negotiating European Directives and implementing and enforcing regulations on medical devices, contributing to standard setting on medical devices, evaluating medical devices and providing consultancy advice to users and purchasers, and providing support services for these activities. Its website enables access to all its publications and notices.[57]

What is a medical device?

The definition used by the MHRA is based on the European Directive definition:[58]

Any instrument, apparatus, material or other article, whether used alone or in combination, including the software necessary for its proper application, intended by the manufacturer to be used for human beings for the purpose of:

- diagnosis, prevention, monitoring, treatment or alleviation of disease
- diagnosis, monitoring, treatment, alleviation of or compensation for an injury or handicap
- investigation, replacement or modification of the anatomy or of a physiological process
- control of contraception

and which does not achieve its principal intended action in or on the human body by pharmacological, immunological or metabolic means, but which may be assisted in its function by such means.

Annex B to safety notice 9801 from the MDA gives examples of medical devices.[59] It covers the following:

- equipment used in the diagnosis or treatment of disease, or monitoring of patients, e.g. syringes and needles, dressings, catheters, beds, mattresses and covers, and other equipment
- equipment used in life support, e.g. ventilators, defibrillators
- equipment used in the care of disabled people, e.g. orthotic and prosthetic appliances, wheelchairs and special support seating, patient hoists, walking aids, pressure care prevention equipment
- aids to daily living, e.g. commodes, hearing aids, urine drainage systems, domiciliary oxygen therapy systems, incontinence pads, prescribable footwear
- equipment used by ambulance services (but not the vehicles themselves), e.g. stretchers and trolleys, resuscitators
- other examples of medical devices include: condoms, contact lenses and care products, intra-uterine devices.

Bed rails also come within the definition of medical devices and the HSE has issued a circular on bed rail risk management.[60] Between 2001 and 2005 RIDDOR identified 10 fatal accidents and a number of major injury incidents in which the use of bed rails was implicated. The HSE circular sets out the major problems, legal considerations and risk management stages and strategy.

The Medical Devices Regulations[61] require that from 14 June 1998 all medical devices placed on the market (made available for use or distribution even if no charge is made) must conform to 'the essential requirements' including safety required by law, and must bear a CE marking as a sign of that conformity. Although most of the obligations contained in the Regulations fall on manufacturers, purchasers who are positioned further down the supply chain may also be liable – for example, for supplying equipment which does not bear a CE marking or which carries a marking liable to mislead people.[62] This is the requirement of the EC Directive on medical devices.[63] The manufacturer who can demonstrate conformity with the regulations is entitled to apply the CE marking to a medical device.

The essential requirements include the general principle that, 'A device must not harm patients or users, and any risks must be outweighed by benefits'.

Design and construction must be inherently safe, and if there are residual risks, users must be informed about them. Devices must perform as claimed and not fail due to the stresses of normal use. Transport and storage must not have adverse effects. Essential requirements also include pre-requisites in relation to design and construction, infection and microbial contamination, mechanical construction, measuring devices, exposure to radiation, built-in computer systems, electrical and electronic design, mechanical design, devices which deliver fluids to a patient, function of controls and indicators.

Exceptions to these regulations include:

- in-vitro diagnostic devices (covered by separate regulations which came into force in 2000)
- active implants (covered by the Active Implantable Medical Devices Regulations[64])
- devices made specially for the individual patient ('custom made')
- devices undergoing clinical investigation
- devices made by the organisation ('legal entity') using them.

In January 1998 the MDA issued a device bulletin[65] giving guidance to organisations on implementing the regulations. The MDA (now the MHRA) has powers under the Consumer Protection Act 1987 to issue warnings or remove devices from the market.

Classification of devices

Devices are divided into three classes according to possible hazards, class 2 being further subdivided: class 1 with a low risk, e.g. a bandage; class 2a medium risk, e.g. simple breast pump; class 2b medium risk, e.g. ventilator; class 3 high risk, e.g. intra-aortic balloon.

Any warning about equipment issued by the MHRA should be acted on immediately. Failure to ensure that these notices are obtained and acted on could be used as evidence of failure to provide a reasonable standard of care.

Adverse incident reporting procedures

In 1998 the MDA issued a safety notice[66] requiring healthcare managers, healthcare and social care professionals and other users of medical devices to establish a system to encourage the prompt reporting of adverse incidents relating to medical devices to the MDA. The procedures should be regularly reviewed and updated as necessary, and should ensure that adverse incident reports are submitted to the MDA in accordance with the notice. The notice was revised in 2007 can be accessed via the MHRA website.[67]

What is an adverse incident?

The safety notice defines an adverse incident as 'an event which gives rise to, or has the potential to produce, unexpected or unwanted effects involving the safety of patients, users or other persons'. It may be caused by shortcomings in:

> the device itself, instructions for use, servicing and maintenance, locally initiated modifications or adjustments, user practices including training, management procedures, the environment in which it is used or stored or incorrect prescription.

Where the incident has led to or could have led to the following:

> Death; life threatening illness or injury; deterioration in health; temporary or permanent impairment of a body function or damage to a body structure; the necessity for medical or surgical intervention to prevent permanent impairment of a body function or permanent damage to a body structure; unreliable test results leading to inappropriate diagnosis or therapy.

Minor faults or discrepancies should also be reported to the MHRA and there should be regular links with the website to keep up to date with their warnings. The MHRA publishes a list of one liners: examples of reported hazards. The One Liner issue in January 2008 gives examples of incidents where things have gone wrong because of user faults. For example a medical air hose attached to an intensive care ventilator ruptured because the hose had been melted by the heat from a reading light placed next to the ventilator. Another example was where a portable examination couch collapsed and folded up during physiotherapy treatment, injuring the patient and the physiotherapist. The couch had been overloaded and had not been regularly maintained. An MHRA warning published in 2008[68] related to the fact that Beatle wheelchairs in front wheel drive configuration have tipped when travelling on slopes. Amended instructions for users were to be distributed. Warnings were issued in 2007 about Invacare Action wheelchairs fitted with a manual ratchet recliner mechanism[69] and Invacare Action 2000 wheelchairs (blue frame).[70]

Liaison officer

The safety notice suggests that organisations should appoint a liaison officer who would have the necessary authority to:

- ensure that procedures are in place for the reporting of adverse incidents involving medical devices to the MDA
- act as the point of receipt for MDA publications
- ensure dissemination within their own organisation of MDA publications
- act as the contact point between the MDA and their organisation.

Guidance from the MHRA (formerly MDA)

The MDA, the predecessor to the MHRA, published guidance on the responsibilities of individuals and organisations.[71] It also published a checklist for health professionals to ask themselves before they use medical devices. The checklist is shown in Figure 15.4.

On 1 April 2003 the Medicines Control Agency merged with the Medical Devices Agency to form the Medicines and Healthcare Products Regulatory Agency (MHRA). The Department of Health considered that this merger would provide the opportunity to build on the undoubted strengths of the MCA and would continue to be a world leader in terms of its scientific expertise.

Figure 15.4   Checklist for health professionals.

- Do I know how to handle the medical devices in my unit?
- What preparation have I been given in how to use a medical device? Was the preparation formalised and recorded or ad hoc?
- How was my competency to use this equipment safely assessed?
- Am I familiar with the instructions on how to use this piece of equipment and any warning labels?
- When was this equipment last serviced?
- Do my junior staff colleagues know how to use this equipment?
- What is the clearing and/or decontamination procedure and my responsibilities?
- Do I know who is responsible for risk management in my organisation?
- Do I know how to report an adverse incident?
- Do I know who my MDA liaison officer is?

Medical Devices Regulations 2002

Additional regulations[72] which came into force on 13 June 2002 cover (a) active implantable medical devices and accessories to such devices and (b) *in vitro* diagnostic medical devices and accessories to such devices. They can be accessed on the Office of Public Sector Information website.[73]

Installation options

Arrangements for installation vary between authorities. We consider below the liability in a range of different installation systems.

A fitter

By far the best arrangement, except where the supplier arranges its own fitting of the equipment, is for the equipment to be fitted by a qualified employee of the social services authority. The fitter should be appropriately qualified and should liaise with the occupational therapy department that has recommended the provision of the equipment. In this way the height of the fitting can be placed appropriate to the client's needs. The fitter would also be able to judge the thickness of the walls and how the equipment should be attached. As an employee the fitter would be responsible to the social services authority and thus the authority would be vicariously liable for any harm occurring as a result of the fitter's negligence.

The person who has the responsibility of instructing the client/carer on the use of the equipment should be identified.

The carer/neighbour

Sometimes the equipment may be supplied by the statutory authority but it is left to the client to arrange installation. If this is so, comprehensive instructions should be given on how the equipment should be installed. If, for example, a bath rail supplied by social services comes away from the wall having been fitted by a neighbour, liability for the harm would depend on whether sufficient information was given to the client to ensure that the equipment was safely installed.

If all that could be reasonably done had been done by the local authority, then the client or the person suffering harm would have no right of action against the social services authority.

Unqualified employee of the social services authority

Unfortunately, in some districts the installation of equipment is left to the van driver/odd job man of the social services authority. If, as a consequence of a lack of training, the equipment is fitted negligently and then harm occurs, the social services authority would be responsible. There might also be some responsibility attached to those community professionals who were aware of the dangers of this practice and who failed to bring it to the attention of senior management.

An independent contractor

Employed by the client

Where the client purchases equipment, or the equipment is supplied by the social services authority and the client undertakes to obtain a contractor to install the equipment, then providing there has been no negligence by the social services in providing the names of potential contractors, they would not be held liable in the event of the equipment being badly installed. The contractor would have to take responsibility. However, if the harm that occurred was not the result of the faulty installation but the result of negligent advice over what equipment was necessary or suitable, then the contractor is unlikely to be responsible.

Paid by the LA

In general this system should ensure that the work of installation is properly and professionally completed and, should this not be the case, the independent contractor would be liable for any harm. However, if there is evidence that the LA should not have chosen that contractor or that the LA failed to give the contractor the relevant information for the equipment to be installed safely, there may be liability on the part of the LA.

Situation

> A local authority has a contract with outside suppliers and installers for fitting adaptations. It is discovered that the contractors have failed to follow the specified requirements. For example, they have put the bath rail at the wrong height. What is the legal situation?

If it can be shown that the LA OT or other employee did all that was reasonable in selecting and instructing the contractor, then it is likely that the contractors would be liable for any harm that occurred as a result of negligence in failing to follow the instructions.

Should the OT check the work of the outside contractor?

The answer depends on the risks of harm, what would be reasonable practice on the part of the OT, and the nature of the equipment and installation. Certainly where the client needs instruction in its use, arrangements should be made to ensure that this instruction is given before the client uses the equipment and suffers possible harm.

Maintenance

Often there is no clarity over who has the responsibility of ensuring that equipment is regularly checked and, if necessary, serviced or maintained. It is essential that there should be procedures to determine this when the equipment is first supplied so that the responsibility is clearly defined. Some equipment must by law be regularly serviced, for example lifts. When this equipment is installed an agreement for the future inspection and servicing of the lift should be arranged.

Responsibility for maintenance would normally reside with the owner of the equipment. If the social services authority remains the owner and the equipment is merely loaned to the client, then the authority should set up an appropriate system for inspection and maintenance. Where equipment is transferred into the ownership of the client or the client purchases it direct, then the client would usually be the one responsible for ensuring inspection and maintenance. However, the authority would have a responsibility to ensure that all the necessary information was passed on to the client. Account would also have to be taken of the physical and mental capacity of the client to undertake this.

Once the responsibility for ensuring inspection and maintenance and the time limits within which any inspection should take place are defined, then should harm result from a failure to inspect and/ or maintain, liability should be clear. When an OT issues equipment to clients, she should ensure that she documents any maintenance requirements and the time schedule and whether any subsequent visit for inspection of the equipment is necessary.

Exemption from liability

Some authorities use a form which is signed by the client in an attempt by the authority to exempt it from liability should harm occur. An example of such a form is shown in Figure 15.5. The notice in Figure 15.5 would not be effective in removing all liability from the Social Services Department

Figure 15.5   Example of notice attempting to exempt from liability.

I ... acknowledge that the following equipment has been provided to me by the ... Social Services Department:

(1) ...
(2) ...
(3) ...

and I agree to be responsible for the installation and maintenance of this equipment and not to hold the ... Social Services Department for any loss, harm or injury caused by the said equipment.

Signature:
Witness:
Date:

if one of their staff had been negligent in carrying out their duties and responsibilities. This is because the provisions of the Unfair Contract Terms Act prohibit evasion of liability for negligence if personal injury or death occurs as a result. If there has been negligence, the notice will be of no effect (see Chapter 10).

Sometimes, however, the notice is not to exempt from liability but to instruct the client on the use of the equipment and to ensure the client will be safe. To provide written instruction may well be a part of the duty of care. However, any attempt to use it as an exemption notice will not be effective if personal injury occurs. An exemption notice may be effective if loss or damage to property occurs (see Chapter 10).

Use of equipment by a non-client

The same principles apply if it is feared that the equipment would be used by someone other than the client. Thus a bath or shower stool may have been provided for the client but is used by another person who suffers harm when the stool breaks under their weight. If written instructions had been given when the equipment was delivered and installed that it should not be used by anyone else, then the local authority should not be liable for that other person's harm, if the equipment was safe for the client. Again the written instructions act not as a disclaimer but as information about the correct use of the equipment. If the OT has given all the necessary information and instructions according to the Bolam test, neither she nor her employer should be found liable in negligence.

Failure by the client to follow instructions

The same principles would apply where the client fails to follow instructions: the OT should not be regarded as negligent if she has used all reasonable care in instructing the client and warning of the dangers of ignoring this advice. However, the OT must take account of any disabilities of the client, in giving this advice, and in some situations would have to explain to a carer how the equipment should be used. OTs may say that they have no time to put instructions to the client or carer in writing, but if this could be done it could prevent a lot of wasted time, make the instructions clearer for client and carer and also give them a document to which they could refer. In addition, of course, in the event of any dispute over what instructions were given, the OT could refer to the document.

Insurance cover

At the same time that responsibility for the inspection and servicing of the equipment is decided, the liability for providing insurance cover should be agreed where this is deemed necessary. It may be that a social services authority has its own group policy for insurance cover which can be used to protect an individual client. It may be that the client is covered by his or her own house or personal insurance cover. The OT should ensure that this question is raised and answered.

Situation

An OT teaches a patient how to fit a raised toilet seat which is subsequently the cause of an accident. Who would provide the compensation?

The answer to this question depends on many different factors. If the OT is not at fault and has done all that she reasonably could to ensure that the client is safe, neither she nor her employer (if she is an employee) will be liable. If, however, the OT is at fault, then she will be personally liable and, if self-employed, her insurance company would pay out compensation to the injured person. If she is employed, the insurers of her employers would pay out compensation (if they are covered); if not the employers would have to pay. If the client has the relevant personal accident cover a claim may be possible under that policy.

A survey carried out by the NHS executive between January and April 1998 concluded that over £55 million a year was being spent on commercial insurance premiums by NHS Trusts. This led to two schemes for non-clinical risks being set up under the NHS Litigation authority: liabilities to third parties (LTPS) and property expenses scheme (PES). Both schemes commenced in April 1999, can be joined by NHS bodies and are known collectively as Risk Pooling Schemes for Trusts (RPST). The LTPS covers employers' liability claims from slips and trips in the work place to serious manual handling, bullying and stress claims. It also covers public and products liability claims, from personal injuries sustained by visitors to NHS premises to claims arising from breaches of the Human Rights Act, Data Protection Act and Defective Premises Act. Cover is also provided for defamation, professional negligence by employees and liabilities of directors. PES provides cover for "first party" losses such as theft or damage to property. Further information on the two schemes can be found on the NHSLA website[74] together with details of the reporting criteria, the fees and the excesses.

Occupational therapists and Medicinal Products

OTs have from 2004 been on the list of registered health practitioners recognised as being able to prescribe under patient group directions. There may also be opportunities for the OT in the future to be recognised as an independent prescriber under the Crown final report recommendations.[75] The College of Occupational Therapists has published a briefing note no 15 on Prescribing, Supply and Administration of Medicines and Occupational Therapists (March 2007) which is to be read in conjunction with briefing note no 14 on Extended scope practice. The briefing note explains that a patient group direction (PGD) is a written instruction for the sale, supply and and/or administration of medication in an identified clinical situation. It applies to groups of patients who may not be individually identified before presenting for treatment but identified by the clinical team e.g. on the ward. The briefing note gives the example of a specialist occupational therapist in rheumatology who can also administer an analgesic to the patient with painful arthritic joints before working with him or her to produce a functional hand splint. The PGD means that there is no need for the patient to make a separate appointment and attendance at another health clinic with another health professional just for the administration of the medication. The briefing note points out that the administration, prescription and supply of medicines is not a basic occupational therapy skill. It is outside the scope of occupational therapy practice and inappropriate to the pre registration education of occupational therapy students. It notes the critical issues which an OT must bear in mind if she is asked to provide medicines under a PGD. The legal background to the prescribing, dispensing and administration of medicinal products is given below.

The prescribing, dispensing and administration of medicinal products has been closely controlled by law. The principle laws are the Medicines Act 1968 and the Misuse of Drugs Act 1971 and regulations made under both Acts. Medicines are grouped in the following categories:

1. *Pharmacy-only products*, (P) i.e. these can be sold or supplied retail only by someone conducting a retail pharmacy business when the product must be sold from a registered pharmacy by or under the supervision of a pharmacist.
2. *General sales list*, (GSL) i.e. medicinal products that may be sold other than from a retail pharmacy, as long as provisions relating to section 53 of the Medicines Act are complied with, i.e. the place of sale must be the premises where the business is carried out; they must be capable of excluding the public; the medicines must have been made up elsewhere and the contents must not have been opened since make-up.
3. *Prescription-only list*, (POM) i.e. these medicines are available only on prescription drawn up by an appropriate practitioner. Schedule 1 of the subsequent regulations lists the prescription-only products and Part II of the schedule lists the prescription-only products that are covered by the Misuse of Drugs Act.

The next paragraphs set out the history of the extension of the prescribing, supply and administering of medicines to other professions. Occupational therapists have not yet achieved the status of being supplementary or independent prescribers. They are able to supply and administer medicines under patient specific directions (see below) and patient group directions (see below).

Groups protocols or patient group directions (PGDs) and patient-specific directions

There has over the last twenty years been an extension of prescribing powers from registered medical practitioners to other health professionals. Community nurses were the first group to be given the legal powers to prescribe certain medicines and medicinal products in the community. In hospitals, patient group directions or group protocols were being used to enable other professionals to prescribe medication for patients who had not been seen by a doctor. The Crown Committee was set up to consider the regulation of the prescribing of medicines. It first considered the arrangements for and legality of group protocols and reported in March 1998 and recommended legislation to ensure that their legal validity was clarified. It was followed by new regulations which came into force on 9 August 2000.[76] These provided for patient group directions to be drawn up to make provision for the sale or supply of a prescription-only medicine in hospitals in accordance with the written direction of a doctor or dentist or other independent prescriber. To be lawful, the patient group direction must cover the particulars that are set out in Part I of Schedule 7 of the Statutory Instrument. These particulars are shown in Figure 15.6. It will be noted from Figure 15.6 that a registered occupational therapist may be one of the professions recognised as able to prescribe under a specific or group patient direction, if the other conditions set out in Figure 15.6 are satisfied.

Independent and Supplementary Prescribing

Following its report on PGDs, the Crown Committee considered the overall regulation of independent and supplementary prescribing. Its final report was published in 1999[77] and it was followed by Health and Social Care Act 2001 which amended section 58 of the Medicines Act 1968 to enable new registered professional groups to be designated by order for the purpose of prescribing medicines for human use. Occupational therapists are not yet specified as supplementary or independent prescribers but may become so in the future. In April 2002[78] the Department of Health announced its intention of introducing supplementary prescribing by a nurse or pharmacist in 2003. The aim was to enable the pharmacists and nurses to work in partnership with doctors and help treat such

Figure 15.6   Regulations on Group Protocols or Patient Group Directions.

Particulars for validity of a patient group direction

- Period during which the direction shall have effect.
- Description or class of prescription-only medicines to which the direction relates.
- Whether there are any restrictions on the quantity of medicine which may be supplied on any one occasion and, if so, what restrictions.
- Clinical situations that prescription-only medicines of that description or class may be used to treat.
- Clinical criteria under which a person shall be eligible for treatment.
- Whether any class of person is excluded from treatment under the direction and, if so, what class of person.
- Whether there are circumstances in which further advice should be sought from a doctor or dentist and, if so, what circumstances.
- Pharmaceutical form or forms in which prescription-only medicines of that description or class are to be administered.
- Strength, or maximum strength, at which prescription-only medicines of that description or class are to be administered.
- Applicable dosage or maximum dosage.
- Route of administration.
- Frequency of administration.
- Any minimum or maximum period of administration applicable to prescription-only medicines of that description or class.
- Whether there are any relevant warnings to note and, if so, what warnings.
- Whether there is any follow-up action to be taken in any circumstances and, if so, what action and in what circumstances.
- Arrangements for referral for medical advice.
- Details of the records to be kept of the supply or the administration of medicines under the direction.

The classes of individuals by whom supplies may be made are set out in Part III of Schedule 7 and include the following:

ambulance paramedics (who are registered or hold a certificate of proficiency)
pharmacists
registered health visitors
registered midwives
registered nurses
registered ophthalmic opticians
state registered chiropodists
state registered occupational therapists
state registered orthoptists
state registered physiotherapists
state registered radiographers.

The person who is to supply or administer the medicine must be designated in writing on behalf of the authorising person (see below) for the purpose of the patient group direction. In addition to compliance with the particulars set out above, a patient group direction must be signed on behalf of the authorising person. This is defined as the Common Services Agency, the (special) health authority, the NHS trust or primary care trust. The Department of Health has developed PGDs for certain chemical and biological countermeasures in emergency situations, such as atropine and these can be downloaded from its website.[1] The Royal Pharmaceutical Society of Great Britain published in September 2007 a resource pack for pharmacists on patient group directions which would also be of interest to registered occupational therapists.

conditions as asthma, diabetes, high blood pressure and arthritis. The doctor would draw up a plan with the patient's agreement, laying out the range of medicines that may be prescribed and when to refer back to the doctor. This early announcement was followed by a press release in November 2002,[79] which gave further details of the patient conditions and the medicinal products that would be the subject of supplementary prescribing. In April 2005 chiropodists and podiatrists, physiotherapists and radiographers were added to list of those who could become supplementary prescribers and restrictions on their prescribing controlled drugs or unlicensed medicines were removed.[80] The supplementary prescriber works within a Clinical Management Plan (CMP) agreed with the independent prescriber. Independent prescribers are clinically responsible for the overall care of the patient and can prescribe without reference to another clinician. In 2007 the HPC published changes to the approval process that education providers have to complete before a stand alone POM programme is approved by the HPC.[81]

Implications for occupational therapists

The power to prescribe under a patient specific or group direction has developed the scope of professional practice of the occupational therapist and at the same time opened up new challenges. As with direct access of the patient to the occupational therapist or self-referral considered in Chapter 10, it is essential to identify the boundaries within which the occupational therapist can safely and competently practice.

Bhanu Ramaswamy in a personal account of experience with supplementary prescribing provides guidance for other physiotherapists who would like to become supplementary prescribers.[82] Her advice may also be of value to occupational therapists in the future. The Department of Health has provided guidance on prescribing, supply and administration of medicines.[83] The College of Occupational Therapists has provided guidance on prescribing, supply and administration of medicines and occupational therapists which was revised in 2007.[84] Reference should be made to Chapter 10 and the discussion of the scope of professional practice.

Legal responsibilities of the prescriber

An occupational therapist is legally responsible for any harm which has been caused by her negligence in prescribing a medicine under a patient group or specific direction. She could face fitness to practice proceedings, criminal proceedings if the patient has died or suffered and disciplinary action. She would also have to give evidence in any civil litigation brought by the patient or his family if the patient has died against the employer who is vicariously liable for the negligence of the employee. It is essential that the occupational therapist works within the parameters of the powers delegated to her and the conditions of the patient group directions which are shown in Figure 15.6. She must also ensure that any concerns or doubts she has about the patient or the medicine are checked with the clinician identified as the independent prescriber and/or the pharmacist. If the patient asks the occupational therapist's advice about medicines, then it is essential that the occupational therapist remains within the scope of her competence. She may for example be able to suggest a medication which is available on the General Sales List (GSL) but only if she is aware of any other medications which the patient may be taking and from her knowledge and training is sure that there are no contra-indications. Nor should an occupational therapist advise a patient to stop or change any medication recommended by a doctor unless that advice is clearly within the scope of her knowledge and competence as the prescriber under a group or specific patient direction or the doctor has been consulted.

Can an occupational therapist in private practice sell GSL medicines?

Medicines which can be sold over the counter in any retail establishment, corner shop or supermarket could be sold by an occupational therapist in private practice, provided of course, that she conforms to the requirements set out in section 53 of the Medicines Act (see above) and she complies with the Trade Descriptions Act and does not hold out herself as being able to give pharmaceutical advice. She must take care where she is treating the patient, that she follows the reasonable practice expected of an occupational therapist in supplying any medicines on the general sales list. It would be illegal for her to sell medicines which are Pharmacy-only products or available only on prescription.

Conclusions

Legal issues relating to equipment are likely to continue to be a constant concern of OTs. Clear record keeping of inventories has become a necessity since the coming into force of the consumer protection legislation and the possibility that an OT department could be held liable for the supply of defective equipment. It is essential that the OT ensures that she is the recipient of any adverse notices issued by the MHRA and that she in turn is familiar with the procedure for making any concerns about the safety of equipment known to the appropriate authority. As the expanded scope of professional practice of the OT grows it is likely that the OT will be increasingly involved in the supply of medication to patients under patient group directions and eventually as a supplementary prescriber.

 Questions and exercises

1 Review the procedure you follow in choosing equipment for a client, taking into account risk assessment factors.
2 Draw up a leaflet to give to the client about the supply of equipment in the home, which covers instruction on use, maintenance, insurance and any other aspects you consider necessary.
3 A client is considering bringing a claim against manufacturers because of faulty equipment. What advice could you give her about her rights?
4 A client complains that a hoist recently provided has broken. What actions lie against the manufacturers?
5 Obtain details of the role and function of the Medicines and Healthcare Products Regulatory Authority (MHRA) and identify its importance for the work of the OT department.

References

1 Mandelstam, M. (2001) Safe use of disability equipment and manual handling: Legal aspects. *British Journal of Occupational Therapy, Part 1, Disability Equipment*, **64**(1), 9–16; *Part 2, Manual Handling*, **64**(2), 73–80.
2 Mandelstam, M. (1997) *Equipment for Older or Disabled People and the Law*. Jessica Kingsley Publishers Ltd, London.

3 College of Occupational Therapists (2008) Position statement on Transforming Community Equipment Services COT, London.

4 Audit Commission (2000) Fully Equipped: The provision of equipment to older or disabled people by the NHS and social services in England and Wales.

5 Audit Commission (2002) Disability Services still cause for serious concern; www.audit-commission.

6 HSC 2001/008; LAC(2001)13 Community Equipment Services.

7 DoH (2001) *Health Guide to Integrating Community Equipment Services*. DoH, London.

8 HSC 2001/01; LAC(2001)1 Intermediate Care Guidance.

9 LAC(2003)14 Changes to Local Authority Charging Regime for Community Equipment and Intermediate Care Services.

10 The Community Care (Delayed Discharges etc) Act (Qualifying Services) (England) Regulations 2003, SI 2003/1196.

11 College of Occupational Therapists (2003 revised 2007) Changes to the LA charging regime for community equipment and intermediate care services.

12 www.dh.gov.uk/en/SocialCare/Socialcarereform/Communityequipment

13 www.csed.csip.org.uk/

14 www.icesdoh.org

15 *Deacon v McVicar and another* (QBD) 7 January 1984, Lexis transcript.

16 *R v Gloucester County Council and another, ex parte Barry* [1997] 2 All ER 1, HL.

17 Wright, C. & Ritson, E. (2001) An investigation into occupational therapy referral priorities within Kensington and Chelsea Social Services. *British Journal of Occupational Therapy*, **64**(8), 393–7.

18 See for example Ashby, M. *et al.* (1995) Snoezelen: Its effects on concentration and responsiveness in people with profound multiple handicaps. *British Journal of Occupational Therapy*, **58**(7), 303–6.

19 van Diepen, E. Baillon, S.F., Redman, J. *et al.* (2002) A pilot study of the physiological and behavioural effects of Snoezelen in dementia. *British Journal of Occupational Therapy*, **65**(2), 61–6.

20 Curtin, M. (1994) Technology for people with tetraplegia: Part 1 (accessing computers) and Part 2 (environmental control units). *British Journal of Occupational Therapy*, **57**(10), 376–80 and (11) 419–24.

21 Curtin, M. (1993) Powered wheelchairs and tetraplegic patients: Improving the service. *British Journal of Occupational Therapy*, **56**(6), 204–6.

22 See for example Pain, H. *et al.* (1994) An evaluation of kettle tippers. *British Journal of Occupational Therapy*, **57**(1), 5–8.

23 Pain Helen, McLellan Linda, Gore Sally, and others (2003) Choosing disability equipment: A guide for Users and Professionals. Jessica Kingsley, London.

24 Sweeney, G.M. & Clarke, A.K. (1992) Easy chairs for people with arthritis and low back pain: Results for an evaluation. *British Journal of Occupational Therapy*, **55**(2), 69–72.

25 Chamberlain, E., Evans, N., Neighbour, K. & Hughes, J. (2001) Equipment is it the answer? An audit of equipment provision. *British Journal of Occupational Therapy*, **64**(12), 595–600.

26 Heaton, J. & Bamford, C. (2001) Assessing the outcomes of equipment and adaptations: Issues and approaches. *British Journal of Occupational Therapy*, **64**(7), 346–56.

27 Jepson, J. (1998) Study into the equipment needs of people with restricted growth. *British Journal of Occupational Therapy*, **61**(1), 22–6.

28 Silcox, L. (1995) Assessment for the prescription of wheelchairs: What training is available to therapists? *British Journal of Occupational Therapy*, **58**(3), 115–18.

29 McColl, I. (1986) *Review of the artificial limb and appliance centre services*, vol. 1 & 2: The report of an independent working party. HMSO, London.

30 Greenfield, E., Lachmann, S. & Wrench, A. (1993) Handing over the controls: Alternative controls for wheelchairs in Cambridge. *British Journal of Occupational Therapy*, **56**(3), 94–6.

31 White, E.A. (1992) Wheelchair stump boards and their use with lower limb amputees. *British Journal of Occupational Therapy*, **55**(5), 174–8.

32 McMahon, M. & Dudley, N.J. (1992) General practitioners and wheelchair prescribing. *British Journal of Occupational Therapy*, **55**(5), 183–5.

33 White, E.A. (1994) Wheelchair referrals in England. *British Journal of Occupational Therapy*, **57**(12), 471–5.

34 *The Times* (news report), 24 February 1996.

35 NHS Executive and Department of Health (2000) York Health Economics Consortium, *Evaluation of the Powered Wheelchair and Voucher Scheme Initiatives*, Final Report. Stationery Office, London.

36 Evans, R. (2000) The effect of electrically powered indoor/outdoor wheelchairs on occupation: a study of users' views. *British Journal of Occupational Therapy*, **63**(11), 547–53.

37 White, E.A. (1998) Effectiveness in wheelchair service provision. *British Journal of Occupational Therapy*, **61**(7), 301–5.

38 www.direct.gov.uk/en/DisabledPeople/HealthAndSupport/Equipment

39 CSP Wales 1st Floor Transport House 1 Cathedral Road Cardiff CF11 9SD 02920 382 429.

40 National Wheelchair Managers Forum (2004) *Healthcare standards for wheelchair services*. National Wheelchair Managers Forum, London.

41 MDA/2005/025 Posture belts fitted to wheelchairs and seating.

42 Medicines and Healthcare Products Regulatory Agency (2004) Stability of Wheelchairs DB 2004 (02).

43 www.mhra.gov.uk/Publications/Safetyguidance

44 Muscular Dystrophy Campaign Wheelchair provision for children and adults with muscular dystrophy and other neurological conditions: best practice guidelines (2006) MDC.

45 www.muscular-dystrophy.org

46 www.csed.csip.org.uk/workstreams/transforming-community

47 www.dh.go.uk/en/SocialCare/Socialcarereform/Community

48 *Smith (Jean) v Northamptonshire County Council* The Times Law Report 24 March 2008.

49 *Donoghue v Stevenson* [1932] AC 562.

50 Dimond, B. (1993) Protecting the consumer. *Nursing Standards*, **7**(24), 18–19.

51 *A and others v National Blood Authority and another*. Times Law Report, 4 April 2001.

52 *Piper v JRI (Manufacturing) Ltd* [2006] EWCA Civ 1344.

53 *Tesco Stores Ltd and another v CFP (a minor by his litigation friend) and LAP* [2006] EWCA Civ 393.

54 *Abouzaid v Mothercare (UK) Ltd* [2006] EWCA Civ 348.

55 *Smithkline Beecham v Horne Roberts* [2001] EWCA Civ 2006.

56 Vincent, C. (2000) Towards the Development of a Policy of Recycling Assistive Technology for People Living with a Disability. *British Journal of Occupational Therapy*, **63**, 35–43.

57 www.medical-devices.gov.uk

58 European Union Directive 93/42/EEC.

59 MDA SN 9801 Reporting Adverse Incidents Relating to Medical Devices, January 1998.

60 www.hse.gov.uk/lau/lac/79-8.htm

61 SI 1994/3017 Medical Devices Regulations 1994 came into force 1 January 1995, mandatory from 14 June 1998. Directive 93/42/EEC.

62 Medical Devices Agency Bulletin, Medical Device and Equipment Management for Hospital and Community-based Organisations. MDA DB 9801 January 1998.

63 93/42/EEC Directive concerning medical devices.

64 Directive 90/385/EEC came into force 1 January 1993 and is mandatory from 1 January 1995.

65 Medical Devices Agency Bulletin, Medical Device and Equipment Management for Hospital and Community-based Organisations. MDA DB 9801 January 1998.

66 MDA SN 9801 Reporting Adverse Incidents Relating to Medical Devices, January 1998.

67 MHRA (2007) Reporting Medical Device Adverse Incidents and Disseminating Medical Device Alerts MDA/2007/001.

68 Medical Healthcare Products Regulatory Agency MDA/2008/029 Beatle and Puma Battery powered wheelchairs manufactured by Movingpeope.net.

69 MDA/2007/075.

70 MDA/2007/074.

71 Medical Devices Agency Bulletin, Medical Device and Equipment Management for Hospital and Community-based Organisations. MDA DB 9801 January 1998.

72   Consumer Protection Medical Devices Regulations SI 2002/618.
73   www.opsi.gov.uk/legislation
74   www.nhsla.com/Claims/Schemes/RPST
75   DoH (1999) Final Report on the Prescribing, Supply and Administration of medicines, chaired by Dr June Crown. Department of Health, London.
76   Prescription-Only Medicines (Human Use) Amendment Order 2000 SI 2000/1917.
77   Department of Health, Review of Prescribing, Supply and Administration of Medicines Final Report (Crown Report), Department of Health, London, March 1999.
78   Department of Health press release 2002/0189, Groundbreaking new consultation aims to extend prescribing powers for pharmacists and nurses, 16 April 2002.
79   Department of Health press release 2002/0488, Pharmacists to prescribe for the first-time nurses will prescribe for chronic illness, 21 November 2002.
80   The National Health Service (Primary Medical Services) Miscellaneous Amendments) Regulations SI 2005/893; The Medicines for Human Use (Prescribing) Order SI 2005/765.
81   www.hpc-uk.org/aboutregistration/educationandtraining/pom/
82   Bhanu Ramaswamy (2006) *An experience of supplementary prescribing.* Agility No 2 9–10.
83   Department of Health (2006) *Medicines Matters: A guide to mechanisms for the prescribing, supply and administration of medicines.* DH, London.
84   College of Occupational Therapists (2007) Prescribing, supply and administration of medicines and the occupational therapist Briefing note 15. COT, London.

16 Transport Issues

Most occupational therapists (OTs) are required to drive a car as part of their duties and many legal problems can arise. Concerns centre on the following areas, which are covered in this chapter:

- In the course of employment
- Transporting other people and equipment
- Insurance issues
- Crown cars and lease cars
- Responsibilities of the employer towards transport and insurance

- Tax situation and private mileage
- Disabled parking and badges
- Clients and driving cessation
- Public transport and taxis

In the course of employment

In Chapter 10 on negligence it was noted that an employer is only vicariously liable for the acts of the employee if the employee was acting in the course of employment. Many community professionals transport others as part of their work – clients, carers, colleagues and others. Where this is clearly indicated in the job description, the employer would have to accept that he is vicariously liable for any harm caused by the employee while driving in the course of employment. The employee, if driving her own car, would have to ensure that all the necessary measures in terms of appropriate insurance cover had been taken. As a consequence of the decision by the House of Lords where it held that a Board of Governors was vicariously liable for the sexual assaults committed by a warden upon pupils since they were committed in the course of employment,[1] the definition of course of employment has been widened and thus may include activities which were expressly forbidden by the employer (see Chapter 10).

Legal Aspects of Occupational Therapy, Third Edition By Bridgit Dimond
© 2010 Bridgit Dimond

Giving lifts

It may for example be that an employee is forbidden to give lifts to others and yet disobeys these instructions.

Situation

An OT is aware that she is not permitted within her job description to give lifts to others. She visits an isolated cottage where the GP has called and left a prescription which the client has not been able to take to a chemist. She realises that the client has no transport and offers to take a carer to the chemist's shop and return with the medication. On the return journey she is involved in an accident. Her insurance company claims that it should not be liable for the injury to her passenger since she had not notified it that she took passengers as part of her job. Her employers claim that she was not acting in the course of employment since she was forbidden to transport persons other than clients and she was employed as an OT not a chauffeur. What is the legal situation?

In the above situation the fact that the OT was forbidden to take passengers will not necessarily take her actions outside the definition of 'in course of employment' (see Chapter 10 and in particular the case of *Lister & Others v Hesley Hall Ltd*[2]). However, she is likely to face disciplinary proceedings. In contrast, if she picked up hitch-hikers this would be unlikely to come within the course of employment. The employer would probably not be liable for any harm caused to the hitch-hikers.

It is of great benefit if employer and employee spell out exactly what use can be made of an employee's car for work purposes, to prevent a dispute arising later. It is also essential to clarify the use for insurance purposes (see below).

Transporting other people and equipment

People

Even where the employer expressly agrees that the OT can use her car for transporting clients, legal issues can arise if the client is injured or causes an accident.

What if the passenger becomes disturbed?

Situation

An OT arranges to take an older mentally infirm patient home to make an assessment visit. On the journey the client becomes very disturbed, tries to get out of the car, succeeds in opening the back door and falls out. Is the OT liable?

This situation is of concern to many community workers, particularly OTs. If the incident is reasonably foreseeable then it could be argued that the OT should have taken the precaution of arranging 'child locks' on the car so that this could not occur. Alternatively, the precautions may have involved taking an assistant with her. Her duty of care to the client would require her to take reasonable precautions against events which are reasonably foreseeable. Before embarking on the journey she should have made an assessment as to whether the client would be safe in the car and whether or not an assistant should have sat with the client. In making this decision she should be aware that she is responsible for taking precautions to meet all reasonably foreseeable risks of harm to the client or to others.

What if the community professional took passengers on the basis that they were taken at their own risk? Such an arrangement is prohibited under road traffic legislation and this device could not be used to exempt the driver from liability for the passenger's safety, but contributory negligence can be a factor. The COT has provided a briefing note on transporting clients or equipment in your own vehicle.[3] The Transport Research Laboratory has published guidance on the safety of child wheelchair occupants in road passenger vehicles.[4]

Case: *Eastman v SW Thames Regional Health Authority*[5]

Damages were awarded against the health authority in respect of injuries which the claimant sustained when travelling in an ambulance without a seat belt. Although the ambulance driver was acquitted of all blame for the accident it was held that a duty of care was owed to advise passengers to wear a seat belt. The defendants appealed to the Court of Appeal and the appeal was allowed. It was held that adult passengers possessed of their faculties should not need telling what to do. The attendant was under no obligation to point out the existence of a seat belt and a notice recommending their use.

It should be noted that this case refers to the duty of care to adults possessed of their faculties. Where a health professional is transporting a client in her own car and the client is frail or mentally incompetent, the courts would probably accept that a duty of care was owed to ensure that the client was reasonably safe. This might in exceptional circumstances require child-proof locks.

What if a passenger causes damage to the OTs car?

It depends on the circumstances as to whether there is likely to be any liability on the part of the employer. It would have to be established that the employer was aware that harm could occur and failed to take reasonable precautions against that harm arising. If such fault could not be found, then the employer would not be liable and the OT would be responsible for paying for the damage to be rectified.

Infectious disease and transport

What if a client carried in the car is suffering from an infectious disease, which another patient picks up while being transported in the same vehicle? There would be a duty on the OT, if she is aware that she is carrying in her car a person suffering from an infectious disease, to ensure that after this use the car was cleaned and disinfected to prevent any cross-infection. If she fails to do this to a reasonable standard then she and her employer could be liable.

Equipment

It is also important that the OT is clear on her duties in relation to the transporting of equipment. To ensure that the client obtains equipment without delay she may be inclined to decide to take equipment herself rather than wait for a van to be provided by her employers. She should take special precautions to ensure that her visibility in the car is not impaired and that she does not suffer injury from the manual handling of equipment on her own. Should such injury occur, and she attempt to bring a claim, she may be met with the defence of contributory negligence – that it was her own responsibility.

If the equipment is stolen, her insurance company may not be prepared to pay compensation for the loss unless there is an express term covering such liability and the OT had made it clear in her application for insurance cover that the carrying of equipment for work purposes was part of her agreed activities. It could well be a requirement of such additional insurance cover that the equipment is only carried out of sight in the boot of the car.

Jennifer Woolloff,[6] in an article looking at issues arising in the transport of equipment, provides a checklist for questioning whether methods of transport are safe, considers the implications of poor practice and provides some suggested solutions.

Even if a taxi were to be hired for the transport of equipment, this may not absolve the OT (and her employer) from liability if the equipment is unsafe and the driver is injured or an accident occurs, though in this case the cab driver may also be contributorily negligent in not ensuring that the equipment was safely stowed.

The test in such cases of liability would be whether there were reasonably foreseeable risks and whether reasonable care had been taken to remove or reduce the risk of harm. If the answer was yes to the first question and no to the second, then there could be liability on the OT and her employer (vicariously) in the event of personal injury or loss or damage to property. If the employer is aware of the risks and fails to agree to reasonably safe transport, then there may also be direct liability for negligence on the part of the employer.

Insurance issues

Absolute disclosure is required in any insurance contract and, therefore, if there is any likelihood that the employee will require to use his car during work, this and the reasons should be disclosed. Should the driver not inform the insurers of a significant fact, this omission could invalidate the cover even though this omission has no relevance to a claim. In the absence of valid cover, the Motor Insurer's Bureau provides compensation for personal injuries suffered by third parties. An interesting recent development has been the suggestion that if a driver uses his car for car boot sales without the consent of the insurance company, this could invalidate his car insurance. If an OT has business cover for her car, she should check with the insurance cover that this would cover transporting patients. "Business" is such a vague term that explicit details of the OT's business should be made known to the insurance company.

Crown cars and lease cars

Crown cars

Where the employee has the use of a crown car, insurance is normally provided through the employer and the crown is exempt from the provisions of the Road Traffic legislation requiring road tax.

Lease cars

Usually the company providing the car would ensure that the appropriate insurance cover is taken out. However, this is not always so and the driver must ensure that she has the correct insurance cover.

Servicing

With both crown and lease cars there may be service agreements which enable the user to have the car serviced at regular intervals as part of the agreement. The responsibility would be upon the user to ensure that the car was regularly maintained and also to ensure that any faults were reported and rectified. Should an accident occur because the user has failed to take action to remedy a defect, the user could face disciplinary proceedings from the employer and in some cases also face criminal prosecution herself.

Responsibilities of the employer towards transport and insurance

What duties does an employer have in relation to transport by an employee?
    The following case illustrates the question.

Case: *Reid v Rush and Tompkins Group plc*[7]

The claimant suffered severe injuries while driving the defendant's Land Rover in Ethiopia in the course of his employment by the defendant. It collided with a lorry. The accident had been caused solely by the negligence of the lorry driver who could not be traced. The claimant contended that the defendant was in breach of its duty of care as employer in failing either to insure him so as to provide suitable benefits in the event of injury resulting from third party negligence, or to advise him to obtain insurance for himself; and that had he been so advised he would have obtained personal accident cover. The basis for these arguments was that there was an implied term in the contract of employment requiring such insurance cover or advice, or that there was a duty of care owed in the law of negligence by the employer to the employee; or that the employer had a duty of care because of the special relationship which existed between them.

None of the arguments put forward by the employee succeeded. The Court of Appeal held that there was no duty on the employer to take all reasonable steps to protect the employee's economic welfare while acting in the course of employment, even if loss was foreseeable. They cited the case of *Edwards v West Hertfordshire Hospital Management Committee*[8] in support of this decision. The duty of the employer was limited to the protection of the employee against physical harm or injury.

If, therefore, the employer fails to warn employees to take out insurance cover, taking out that cover is the responsibility of the employee even if the car is used solely for work purposes. Where the employer assists the employee in the purchase of the car or provides the transport, it should be made clear what are the respective duties of employer and employee in relation to the transport, to prevent any misunderstanding or omissions.

Tax situation and private mileage

It is impossible in a book of this sort to cover the details of the law relating to the taxation of the benefit obtained from the use of cars provided by employers, and the way in which private mileage is treated by the Inland Revenue. However, it is important that those employees who have the use of a car provided by the employer keep accurate records of their use of the car for private purposes, as well as their use of the car for work. Records should be made as soon as possible after the journey.

    OTs in independent practice will also need to keep comprehensive records of all costs associated with the car in calculating their profit and income tax (see Chapter 28).

Disabled parking and badges

OTs may be involved in the assessment of the eligibility of disabled persons to have badges which will entitle them to park in parking bays designated for disabled persons. Each local authority has a duty to implement the provisions of the Chronically Sick and Disabled Persons Act 1970 and assist in travelling arrangements for disabled persons.

Regulations providing exemptions from parking restrictions for disabled persons have been revised in 2000 and 2007.[9] The Regulations require that orders made by local authorities prohibiting vehicles from waiting on roads marked by yellow lines or which prohibit the waiting of vehicles in roads or in street parking places, include an exemption from waiting prohibitions in certain circumstances and from charges and time-limits at places where vehicles may park or wait, in respect of vehicles displaying a disabled person's badge.

The Department of Transport devised a scheme known as the orange badge scheme which provided parking concessions for disabled persons and has been in operation since 1971. That scheme has been superseded as a result of a recommendation of the European Union to introduce a standard design of parking badge across Europe. The new blue badge was introduced throughout the UK in April 2000 and the use of orange badges expired on 31 March 2003. Details about the blue badge scheme are available from the Department of Transport.[10] Traffic signs which show the wheelchair symbol on an orange background will gradually be replaced by the symbol against a blue background. In Wales, regulations have been passed to introduce the blue badges for disabled people[11] (see below).

Eligibility for the blue badge

The following are automatically entitled to apply for a badge:

- Over two years and either
  - Receive the higher rate of the mobility component of the disability living allowance or
  - Are registered blind or
  - Receive a war pensioner's mobility supplement.

Others may be eligible for a badge if:

- Over two years and either:
  - Have a permanent and sustainable disability which means you cannot walk, or which makes walking very difficult or
  - Drive a motor vehicle regularly, have a severe disability in both arms, and are unable to operate all or some types of parking meter (or would find it very difficult to operate them) (This may require answering further questions so that the local authority can determine eligibility for a badge.)

The parent of a child who is less than two years old, may apply for a badge for the child, if they have a specific medical condition which means that they either:

- Must always be accompanied by bulky medical equipment which cannot be carried around without great difficulty or
- Need to be kept near a vehicle at all times, so that they can, if necessary, be treated in the vehicle, or quickly driven to a place where they can be treated, such as a hospital.

The badges can be used throughout the UK and whilst travelling abroad through the European Union (EU). Further information on the use of the Blue Badge in EU countries can be obtained from the Institute of Advanced Motorists (IAM).[12]

Local authorities are responsible for issuing Blue Badge parking permits and applications should be addressed to them. It is an offence to park a vehicle which is not displaying a badge in a Blue Badge parking bay. It is also an offence to refuse or fail to produce a badge for inspection by police officers, traffic wardens, local authority parking attendants and civil enforcement officers. Blue Badge holders qualify for a 100 per cent exemption from the London Congestion Charge, but holders must register with Transport for London (TfL) at least 10 days before the journey and pay a one-off £10 registration fee. A registration form can be down loaded from the TfL website.[13]

It should be noted that entitlement to receive a blue badge does not necessarily mean that the disabled person is fit to drive and any change in the physical or mental condition of the driver which impairs driving ability should be reported to the Driver and Vehicle Licensing Agency.[14]

Administration of the blue badge scheme

The scheme is administered by the local authority Social Services Department. It does not apply to private roads, off-street car parks (unless disabled parking is provided), in certain town centres, in Central London (see below) and at some airports. If the disabled person is refused a permit, an appeal mechanism should be in place. An OT who has carried out the assessment must be prepared to justify both her findings and her conclusions and should follow the guidance given in Chapter 13 on impartiality and professional integrity in report writing and giving evidence.

Central London

Central London has an independent concessionary scheme operated by the City of London, the City of Westminster, the Royal Borough of Kensington and Chelsea and part of the London Borough of Camden. Details of the concessions are available from the relevant London councils (see Department for Transport for further details[15]).

Entitlements

The blue badge scheme allows a holder to park free of charge and without time limit at parking meters, without a time limit at other places where non-holders' time is limited, and up to three hours on single or double yellow lines. The blue badge must be displayed. Some routes are designated as 'red routes' and are subject to special controls on stopping, loading and unloading, but some concessions may be made for blue badge holders (such as stopping to pick up or set down). There is a list of places where a blue badge holder cannot park, which includes where there is a ban on loading or unloading, all pedestrian crossings (including Zebra, Pelican, Toucan and Puffin), where there are double white lines in the centre of the road, in a bus or tram lane during its hours of operation, on any clearway, double or single red lines during their hours of danger, in parking bays reserved for specific users, on a residents parking bay, where temporary restrictions on parking are in force, and on school 'keep clear' markings during the set hours. In addition, disabled parking is not permitted where it would be obstructive or cause a danger to others.

A vehicle must be moved if a police officer or a traffic warden in uniform requests it.

Misuse of the Blue Badge

Local authorities can take away a badge if the badge holder misuses it such as by allowing other people to use it or if a disabled person's condition improves so that they are no longer eligible for the scheme. New measures are to be taken to prevent abuse of the disabled parking schemes.[16] The most frequent abuses are by friends and relatives misusing the badge. The Department of Transport is tightening eligibility criteria and making it harder to forge blue badges. Mobilise, a charity for disabled drivers and passengers, has urged the Government to tighten the procedure for issuing badges. The Commons Transport Select Committee in June 2008 found that some councils were ignoring the Department for Transport's guidelines and not ensuring that applicants for blue badges had an independent assessment of their mobility and instead taking recommendations from applicants' GPs which were given out under pressure from the patient. The parking concession is estimated to be worth up to £5,000 per year.[17]

Wales and the Blue Badge scheme

Wales has its own Blue Badge scheme which came into force in July 2000 replacing the orange badge scheme. Blue badge holders qualify for free toll across the Severn bridge. Eligibility is similar to the English scheme and applications should be made to the local authority in which the applicant lives. Further information can be obtained from the Welsh Assembly Government website.[18]

The Motability Scheme

Motability, an independent not-for-profit organisation, runs a scheme for disabled people to buy or lease an adapted car. Applications can be made by those who receive the war pensioner's mobility supplement or the higher rate of the mobility component of the disability living allowance. It is also possible for a person in receipt of either of those benefits to apply for a car as a passenger and nominate two other people as the driver. Through the care hire scheme a new car is supplied for lease by a Motability Accredited dealer for at least three years. Comprehensive insurance, routine servicing and breakdown assistance are included. Hire purchase can also be arranged. Motability also offers a hire purchase scheme for powered wheelchairs or scooters. Disabled people do not have to pay VAT on the cost of hiring a car through the Motability scheme. Further information is available on the Motability website.[19] Countrywide Publications provides useful information on motoring for disabled people and holidays and courses for disabled people[20]

Clients and driving cessation

Situations have been considered in other chapters (for example, Chapter 8, pp. 113 and 116), where legal issues arise when patients are advised that they should not be driving and they fail to obey those instructions. Under the Road Traffic Acts it is an offence for an individual to drive a car if they are suffering from a physical or mental defect which impairs their driving safely. Occupational therapists may be confronted with patients very anxious to drive when it is medically contra-indicated. Help in determining a client's ability to drive may in the future be available from a driving simulator on a lap top, which could save the expense of a road test.[21] The College of Occupational Therapists revised its guidance on Fitness to Drive in 2007.[22]

Situation: Insisting on driving

An occupational therapist is treating a patient who has suffered a stroke. Movement on the left side is restricted but the patient is anxious to drive since he acts as the sole carer for his wife who has motor neurone disease. The occupational therapist suspects that he is driving contrary to clinical advice. What is the legal position of the occupational therapist?

This is not an uncommon situation since the inability to drive can be seen as a considerable hardship for many people who have suffered neurological damage or physical injuries. Many patients may therefore be tempted to commence driving before they are physically or mentally fit to do so. The occupational therapist can advise such patients that they are committing a criminal offence. In serious cases where the occupational therapist considers that there is a grave danger of serious harm to other people, it would probably be an exception to her duty of confidentiality to advise the DVLA or others of the dangers (see Chapter 8 on confidentiality). However it would be preferable to attempt to persuade the driver to cease to drive or to notify the DVLA himself and show him any appropriate literature. Those suffering from diabetes which requires insulin are required to inform the Driver and Vehicle Licensing Agency. Those diabetics who take tablets but also have a complication such as retinopathy must also inform the DVLA. The charity Diabetes UK has called for the law to be changed following research in the USA that people with diabetes are unfairly being prevented from driving since the rate of road collisions is no higher among diabetics who controlled their condition with insulin than among non-diabetics.[23] A train driver who suffered from epilepsy was jailed for 8 years after killing a young woman in a car crash. He had been advised by doctors not to drive.[24]

Jacki Liddle and Kryss McKenna[25] consider the issues relating to older drivers and cessation in a fully referenced article, with a table illustrating the international differences in licensing regulations for older drivers and the role of the occupational therapist. Research by Robyn Lister,[26] albeit in a small-scale study, is useful in indicating how OTs can develop effective ways of supporting those who can no longer drive following a stroke, and assist them in adapting to their new circumstances. The life changing traumatic effects of having to cease driving cannot be overestimated and research conducted into the experience of those who have had to cease driving can be of great assistance in planning driving cessation[27]

Situation: Scooter, wheelchair or car?

An OT refers a client who has motor neurone disease to a wheelchair unit for an indoor/outdoor scooter. The unit has recommended an attendant propelled chair due to his marked deteriorating condition. The OT who is not employed by the wheelchair unit is wondering whether she can legally advise the client on the self-purchase of a scooter.

In this situation the wheelchair service has assessed the patient and concluded that he is not competent to manage a wheelchair on his own. The OT must therefore assess whether the client is capable of managing a scooter. She might need to obtain specialist help. A driving assessment centre may be able to advise on driving a scooter as well as a car.

Public transport and taxis

Public transport and taxis are subject to the provisions of the Disability Discrimination Act 1995 and the Accessibility Regulations drawn up under the Disability Discrimination Act. Under these regulations improved accessibility to buses, coaches and trains must be provided. Taxis are also covered by similar regulations. The Act is considered in Chapters 19 and 20.

Conclusion

Whether an OT is provided with a car from her employer or a lease car, or uses her own transport, it is essential that she makes inquiries as to any conditions laid down in relation to insurance cover and the exact terms on which she is allowed to use the car in connection with work. Her duty of care also extends to ensuring that disabled persons are treated fairly in obtaining parking badges and that patients who are not medically fit to drive are warned of the consequences.

 Questions and exercises

1   While giving a lift to a carer, contrary to the instructions of your employer, you are involved in an accident which leads to the carer being injured. What is the situation in law?
2   Draw up a procedure which can cover the use of crown, lease or employee-owned cars.
3   Advise a client on how to obtain a parking permit for disabled persons.
4   What action would you take if a stroke patient, not yet fully recovered, was adamant that he would drive, contrary to clinical advice?

References

1   *Lister & Others v Hesley Hall Ltd*, [2001] UKHL 22 [2002] 1 AC 215; The Times Law Report, 10 May 2001; [2001] 2 WLR 1311.
2   *Lister & Others v Hesley Hall Ltd*, [2001] UKHL 22 [2002] 1 AC 215; The Times Law Report, 10 May 2001; [2001] 2 WLR 1311.
3   College of Occupational Therapists (2009) Transporting clients or equipment in your own vehicle Briefing note no 117. COT, London.
4   Visikis C, Le Claire M, Goodacre O, Thompson A and Carroll J (2008) *The safety of child wheelchair occupants in road passenger vehicles*. Transport Research Laboratory, Wokingham.
5   *Eastman v S.W. Thames Regional Health Authority* (CA) Times Law Report, 22 July 1991.
6   Woolloff, J. (2003) Is the cost of transporting equipment too high. *British Journal of Occupational Therapy*, **66**(1), 31–2.
7   *Reid v Rush and Tompkins Group plc*, Times Law Report, 11 April 1989.
8   *Edwards v West Hertfordshire Hospital Management Committee* [1957] 1 WLR 1415.
9   Local Authorities' Traffic Orders (Exemptions for Disabled Persons (England)) Regulations 2000 SI 2000/683 (replacing Regulations 1986 SI 1986/178); The Disabled Persons (Badges for Motor Vehicles) (England) (Amendments) Regulations 2007 SI 2007/2531.
10   www.dft.gov.uk; Department for Transport, Mobility and Inclusion Unit Zone 1/18, Great Minster House, 76 Marsham Street, London SW1P 4DR; blue.badge@dft.gov.uk.
11   Disabled Persons (Badges for Motor Vehicles) (Wales) Regulations 2000 SI 2000/1786 made under the Chronic Sick and Disabled Persons Act 1970 section 21; Local Authorities' Traffic Orders (Exemptions for Disabled Persons) (Wales) Regulations 2000 SI 2000/1785.
12   www.iam.org.uk
13   www.tfl.gov.uk
14   Driver and Vehicle Licensing Agency (DVLA), Swansea, SA99 1TU.
15   Department for Transport, Mobility and Inclusion Unit Zone 1/18, Great Minster House, 76 Marsham Street, London SW1P 4DR.
16   Ben Webster. Clampdown on blue badge parking cheats The Times 24 January 2008.

17 Ben Webster. Disabled badges given too easily, say MPs The Times 10 June 2008 page 12.

18 http://new.wales.gov.uk/topics/IntegratedTransport/BlueBadge.

19 www.motability.co.uk

20 Countrywide (no date) Motoring for disabled people – an independent guide for disabled people Countrywide publications Peterborough.

21 Lee Hoe C (2006) Virtual driving tests for older adult drivers. *British Journal of Occupational Therapy*, **69**(3), 138–41.

22 College of Occupational Therapists (2007) Fitness to Drive Briefing note no 26. COT, London.

23 News item Road Ban for diabetics 'unfair' The Times 12 May 2008.

24 News item Epileptic's fatal crash The Times 13 December 2008.

25 Liddle, J. & McKenna, K. (2003) Older drivers and driving cessation. *British Journal of Occupational Therapy*, **66**(3), 125–32.

26 Lister, R. (1999) Loss of ability to drive following a stroke: The early experiences of three elderly people on discharge from hospital. *British Journal of Occupational Therapy*, **62**(11), 514–20.

27 Liddle Jacki, Turpin Merril, Carlson Glenys and Mckenna Kryss (2008) The needs and experiences related to driving cessation for older people. *British Journal of Occupational Therapy*, **71**(9), 379–88.

17 Statutory Organisation of Health and Social Services

This chapter considers the statutory duties placed upon the Secretary of State for Health and the social services authorities in the provision of health, community and social services. It considers the organisations which are involved in the commission and provision of health and social care. It also looks at the developments under the NHS White Paper and NHS Plan to modernise the NHS, and the organisations which have been established to ensure that standards are set and maintained. The following topics are covered:

- Statutory framework of the NHS
- Social services organisations
- White Paper on the NHS 1997
- Abolition of the internal market and GP Fundholding
- Department of Health and strategic health authorities
- Establishment of primary care trusts
- Care trusts
- Partnership arrangements
- Standards
- Clinical Governance and the duty of quality
- Care Quality Commission (replacing the Commission for Health Audit and Inspection (CHAI); Commission for Social Care Inspection (CSCI) and the Mental Health Act Commission (MHAC))
- Audit Commission
- National Council for Health and Clinical Excellence (NICE)
- National Service Frameworks (NSF)
- NHS Direct
- Walk-in clinics
- Additional funding of £20 billion
- National Plan for the NHS
- NHS Modernisation Agency and Board
- Bristol paediatric heart surgery inquiry
- Health and Social Care (Community Health and Standards) Act 2003
- Services Quality and Governance

Legal Aspects of Occupational Therapy, Third Edition By Bridgit Dimond
© 2010 Bridgit Dimond

Statutory framework of the NHS

The NHS was established on 5 July 1948 under the National Health Service Act 1946. This legislation was re-enacted in the National Health Service Acts of 1977 and 2006 and placed the duties shown in Figure 17.1 on the Secretary of State.

Section 2 of the 2006 Act is subject to section 3(3) which is shown in Figure 17.2.

Part II of the Act covers the provision of services by general practitioners, dental practitioners, pharmacists and others who provide services under a contract for services with the Health Authorities (which took over responsibilities from the Family Health Service Authorities in 1996) and now come under primary care trusts.

Figure 17.1   Duty under NHS Act 1977 sections 1 and 2 as reenacted in sections 1 and 2 of the NHS Act 2006.

1(1)   The Secretary of State must continue the promotion in England of a comprehensive health service designed to secure improvement—
  (a)   in the physical and mental health of the people of England, and
  (b)   in the prevention, diagnosis and treatment of illness.
(2)   The Secretary of State must for that purpose provide or secure the provision of services in accordance with this Act.
(3)   The services so provided must be free of charge except in so far as the making and recovery of charges is expressly provided for by or under any enactment, whenever passed.
2(1)   The Secretary of State may
  (a)   provide such services as he considers appropriate for the purpose of discharging any duty imposed on him by this Act, and
  (b)   do anything else which is calculated to facilitate, or is conducive or incidental to, the discharge of such a duty.

Figure 17.2   Duties under section 3 of the NHS Act 1977 reenacted in section 3 of the NHS Act 2006.

3(1)   The Secretary of State must provide throughout England to such extent as he considers necessary to meet all reasonable requirements –
  (a)   Hospital accommodation;
  (b)   Other accommodation for the purpose of any service provided under this Act;
  (c)   Medical, dental, ophthalmic, nursing and ambulance services;
  (d)   Such other services or facilities for the care of pregnant women, women who are breastfeeding and young children as he considers are appropriate as part of the health service,
  (e)   such other services or facilities for the prevention of illness, the care of persons suffering from illness and the after-care of persons who have suffered from illness as he considers are appropriate as part of the health service,
  (f)   such other services or facilities as are required for the diagnosis and treatment of illness.

Since 1948 the NHS has been subject to many reorganisations and one of the most significant came into being as a result of the NHS and Community Care Act 1990.

This Act led to the establishment of NHS Trusts and Group Fund Holding Practices. The NHS Trusts were to be the principal providers of NHS secondary and community healthcare. Purchasers were either GPs who were approved as fundholders to hold a budget to purchase secondary and community healthcare services for their patients, or were health authorities. In April 1996 health authorities were reorganised: the former district health authorities (DHAs) and family health services authorities (FHSAs) were abolished and in their place were established new health authorities which had the responsibility of commissioning and, in conjunction with GP fundholders, purchasing services from providers as well as carrying out responsibilities in relation to the primary healthcare services formerly undertaken by FHSAs. In this way, the internal market was created and the purchase and provision of healthcare was agreed in NHS contracts. However, this organisation was radically changed following the White Paper[1] on the NHS and the Health Act 1999. Further changes have been brought about by the National Health Service (Primary Care) Act 1997, Health and Social Care Act 2001, NHS Reform and Health Care Professions Act 2002 and the Health and Social Care (Community Health and Standards) Act 2003, National Health Service Act 2006, Health and Social Care Act 2008 and Health Act 2009

Social services organisations

Local authorities have the statutory responsibility of providing social services and are able to charge for the services they provide. The main statutes are the National Assistance Act 1948, the Local Authority Social Services Act 1970 and the Local Government Act 1972. Under the Local Government Act 2000 local authorities have a statutory duty to promote economic, social and environmental well-being in their areas. This will increase their involvement in health service provision (see below). A basic principle of the provision of health services is that they are provided without charge at the point of delivery (unless there is specific statutory provision, as there is for prescription charges). Local authority services can be provided on the basis of means testing. (This does not apply to services provided under section 117 of the Mental Health Act 1983; see Chapter 21). A White Paper was published in 1998 which set a strategy for the development of social services[2] (see Chapter 18).

The effect of the NHS and Community Care Act 1990 was to place responsibilities on local authorities for the funding of residential and nursing home accommodation on a means tested basis. Previously residents had secured their income and payment of their fees from the Department of Social Security (DSS). (Those residents who were already receiving payments through the DSS had preserved rights to continue receiving them from the DSS. However, these preserved rights were abolished in 2001.[3]) The National Health Service and Community Care Act 1990 also placed responsibilities on local authorities to assess clients for community care services. These duties are considered in Chapter 18.

Increasingly legislation has facilitated and encouraged joint working between health and social services, and transfers of funds between the authorities. The Health Act 1999 created a statutory duty for co-operation between NHS bodies (section 26) and between NHS bodies and local authorities:

> In exercising their respective functions NHS bodies (on the one hand) and local authorities (on the other) shall co-operate with one another in order to secure and advance the health and welfare of the people in England and Wales. (section 27) (Re-enacted in section 82 of the NHS Act 2006).

The powers given by section 28A of the NHS Act 1977 for transfers of funds between local authorities and health bodies were strengthened by sections 29 and 30 of the Health Act 1999.[4]

Under section 7 of the Health and Social Care Act 2001 the extent of the overview and scrutiny committees set up under section 21 of the Local Government Act 2000 is extended

To review and scrutinise, in accordance with regulations under that section, matters relating to the health service (within the meaning of that section) in the authority's area, and to make reports and recommendations on such matters in accordance with the regulations.

Local authorities are also represented on primary care trust boards (see below).

White Paper on the new NHS 1997

The White Paper[5] on the NHS envisaged that the internal market would be abolished. The main features of the White Paper are shown in Figure 17.3.

Abolition of the internal market and GP fundholding

The NHS agreements between health authorities or GP fundholders and NHS trusts were replaced by long-term, three-year arrangements for the provision of services. Extra contractual referrals no longer existed. GP fundholding was abolished. GPs were expected to participate in the new arrangements for primary healthcare[6] (section 6 NHS Reform and Health Care Professions Act 2002). (In Wales known as local health groups which eventually became local health boards)

Department of Health and strategic health authorities

The Department of Health now works through four Regional Directorates of Health and Social Care (London, the South, the North, and the Midlands and Eastern). Under the NHS Reform and Health Care Professions Act 2002, strategic health authorities have been set up for England which have the responsibility for commissioning and planning the provision of health services. They were established in 2003 as a result of the amalgamations of the existing health authorities under section 1 of the NHS Reform and Health Care Professions Act 2002. (In Wales health authorities were abolished.) The new strategic health authorities have the responsibility of planning, in co-ordination with other agencies, the implementation of the strategy of the Department of Health. They are responsible for the planning and commissioning of health services, agreeing performance agreements with PCTs and NHS trusts, and monitoring their performance. A Health Improvement Plan is agreed as the local strategy and implemented through a Service and Financial Framework.

Figure 17.3   Main features of the White Paper.

(1)   Abolition of the internal market and GP fundholding
(2)   Establishment of primary care groups leading to primary care trusts
(3)   Establishment of the National Council for Health and Clinical Excellence
(4)   Establishment of the Commission for Health Improvement (now Care Quality Commission)
(5)   Setting up of National Service Frameworks
(6)   Introduction of NHS Direct
(7)   Introduction of clinical governance

The strategic health authorities are responsible for contracting for the provision of health services in a given area and ensuring that the health needs within their catchment area are met and that they work with the Secretary of State to an agreed plan and under his directions. Their constitution, powers functions and duties are set out in the National Health Service Act 2006 sections 13–17 and Schedule 2. Each SHA is a corporate body which consists of a chairman and members appointed by the Secretary of State. Each Strategic Health Authority is required to make arrangements to ensure that it receives advice from persons with professional expertise relating to the physical or mental health of individuals to enable it to exercise its functions effectively. (S.17 of NHS Act 2006) Members of the strategic health authority are required to comply with a Code of Accountability and a Code of Conduct, drawn up by the Department of Health.

Establishment of primary care trusts (PCTs)

Primary care groups were envisaged in the NHS White Paper as bringing together GPs and community nurses in each area. Their role was to improve the health of local people and they would have strong support from their health authority and the freedom to use NHS resources wisely, including savings. The White Paper envisaged that primary care groups could become primary care trusts, i.e. free-standing organisations. Such trusts could include community health services from existing trusts. All or part of an existing community NHS trust could combine with a primary care trust in order to integrate better services and management support. The White Paper specifically stated that these new trusts would not be expected to take responsibility for specialised mental health or learning disability services.

Earlier statutes such as the NHS and Community Care Act 1990, the National Health Service Act 1977 and the National Health Service (Primary Care) Act 1997 were amended by sections 1 to 12 and Schedule 1 of the Health Act 1999 to regulate the establishment of primary care trusts. The main functions of the primary care trust, as set out in section 2 of the Health Act 1999, were:

- providing or arranging the provision of services under Part 1 of the NHS Act 1977
- exercising functions in relation to the provision of general medical services under Part 11 of the NHS Act 1977
- providing services in accordance with section 28C arrangements.

Schedule 1 to the 1999 Act provides for the more detailed regulation including the Primary Care Trust Orders, the trusts' constitution and membership, and staff, and their powers and duties. Rules also cover the transfer of property and the transfer of staff. Statutory Instruments provide further regulations for PCTs.[7]

It is a specific requirement of the PCT that as soon as practicable after the end of each financial year, every PCT shall prepare a report of the trust's activities during that year and shall send a copy of the report to the health authority within whose area the trust's area falls, and to the Secretary of State. Official guidance has been provided by the Department of Health covering the financial framework,[8] the arrangements for staff transfer[9] and arrangements for estates and facilities management.[10] All these documents are available from the Department of Health website.[11] The NHS Confederation provided a briefing note on the primary care trusts[12] and expressed concerns about the lack of clarity of accountability within the primary care trusts and the internal governance arrangements outlined in the Department of Health guidance. More robust arrangements for accountability of the primary care trusts were put in place.[13]

The Secretary of State has the power (S.7 of the 2006 Act) to direct a strategic health authority, primary care trust or Special health authority to exercise any of his functions relating to the heath service which are specified in the directions. The Secretary of State may also give directions to strategic health authorities, primary care trusts, NHS trusts and special health authorities about their exercise of any functions.

An NHS contract is an arrangement under which one health service body (the commissioner) arranges for the provision to it by another health service body (the provider) of goods or services which it reasonably requires for the performance of its functions. Such a contract does not give rise to contractual rights and liabilities but any disputes over such arrangements may be referred to the Secretary of State for his determination.

The Secretary of State also has the power to make arrangements with other bodies or individuals or voluntary organisations to assist in the provision of any services under the Act.

The NHS Reform and Healthcare Professions Act 2002 replaced the permissive power on the Secretary of State to establish PCTs by a statutory duty to establish PCTs across the whole of England.

Recent developments for Primary Care Trusts (Local Health Boards in Wales)

Recent years have seen a devolution of funding and powers to primary care with more services being available from primary care trusts. Sections 18–24 and Schedule 3 of the NHS Act 2006 reenacts the constitution, function and powers of the PCTs. They were established by the Secretary of State who has the power to vary their areas, abolish them or establish a new PCT. A Strategic Health Authority may give directions to a PCT about the exercise of its functions. The PCT may provide services under an agreement for primary medical services and primary dental services and premises for pharmaceutical services and primary medical, dental and ophthalmic services. They can also manage health service hospitals. They have a duty, to enable them effectively to exercise their functions, to make arrangements to secure appropriate advice from persons with professional expertise about the physical and mental health of individuals. They are required to prepare and keep under review a plan which sets out the strategy for improving the health of the people for whom they are responsible and the provision of health services to them. Each local authority in the PCT catchment area must participate in the preparation or review of the plan. PCTs, SHAs and LAs must have regard to these plans in the exercise of their functions. The National Audit Office reviewed the progress in implementing clinical governance in primary care and drew lessons for the new PCTs in January 2007.[14] It urged the NHS to ensure that a focus on quality and safety was at the top of the agenda in primary care. It noted that progress in implementing clinical governance was not uniform and the independence of primary care contractors, such as GPs, community pharmacists, dentists and practice nurses was a major challenge. The PCT did not have direct line management authority over individual contractors. PCTs needed to develop a strategy for engaging their independent contractors in improving quality and safety and create a professional culture within their organisations.

Section 139 of the Health and Social Care Act 2008 (by inserting section 23A into the National Health Service Act 2006) placed a duty on primary care trusts to make arrangements to secure continuous improvement in the quality of healthcare provided by it and by other persons pursuant to arrangements made by it. In discharging this duty a Primary Care Trust must have regard to the standards set out in statements under section 45 of the Health and Social Care Act 2008:

"Health care" means—

(a) services provided to individuals for or in connection with the prevention, diagnosis or treatment of illness, and

(b) the promotion and protection of public health.

Care trusts

Following the implementation of Part 3 of the Health and Social Care Act 2001, care trusts have been established which enable social services as well as health services to be provided by the same trust. Section 45 enables an organisation to be designated as a care trust (following an application by a local partnership of primary care trust and LA), where:

- A primary care trust or an NHS trust is, or is to be, a party to any existing or proposed LA delegation arrangements, and
- The relevant authority is of the opinion that designation of the trust as a care trust would be likely to promote the effective exercise by the trust of prescribed health-related functions of a local authority (in accordance with the arrangements) in conjunction with prescribed NHS functions of the trust.

The Secretary of State has the power to dissolve the PCT or NHS trust and designate a care trust. (S.77 of the 2006 NHS Act). Under section 45(9) of the 2001 Act (now reenacted in section 77(10) of the NHS Act 2006), the designation of a body as a care trust shall not affect any of the functions, rights or liabilities of that body in its capacity as a primary care trust or NHS trust.

Partnership arrangements

Section 31 of the Health Act 1999 enables partnerships arrangements to be set up[15] to improve services for users, through pooled funds and the delegation of functions (lead commissioning and integrated provision). Guidance sets out details on who can make use of these arrangements and the conditions necessary.[16] Partnership arrangements can be directed under section 46 of the Health and Social Care Act 2001 when it is considered that an NHS body or local authority is failing in the exercise of its functions.

Standards

Following the White Paper there has been greater emphasis on standard setting in the light of research findings on clinical effectiveness and excellence. Standard setting and monitoring have become an even more significant part of the practitioner's professional responsibilities. Standards in relation to the law are discussed in Chapter 10 on the law of negligence. The extent to which clinical guidelines, protocols, procedures and practices are enforceable through the courts is considered in a fascinating work by Brian Hurwitz.[17] Statutory standards may be imposed as a result of section 46 of the Health and Social Care (Community Health and Standards) Act 2003.

Clinical Governance and the duty of quality

One of the most significant changes envisaged by the Government in its White Paper was the concept of clinical governance, defined as:

> A framework through which NHS organisations are accountable for continuously improving the quality of their services.[18]

The idea of clinical governance[19] is basically simple. In the past, the trust board and its chief executive have been responsible for the financial probity of the organisation; there has been no statutory

Figure 17.4   Section 45 Health and Social Care (Community Health and Standards) Act 2003.

'It is the duty of each NHS body to put and keep in place arrangements for the purpose of monitoring and improving the quality of healthcare provided by and for that body.'

(2)   Healthcare means the services provided to individuals for or in connection with the prevention, diagnosis or treatment of illness and the promotion and protection of public health.

responsibility of the trust for the overall quality of the organisation. Under the concept of clinical governance the board and its chief executive are responsible for the quality of clinical services provided by the organisation. In theory this could mean that a board is removed or a chief executive dismissed if a baby suffers brain damage at birth or a mother dies in childbirth as a result of negligence.

An information guide for OTs and a position statement on clinical governance were published in June 1999[20] by the COT. The November 2000 issue of the *British Journal of Occupational Therapy* included several articles on different aspects of clinical governance and occupational therapy.[21] It looked at the key elements in the Department of Health's strategy:[22] setting, delivering and monitoring quality standards. The COT information leaflet also provided guidance for OTs working within social services and in the independent and voluntary sectors.

The concept of clinical governance is based on the statutory duty of quality under section 18 of the Health Act 1999. For the first time in its history there was a statutory duty on the NHS to promote quality. The duty was re-enacted in 2003. Section 45 of the Health and Social Care (Community Health and Standards) Act 2003 is shown in Figure 17.4.

The duty falls primarily on the chief executive of each strategic health authority, PCT and NHS trust to implement. In practice, each chief executive designates officers to be responsible for quality or clinical governance in specified areas of clinical practice. Government guidance was published in 1999.[23] This follows on from the original consultation document *A First Class Service: Quality in the new NHS.*[24] The aim to develop quality within the NHS was to be secured in three ways:

- setting clear national quality standards
- ensuring local delivery of high quality clinical services
- effective systems for monitoring the quality of services.

The Commission for Health Improvement (CHI) and the Healthcare Commission/Commission for Health Audit and Inspection (CHAI))

Sections 19–24 of the Health Act 1999 established the Commission for Health Improvement (CHI) and set out its functions and powers. It was a body corporate, i.e. it could sue and be sued on its own account.

Section 19(2) of the Health Act 1999 gave powers to the Secretary of State to make regulations covering the exercise of its functions. Under section 19(3) the Secretary of State could give directions with respect of the exercise of any functions of the Commission and it was the legal duty of the Commission to comply with any such directions (section 19(4)).

Additional powers were given to the Secretary of State under section 23 of the Health Act 1999 by regulations to confer a right by authorised persons to enter NHS premises to inspect those premises and/or take copies of prescribed documents or require persons to produce documents or other information or reports, and to interview persons. Regulations could also be made (section 23(2)) on the disclosure of confidential information and the identification of a living individual. Section 24(1) made it a criminal offence to disclose, without lawful authority, knowingly or recklessly, confidential information obtained by the Commission. Further provisions relating to the functions and constitution of CHI were added by sections 12, 13 and 14 of the NHS Reform and Health Care Professions Act 2002.

Under the Health and Social Care (Community Health and Standards) Act 2003 CHI amalgamated with the National Care Standards Commission to become the Commission for Healthcare Audit and Inspection (CHAI), which became fully operational in April 2004. In addition, a new body called the Commission for Social Care Inspection became responsible for the monitoring of standards in social services and in care homes and other organisations (see Chapter 18).

Care Quality Commission (CQC)

In April 2009 the Care Quality Commission replaced the Healthcare Commission, the Commission for Social Care Inspection and the Mental Health Act Commission and became fully operational in 2010. Its basic functions are:

1. registration functions (as set out in sections 8 to 44 of the Health and Social Care Act 2008),
2. review and investigation functions (as set out in sections 45 to 51 of the Health and Social Care Act 2008) and
3. functions under the Mental Health Act 1983 (formerly carried out by the Mental Health Act Commission)

Section 3(1) of the 2008 Act states that:

> The main objective of the Commission in performing its functions is to protect and promote the health, safety and welfare of people who use health and social care services.

Section 3 (2) requires the Commission to perform its functions for the general purpose of

encouraging—

(a) the improvement of health and social care services,
(b) the provision of health and social care services in a way that focuses on the needs and experiences of people who use those services, and
(c) the efficient and effective use of resources in the provision of health and social care services.

'Health and social care services' means the services to which the Commission's functions relate. The Commission is to have regard to the following matters:

(1) In performing its functions the Commission must have regard to—
  (a) views expressed by or on behalf of members of the public about health and social care services,
  (b) experiences of people who use health and social care services and their families and friends,
  (c) views expressed by local involvement networks about the provision of health and social care services in their areas,
  (d) the need to protect and promote the rights of people who use health and social care services (including, in particular, the rights of children, of persons detained under the Mental Health Act 1983, of persons who are deprived of their liberty in accordance with the Mental Capacity Act 2005 and of other vulnerable adults),

(e)   the need to ensure that action by the Commission in relation to health and social care services is proportionate to the risks against which it would afford safeguards and is targeted only where it is needed,

(f)   any developments in approaches to regulatory action, and

(g)   best practice among persons performing functions comparable to those of the Commission (including the principles under which regulatory action should be transparent, accountable and consistent).

In performing its functions the Commission must also have regard to such aspects of government policy as the Secretary of State may direct (section 4(2)).

The CQC is required to publish a statement on user involvement. This must describe how it proposes to:

(a)   promote awareness among service users and carers of its functions,

(b)   promote and engage in discussion with service users and carers about the provision of health and social care services and about the way in which the Commission exercises its functions,

(c)   ensure that proper regard is had to the views expressed by service users and carers, and

(d)   arrange for any of its functions to be exercised by, or with the assistance of, service users (i.e. people who use health or social care services) and carers (people who care for service users as relatives or friends).

From time to time the Commission may revise the statement and must publish any revised statement. Before publishing the statement (or revised statement) the Commission must consult such persons as it considers appropriate.

Further functions are set out in sections 53 to 59. These include:

- The provision of information and advice to the Secretary of State
- Studies on improving economy, efficiency and effectiveness and their publication

Powers of the CQC

The CQC is given powers of inspection for registration purposes (S.60) and in accordance with Regulations, entry and inspection if it considers it necessary or expedient for the purposes of any of its regulatory functions (S62). The individual making the inspection must if so required produce some duly authenticated document showing the person's authority to exercise the power. The powers of the inspector under S.63 are shown in Figure 17.5. Anyone obstructing the inspector in the carrying out of these powers can be prosecuted. The CQC also has powers under S. 64 to require the provision of any information, documents, records (including personal medical records) or other items which the Commission considers it necessary or expedient to have for the purposes of any of its regulatory functions. Those who must provide this information are:

(a)   an English NHS body,

(b)   a person providing healthcare commissioned by a Primary Care Trust,

(c)   an English local authority,

(d)   a person providing adult social services commissioned by an English local authority, or

(e)   a person who carries on or manages a regulated activity.

Where the information is on computer, then the CQC has the power to require the provision of information, documents or records in legible form.

Failure to comply with the request without reasonable excuse is a criminal offence.

Under S 65 the CQC has the power to require an explanation. The CQC is also required to comply with the rules relating to interaction with other bodies as laid down in Schedule 4 (S.66). These

Figure 17.5   Powers of the CQC Inspector S 63 of Health and Social Care Act 2008.

The inspector may if he or she considers it necessary or expedient for relevant purposes:

(a) make any examination into the state and management of the premises or the treatment of persons receiving care there,

(b) inspect and take copies of any documents or records,

(c) have access to, and check the operation of, any computer, and any associated apparatus or material, which is or has been in use in connection with any documents or records,

(d) inspect any other item,

(e) seize and remove from the premises any documents, records or other items,

(f) interview in private—

   (i) any person who carries on or manages a regulated activity, or who manages the provision of NHS care or adult social services, at the premises,

   (ii) any person working at the premises, and

   (iii) any person receiving care at the premises who consents to be interviewed, and

(g) if the conditions in subsection (3) are met, examine in private any person receiving care at the premises.

(3) The conditions are—

(a) A is a registered medical practitioner or registered nurse,

(b) A has reason to believe that the person to be examined is not receiving proper care at the premises, and

(c) the person to be examined—

   (i) is capable of giving consent to the examination and does so, or

   (ii) is incapable of giving consent to the examination.

(4) The power under subsection (2)(b) includes power—

(a) to require any person holding or accountable for documents or records (whether or not kept at the premises) to produce them for inspection at the premises, and

(b) to require any records which are kept by means of a computer to be produced in a form in which they are legible and can be taken away.

(5) The power under subsection (2)(f)(i) to interview a person in private includes power, in the case of a body corporate, to interview in private—

(a) any director, manager, secretary or other similar officer of the body corporate, and

(b) where the body is an English NHS body or English local authority, any officer or member of the NHS body or local authority.

(6) A may—

(a) require any person to afford A such facilities and assistance with respect to matters within the person's control as are necessary to enable A to exercise powers under section 62 and this section, and

(b) take such measurements and photographs, and make such recordings, as A considers necessary to enable A to exercise those powers.

(7) A person who without reasonable excuse—

(a) obstructs the exercise of a power conferred by section 62 or this section, or

(b) fails to comply with a requirement imposed under this section,

is guilty of an offence and liable on summary conviction to a fine not exceeding level 4 on the standard scale.

enable the CQC to delegate its inspection powers to another public body, provide advice and assistance, co-operate and take joint action with other public bodies.

The CQC is also required under S.67 to promote the effective co-ordination of reviews or assessments carried out by public bodies or other persons in relation to the carrying on of regulated activities. The Secretary of State may publish guidance about steps which regulatory authorities may take in exercising relevant powers with a view to avoiding the imposition of unreasonable burdens on those in respect of whom the powers are exercisable (S.68). The CQC and the Welsh Ministers must co-operate with each other for the efficient and effective discharge of their corresponding functions (S.69), as must the CQC and the Independent Regulator of NHS Foundation Trusts (S.70). Under S.75 the Secretary of State may cause an inquiry to be held into any matter connected with the exercise by the Commission of any of its functions. It is an offence, (subject to specified statutory defences) under S.76 if information, which has been obtained by the CQC on terms or in circumstances requiring it to be held in confidence, and it relates to and identifies an individual, is knowingly or recklessly disclosed during the lifetime of the individual. The CQC is required to prepare and publish a code in respect of the practice it proposes to follow in relation to confidential personal information (S.80). The Secretary of State has the power to issue a direction to the CQC if he considers that it is failing to discharge its functions (S.82). It is required to publish an annual report. The CQ C has the power to issue a fixed penalty notice.

The CQC has published a booklet *About the Care Quality Commission*, which explains its functions and another setting out full details of its enforcement policy. Both are available on its website.[25] Its intention in its enforcement policy is that the CQC should

- Harness a range of regulatory approaches
- Prioritise on the basis of risk
- Be transparent and open and
- Be proportionate.

Audit Commission

The Audit Commission is a non-departmental public body sponsored by the Office of the Deputy Prime Minister with the Department of Health and the National Assembly for Wales. It is responsible for ensuring that public money is used economically, efficiently and effectively. Its reports are available from its website. The Audit Commission covers local government, housing, health, criminal justice and community safety, working in audit, inspection, collecting information to measure performance, assessing local authorities and carrying out national studies. It has 18 commissioners and a chairman and employs 2500 people led by a chief executive. Its income is the fees charged for its work, and government grants. In 2003–4 its annual income was £218 million. Under section 56 of the Health and Social Care Act 2008, the Care Quality Commission and the Audit Commission may exercise jointly their respective functions under section 54 of the Health and Social Care Act 2008 and under sections 33 and 34 of the Audit Commission Act 1998. The two Commissions are to agree terms and payment and must have regard to any guidance issued by the Secretary of State.

The Audit Commission in Wales merged with the Welsh part of the National Audit Office to create a new, independent, unified audit and inspection organisation in April 2005.

National Institute for Health and Clinical Excellence (NICE)

This statutory body was established on 1 April 1999 to promote clinical and cost-effectiveness. The then Secretary of State stated that its task would be to abolish postcode variation in the country, so that there would be national standards for the provision of healthcare such as medicines. One of the functions of NICE is to issue clinical guidelines and clinical audit methodologies and information on good practice. NICE has a major role to play in the setting of standards of practice, by disseminating the results of research on what is proved to be clinically effective, research-based practice. One of its first activities was to recommend to the Secretary of State that the expense of Relenza, a drug developed by Glaxo Welcome for preventing 'flu, did not justify funding through the NHS since it appeared to have little benefit for those groups most at risk – older people and asthma sufferers. NICE's recommendations were accepted by the Secretary of State. Subsequently, following further research, it recommended the use of Relenza in the NHS.

One of the results of NICE guidance is that patients who claim to have suffered as a result of a failure to provide a reasonable standard of care, are able to use evidence of clinical effectiveness and research-based practice to illustrate failings in the care provided to them. It could be argued that failure to follow the recommendations of NICE will be prima facie evidence of a failure to follow a reasonable standard of care according to the Bolam test.[26] NICE grades its recommendations from level 1 to 3. Level 1 is a generally consistent finding in a majority of multiple acceptable studies; level 3 is limited scientific evidence which does not meet all the criteria of acceptable studies. (It is interesting to note that in the NICE guidelines on pressure ulcer risk management and prevention[27] the only level 1 guideline is: 'risk assessment tools should only be used as an aide-mémoire and should not replace clinical judgment'.)

In more recent years NICE has been concerned at the failure by NHS trusts and PCTs to follow clinical guidance and has looked at ways of securing the implementation of its guidance. It has faced several legal challenges. For example the drug manufacturers Eisai Ltd sought judicial review of the guidance issued by NICE on restricting the use of drugs for the treatment of Alzheimer's Disease.[28] The judge held that the processes of NICE were not flawed, but there were breaches of discrimination legislation As a consequence of the case, NICE was asked to revise its guidance within 28 days and the revised guidance can be seen on its website.[29] Subsequently Eisai Ltd won its appeal in the Court of Appeal[30] and the House of Lords refused NICE permission to appeal. As a consequence of the Court of Appeal decision NICE made further information available and received further comments, but eventually did not change its decision that specific drugs were only effective for those with moderate Alzheimer's. It stated that because of the distressing and debilitating nature of Alzheimer's it "has published a clinical guideline on the management of dementia (including Alzheimer's disease) which outlines the package of medical and social care that should be available for people with dementia and their carers, including social, medical and psychological treatment from early detection through to end of life."

The full list of completed guidelines, guidelines in development, completed interventional procedures covering clinical areas, public health and patient safety can be seen on the NICE website.[31]

Draft guidance from NICE on the treatment of osteoporosis was challenged by patients by judicial review. On 19 February 2009 Mr Justice Holman ruled that NICE wrongly failed to disclose the economic reasoning behind a decision in October to restrict the supply of strontium ranelate, a drug manufactured by Servier laboratories under the brand name Protelos. Nice should have disclosed to the drug's manufacturers and other interested parties the economic model underpinning its decision.

NICE has not yet abolished the postcode lottery: for example more than half of couples seeking embryo screening to protect their offspring from inherited genetic diseases such as breast cancer are being prevented from doing so. The technique of pre-implantation genetic diagnosis has not yet been considered by NICE.[32]

In December 2008 NICE announced that it intended to speed up decision making on guidance relating to several cancer drugs by increasing the number of its advisory committees and by starting the evaluation process more than a year before a drug company expects to obtain a licence.

Some of the achievements of NICE in its 10-year history were set out by the chairman in an article.[33] He described the setting up of a Citizens Council which has presented 11 reports on topics as diverse as health inequalities an 'only in research' recommendations and whose conclusions have been incorporated into Social Value Judgments, a guideline to help NICE's advisory bodies develop guidance that incorporates the public's values. In 2005 NICE was given the responsibility of developing guidance for all those with a role to play in the general health of communities. Public health guidance makes recommendations on activities, policies and strategies that can prevent disease or improve health (see Chapter 11).

Following the Darzi Report High Quality Care For All in June 2008 four new areas of work have been taken forward by NICE. These include:

- Advising on indicators for the Quality and Outcomes Framework (NICE is now responsible for producing an annual "menu" of new, evidence-based clinical and cost-effective indicators where there is a strong case for encouraging uptake of good practice.)
- Developing a fellowship programme to reward contributions to quality care. The fellowship programme will recognise clinicians who have made a major contribution to improving the quality of healthcare in areas related to NICE activities. 20 NICE Fellows drawn from senior NHS healthcare professionals will be appointed in 2009–10 who will be actively involved with NICE and will help drive up the quality of clinical care delivered and encourage the introduction of cost-effective innovation into clinical practice by:
  - Acting as ambassadors for NICE
  - Promoting the use of NICE guidance (including NICE quality standards) within their own specialty
  - Engaging with commissioners in order to ensure that the commissioning of local services is aligned with NICE guidance.
- Setting quality standards (A new National Quality Board will offer advice to Ministers on what the priorities should be for NICE's clinical standard setting. It's envisaged that NICE quality standards will be produced in collaboration with the NHS, its partners, and patients.)
- Setting up NHS Evidence (NHS Evidence was launched by NICE in April 2009. It is a web-based search portal offering reliable information for clinicians and commissioners.[34] It will include not only NICE guidance but content from other validated national and international sources).

Further information on all of these can be found on the NICE website.

National Service Frameworks (NSFs)

The White Paper envisages the setting up of evidence-based National Service Frameworks which identify what patients can expect to receive from the NHS in major care areas or disease groups. One of the first NSFs to be published was that for mental health and older people.[35] Some of the problems of implementing these frameworks in the context of traditional professional attitudes and views of organisations are discussed in a research paper by Edward Peck and others.[36] They discuss three models for organisational development. Eventually NSFs will cover most of the main spheres of clinical practice. They will doubtless assist managers and clinicians in obtaining the resources to ensure a reasonable standard of care for the patients. Inevitably, however, they are also likely to support litigation where patients who have suffered personal injuries are able to compare local facilities unfavourably with the norm laid down in the NSF. NSFs at present cover the following areas: cancer; children; coronary heart disease; diabetes; long-term health conditions; mental health; older people; paediatric intensive care; renal service and chronic obstructive pulmonary disease. The NSF on care of older people is considered in Chapter 24 and the children's NSF in Chapter 23.

It is hoped that eventually, as a result of the work of NICE, the NSFs and the CQC, in contrast to the existing situation, most OT practice and procedures will be based on research-based clinically effective practice (see Chapter 26 on research-based practice).

NHS Direct

The White Paper on the NHS[37] proposed the establishment of NHS Direct and, following a pilot scheme whereby patients could phone direct to a 24-hour phone line and get immediate advice from a registered nurse, NHS Direct was implemented across the country. The service aims to provide both clinical advice to support self-care and appropriate self-referral to NHS services, as well as access to more general advice and information. It was hoped that NHS Direct, through linking up with out-of-hours services, would provide a triage assessment for out-of-hours visits by doctors. NHS Direct was used as the main link for the relatives of children who had received post-mortems, to obtain information as to whether any organs had been removed and retained. An improved NHS Direct Online website, including a new interactive enquiry service, was launched in November 2001.[38] In April 2003 it was announced[39] that the success of NHS Direct had led to plans for considerable expansion over the following three years and a strategy document was published.[40] Its call capacity was to be doubled to 16 million calls annually, with an 80% increase in funding. The intention was to enable NHS Direct to:

- Provide a single access point to the NHS out-of-hours services
- Handle all low priority 999 ambulance calls
- Establish a new national NHS Direct digital TV service
- Become a distinct national organisation, independent of the Department of Health, with funding devolved from Whitehall direct to PCTs.

In October 2008 NHS Direct and NHS Choices joined forces to create a single website for access to NHS information.[41] NHS Direct continues to provide a telephone service on 0845 4647.

Walk-in clinics

A press announcement[42] publicised the setting up of more direct access clinics run by nurses, to which any person can go for assistance and advice on healthcare. They aim, in the words of the press release:

> to offer quick access to a range of NHS services including free consultations, minor treatments, health information and advice on self-treatment. They are based in convenient locations that allow the public easy access and have opening hours tailored to suit modern lifestyles, including early mornings, late evenings, and weekends. The centres will have close links with local GPs ensuring continuity of care for their patients.

The advantages to the public are clearly apparent: fast service, no wait, close to work, easy access, immediate advice, speedy prescriptions. Many of the clinics were planned to be linked with GP surgeries through information technology. At present there appears to be little OT involvement in the walk-in centres, but this may in the future be seen as a useful addition to the service.

Additional funding of £20 billion

In March 2000 the Chancellor of the Exchequer announced that an additional £20 billion was to be given to the NHS over the next four years. Following this, the Prime Minister set up a Cabinet Committee to agree and monitor the standards for performance within the NHS. He identified five challenges:

- All parts of the NHS would be required to work to end bed-blocking and unnecessary hospital admissions.
- They would have to put systems in place to identify and root out poor clinical practice.
- More flexible training and working practices should be introduced and efforts made to ensure doctors do not waste time dealing with patients who could be treated by other care staff.
- Booking systems should be adopted to ensure that patients with the most serious conditions get treated as quickly as possible.
- Prevention, with better health awareness programmes, should be addressed.

National Plan for the NHS

On 22 March 2000 the Prime Minister announced to the House of Commons that there were five challenges to be faced in the NHS. These are shown in Figure 17.6.

Following the Prime Minister's announcement, the Secretary for Health announced that he was setting up discussions with key professionals in the NHS to develop a National Plan based on these five challenges. He intended to establish six modernisation action teams with a specific remit to address variations in performance and standards across the care system. The NHS Plan was published in July 2000[43] and had the aim of increasing investment into the NHS and at the same time meeting the five challenges shown in Figure 17.6. Since then new organisations and bodies have been established to implement the significant changes envisaged in the plan (see Chapter 14 for the establishment of the Commission for Patient and Public Involvement, Patient Advocacy and Liaison Services (PALS), Independent Complaints and Advice Services (ICAS) and Patients' Forums, Chapter 4 for the Council for the Regulation of Healthcare Professions, Chapter 3 for the setting up of the Health Professions Council).

Figure 17.6 Challenges for the NHS.

- Partnership – making all parts of the health and social care system work better together and ensuring the right emphasis at each level of care
- Performance – improving both clinical performance and health service productivity
- Professions – increasing flexibility in training and working practices and removing demarcations, in the context of major expansion of the healthcare workforce
- Patient care – which has two components: ensuring fast and convenient access to services, and empowering and informing patients so that they can be more involved in their own care
- Prevention – tackling inequalities and focusing the health system on its contribution to tackling the causes of avoidable ill-health

NHS Modernisation Agency

This was envisaged in the NHS Plan as an organisation which would spread best practice. Chapter 6 of the NHS Plan stated:

> We will create a new Modernisation Agency to help local clinicians and managers redesign local services around the needs and convenience of patients. It will encompass the existing National Patients' Action Team, the Primary Care Development Team, the 'Collaborative Programmes' and the clinical governance support unit. The NHS Leadership Centre will also become the responsibility of the new Modernisation Agency, as will the Beacon Programme and the NHS annual awards programme. The Agency will work with all Trusts to support continuous service improvements.

The staff of the NHS Modernisation Agency were mostly drawn from professionals on secondment from the NHS. In April 2005 a new much smaller central organisation replaced the Modernisation Agency with 150 staff compared to 760. It focused on innovation and could commission support for its activities from a range of public and private sector providers.

The NHS Modernisation Board

The NHS Modernisation Board was chaired by the Secretary of State and includes the Department of Health's permanent secretary, the NHS Chief Executive and representatives from leading health-care organisations, people who work in the NHS and patient and citizen representatives. Its role is to ensure that those involved in the implementation of the NHS Plan are making real and speedy progress. It also oversees the progress of the Department of Health, the Modernisation Agency, the taskforces, the NHS and the social care community. It publishes an annual report.[44] The Modernisation Board was replaced in April 2005.

A review of arm's length bodies was carried out between 2005 and 2007 to determine how the organisations should be rationalised and functions transferred to others. The NHS Modernisation Agency was abolished. Subsequently as part of the Darzi review a National Quality Board was established.

The National Quality Board (NQB)

The NQB (in the words of the Department of Health) is 'a multi-stakeholder board established to champion quality and ensure alignment in quality throughout the NHS. The Board is a key aspect of the work to deliver high quality care for patients'.

The aim of the Board is to bring together all those with an interest in improving quality, to align and agree the NHS quality goals, whilst respecting the independent status of participating organisations.

Its role is to provide strategic oversight and leadership in quality across the NHS.

The key functions of the Board are to:

- ensure the overall alignment of the quality system
- deliver on specific technical responsibilities including those set out in the Next Stage Review, namely to oversee the work to improve quality indicators, advise the Secretary of State on the priorities for clinical standards set by NICE and make an annual report to the Secretary of State on the state of quality in England using internationally agreed comparable measures

- assume a wider leadership responsibility for driving the quality agenda and acting as a power-house for change.

The membership includes representatives from some of the national organisations including: the chairs of the Care Quality Commission, NICE, NPSA, and Monitor. Also on the Board are the NHS medical director, the Chief Nursing Office and the Chief Medical Officer and the Director General for Social Care, Local Government and Care Partnerships. Expert and lay members from a variety of disciplines have also been appointed. Its annual report for 2009 is available from the DH website.

Lord Darzi's other recommendations are considered in Chapter 29.

The National Patient Safety Agency

This was set up in 2001 and is discussed in Chapter 11.

Bristol paediatric heart surgery inquiry

The report of this Inquiry,[45] chaired by Professor Ian Kennedy, into the deaths of children during heart surgery in Bristol should have had a major impact on standards and procedures within the NHS. Some commentators have suggested that in future, people will talk about before and after Bristol. The Inquiry has made significant and strong recommendations across a wide field of professional practice including:

- respect and honesty
- a health service which is well led
- competent healthcare professionals
- the safety of care
- care of an appropriate standard
- public involvement through empowerment
- the care of the child.

These recommendations have become the starting point for further reform of standards within healthcare, and the Healthcare Commission (Commission for Healthcare Audit and Improvement) has had them in mind in carrying out its inspections. The Care Quality Commission has now replaced the Healthcare Commission.

Health and Social Care (Community Health and Standards) Act 2003

This Act enabled the establishment of NHS Foundation Trusts and defined their functions, powers and controls over them. It also abolished the Commission for Health Improvement (CHI), replacing it with the Commission for Health Audit and Inspection (CHAI), and abolished the National Care Standards Commission, replacing it with the Commission for Social Care Inspection. Section 46 of the Health and Social Care (Community Health and Standards) Act 2003 gave power to the Secretary of State to prepare and publish statements of standards in relation to the provision of healthcare by and for English NHS bodies and cross-border SHAs (strategic health authorities). Failure to comply with these statements of standards could lead to inspection by CHAI, action by the Secretary of State to remove the NHS trust board or possibly (and this remains to be seen) legal action for breach of statutory duty by the patient. Certainly the patient could use failure to comply with the standards as evidence of a breach of the duty of care, which has caused harm, in an action for compensation in the law of negligence. Under section 46(4) the standards set out in statements are to be taken into account by every English NHS body and cross-border Strategic Health Authorities in discharging their duties under section 45. These provisions were reenacted in Section 45 of the Health and Social Care Act 2008.

Under section 45(1) the Secretary of State may prepare and publish statements of standards in relation to the provision of NHS care and under 45(2) the Secretary of State must keep the standards under review and may publish amended statements whenever the Secretary of State considers it appropriate. In addition the Secretary of State may direct a person:

(a) to prepare a draft statement of standards for the purposes of subsection (1), submit it to the Secretary of State for approval and publish it in the form approved or modified by the Secretary of State;

(b) to keep standards under review for the purposes of subsection (2) and, whenever the person considers it appropriate, submit a draft amended statement to the Secretary of State for approval and publish it in the form approved or modified by the Secretary of State.

(4) The Secretary of State must consult such persons as the Secretary of State considers appropriate—

(a) before publishing a statement under subsection (1) or approving a statement under subsection (3)(a);

(b) before publishing under subsection (2), or approving under subsection (3)(b), any amended statement which in the opinion of the Secretary of State effects a substantial change in the standards.

The Care Quality Commission (CQC) (see below) undertakes reviews of health and social services providers using the indicators set by the Secretary of State to assess their performance.

The Health and Social Care (Community Health and Standards) Act 2003 made provision for:

Part 1 NHS Foundation Trusts and the Independent Regulator
Part 2 Standards: Regulatory Bodies: Commission for Health Audit and Inspection
Commission for Social Care Inspection
Quality standards in NH
Functions under the Care Standards Act 2000

Part 3 Recovery of NHS charges
Part 4 Dental and medical services
Part 5 Miscellaneous, including abolition of Public Health Laboratory Service Board
Part 6 Final provisions

Schedules specifying constitution of various bodies and providing details of the new legislation in the Act

NHS foundation trusts

An NHS foundation trust is defined in the Health and Social Care (Community Health and Standards) Act 2003 (re-enacted in section 30 of the NHS Act 2006) as

a public benefit corporation which is authorised to provide goods and services for the purposes of the health service in England.

A public benefit corporation is a body corporate which following an application under this Chapter is constituted in accordance with Schedule 7.

Statutory provisions relating to NHS Foundation Trusts were re-enacted in Chapter 5 of the NHS Act 2006 sections 30 to 65 and the section numbers below refer to the 2006 Act.

An NHS Foundation Trust is a body corporate and rules relating to its constitution are set out in Schedule 7 of the 2006 Act. A body corporate, known as the Independent Regulator of NHS Foundation Trusts (called the regulator[46]), is set up under section 31 of the Act with additional provisions relating to membership, tenure of office, general and specific powers, finance, and reports set out in Schedule 8. The regulator has a duty to exercise its functions in a manner that is consistent with the performance by the Secretary of State of the duties under sections 1, 3 and 258 of the NHS Act 2006 (Duty as to health service and services generally and as to university clinical teaching and research). NHS trusts can apply to the regulator for authorisation to become an NHS foundation trust. The application must describe the goods and services it intends to provide together with a copy of the proposed constitution of the trust. The main differences between an NHS foundation trust and an NHS trust are:

- An NHS foundation trust is an independent public benefit corporation, not under the direct control of the Secretary of State.
- An NHS foundation trust comes under the control of an Independent Regulator which gives an authorisation for the establishment of the NHS foundation trust and must secure that the principle purpose of the trust is the provision of goods and services for the purposes of the health service in England. (These include education and training, accommodation and other facilities and carrying out research.) An authorisation can restrict the provision of private healthcare by the NHS foundation trust.
- The NHS foundation trust has a general duty to exercise its functions effectively, efficiently and economically (section 63 of the National Heath Service Act 2006) comparable to the duty of an NHS Trust under section 26 of the NHS Act.
- Ownership and accountability for the NHS foundation trust are in the hands of the local community rather than the Secretary of State.
- NHS foundation trusts can raise capital (section 46) (within overall limits and according to a prudential borrowing code (PBC) (section 41) and retain any operating surplus. (The PBC is to be drawn up by the Regulator and placed before Parliament.).[47]
- NHS foundation trusts will be expected to comply with national standards and targets, but will not be subject to directions from the Secretary of State or performance management by strategic health authorities and the Department of Health. (They will however be subject to inspections and inquiries carried out by CQC, which must report to the Regulator.)
- Individuals with an interest in the development and well-being of an NHS foundation trust can register as members. These members become responsible as owners of the trust.
- Each NHS foundation trust will establish a board of governors who will ensure that the local community is directly involved in the governance of the trust. Regulations may make provision for the conduct of elections for membership of the board of governors.
- Primary care trust (PCT) Patient Forums for any PCT area served by an NHS foundation trust will have the right to inspect the NHS foundation trust's services, commission independent advocacy in relation to services provided by the NHS foundation trust, promote the involvement of members of the public in consultations, decisions and policy development by the NHS foundation trust, advise the trust on encouraging public involvement and monitor its success in achieving public involvement. (Patient Forums have been replaced by LINKs; see Chapter 4.)

- An NHS foundation trust may do anything which appears to it to be necessary or desirable for the purpose of or in connection with its functions (section 47), including the acquiring and disposing of property, entering into contracts, and accepting gifts of property.
- The authorisation must require an NHS foundation trust to disclose such information as the Secretary of State specifies to the regulator and may require an NHS foundation trust to allow the regulator to enter and inspect premises owned or controlled by the trust.
- Sections 56 and 57 provide for the mergers of NHS foundation trusts with NHS foundation trusts and/or NHS trusts.

Bill Moyes was appointed in December 2003 as chair of the Independent Regulator of NHS Foundation Trusts. He has the responsibility of authorising, monitoring and regulating NHS Foundation Trusts and works with a board of up to five members including the chair and a deputy chair. The Regulator has the power to serve notice on a failing trust to order it to carry out specific functions. Ultimately the regulator has the power to make an order providing for the dissolution of the trust. Regulations were published in April 2003 to cover the dissolution of an NHS foundation trust under section 25. A short guide to foundation trusts was published in 2005.[48]

NHS Constitution and the Darzi Plan

The final report of Professor Lord Darzi, *High Quality of Care for All* on the future of the NHS was published in 2008.[49] It set out a strategy to secure high quality care across the NHS and identified the measures both immediate and long term which would be taken. An NHS Constitution was also published and is reproduced as Appendix 2 to this book. Both the Strategic plan and the NHS Constitution are discussed in Chapter 29.

Service quality and governance within OT

In July 2003 the College of Occupational Therapists published its Professional Standards for occupational therapy practice.[50] The standard for service quality and governance applies the principle of clinical governance to the OT and states:

> The principles of quality and governance apply equally to all occupational therapists, in all settings. Individual therapists and services have a duty to provide an occupational therapy service of the highest competence, safety, quality and value.

Four standard statements are then set out:

(1) Occupational therapists should maintain and develop their knowledge, skills and behaviour, and therefore their competence to practise.
(2) Occupational therapists should protect and maintain the safety of those who use their service.
(3) Occupational therapists should provide a service of consistent quality, in line with local, professional and national standards.
(4) Occupational therapists should provide a service that is of the highest quality and the best value for money.

The COT revised the professional standards and the standard statements in 2007 but no amendments were made to those quoted above.

These standards, together with the statutory duty of quality which section 45 of the Health and Social Care (Community Health and Standards) Act 2003 places upon the NHS organisation, should assist the OT if she is aware that resource or other pressures are leading to an unacceptable level of service. She would have a professional responsibility to raise this issue with her senior managers (see section on whistleblowing in Chapter 19). There is a statutory duty on NHS trusts to ensure that they exercise their functions effectively, efficiently, and economically (S.26 NHS Act 2006). In applying this duty to occupational therapy departments, OTs might find the work at Newham Children's Services Occupational therapy Department in reducing complaints and the length of the waiting list for OT services by using the business process redesign (BPR) of considerable interest.[51]

Conclusion

There is no doubt that clinical governance, clinical effective practice, evidence-based medicine, and the National Service Frameworks are playing an increasingly major role in healthcare. The future challenge for the Government is to ensure high national standards across the country in the provision of healthcare at a time of considerable pressure on public expenditure as a result of the credit crunch and recession and also foster local decision making and local initiatives to ensure high morale and enterprise upon which developments within healthcare depend. In addition, as new forms of co-operation between local social services authorities and primary care trusts, NHS trusts and care trusts develop, new opportunities will be presented to OTs to ensure more effective care for their clients. Statutory changes to organisational structure in the NHS present OTs with many challenges, and Alice Godfrey[52] points out the importance of OTs recognising the significance of these changes to their practice.

Statutory developments within social services and the establishment of care trusts are considered in the next chapter, which also discusses legal issues arising in community care and disability discrimination.

 Questions and exercises

1   Discuss the impact of clinical governance on the work of the OT.
2   What benefits does the establishment of primary care trusts and care trusts bring to the OT department?
3   Obtain a copy of the local health improvement plan for your area and a copy of the Service and Financial Framework and consider their implications for your department.
4   Access the NICE website and consider guidance which is relevant to your particular work as an OT. To what extent have its recommendations been implemented?
5   To what extent are your professional actions supported by research as being clinically effective?
6   What national standards or Audit Commission reports have been published in relation to your work? To what extent have their recommendations been implemented?
7   Do you consider that litigation and complaints have been reduced as a result of quality monitoring and audit in your department?
8   Obtain a copy of the report of the Bristol Inquiry and identify the extent to which your department works in accordance with its recommendations.

References

1 DoH (1997) *A New NHS: Modern Dependable*. HMSO, London.
2 DoH (1998) White Paper, *Modernising Social Services*.
3 Health and Social Care Act 2001 sections 50–52; The Preserved Rights (Transfer of Responsibilities to Local Authorities) Regulations 2001 SI 2001/3776; LAC(2002)7.
4 HSC 2000/11 LAC(2000)10 Commencement of sections 29 and 30 of the Health Act 1999.
5 DoH (1997) *A New NHS: Modern Dependable*. HMSO, London.
6 DoH (1996) *Primary Care: Delivering the Future*. DoH, London.
7 Primary Care Trusts (Membership, Procedure and Administration Arrangements) Regulations 2000 SI 2000/89, as amended by SI 2001/3787; 2002/38, 557, 880, 881, 2469 and 2861; SI 2003/1616; NHS Reform and Health Care Professions Act 2002 (Supplementary, Consequential etc. Provisions) Regulations 2003 SI 2003/1937.
8 NHS Executive (1999) *Primary Care Trusts: Financial Framework*. Catalogue No. 10389.
9 NHS Executive (1999) *Working Together: Human resources guidance and requirements for Primary Care Trusts*. Catalogue No. 10390.
10 NHS Executive (1999) Primary Care Trusts: A guide to estate and facilities matters. Catalogue No. 10393.
11 www.doh.gov.uk/coin.htm or they can be viewed at http://tap.ccta.gov.uk/doh/coin4.nsf.
12 NHS Confederation *Briefing Primary Care Trusts – new guidance*, Issue No. 39, February 2000.
13 DoH (2001) *Shifting the Balance of Power within the NHS: Securing Delivery*. DoH, London.
14 National Audit Office (2007) Improving quality and safety – progress in implementing clinical governance in primary care: Lessons for the new Primary Care Trusts. HC 100 2006–7. Stationery Office, London.
15 The Health Act 1999 Partnership Arrangements SI 2000/617.
16 HSC 2000/010; LAC (2000)9 Implementation of the Health Act 1999 Partnership Arrangements.
17 Hurwitz, B. (1998) *Clinical Guidelines and the Law*. Radcliffe Medical Press, Oxford.
18 DoH (1998) *A First Class Service: Quality in the new NHS*. HSC 1998/113.
19 DoH (1999) *NHS Executive Clinical Governance: Quality in the new NHS*. HSC 1999/065.
20 Seeley, C. (1999) Clinical Governance An information guide for occupational therapists. *British Journal of Occupational Therapy*, **62**(6), 263–8; College of Occupational Therapists Position Statement on Clinical Governance. *British Journal of Occupational Therapy*, **62**(6), 261–2.
21 www.audit-commission.gov.uk/aboutus/index.asp
22 HSC 2000/010; LAC (2000)9 Implementation of the Health Act 1999 Partnership Arrangements.
23 DoH (1999) *NHS Executive Clinical Governance: Quality in the new NHS*. HSC 1999/065.
24 DoH (1998) *A First Class Service: Quality in the new NHS*. HSC 1998/113.
25 www.cqc.org.uk
26 *Bolam v Friern Barnet Hospital Management Committee* [1957] 1 WLR 582.
27 National Institute for Clinical Excellence (2001) NICE guideline on pressure ulcer risk management and prevention.
28 *Eisai Ltd v National Institute for Health and Clinical Excellence (Alzheimer's Society and Shire Pharmaceuticals Ltd Interested parties)* [2007] EWHC 1941.
29 http://guidance.nice.org.uk/TA111.
30 *R (on the application of Eisai) v National Institute for Health and Clinical Excellence and Shire Pharmaceuticals Ltd and the Association of the British Pharmaceutical Industry* [2008] EWCA Civ 438.
31 www.nice.org.uk
32 Rose David 'Postcode lottery' for gene screening funds The Times 15 January 2009.
33 Rawlins Michael (Sir) (2009) The NICE decade. *British Journal of Healthcare Management*, **15**(4), 197.
34 www.evidence.nhs.uk/
35 DoH (1999) National Service Framework for mental health services.
36 Peck, E., Grove, B. & Howell, V. (2000) Upsetting the apple cart whilst pulling it along the road: Implementing the National Service Framework for Mental Health. *Managing Community Care*, **8**(2).
37 DoH (1997) White Paper *The New NHS – Modern – Dependable*.

38   DoH (2001) Press Release 2001/0573 Personalised Health Information at the touch of a button.
39   DoH (2003) Press Release 2003/0165 *NHS Direct to more than double in size.*
40   DoH (2003) *Developing NHS Direct.*
41   www.nhs.uk
42   DoH (1999) Press Release Frank Dobson announces more NHS walk-in clinics.
43   DoH (2000) *The NHS Plan for investment A plan for reform*, Cm 4818-1; www.nhs.uk/nhsplan/contents/pdf.htm
44   DoH (2003) *The NHS Modernisation Board's annual report*; www.doh.gov.uk/modernisationboardreport/index.htm
45   *Bristol Royal Infirmary Inquiry Learning from Bristol*: the report of the public inquiry into children's heart surgery at the Bristol Royal Infirmary 1984–1995, Cm 5207.
46   www.doh.gov.uk/nhsfoundationtrusts/independentregulator.htm
47   www.doh.gov.uk/nhsfoundationtrusts/fmance.htm
48   Department of Health (2005) *A Short Guide to NHS Foundation Trusts*. DH, London.
49   Department of Health (2008) High Quality of Care for All CM 7432 DH, London.
50   College of Occupational Therapists (2003) *Professional Standards for Occupational Therapy Practice*. COT, London.
51   Horton Ayana and Hall Jennifer (2008) Redesigning occupational therapy service provision to increase efficiency, effectiveness and stakeholder satisfaction. *British Journal of Occupational Therapy* April 2008 Vol **71**(4), 161–4.
52   Godfrey, A. (2000) Policy changes in the National Health Service: Implications and opportunities for occupational therapists. *British Journal of Occupational Therapy*, **63**(5), 218–24.

18 Community Care and the Rights of the Disabled

In the last chapter we looked at the statutory organisation of the NHS and social services provision and recent legal changes. This chapter considers the legal issues which can arise in community care and the effect of recent statutory changes on the role of the occupational therapist (OT). It also considers the impact of the Disability Discrimination Act 1995. Luke Clements' book *Community Care and the Law*[1] provides a good overview of the basic statutory provisions relating to community care. The COT published a strategy for modernising OT services in local health and social care communities in 2000[2] which was launched in 2002 (see Chapter 1). Jill Riley[3] is concerned that this strategy may reveal a missed opportunity for the COT to establish a firm foundation for occupational therapy in social services departments. The COT published a position statement on the value of OT and its contribution to adult social service users and their carers in 2008[4] and also combined with the DH in 2008 in publishing a book on sustaining a high quality workforce for adult social care.[5]

This chapter seeks to cover the implications of the law for all OTs whatever their focus of interest. Reference should be made to Chapter 15 for equipment issues, to Chapter 16 for transport issues and to Chapters 20–24 covering individual client groups. The following topics are covered in this chapter:

Community Care	Disability Discrimination
• Introduction	• Disability Discrimination Act 1995
• The White Paper *Caring for People*	• Discrimination in the provision of goods, facilities and services
• The NHS and Community Care Act 1990	• Discrimination in education
• The Duty to Assess	• Special Educational Needs and Disability Act 2001
• Community care plans	• Public transport
• Care management approach	• National Disability Council
• Carers	• Disability Rights Commission

Legal Aspects of Occupational Therapy, Third Edition By Bridgit Dimond
© 2010 Bridgit Dimond

Developments in community care

The debate on the value of developing community care goes back to the late 1950s and the 1960s and progress was made to a limited extent in reducing the size of long-stay NHS institutions, both for the mentally disturbed and older people. The greatest impetus to the recent changes, however, was the report prepared by Sir Roy Griffiths, who was invited in December 1986 by the then Secretary of State, Norman Fowler, to carry out a review of community care policy.[6] The report was presented in February 1988 and contained radical suggestions for a significant change in the funding of accommodation in the community and greater emphasis on clear lines of managerial accountability. Provision in future had to be on the basis of an assessment of need and the development of local plans, drawn up by the local authorities (LAs) in conjunction with health authorities and the voluntary sector.

The White Paper *Caring for People*

In November 1989 a White Paper was published, *Caring for People; Community Care in the next decade and beyond*,[7] which set out the following key objectives in community care:

- to promote the development of domiciliary, day and respite services to enable people to live in their own homes wherever feasible and sensible
- to ensure that service providers make practical support for carers a high priority
- to make proper assessment of need and good care management the cornerstone of high quality care
- to promote the development of a flourishing independent sector alongside good quality public services
- to clarify the responsibilities of agencies and so make it easier to hold them to account for their performance
- to secure better value for taxpayers' money by introducing a new funding structure for social care.

These objectives of the White Paper envisaged that certain key changes would be required, including:

- LAs becoming more responsible, in collaboration with other agencies, for making assessments and meeting individual community care needs
- LAs being required to publish clear plans for the development of community care services
- LAs making maximum use of the independent sector
- a new funding structure for provision of residential and nursing home accommodation
- eligibility for income support and housing benefit to be made irrespective of whether the person is living in their own home or in residential accommodation
- LAs being required to establish inspection and registration units
- a specific grant to promote the development of social care for seriously mentally ill people.

The White Paper explained how these key changes would work in practice and outlined the roles and responsibilities of the social services authorities and also those of the health services. Emphasis was placed on quality control and achieving high standards of care, collaborative working and service for people with a mental illness. It also considered the issue of resources and the links with social security. Separate chapters covered Wales and Scotland.

The NHS and Community Care Act 1990

Many of the recommendations of the White Paper were incorporated in the NHS and Community Care Act 1990. The main provisions of this Act in relation to community care are listed in Figure 18.1.

It should be noted that section 7 of the Local Authority Social Services Act 1970 requires an LA to act under the guidance of the Secretary of State in exercising its social services functions. Section 46(3) provides the first statutory definition of community care services, given in Figure 18.2.

Four main topics of the community care provisions will be considered in the first part of this chapter: the duty to assess, the duty to prepare community care plans, the care management approach and long-term care and NHS/social services responsibilities.

Figure 18.1   The community care provisions of the NHS and Community Care Act 1990.

Section 46(3): Statutory definition of community care

Sections 42 to 45: The provision of accommodation and welfare services, charges for accommodation and the recovery of charges provided by LAs

Section 46: The provision of a community care plan by each LA

Section 47: Assessment of needs for community care services

Section 48: Inspection of premises used for provision of community care services

Section 49: Transfer of staff from health service to LAs

Section 50: Power of Secretary of State to give directions and instruct LAs to set up complaints procedures

Sections 51 to 58: Provisions for Scotland.

Figure 18.2   The NHS and Community Care Act 1990 – section 46(3).

'Community care services' means services which a local authority may provide or arrange to be provided under any of the following provisions—

(a)   Part III of the National Assistance Act 1948 [provision of accommodation for those over 18 who need it because of age, illness, disability or any other circumstances];
(b)   section 45 of the Health Services and Public Health Act 1968 [covers arrangements for promoting the welfare of 'old people'];
(c)   section 21 of and Schedule 8 to the National Health Service Act 1977 [the provision of services for the care of mothers and young children; prevention, care and after care; home help and laundry facilities]; and
(d)   section 117 of the Mental Health Act 1983 [the duty of the health authority and local social services authority to provide, in co-operation with relevant voluntary agencies, after care services for any person who has been detained under specified sections of the Mental Health Act 1983].

The duty to assess

Section 47 of the NHS and Community Care Act 1990 places upon the LA a duty to carry out an assessment for any individual who would appear to be eligible for its services. The actual wording is set out in Figure 18.3.

These subsections are subject to the emergency provisions which are shown in Figure 18.4.

Disabled persons

There is a statutory requirement (section 47(2)) upon LAs in carrying out an assessment to proceed under the Disabled Persons (Services, Consultation and Representation) Act 1986 if, at any time during the assessment of needs, it appears that the client is a disabled person. They need not wait for a request from the person but must inform him that they will be doing so and inform him of his rights under the 1986 Act (see Chapter 20). Section 47(7) states that the section is 'without prejudice' to section 3 of the Disabled Persons (Services, Consultation and Representation) Act 1986. This means that it does not affect the provisions of the 1986 Act which exist in parallel with the provisions for giving information under the 1990 Act. 'Disabled person' has the same meaning as that used in the 1986 Act.

Figure 18.3   The NHS and Community Care Act 1990 – section 47(1).

Assessment of needs for community care services

Subject to subsections (5) and (6) below [see Figure 18.4], where it appears to a local authority that any person for whom they may provide or arrange for the provision of community services may be in need of any services, the authority—

(a)   shall carry out an assessment of his needs for those services; and
(b)   having regard to the results of that assessment, shall then decide whether his needs call for the provision by them of any such services.

Figure 18.4   Emergency provisions – subsections 47(5) and (6).

(5)   Nothing in this section [47] shall prevent a local authority from temporarily providing or arranging for the provision of community care services for any person without carrying out a prior assessment of his needs in accordance with the preceding provisions of this section if, in the opinion of the authority, the condition of that person is such that he requires those services as a matter of urgency.
(6)   If, by virtue of subsection (5) above, community care services have been provided temporarily for any person as a matter of urgency, then, as soon as practicable thereafter, an assessment of his needs shall be made in accordance with the preceding provisions of this section.

Involvement of health and housing authorities

Under section 47(3)(a) the LA must notify the relevant health authority if at any time during the assessment it appears to the LA that there may be a need for the provision to that person of any services under the National Health Service Act 1977. Under section 47(3)(b) a similar provision exists if there is seen to be a need for the provision of any services which fall within the functions of a local housing authority. In such circumstances the LA has a duty not only to notify the health authority and/or housing authority but also to invite them to assist, to such extent as is reasonable in the circumstances, in the making of the assessment. In making a decision as to the provision of the services needed for the person in question, the LA shall take into account any services which are likely to be made available to him by the health authority or housing authority.

Central government directions and guidance

The Secretary of State has the power to make directions relating to assessments (section 47(4)). Subject to this the LA shall carry out the assessment in such manner and take such form as it considers appropriate. Directions were issued by the Department of Health in 2004[8] about the involvement of carers in the assessment (see below) and can be obtained from the DH website which required the local authority to consider whether the person being assessed has any carers and, where they think it appropriate consult those carers. In addition the LA must take all reasonable steps to reach agreement with the person and, where they think it appropriate, any carers of that person, on the community care services which they are considering providing to him to meet his needs. The LA must provide information to the person and, where they think it appropriate, any carers of that person, about the amount of the payment (if any) which the person will be liable to make in respect of the community care services which they are considering providing to him.

Guidance has been issued to local and other authorities for use in carrying out the assessments.[9] In addition, the Social Services Inspectorate (SSI) has prepared several handbooks on guidance in care management and assessment for managers and practitioners.

Entitlement to assessment

Entitlement is not defined in the section other than in terms of eligibility for service provision. This is determined by residence (see below). Could it be argued that if the LA does not provide specific services then the assessment for those services need not be carried out?

The words 'any person for whom they may provide or arrange for the provision of community care services' cover all those services under the Acts specified in section 46(3), which defines what is meant by community care services. The fact that the LA does not supply all the services the client may require cannot be a justification for not carrying out the assessment. After all, it could be argued that until the assessment has been carried out it cannot be certain which services the client will or will not require. The duty to assess is owed to those who are ordinarily resident within the LA area. Guidance on the possibility of making arrangements with other LAs for the provision of services stresses the need to take into account the desirability of providing services in the locality.

Carrying out the assessment

Stages in the process

The summary of practice guidance included in both the *Managers' Guide*[10] and the *Practitioners' Guide*[11] sets out the stages which should be followed in implementing the care management and assessment process. These stages are shown in Figure 18.5.

Levels of assessment

The *Practitioners' Guide* suggests that stage one requires an initial identification of the need and the determination of the level of assessment required in the light of that assessment. For example it sets out six possible levels of assessment:

1. simple assessment
2. limited assessment
3. multiple assessment
4. specialist assessment either simple or complex
5. complex assessment
6. comprehensive assessment.

An example of an outcome from a level one assessment is a bus pass or badge for a disabled car driver. An example of an outcome from a level six assessment could be family therapy, substitute care or intensive domiciliary support.

Figure 18.5   Care management and assessment process.

Stage 1: Information to carers and prospective clients on needs for which the agencies accept responsibility and the range of services currently available.

Stage 2: The level of the assessment required is decided.

Stage 3: A practitioner is allocated to assess the needs of the individual and of any carers.

Stage 4: The resources available from statutory, voluntary, private or community sources that best meet the individual's requirements are considered. The role of the practitioner is to assist the user in making choices from these resources and to put together an individual care plan.

Stage 5: The implementation of the plan, i.e. securing the necessary financial or other identified resources.

Stage 6: Monitoring of implementation of the care plan.

Stage 7: Review of the care plan with the user, carers and service providers, firstly, to ensure that services remain relevant to needs and, secondly, to evaluate services as part of the continuing quest for improvement.

Differing perceptions of need

The assessment of need is described in the *Practitioners' Guide* as being undertaken to 'understand an individual's needs, to relate them to agency policies and priorities, and to agree the objectives for any intervention'.

The practitioner is required by the guidance 'to define, as precisely as possible, the cause of any difficulty'. It recognises that need is unlikely to be perceived and defined in the same way by users, their carers, and any other care agencies involved. It suggests that 'the practitioner must, therefore, aim for a degree of consensus but, so long as they are competent, the users' views should carry the most weight. Where it is impossible to reconcile different perceptions, these differences should be acknowledged and recorded'.

Who carries out the assessment?

There is an emphasis on a multi-disciplinary approach to the task of assessment, with local authorities bringing in relevant professionals where necessary. The White Paper, *Caring for People; Community care in the next decade and beyond* suggests:

> 3.25 All agencies and professions involved with the individual and his or her problems should be brought into the assessment procedure when necessary. These may include social workers, GPs, community nurses, hospital staff such as consultants in geriatric medicine, psychiatry, rehabilitation and other hospital specialties, nurses, physiotherapists, occupational therapists, speech therapists, continence advisers, community psychiatric nurses, staff involved with vision and hearing impairment, housing officers, the Employment Department's Settlement Officers and its Employment Rehabilitation Service, home helps, home care assistants and voluntary workers.

> 3.26 Assessments should take account of the wishes of the individual and his or her carer, and of the carer's ability to continue to provide care, and where possible should include their active participation. Effort should be made to offer flexible services which enable individuals and carers to make choices.

Where the client is in hospital, the lead agency for carrying out the assessment will be the health services; where the client is in the community or in residential accommodation, the lead agency will be the local authority.

What if the client refuses to co-operate in the assessment?

It would seem that there is a duty under section 47(l)(a) of the 1990 Act for the assessment to be made even if the client refuses. Clearly, however, this may lead to a less than satisfactory assessment and any later objection by the client to the assessment should take account of her lack of co-operation. Where the client is incapable of assisting in the assessment, e.g. as a result of mental disability, the co-operation of relatives, carers or other representatives should be sought. The Mental Capacity Act 2005 now ensures that where decisions are required on behalf of a mentally incapacitated adult, then they must be made in his or her best interests. There are provisions for the appointment of an independent mental capacity advocate, where a relative cannot be consulted, where decisions relating to serious medical treatment, NHS or local accommodation arrangements are being made or other specified decisions are being made (see Chapters 22 and 24).

Disputes over care plans

In a case discussed in chapter 23[12] a single mother failed in her application for judicial review of the Council's care plan for her disabled daughter on the grounds that its rejection of an independent review was both unreasonable according to the Wednesbury principle and a breach of article 8 of the European Court of Human Rights.

In the following case the claimant alleged that the Council was failing to provide services according to the existing care plan, had failed to complete a lawful assessment on the claimant's accommodation and care needs and was failing to make arrangements for the provision of suitable accommodation pending the completion of an assessment of her accommodation under S 47(5) of the 1990 Act.

Case: *R (on the Application of Irenschild) v London Borough of Lambeth 2006*[13]

Mrs Irenschild suffered an accident which left her with serious back and neck injuries and she had lost the ability to stand and move about unsupported, in constant pain and suffering from urinary and faecal incontinence. The Judge allowed the application holding that the LA's community care assessment was unlawful: it had failed to take into account significant matters contained in the occupational therapist's report; it had not followed the guidance issued by the Department of Health in its Fair Access to Services paper and it was procedurally unfair in that certain issues had not been raised with the claimant (e.g. that the claimant had not had a fall in 8 years – which was contested by the claimant).

GPs and primary care trusts

In the community

From April 1990 General Practitioners have had, as part of their terms of service, the duty to carry out an annual assessment of every patient on their list who is aged 75 years or more. This work is increasingly delegated to practice nurses but there is no reason why occupational therapists should not take a greater responsibility in the assessment of these groups. From 2004 significant changes have taken place in the role of the primary care trust and its relationship with general practitioners. PCTs receive a cash-limited allocation for the provision of primary care. They commission six directed enhanced services and other enhanced services. GPs have new contractual terms with the PCTs. Under contracts to provide general medical services GPs must provide essential services, have the expectation and right to provide additional services and the right to provide certain of the directed enhanced services.[14] Contractors are subject to statutory requirements relating to quality, including a new duty of clinical governance (see chapter 17 for further discussion on PCTs).

The OT and the assessment

The OT has a major role to play in the multi-disciplinary team which is concerned with making the assessment. This would apply whether the OT works in the health or social services or housing sector. As has been seen, the local authority has a duty to involve the health service and/or the housing authority should it appear that there may be need for their services to be provided.

The COT standards for practice in home assessment with hospital in-patients were published in September 2000.[15] This core standard covers the referral procedure, preparation for home assessments, roles and responsibilities, assessment and treatment and health and safety. They should be read in conjunction with the OT professional standards and statements published in 2007.[16]

Assessment and goal setting is one of the professional standards for OT practice set by the COT in 2007.[17] It states that:

> Assessment provides the foundation for effective treatment and it is crucial to undertake a thorough and reliable assessment at several stages during the occupational therapy process, because without thorough and accurate assessment the intervention selected may prove inappropriate and/or ineffective.

There are five standard statements as follows:

1. Occupational therapists should prepare for an assessment by ensuring that it is appropriate and safe, and that the person being assessed has given their consent.
2. A decision not to carry out, or to discontinue, assessment should be based on identifiable and justifiable reasons.
3. The assessment tool should be fit for purpose, and should be used appropriately by the occupational therapy service and its staff.
4. The assessment should be carried out under conditions that recognise and value the needs of the service user and their main carer/s.
5. The goals for intervention should be agreed in discussion with the service user and/or their carer, based on their priorities and the needs as indicated by the assessment.

As with all standards, monitoring forms are provided. The standards apply, of course, to all assessments and not just community care ones.

Michael Mandelstam has provided a detailed review of the role of the OT in carrying out community care assessments[18] and has updated his textbook.[19]

Phillips and Renton conclude that assessment of function is the core of occupational therapy[20] only when placed in conjunction with other central aspects of the profession which include the resolution of problems through intervention and reassessment.

The impact of resource issues on assessments as considered by the House of Lords in the *Gloucester* case[21] is discussed in Chapter 20.

The use of activities of daily living (ADL) indices by OTs

In the first edition of this book, the research of OTs in the use of specific assessment tools was discussed. Various models of occupational therapy are in current use and many different assessment aids are used by OTs and it is important for the future to ensure that whatever tools are used, they are based on research findings, and that professional judgement is used in determining their appropriateness for the individual client. For example, Lori Letts and colleagues[22] consider the reliability and validity of the safety assessment of function and the environment for rehabilitation (SAFER tool) to assess people's abilities to manage functional activities safely within their homes. The authors conclude that whilst the SAFER tool does appear to be a reliable instrument that focuses on a person's ability to function safely in the home environment and could therefore be used by OTs in community practice, it did not demonstrate a link between the SAFER tool scores and independence in ADL and IADL. The National Institute for Health and Clinical Excellence (NICE), as its work progresses, is likely to review various models of assessment currently in use and advise on the clinical effectiveness of each as established by research (see Chapter 17 for the work of NICE).

Assessment of OT needs by non-occupational therapists

Sometimes assessment of the need for occupational therapy services is made by other practitioners. Thus Sparling and colleagues[23] surveyed GPs to establish the extent to which they would use the service of a community psychiatric occupational therapy service if one were available. It was clear that many required more information on what such a service could provide. There is a lesson here in terms of education of other professionals to ensure that they understand the role which OTs can play in different specialties. This also applies to the use of unregistered support workers (see Chapter 10). From April 1990 GPs have had, as part of their terms of service, the duty to carry out an annual assessment of every patient on their list who is aged 75 years or more. In a follow-up survey of the implications of this duty, Nocon[24] found that there were more referrals to community occupational therapy than to any other service. However, nurses identified significantly more needs for occupational therapy and other help than GPs and the study concluded that the assessments should be carried out by nurses rather than GPs. The survey also highlighted the resource implications of full assessments being undertaken.

Community care plans

Section 46 of the 1990 Act required each LA to prepare and publish a plan for the provision of community care in their area. The section also required the LA to keep the plan, and any further plans prepared by them under this section, under review, and empowered the Secretary of State to direct the intervals at which the LA must prepare and publish modifications to the current plan or a new plan. Section 46 was disapplied in relation to England from 9 July 2003.[25]

Consultation

Statutory duties under section 46(2) are placed upon the LA to consult other organisations in the development of community care plans. Directions on Consultation were issued by the Secretary of State for Health on 25 January 1993 and for the Welsh Office on 22 February 1993.[26] The Directions are intended to ensure that there is full and proper consultation between LAs and independent sector providers on community care plans by requiring LAs to consult with organisations which have declared themselves as representing independent sector providers. The second direction requires that LAs state in their plans the arrangements for consulting all those parties with a statutory right to be consulted.

Initial policy guidance on the preparation of community care plans was given[27] which advised LAs on:

- the statutory requirements on LAs to consult in the planning process
- the statutory requirements for publishing plans
- the arrangements for monitoring plans
- the scope and content of the plans of social services departments (SSDs).

The OT and community care plans

Community care plans are central to the effective development of community care in partnership with all relevant statutory, voluntary and independent organisations. If carefully revised and monitored they can highlight deficiencies and surpluses in the provision and ensure that the assessed needs of clients are being met. It is therefore essential that the OT should have a significant role in the preparation and revision of these plans, and ensure that weaknesses which she is aware of in the provision of community care services are brought to the attention of those responsible for finalising the plans.

Care management approach

Care manager

The post of care manager was described as follows in an affidavit evidence to court by the Director of Social Services for Newcastle-upon-Tyne City Council:[28]

> The role of the Care Manager can be traced back to the report of Sir Roy Griffiths which advised the Government on changing community care policy. This role is intended to be held by a social worker, community nurse, occupational therapist or some other person with a professional relationship with the client who needs help. The Care Manager is an advocate on behalf of the client, and as the title suggests, manages the resources available from the Social Services Department or the voluntary sector to the best advantage of the client. It is not a statutory post but is recognised, I understand, by all social services authorities, as good practice to ensure that all available resources and agendas are working in proper co-ordination to meet the needs of the client. The Care Manager has no managerial role in a residential home but will ensure that whatever resources, whether home care or residential care in nature, are properly and most effectively used on the client's behalf.

The role of the care manager is set out in the guidance published by the Department of Health Social Services Inspectorate. Annex A of the Practitioners' Guide[29] gives an example of the various stages of care management:

- publishing information
- determining the level of assessment
- assessing need
- care planning
- implementing the care plan
- monitoring
- reviewing.

The status of the claimant's case manager was considered in a case in 2005.

Case: *Wright v Sullivan*[30]

> The claimant was born in 1984 and was 20 at the time of the hearing. She had problems in learning and had one to one tuition. She was badly beaten up when she was 14 years old. 11 months later she was knocked down by a car when crossing the road. Liability was eventually accepted by the defendant as 70% with 30% contributory negligence. A dispute arose as to the amount of compensation. She had suffered a very severe concussive head injury resulting in brain damage with physical and mental symptoms. She developed post-traumatic epilepsy for which there was a 70% chance of bringing under control, poor concentration and memory reduction in her powers of literacy and a personality change. It was said that she was fully capable of all acts of daily living, but she required daily supervision of her behaviour by others and daily care in the absence of her mother. It was considered that she would be incapable of managing and administering her

own financial affairs or of independent living. Her chances of finding work were severely jeopardised and her affairs were managed by the Court of Protection. The daughter got into trouble and was placed under the probation service. She was evicted from a hostel for rule-breaking. She became pregnant and the mother was providing care for her and the child. The mother had failed to obtain help from social services or other agencies. An application for an interim payment was made to enable a clinical case manager to be appointed. The defendants asserted that damages would be reduced because of the 30% contributory negligence and the fact that some of the symptoms were the result of the beating prior to the RTA and not attributable to the road accident and there was a dispute about her earning capacity. The defendants insurers proposed that a clinical case manager should be instructed jointly to consider the claimant's needs and to prepare a report. Until the report was available the interim payment should be deferred. The claimant objected to the joint instruction, stating that the clinical case manager is a person engaged on behalf of the claimant and whose relationship with the claimant is therapeutic. Although an expert in her field, she would not be called on behalf of the claimant to give evidence in her capacity as an expert witness, but as a witness of fact. The judge ordered the payment of the interim sum of £50,000 with no conditions on the order. The defendant appealed and the claimant cross-appealed submitting that the clinical case manager should be seen as a witness of fact. The Court of Appeal considered the role of the clinical case manager as set out in the British Association of Brain Injury Case Managers in 2005 (see Figure 18.6) The court was told that an occupational or physiotherapist often fulfilled the role of clinical case manager. The Court of Appeal rejected the submission of the defendant that the clinical case manager should be seen as an expert witness. It said that the clinical case manager may receive suggestions from other experts, but ultimately she must make decisions in the best interests of the patient and not be beholden to two different masters. The Court rejected the defence

Figure 18.6 Principles and guidelines for case management best practice from the British Association of Brain Injury.

(a)   A clinical manager must have a relevant professional qualification.
(b)   The responsibilities of a clinical case manager include:
    (i)   Advocating for and on behalf of a client
    (ii)   Protecting a client from vulnerability and abuse
    (iii)   Maintaining effective communication systems for, amongst others, the client
    (iv)   Co-ordinating a package of rehabilitation and care/support relevant to his/her needs
    (v)   Managing such package using evidence-based practice and in line with National standards
    (vi)   Undertaking an appropriate full needs and risk assessment
    (vii)   Designing a case management plan to meet the assessed needs
    (viii) Implementing the plan taking account of quality, safety, efficiency and cost-effectiveness
    (ix)   Monitoring progress/deterioration and updating goals and related documentation.
(c)   The relationship between clinical case manager and his/her client (injured party) is therapeutic and professional.
(d)   The clinical case manager owes a duty of care to the injured party.
(e)   The instruction to the clinical case manager should be from the client or from a representative of his or her behalf (e.g. a receiver).
(f)   Joint instructions can lead to conflict and are not recommended.
(g)   The clinical case manager should be responsible for providing factual evidence as to work completed and the underlying reason for this, if so required.
(h)   The clinical case manager should only act as a witness of fact as regards the service provided for a case management client.

submission that the instruction of the clinical case manager should be joint instruction and neither party should be permitted to have "behind closed doors" access to her. It held that the role of the clinical case manager, if she is called to give evidence at the trial, will clearly be one of a witness of fact. She is there to give evidence of what she did and why she decided to do it. She will not be giving evidence of expert opinion. The Civil Procedure Rules on expert witnesses do not therefore apply to her.

Multi-disciplinary working

The more complex the needs of the client, the more likely it is that the care manager will be involved in inter-agency, multi-disciplinary co-operation in the assessment. Different inter-agency models of assessment are discussed in the Managers' Guide[7] (pp. 58–60). The delivery of the service will often be by means of a multi-disciplinary team. Community mental health teams, for example, include both health and social services staff working together with the voluntary and independent sector to provide mental health services for the client. Similar teams are now being developed across all sectors of social services provision. In arranging the most appropriate purchasing contract it is essential that the care manager has a clear understanding of the role of each team member and the function of the key worker. The legal liability of the key worker is discussed in Chapter 10.

Modernising social services

The White Paper *Modernising Social Services* in 1998 which set a strategy for the development of social services[31] covered the following areas:

- services for adults: independence, consistency, meeting people's need
- services for children: protection, quality of care, improving life's chances
- improving protection: new inspection systems, stronger safeguards
- improving standards in the workforce: creating a General Social Care Council, improving training
- improving partnerships: better joint working for more effective services
- improving delivery and efficiency: making sure it happens.

The Care Standards Act 2000 saw the implementation of many of the proposals contained in the White Paper, including the establishment of the General Social Care Council (see Chapter 5) the National Care Standards Commission (NCSC) and the repeal of the Registered Homes Act 1984. The NCSC has been replaced by new bodies following the Health and Social Care (Community Health and Standards) Act 2003 and the Health and Social Care Act 2008 (see below).

Long-term care and NHS/social services responsibilities

In the Parliamentary debates on the community care provisions of the 1990 Act much emphasis was placed upon the need to secure a seamless provision of services from one organisation to another. Considerable difficulties have, arisen, however, in the implementation of a seamless service and in ensuring close co-operation and collaboration between the various providers.

One difficulty is that of defining where the NHS statutory duty to provide ends, and the statutory duty of the LA begins. Whilst local arrangements could resolve many disputes, the fact that the NHS care must be provided free at the point of delivery (unless charges are specifically statutorily stipulated, e.g. prescription charges) but that most social services can be means tested, means that the distinction is extremely important from the client or patient's point of view.

There have been several cases brought before the Health Service Commissioner (HSC) about the failures of health authorities to make provision for the continuing care needs of their patients. Department of Health and Welsh Office advice was issued,[32] setting the principles on which continuing care should be provided by the different statutory authorities. Each LA was asked to prepare, in conjunction with the health authority and voluntary groups, local eligibility policies for continuing care.

Many commentators agree that, as long as there is a distinction between the authorities in terms of payment, it is essential to have national criteria on the responsibilities of each so that an individual in one part of the country does not obtain free a service which a person in another part of the country has to pay for (i.e. a postcode lottery). Each health authority in conjunction with LAs and other agencies is required to establish a procedure for reviewing decisions in relation to the provision of continuing care. Guidance was published in 1995.[33] It sets out a recommended review procedure to be established in the context of high quality discharge policies based on proper assessment and the provision of all relevant information and sensitivity to the needs and concerns of patients and their families. The working of the review procedures was to be monitored as part of the overall evaluation of the community care provisions (see below).

Eligibility and *Fair Access to Care Services*

The White Paper in 1998[34] (see above) identified the need for guidance on eligibility criteria for adult social care. This was provided in the *Fair Access to Care Services (2002)* for councils with social services responsibilities, for them to achieve fair access to care services through reviewing and revising their eligibility criteria for adult social care.[35] The guidance provides a national framework for councils to use when setting their eligibility criteria. The Department of Health stated[36] that it was not its intention

> that individuals with similar needs receive similar services up and down the country. This is because although councils should use the same eligibility framework to set their local criteria, the different budgetary decisions of individual councils will mean that some councils will be able to provide services to proportionately more adults seeking help than others.

Whilst it is clear that as long as there are different social services authorities with varying levels of resources there will be wide differences between the social services offered to those in need, this inequality will not always seem justifiable to those who are seeking the provision of those services. An analysis by Karen Lett and others suggested that the implementation of the FACS eligibility criteria for equipment provision had not achieved its goal in ending postcode variability.[37] Inconsistencies between colleagues still existed. The College of Occupational Therapist provided guidance on Fair Access to Care Services which was revised in 2006 in briefing note 16 which incorporated briefing note no 12.[38] Draft revised guidance for Fair Access to Services was published in 2007[39] which was intended to replace the 2003 FACS guidance. A consultation paper on the draft guidance, based on the comments by the CSCI on the Fair Access Guidance[40] took place in 2009.[41] The revised guidance on Fair Access to Services had 2 key objectives:

- to situate the application of eligibility criteria firmly within the new policy context of personalised provision of care and support and

- to ensure that the process for determining eligibility is as fair, transparent and consistent as possible, leading to high-quality outcomes for people seeking support.

The aim of the revised guidance was to:

- Assist councils to determine eligibility in a way that is fair, transparent and consistent, ensuring that all their citizens can expect some level of support, whether or not they receive statutory funding;
- Emphasise the benefits of early intervention and prevention and greater access to universal services, including high quality information and advice enabling people to make choices;
- Ensure that eligibility criteria for social care are applied in a way that is consistent with the personalisation agenda set out in *Putting People First*, based on choice and control, enabling people to live independently within strong and supportive local communities.

For a consideration of Intermediate Care see Chapter 24.

The provision of community equipment must be provided free of charge, regardless of the operational name of the service[42] (see Chapter 15).

Recent developments in long-term care

The use of local eligibility criteria for access to continuing care (and therefore non-means tested services from the NHS) has led to considerable diversity between different PCTs and local authorities, and many disputes over a refusal to provide NHS care. In July 2001 the Department of Health published a consultation document 'Guidance on Fair Access to Care Services' to ensure greater consistency in the use of eligibility criteria for access to care services. However this failed to meet the problem and in 2006 the following case was heard:

Case: *R (on the application of Grogan) v Bexley NHS Care Trust* [2006][43]

G. applied for judicial review of a decision by an NHS trust that she did not qualify for continuing NHS healthcare. If the NHS provided care it would be free; if it were the social services, she would be means tested. The high court held that an NHS trust should apply a primary health need test to determine whether accommodation should be provided by the NHS or social services. The criteria of the NHS trust for determining whether the patient had continuing care needs were fatally flawed and it failed to give reasons why it considered that the patient's continuing care needs were neither complex nor intense. The court ordered the trust's decision to be set aside and remitted for fresh consideration. The Court of Appeal held that it was for the primary care trust, acting on behalf of the Secretary of State, to determine whether the care needs of a woman who required constant and expensive care should be met by the health service or by social services.[44] Sections 1–3 of the National Health Service Act 2006 gave the care trust the power to decide where to draw the line. The social services authority did not have the power to reach its own decision.

Following the decision in the Grogan case, the DH announced that a national framework for continuing care would be implemented in October 2007. Assessments for continuing NHS care were to be carried out by a multi-disciplinary team using the concept of 'a primary health' need as the criteria for the receipt of continuing healthcare.[45] New eligibility criteria were introduced in 2007 in a National Framework for NHS Continuing Healthcare which was designed to resolve the disputes over whether it was an NHS or social services duty to provide care. This is considered in Chapter 24.

Inspection

LAs had the responsibility under the Registered Homes Act 1984 of inspecting residential care homes. These duties in respect of inspection were extended under the NHS and Community Care Act 1990. Subsequently, under the Care Standards Act 2000, the National Care Standards Commission was established to take over from health authorities and local authorities responsibilities for the registration and inspection of independent hospitals and registered care homes. Care standards were published which all premises registered under the Act were obliged to implement. Subsequently, under the Health and Social Care (Community Health and Standards) Act 2003 the National Care Standards Commission was abolished and its responsibilities of registration and inspection were taken over in respect of independent hospitals by the newly established Commission for Healthcare Audit and Inspection (CHAI) and in respect of the registered care homes by the Commission for Social Care Inspection (CSCI). Both CHAI and the CSCI were absorbed into the Care Quality Commission in April 2009 (see below).

CSCI reported that one in five residential care homes in England flouts the national minimum standards and could face fines of up to £50,000 when the new regulator took over in April 2009 (see below). In addition one third were judged to be only adequate or poor by inspectors over the past year. CSCI was also concerned at the high level of vacancies and the rapid turnover of staff in some homes and untrained helpers being sent to elderly people's homes.[46] In 2006 CSCI published lessons from its inspections.[47]

On 1 April 2009 the Care Quality Commission (CQC) was established taking over the work of CSCI, the Mental Health Act Commission and the Healthcare Commission (see Chapter 17 for further details of its powers). The then Chairman of CQC, Baroness Young of Old Scone, in an interview with the Times,[48] stated that she was most worried about the quality of social care services as large care home providers or family run businesses might cut corners because of the recession. Unlike CSCI the CQC will have the power to levy fines, suspend new admissions and close homes temporarily.

The COT has developed benchmarking of good practice in care homes enabling OTs to evaluate current practice and promote excellence in activities in care homes.[49]

Carers

The Carers (Recognition and Services) Act 1995 which came into force on 1 April 1996 placed a duty on local authorities to provide for the assessment of the ability of carers to provide care and for connected purposes. The basic provisions are shown in Figure 18.7. The duty to assess the carer on request also applies where the local authority makes an assessment of the needs of a disabled child for the purposes of Part III of the Children Act 1989, or a disabled person under section 2 of the Chronically Sick and Disabled Persons Act 1970, and a carer provides or intends to provide a substantial amount of care on a regular basis for the disabled child or disabled person (see Chapters 20 and 23).

Excluded from those carers entitled to be assessed are those providing care by virtue of a contract of employment or other contract with any person, or as a volunteer for a voluntary organisation.

Directions can be given by the Secretary of State as to the manner in which an assessment under subsection (1) or (2) is to be carried out or the form it is to take. Subject to such directions, the assessment shall be carried out in such manner and take such form as the LA consider appropriate. The Act applies to the appropriate provisions in Scotland but does not extend to Northern Ireland.

Figure 18.7   The Carers (Recognition and Services) Act 1995 – section 1(1).

[I]n any case where—

(a)   a local authority carry out an assessment under section 47(l)(a) of the [1990] Act of the needs of a person ('the relevant person') for community care services, and

(b)   an individual ('the carer') provides or intends to provide a substantial amount of care on a regular basis for the relevant person,

the carer may request the local authority, before they make their decision as to whether the needs of the relevant person call for the provision of any services, to carry out an assessment of his ability to provide and to continue to provide care for the relevant person; and if he makes such a request, the local authority shall carry out such an assessment and shall take into account the results of that assessment in making that decision.

The situation of young carers may give rise to considerable concerns and could even become a child protection issue, for example if the youngster is missing school because of caring responsibilities. Reference should be made to guidance from the Chief Inspector.[50]

Carers and Disabled Children Act 2000

This Act, which was passed to make up for some of the shortcomings in the Carers (Recognition and Services) Act 1995, gives a right to carers to be assessed, enables the local authority to provide services to carers following such an assessment and authorises the provision of vouchers. The Act is considered further in Chapter 23. The Carers (Equal Opportunities) Act 2004 amended the 1995 and 2000 Acts to ensure that an assessment under Section 1(2) must include consideration of whether the carer works or wishes to work, and whether the carer is undertaking, or wishes to undertake, education, training or any leisure activity.

Directions were issued by the Department of Health in 2004[51] about the involvement of carers in the assessment, which required the local authority to consider whether the person being assessed has any carers and, where they think it appropriate, consult those carers. In addition the LA must take all reasonable steps to reach agreement with the person and, where they think it appropriate, any carers of that person, on the community care services which they are considering providing to him to meet his needs. The LA must provide information to the person and, where they think it appropriate, to any carers of that person, about the amount of the payment (if any) which the person will be liable to make in respect of the community care services which they are considering providing to him.

The duty to assess the carer on request also applies where the local authority makes an assessment of the needs of a disabled child for the purposes of Part III of the Children Act 1989 or section 2 of the Chronically Sick and Disabled Persons Act 1970 and a carer provides or intends to provide a substantial amount of care on a regular basis for the disabled child or person. The LA may take into account an assessment made under section 1 or 6 of the Carers and Disabled Children Act 2000 in carrying out its assessment (S.1(2)(A) of 1995 Act).

Excluded from those carers entitled to be assessed are those providing care by virtue of a contract of employment or other contract with any person, or as a volunteer for a voluntary organisation. The cases of *R (on the application of B) v London Borough of Newham*[52] and of *R (on the application of LH) v London Borough of Lambeth*[53] illustrate the working of the 1995 and 2000 Acts. The former is discussed in full.

R (on the application of B) v London Borough of Newham

Mr B was 64 years of age and suffered from depression and high blood pressure, a shoulder problem and other more minor medical problems. He left work to become a full-time carer for his family. His wife, the claimant was 38 years old, registered blind and suffered from osteoarthritis and asthma. Their eldest child C was aged 18 and lived at home. He was partially sighted and described as being in danger of social isolation if not given support and encouragement. He attended college and the Chicken Shed Theatre Company. A daughter of 13 was partially sighted and suffered from urinary incontinence. A brother of 8 suffered from Attention Deficit Hyperactive Syndrome (ADHS) and his behaviour demanded constant attention and was very disruptive to the family and was described as the principal cause of the family's stress. The youngest child was 3 and with no substantial disability but beginning to copy the behaviour of her ADHS brother. The defendants carried out a number of assessments which the claimant alleged were incomplete and unsatisfactory. An interim consent order whereby the family had 6 hours a day and 2 days nursery was agreed as a temporary measure. The issues between the claimant and defendant related mainly to the extent of services provided i.e. the extent of home care support, the extent of nursery provision for H, the girl of 3, and the issue of respite care for H. The claimant alleged that there was criticism of the inadequacy of Mr B's contribution to the support of his wife and his role vis-à-vis the children and also criticism that the behaviour of the boy with ADHS should have been treated by medication, when he was in fact on medication. The judge held that the LA's approach on the issue of home care support and on nurse provision was fatally flawed. The LA had a duty to exercise its discretion and the statutory provisions (e.g. section 2 of the 2000 Act) rationally and in a way which takes important relevant matters into account. Because the family had been so recently assessed it was suggested between the counsel before the judge that a round table meeting should resolve the issues and if another assessment was necessary it should be undertaken by a different person than before.

The legal situation of carers should benefit from the decision of the European Court of Justice in the *Coleman* case[54] where the ECJ held that the EU Directive against discrimination on the grounds of disability applied to the carers of disabled persons as well as to the disabled themselves. The case is considered in chapter 19 in the section on disability discrimination and employment.

The Princess Royal has established an Association for Carers which provides advice and guidance.[55]

Chapter 10 is relevant to legal issues relating to the carer's liability in negligence.

Reference should also be made to a recent case where the High Court accepted that the local authority owed a duty of care to a couple with learning disabilities who were being bullied, assaulted and abused by a gang of youths.[56] However, this decision was overruled by the Court of Appeal.[57] The facts are set out in chapter 22.

The Department of Health published in 2008 a strategy for carers.[58] This emphasises a more integrated and personalised support service for carers. The role of carers in looking after those with dementia and the lack of support provided for them is considered in chapter 24.

Stress and carers

Stress management for carers is discussed by Gregory[59] who describes the setting up and running of a stress management group designed for people who are caring for an older confused person at home. She shows the value that the participants placed on the sessions but

> from the facilitator's point of view it was difficult to know where to set the boundaries for a session. The sessions need to find a point somewhere between a 'chat' and a defined psychotherapeutic structure for them to be effective.

The group also provided valuable insight into the nature of caring at home, what causes most stress and what needs are unfulfilled. In a more recent review, of a stress management programme for carers, Eileen Mitchell[60] found that the findings confirmed that stress management can reduce carer burden and offer coping strategies for those whose task is often underestimated. (See Chapter 11 for law relating to stress and the employee. Chapter 10 is relevant to legal issues relating to carers' liability in negligence.)

Choice of accommodation

It is important to the rights of individuals that they are not transferred against their will to accommodation over which they have had no choice. The assessment process should take into account the views as well as the needs of clients and the right of the client to choose has been the subject of Directions.[61]

Choice of accommodation Directions

These Directions permit the resident a choice of a home, and also cover the situation when an LA decides to make arrangements for residential accommodation for someone with preserved rights (i.e. generally a person who was in residential accommodation on 31 March 1993 and was receiving social security benefits for that accommodation). However, the choice is subject to the regulations and these Directions could not be used by a resident to require the LA to make a placement in the same home from which he is threatened with eviction. (Preserved rights were subsequently abolished).

Guidance accompanied the Directions.[62] This made it clear that the purpose behind the Directions was to ensure that when SSDs made placements in residential and nursing home care, people were able to exercise a genuine choice over where they live. The Guidance covered the suitability of the accommodation, the cost, the availability, the conditions and the possibility of more expensive accommodation where a third party is paying. The Guidance also suggested that, where prospective residents were unable to express a preference for themselves, it would be reasonable to expect authorities to act on the preferences expressed by their carers – unless exceptionally that would be against the best interests of the resident. The client was able to select a place outside the LA's financial limit, if the client or a third party paid the difference between what the LA would pay and the actual cost of the accommodation.

An amendment to these Directions was made in August 1993,[63] so that LAs were only required to place people in their preferred accommodation within England and Wales. The Secretary of State nonetheless expected LAs to assist people if they wished to enter the home of their choice in Scotland, in accordance with this Guidance.

Charges for residential accommodation

Local authorities have a duty to provide accommodation and are able to charge for places in residential accommodation on a means tested basis under sections 21 and 22 of the National Assistance Act 1948. Regulations set out the contributions which are to be made.[64] These enable capital under a specified limit (at present £13,500) to be ignored in the assessment and those with capital over a specified limit (at present £22,250 in England and £22,200 in Wales) to pay the full amount, and those with capital between the two sums would, subject to income, pay on a sliding scale towards the fees. Sefton Borough Council set up a scheme whereby those who were entitled to be provided with accommodation under section 21 could have their capital taken into account unless it was or fell below £1500 (instead of £16,000) (The figure of £1500 was chosen since it would usually leave sufficient for a funeral). The High Court judge[65] dismissed the application on the grounds that those who had capital below £16 000 could not be said to be in need of care and attention which was not otherwise available to them. The Court of Appeal[66] allowed the application for judicial review and held that Sefton had behaved unlawfully.[67] Subsequently, the Community Care (Residential Accommodation) Act 1998 was passed to put the decision of the Court of Appeal on a statutory basis. Section 1 of the 1998 Act states that in determining whether care and attention are otherwise available to a person, a local authority shall disregard so much of the person's capital as does not exceed the capital limit for the purposes of section 22 of the National Assistance Act 1948. The regulations on capital disregard must be followed by local authorities in means testing.[68] The House of Lords[69] has held that in carrying out assessments under the Chronic Sick and Disabled Persons Act 1970 the social services authority can take its resources into account (see Chapter 20).

Monitoring of community care provision

The Audit Office and the Department of Health itself are continually monitoring the effects and implementation of the community care programme. Reports in 1995[70] show failures in providing the benefits of community care to many users and carers, including those with learning disabilities. The Audit Commission carries out joint reviews of social services with the Department of Health's Social Services Inspectorate (SSI) and its equivalent in Wales (Social Services Inspectorate for Wales). The Audit Commission uses a comprehensive performance assessment (CPA) to analyse the efficiency of social services department's activities. In 2003 the Audit Commission published a consultation paper on the future development of CPA[71] which was followed by its strategy for a new CPA framework for 2005–6 and for 2010.[72] Further information can be obtained from the Audit Commission website on which the reports of its inspections of social services' departments can also be viewed.[73]

Community Care (Direct Payments) Act 1996

On 1 April 1997 the Community Care (Direct Payments) Act came into force which enabled social services departments to make payments in cash instead of kind to certain groups in receipt of community care. This enables a person to purchase their own care. However the local authority originally retained its discretion and could not be compelled to offer cash rather than services. The level of payment must be sufficient to enable the recipient to buy the services the payments are intended to cover. New regulations came into force in 2003[74] under which there is now a duty to make direct payments to eligible individuals who appears to be capable of managing a direct payment by himself or with such assistance as may be available to him. (Persons listed in Regulation 2 were ineligible but these regulations were changed in 2009[75] which reduced the categories of exclusion. Schedule 2 to the 2009 Regulations excludes those under drug or alcoholic treatment or rehabilitation regimes imposed under criminal justice legislation) If a person meets the criteria for direct payments and has had a community care assessment then the services needed are identified and he or she then has the choice of using the local social services or using the money provided to buy services from an alternative provider. In the DH circular Transforming Social Care in January 2008[76] it was estimated that only 54,000 out of a potential million recipients were receiving direct payments. The circular aimed at increasing the numbers of persons receiving direct payments or individual budgets (see below). Further information on direct payments is available from the DH publication in March 2008[77] which can be downloaded from its website. An analysis of the purchase of assistive devices by older people who had fallen and called 999 ambulance showed that 54% had purchased their own devices such as walking frames and bath boards spending on average £700 each. The authors concluded that as social services direct payments allow people to manage their own care packages, more people will be buying direct and may be looking for advice.[78]

Amendments were made to the direct payment scheme under the Health and Social Care Act 2008 and subsequent regulations.[79] The Department of Health published guidance in September 2009 on obtaining direct payments which included the amendments introduced by the Health and Social Care Act 2008 and the new regulations.[80] It covers getting direct payments (including: Assessment of your social care needs; Entitlement to direct payments; Spending your direct payments; and Getting enough money; Becoming an employer; Contracting with someone who is self-employed; contracting with an agency; Now you are receiving direct payments: what happens if your needs change?; keeping records and local council checks and complaints). Useful appendices provide further information on the responsibilities of an employer together with other sources of help. The DH also published in 2009 a list of key documents relating to direct payments which is available on its website.

In the following case the defendant in a road traffic accident argued unsuccessfully that the amount of direct payments should be taken into account in calculating the compensation for future care costs.

Case: *Morgan v Phillips*[81]

The claimant was 19 years when she suffered very severe injuries in an RTA when she was knocked down by a car driven by the defendant. She suffered severe brain damage which led to spastic tetraparesis. Her father acted as her litigation friend and receiver. The defendant was held liable for 55% of the damages. Following a community care assessment, the LA offered the claimant a weekly sum to fund a certain level of support. The defendant argued that the claimant's father on behalf of the claimant was bound to accept the offer of the direct payment and that the sum fell to be deducted from the multiplicand in respect of the claimant's future care costs. The court held that the actual consent of the person was required under section 57(1) of the Health and Social Care Act 2001 and her father as receiver did not have the power to give consent on her behalf. The defendant had not shown that there would be any direct payments and therefore the amount of direct payments should not be taken into account in calculating the compensation for future care costs.

Direct payments and liability for support workers

The following situation is of concern to occupational therapists.

Situation: accountability for the support worker?

Hugh has received from social services a care package which enables him to select and pay for his own support workers. His mobility is severely compromised and he needs to be hoisted into and out of his wheelchair. He employed carers sent to him from an independent care agency. Unfortunately they had not been trained in manual handling and in attempting to transfer Hugh from his bed to the wheelchair, he fell to the floor, fracturing his pelvis. Who if anyone is accountable for this accident?

On the few facts given here, it would appear that the care agency did not hold itself out as being the employer of the carers. However if the agency was recommending persons who could be employed as carers by Hugh, it should have ensured that the carers were trained in manual handling. It could be said that the agency owed a duty of care to Hugh, by failing to provide the necessary training, it was in breach of that duty and as a consequence reasonable foreseeable harm to Hugh has occurred (see chapter 10 and the principles of negligence). It would therefore be liable to Hugh. If on the other hand, Hugh had employed a support worker who did not come via an agency, and this was known to health and social care professionals visiting Hugh, then they might have a duty of care to Hugh to advise him that any support worker should have a minimum training in manual handling. Such advice should be put in writing. If Hugh ignores that advice, then he could not hold the health or social care professionals liable (see Chapter 11 for manual handling). (Different principles would apply if Hugh lacked the mental capacity to make such choices – see Chapter 22 and the Mental Capacity Act 2005.)

Strategic planning and community services

Green Paper on the future of social care for adults (2005)

In 2005 the Department of Health published a Green paper on Independence, Well-being and Choice.[82] This aimed to develop a new vision for social care underlain by the principles that everyone has a positive contribution to make to society and they should have the right to control their own lives. Key proposals to deliver this vision include:

- wider use of direct payments and the piloting of individual budgets to stimulate the development of modern services delivered in the way people want
- greater focus on preventative services
- a strong strategic and leadership role for local government, working in partnership with other agencies particularly the NHS
- encouraging the development of new and exciting models of service delivery and harnessing technology to deliver the right outcomes for adult social care.

The Report[83] on the responses to the Government's Green paper stated that the 5 top areas of interest were direct payments/individual budgets; shift to prevention; risk management; vision and assessment.

White Paper: *Our health, our care, our say: A new direction for community services*

Following the Green paper *Independence, well-being and choice*[84] in 2005, a White Paper on Community Health and Social Care was published in 2006[85] which set 4 main goals:

1. better prevention services with earlier intervention
2. more choice and a louder voice for patients
3. improving access to community services and tackling inequalities
4. support for people with long-term conditions.

Achieving these goals would include an expansion of the Expert Patients Programme, support for carers including emergency home-based respite care services the provision of care closer to home, including moving services out of acute hospitals for out-patients, day case surgery and intermediate care and greater partnership working including co-location of services, including health and care services. In addition different providers would be allowed to compete for services. The White paper can be accessed on the DH website.

The 2006 White Paper was followed by the DH circular[86] *Transforming Social Care* which set out the information to support the transformation of social care signified in the Green Paper of 2005 and the White Paper of 2006. It describes the vision for the development of a personalised approach to the delivery of adult social care. The circular anticipated a rise in the numbers of persons over 85 to rise from 1 million in 2006 to 2.9 million in 2036. Direct payments and individual budgets were seen as enabling people to take control of their care. Further information is available on the DH website.[87] The social care reform agenda also envisaged further development of the care services efficiency delivery programme[88] (which was established in 2004) to implement the recommendations of independent reviews of public sector efficiency) that works in partnership with local councils, the NHS, and service providers to deliver efficiency improvements. Six major interconnected and inter-dependent workstreams were developed to deliver end-to-end efficiency improvements to all councils with social services responsibilities. The six workstreams are:

- effective monitoring and modernisation of home-based care
- assessment and care management
- demand forecasting and capacity planning
- homecare re-enablement
- improved procurement practices
- transforming community equipment and wheelchair services (TCEWS) (see Chapter 15).

Personalisation of social services

In supporting this principle objective of personalising social services, a ministerial concordat was launched in December 2007 called *Putting People First a Shared Vision and commitment to the transformation of adult social care*. The concordat set out the shared aims and values (of the central and local government, professional leaders, providers and the regulator) which would guide the transformation of adult social care. The concordat was followed by a toolkit published in June 2008 to assist councils and partners in implementing the necessary changes. These publications can be down loaded from the DH website.[89] Additional information is also available on individual budgets and the documents related to the commitment to individual budgets.

In July 2009 a Green Paper[90] on the funding of long term care was published. The options put forward are discussed in Chapter 24. The National Service Frameworks for Long-term care and for older people are discussed in Chapter 24.

Disability discrimination

The OT is concerned with disabilities and discrimination in several respects:

- She will be caring for many clients who suffer from physical and mental disabilities and will be concerned to ensure that accurate advice is given to them about their right not to be discriminated against
- If a disabled person herself, she may be concerned about her rights in employment, her right to access services and education
- As a manager she may be concerned about the rights of disabled persons and her rights if disabled employees are unable to undertake their work effectively.

Disability discrimination in employment is considered in Chapter 19.

Disability Discrimination Act 1995

The provisions of the Disability Discrimination Act 1995 are set out in Figure 18.8. The Disability Discrimination Act 1995 section 1(1) defines a person as having a disability if

> he has a physical or mental impairment which has a substantial and long-term adverse effect on his ability to carry out normal day-to day activities.

A 'disabled person' is therefore 'a person who has a disability' (section 1(2)). Regulations made under the Act[91] exclude certain conditions from the definition of disability, including addiction to alcohol, nicotine or any other substance (unless the result of medical treatment); tendency to set fires, steal, and to physically or sexually abuse other persons; exhibitionism and voyeurism; and seasonal allergic rhinitis. Most of the words in the statutory definition of disabled require further interpretation and therefore further definitions are given in Schedule 1 to the Act. See also recent statutory instruments covering blind and partially sighted persons.[92]

> 'Mental impairment' includes an impairment resulting from or consisting of a mental illness only if the illness is a clinically well-recognised illness. (Sched. 1 para. 1(2)) (Amended by 2005 Act; see below.)
>   The effect of an impairment is a long term effect if

(a)   it has lasted at least 12 months;
(b)   the period for which it lasts is likely to be at least 12 months; or
(c)   it is likely to last for the rest of the life of the person affected.

Where an impairment ceases to have a substantial adverse effect on a person's ability to carry out normal day-to-day activities, it is to be treated as continuing to have that effect if that effect is likely to recur. (Sched. 1 para. 2.)

Figure 18.8   Disability Discrimination Act 1995.

(1)   Definitions of disability and disabled person
(2)   Employment: discrimination by employers, enforcement provisions, discrimination by other persons, occupational pension schemes and insurance services
(3)   Discrimination in other areas: goods, facilities and services, premises, enforcement
(4)   Education
(5)   Public transport: taxis, public services vehicles, rail vehicles
(6)   National Disability Council
(7)   Supplemental: Codes of Practice, victimisation, help
(8)   Miscellaneous

Severe disfigurement is to be treated as having a substantial adverse effect on the ability of the person concerned to carry out normal day-to-day activities. (Sched. 1 para. 3)

An impairment which affects normal day-to-day activities must affect one of the following:

(a) mobility
(b) manual dexterity
(c) physical co-ordination
(d) continence
(e) ability to lift, carry or otherwise move everyday objects
(f) speech, hearing or eyesight
(g) memory or ability to concentrate, learn or understand
(h) perception of risk of physical danger. (Sched. 1 para. 4(1))

Guidance has been issued by the Secretary of State about the matters which must be taken into account in the application of this definition. It considers what is meant by a substantial adverse effect, and by long-term and normal day-to-day activities. Reference could also be made to Brian Doyle's book on an overview of the Act which includes the statute itself,[93] and also a book edited by Jeremy Cooper.[94]

Discrimination in employment is covered by Part II of the Act and this is considered in Chapter 19 of this book in relation to employee OTs. However, it is also relevant to the employment possibilities of disabled clients. Reference can be made to a guide by Judy Thurgood[95] for the employment implications of the Act for disabled people and the duties placed upon the employer.

Discrimination in the provision of goods, facilities and services

Part III covers discrimination in the provision of goods, facilities and services and makes it unlawful for a provider of services to discriminate against a disabled person in the ways illustrated in Figure 18.9.

Discrimination for the purposes of Part III of the Act is defined in section 20 which states that a provider of services discriminates against a disabled person if:

(a) for a reason which relates to the disabled person's ability, he treats him less favourably than he treats or would treat others to whom that reason does not or would not apply, and
(b) he cannot show that the treatment in question is justified.'

Figure 18.9 Part III Discrimination in the provision of goods, facilities and services – section 19.

It is unlawful for a provider of services to discriminate against a disabled person:

(a) in refusing to provide, or deliberately not providing, to the disabled person any service which he provides, or is prepared to provide, to members of the public
(b) in failing to comply with any duty imposed on him by section 21 in circumstances in which the effect of that failure is to make it impossible or unreasonably difficult for the disabled person to make use of any such service
(c) in the standard of service which he provides to the disabled person or the manner in which he provides it to him; or
(d) in the terms on which he provides a service to the disabled person.

Section 21(1) places a duty upon a provider of services to make adjustments:

> Where a provider of services has a practice, policy or procedure which makes it impossible or unreasonably difficult for disabled persons to make use of a service which he provides, or is prepared to provide, to other members of the public, it is his duty to take such steps as it is reasonable, in all the circumstances of the case, for him to have to take in order to change that practice, policy or procedure so that it no longer has that effect.

Under section 21(2), where a physical feature of a building makes it impossible or unreasonably difficult for disabled persons to make use of such a service, it is the duty of the provider of that service to take such steps as it is reasonable, in all the circumstances of the case, for him to have to take in order to:

(a) remove the feature
(b) alter it so that it no longer has that effect
(c) provide a reasonable means of avoiding the feature; or
(d) provide a reasonable alternative method of making the service in question available to the disabled person.'

Section 19(3) gives examples of services covered by section 20 and 21 and includes:

(a) access to and use of any place which members of the public are permitted to enter
(b) access to and use of means of communication
(c) access to and use of information services
(d) accommodation in a hotel, boarding house or other similar establishment
(e) facilities by way of banking or insurance or for grants, loans, credit or finance
(f) facilities for entertainment, recreation or refreshment
(g) facilities provided by employment agencies or under section 2 of the Employment and Training Act 1973
(h) the services of any profession or trade, or any local or other public authority.'

Part III has been implemented in stages:

- Since 2 December 1996 it has been illegal for service providers to treat a disabled person less favourably because of his or her disability.
- Since 1 October 1999 service providers have had to make reasonable adjustments for a disabled person such as giving extra help or changing the way they provide the service.
- From 1 October 2004 service providers must make other reasonable adjustments to their premises so that there are no physical barriers stopping or making it unreasonably difficult for a disabled person to use the services.

Regulations determine what is reasonable and give guidance on the implementation of the duty[96] under Part III. A Code of Practice for service providers was issued in 1996 and was revised in 1999. A new Code was published in 2002 which replaces the revised Code. It takes account of the further duties on service providers to make adjustments when the physical features of their premises make it impossible or unreasonably difficult for disabled people to use their services. Although these remaining duties do not come into force until 1 October 2004, this Code was issued in 2002 with a commencement date in May 2002 in order to encourage service providers to be proactive and to assist them in preparing for their extended obligations.

The Code covers:

- the statutory duties under Part III of the Act
- the service provider's duty not to treat a disabled person less favourably

- making changes for disabled people: the service provider's duty to make reasonable adjustments, reasonable adjustments in practice
- how building regulations and leases affect reasonable adjustments
- whether a service provider can justify less favourable treatment or failure to make reasonable adjustments
- special rules affecting insurance, guarantees and deposits
- selling, letting or managing premises.

Guidance was provided by the Disability Rights Commission (DRC) on Part III of the Act which came into effect completely in 2004.[97] The Guidance suggested that in the event of a disabled person having a difficulty in accessing a service, he should first talk to the service provider and if this failed, then discuss the difficulty with a local disability organisation or the DRC helpline. A conciliation service was provided by the DRC and it was recommended that conciliation was attempted before an application was made to the court.

Discrimination in education

Part IV of the Act covers discrimination in education and has been amended by the Special Educational Needs and Disability Act 2001. (This is considered in Chapter 23 on children.)

Public transport

Part V of the Disability Discrimination Act covers taxis, hire car services, passengers in wheelchairs, the carrying of guide dogs and hearing dogs, public service vehicles and rail vehicles. Taxi accessibility regulations[98] ensure that disabled persons and persons in wheelchairs can get into and out of taxis safely and can be carried in safety and in reasonable comfort. Taxi drivers also have a duty to carry the guide dogs and hearing dogs of passengers without making an additional charge. Regulations also cover public service vehicles and the access and carriage of disabled persons and wheelchairs.

The Disability Discrimination Act 2005

This Act puts into law some of the recommendations of the Disability Rights Task Force which was set up by the Government in 1997. Section 18 of the Act extends the definition of disability in respect of those with a mental illness (It is no longer a requirement that mental illness must be clinically well-recognised if it is to be the basis of "mental impairment") and includes those diagnosed with cancer, multiple sclerosis and HIV infection from the point at which the disease was diagnosed rather than from the point at which their illness had an adverse effect on them. It also brings councillors, and members of the Greater London Authority within the scope of the DDA, places a new duty on public authorities to have due regard to the need to eliminate harassment of and unlawful discrimination against disabled person, to promote positive attitudes to disabled persons and encourage participation by disabled people in public life and promote equality of opportunity for them. New provisions are introduced in relation to rail vehicles.

National Disability Council

Part VI established the National Disability Council. This Council, following consultation, advised the Secretary of State on relevant matters as requested, and prepared Codes of Practice. Unlike the Equal Opportunity Commission, it did not have the power to take cases to an employment tribunal. The National Disability Council was replaced by the Disability Rights Commission (and subsequently by the Equality and Human Rights Commission).

Disability Rights Commission (DRC)

The Disability Rights Commission was established in April 2000 as a result of the Disability Rights Commission Act 1999. The DRC aimed to resolve disputes through mediation, but it could bring cases to the courts and thereby a body of case law on the rights of disabled people was being established. The DRC also provided information and advice to employers about how to meet their responsibilities under the Disability Discrimination Act 1995. It estimated that there were about 8.5 million disabled people in Britain, of whom about 2.6 million are unemployed or on benefits.[99] The DRC was asked by the Government to draw up a Code of Practice to guide businesses on complying with the 2004 provisions on the part 111 laws relating to the provision of goods and services (see above).

The Equality and Human Rights Commission

A White Paper[100] recommended the establishment of a single body to protect human rights and prevent discrimination. The Equality and Human Rights Commission was established on 1 October 2007 under the Equality Act 2006 replacing the Equal Opportunities Commission, the Disabilities Rights Commission and the Commission for Racial Equality. It also assumes responsibility for promoting equality and combating unlawful discrimination in three new areas: sexual orientation, religion or belief and age. It also has responsibility for the promotion of human rights. The Commission has a general duty under section 3 to exercise its functions with a view to encouraging and supporting the development of a society in which:

a.   people's ability to achieve their potential is not limited by prejudice or discrimination
b.   there is respect for and protection of each individual's human rights
c.   there is respect for the dignity and worth of each individual
d.   each individual has an equal opportunity to participate in society and
e.   there is mutual respect between groups based on understanding and valuing of diversity and on shared respect for equality and human rights.

More specific duties relate to equality and diversity (section 8), human rights (section 9), groups (section 10), monitoring the law (section 11) and monitoring progress (section 12). It has powers to publish or disseminate ideas or information, undertake research, provide education or training, give advice or guidance, and issue codes of practice. It also has the power to carry out an investigation, to apply to court for an injunction against a person who it believes to be committing an unlawful act, to bring proceedings in its own name and to give legal assistance to an individual who alleges that he is a victim of behaviour contrary to the equality enactments. Further information can be obtained from the EHRC website.[101] The scope of the EC Directive on equal treatment in employment and occupation[102] was considered in a significant case. The EHRC supported Sharon Coleman who had a disabled son in claiming that she was discriminated against at work because of her child. She said that she was forced to resign from the law firm because it would not accommodate her responsibility to care for a disabled child. The case was heard by the European Court of Justice's (ECJ) advocate general who decided in her favour.[103] On 17 July 2008 the ECJ[104] ruled that the EU directive which outlawed discrimination or harassment at work on the ground of disability is not limited to disabled people themselves but extends to those caring for them. It is described as a landmark case, which could bring new rights for the 6 million carers in the UK. It is also considered in Chapter 19.

Equality Act 2010

The Equality Act aims to simplify and strengthen rights to equality by updating and existing anti-discrimination laws. It places a duty upon the public sector organisations to have regard to socio-economic inequalities in their strategic planning. It also identifies the following personal characteristics as being protected against discrimination: age; disability; gender reassignment, marriage and civil partnerships; race religion or belief; sex and sexual orientation. The preamble to the Bill set out the following purposes:

Make provision to require Ministers of the Crown and others when making strategic decisions about the exercise of their functions to have regard to the desirability of reducing socio-economic inequalities;
to reform and harmonise equality law and restate the greater part of the enactments relating to discrimination and harassment related to certain personal characteristics;
to enable certain employers to be required to publish information about the differences in pay between male and female employees; to prohibit victimisation in certain circumstances;
to require the exercise of certain functions to be with regard to the need to eliminate discrimination and other prohibited conduct;
to enable duties to be imposed in relation to the exercise of public procurement functions;
to increase equality of opportunity;
to amend the law relating to rights and responsibilities in family relationships; and for connected purposes.

Discrimination

Protection from discrimination on grounds of age came into force in October 2006 as a result of a European Directive[105] which was implemented by the Employment Equality (Age) Regulations 2006.[106] The Regulations only apply to employment and vocational training and only protect employees up to 65 years who can be dismissed after that age provided the employer satisfies the specified procedure set out in the regulations. They are considered in Chapter 19 on employment. The Equality Act 2010 recognises "Age" as a characteristic to be protected from discrimination, not just in employment.

The Occupational Therapist and discrimination

The OT may be involved in litigation relating to discrimination as a result of disputes following her assessment. For example in one case[107] the claimant argued that the defendants' refusal of consent to the installation of a stair-lift (at the claimant's expense) constituted "discrimination within section 22(3) of the Disability Discrimination Act 1995." The facts of the case were that:

In December 2002 Mrs Williams was stuck in her bath for about five hours. On 11 February 2003 an occupational therapist employed by the local authority went to Richmond Court to assess whether she needed adaptations to her flat. He recommended to the director of housing that she did. The recommended work included provision of a shower and a stair-lift that was to go all the way up to her flat from the ground floor. It has been decided she was eligible for a disabled facilities grant. The landlords however refused permission for the construction of a stair lift even though there would be no cost to them. The judge held them to be discriminating against her and they appealed against his decision. The Court of Appeal allowed the appeal on the grounds that as the law stood at that time the managers of the premises were not under any positive obligation to make adjustments or to agree to tenants making adjustments to the common parts of the premises so as to make them more suitable for disabled people. This was in sharp distinction to other provisions in the 1995 Act where positive obligations are imposed.

Law Commission Review

Law Commission is reviewing the law relating to adult social care and published in November 2008, a scoping report to identify the issues. It considered the legislative framework for adult residential care, community care, adult protection and support for carers to be inadequate, often incomprehensible and outdated. It remains a confusing patchwork of conflicting statues enacted over a period of 60 years. There is no single, modern statute to which service providers and service users can look to understand whether (and, if so, what kind of) services can or should be provided. The overall aim of the Law Commission project is to provide a clearer and more cohesive framework for adult social care. This would help to ensure that service users, carers, social care staff, health professionals and lawyers are clear about rights to services and which services are available. It will also aim to modernise the law to ensure that it is no longer based on out-dated principles. The topics which it will consider include:

- statutory principles
- community care assessments
- carers' assessment
- hospital discharge
- eligibility for services
- ordinary residence
- provision of services
- service provision and client groups
- direct payments
- charging for services
- health/social care divide
- safeguarding adults from abuse and neglect
- strategic planning and information to the public
- care standards and regulation
- complaints and redress.

The final stage in the Law Commission process will be the drafting of new legislation, hopefully to replace all the existing social care legislation. The project is much needed.

Conclusions

There have been many statutes, reports, white and green papers, reviews and recommendation over the past 20 years on care in the community and health and social services obligations. Hopefully the outcome of the Law Commission's review will clarify the rights and responsibilities of clients and health and social care professionals in the provision of care in the community. The past years have seen a change of focus of the OT which has been supported by strategic papers from the College of Occupational Therapists. The implications of the establishment of the Equality and Human Rights Commission on reducing discrimination and supporting human rights has yet to be assessed. It appears that many organisations have still not taken on board the full weight of their legal responsibilities. There are many challenges for the OT in this field.

 Questions and exercises

1   What impact have the developments in community care had upon your practice? Are there any specific problems which have arisen and how can these be resolved?
2   An NHS OT carries out an assessment for a client being discharged to his home and prescribes certain equipment including a chemical toilet. She then discovers that her recommendation has been changed by a disability officer employed by social services who is not a registered OT. What action, if any, should she take?
3   Community care plans must be revised annually. What part should the OT play in the preparation of the plan and its revision?
4   Identify the extent to which an OT requires a knowledge of the Disability Discrimination Act 1995 in order to assist her clients.

References

1   Clements, Luke and Thompson Pauline. (2007) *Community Care and the Law*, 4th edn. Legal Action Group, London.
2   College of Occupational Therapists (2000) From Interface to Integration: A strategy of modernising occupational therapy services in local health and social care communities. A consultation. COT, London.
3   Riley, J. (2002) Occupational Therapy in Social Services – A Missed Opportunity? *British Journal of Occupational Therapy*, **65**(11), 502–8.
4   College of Occupational Therapists (2008) Position statement: The value of Occupational Therapy and its contribution to adult social service users and their carers. COT, London.
5   Riley Jill and Whitcombe Steven (2008) *OT in adult social care in England: sustaining a high quality workforce for the future*. COT and DH, London.
6   Griffiths Report (1988) *Community Care, an agenda for action: a report to the Secretary of State for Social Services by Sir Roy Griffiths*. HMSO, London.
7   Secretary of State for Health (1989) *Caring for People; Community Care in the next decade and beyond*. White Paper, 849. HMSO, London.
8   Department of Health Community Care Assessment Directions 2004; LAC (2004) 24.
9   DoH (1990) Caring for People: Community Care in the next decade and beyond. Policy Guidance. HMSO, London.
10 HMSO (1991) *Care Management and Assessment: Managers' Guide*. HMSO, London.

11 HMSO (1990) *Care Management and Assessment: Practitioners' Guide*. HMSO, London.

12 *R (on the application of W.) v Lincolnshire County Council* [2006] EWHC Admin 2365.

13 *R (on the Application of Irenschild) v London Borough of Lambeth* [2006] EWHC 2354.

14 Department of Health (2003),*Delivering Investment in General Practice: implementing the new GMS contract*, DH, December 2003.

15 College of Occupational Therapists (2000) Standards for Practice: Home assessment with hospital in-patients. COT, London.

16 College of Occupational Therapists (2007) *Professional Standards for Occupational Therapy Practice*. COT, London; College of Occupational Therapists (2007) Standard Statements. COT, London.

17 College of Occupational Therapists (2003 revised 2007) *Professional Standards for Occupational Therapy Practice*. COT, London.

18 Mandelstam, M. (1998) A Question of Good Practice? Community care law and occupational therapists. *British Journal of Occupational Therapy*, **61**(8), 351–8.

19 Mandelstam, M. (2009) *Community Care Practice and the Law*, 4th edn. Jessica Kingsley, London.

20 Phillips, N. & Renton, L. (1995) Is assessment of function the core of occupational therapy? *British Journal of Occupational Therapy*, **58**(2), 72–4.

21 *R v Gloucester County Council, ex parte Barry* [1997] 2 All ER 1, HL.

22 Letts, L., Scott, S., Burtney, J., Marshall, M. & McKean, M. (1998) The reliability and validity of the safety assessment of function and the environment for rehabilitation (SAFER tool). *British Journal of Occupational Therapy*, **61**(3), 127–32.

23 Sparling, E., Clark, N. & Laidlaw, J. (1992) Assessment of the demands by general practitioners for a community psychiatric occupational therapist service. *British Journal of Occupational Therapy*, **55**(5), 193–6.

24 Nocon, A. (1993) GPs' assessments of people aged 75 and over: Identifying the need for occupational therapy services. *British Journal of Occupational Therapy*, **56**(4), 123–7.

25 The Community Care Plans (Disapplication)(England) Order 2003 SI 1716.

26 LAC(93)4, WOC 16/93.

27 DoH (1990) Caring for People: Community Care in the next decade and beyond. Policy Guidance (pp. 13–20). HMSO, London.

28 *R v Newcastle-upon-Tyne City Council, ex parte Dixon* (1993) 92 LGR 168 (QBD).

29 HMSO (1990) *Care Management and Assessment: Practitioners' Guide*. HMSO, London.

30 *Wright v Sullivan* [2005] EWCA Civ 656.

31 DoH (1998) White Paper *Modernising Social Services*, Cmd 4169. Stationery Office, London.

32 HSG(95)8, LAC(95)5, WHC(95)7 and WOC 16/95.

33 HSG(95)39, LAC(95)17.

34 DoH (1998) White Paper *Modernising Social Services*, Cmd 4169. Stationery Office, London.

35 LAC(2002)13 *Fair Access to Care Services. Guidance on eligibility criteria for adult social care*.

36 DoH (1998) White Paper *Modernising Social Services*, Cmd 4169. Stationery Office, London.

37 Lett Karen, Sackely Cath and Littlechild Rosemary (2006) The use of Fair Access to Care Services eligibility criteria for equipment provision within local authorities in England. *British Journal of Occupational Therapy*, **69**(9), 420–2.

38 College of Occupational Therapists (2006) Fair Access to Care Services Briefing note no 16.

39 Department of Health (2007) *Prioritising need in the context of Putting People First: A whole system approach to eligibility for social care*. DH, London.

40 Commission for Social Care Inspection (2008) *Cutting the Cake Fairly: CSCI review of eligibility criteria for social care*. DH, London.

41 Department of Health (2009) *Prioritising need in the context of Putting People First: A whole system approach to eligibility for social care*. Consultation on the revision of the Fair Access to Care Services guidance to support councils to determine eligibility for social care services. DH, London.

42 LAC(2003)14 Changes to Local Authority Charging Regime for Community Equipment and Intermediate Care Services.

43 *R (on the application of Grogan) v Bexley NHS Care Trust* [2006] EWHC 44 (2006) 9 CCL 188.

44   *R (St Helens Borough Council) v Manchester Primary Care Trust and Another* The Times Law Report 6 October 2009.

45   DH (2007) The National Framework for NHS Continuing Healthcare and NHS-funded Nursing Care. DH, London.

46   Bennett Rosemary Thousands of homes face £50,000 fine over failure to reach basic standard. The Times 28 January 2009.

47   Commission for Social Care Inspection (2006) *Supporting People – promoting indepdence- lessons from Inspections.* CSCI, London.

48   Rose David Watchdog warns care homes not to cut corners in recession The Times 1 April 2009.

49   College of Occupational Therapists (2007) *Activity Provision Benchmarking good practice in care homes.* COT, London.

50   Social Services Inspectorate. *Young Carers.* Chief inspector of SSI CI(95)12. DoH, London.

51   Department of Health Community Care Assessment Directions 2004; LAC (2004) 24; available on DH carers' website: www.carers.gov.uk/

52   *R (on the application of B) v London Borough of Newham* [2004] EWHC 2503 (Admin).

53   *R (on the application of LH) v London Borough of Lambeth* [2006] EWHC 1190 Admin; [2006] All ER (D) 83 June.

54   Coleman (Social Policy) [2008] EUECJ C-303/06 17 July 2008.

55   www.carers.org/

56   *X and Y v London Borough of Hounslow* [2008] EWHC 1168 (QB) 23 June 2008.

57   *X and Y v London Borough of Hounslow* [2009] EWCA Civ 286.

58   Department of Health (2008) *The Carers' Strategy: Carers at the Heart of 21st Century Families and Communities.* DH, London.

59   Gregory, S. (1991) Stress Management for Carers. *British Journal of Occupational Therapy,* **54**(11), 427–9.

60   Mitchell, E. (2000) Managing carer stress: an evaluation of a stress management programme for carers of people with dementia. *British Journal of Occupational Therapy,* **63**(4), 179–84.

61   National Assistance Act 1948 (Choice of Accommodation) Directions 1992; Choice of Accommodation Directions LAC(92)27 as amended by LAC(93)18.

62   LAC(92)27.

63   LAC(93)18.

64   National Assistance (Assessment of Resources) Regulations SI 1992/2977 as amended.

65   *R v Sefton Metropolitan Borough Council, ex parte Help the Aged* [1997] 3 FCR 392 High Court.

66   *R v Sefton Metropolitan Borough Council ex parte Help the Aged* [1997] 3 FCR 573 Court of Appeal.

67   LASSL(97)13 Responsibilities of Local Authority Social Services Departments: Implications of recent legal judgments.

68   LAC(98)19 Community Care (Residential Accommodation) Act 1998.

69   *R v Gloucester County Council, ex parte Barry* [1997] 2 All ER 1, HL.

70   EL(95)39 and CI(95)7; MENCAP (1995) Britain's other Lottery: A report on the practice of Care Management and Assessment for people with learning disabilities MENCAP, London.

71   Audit Commission (2003) *Patterns for Improvement.*

72   Audit Commission (2003) *CPA the way forward.*

73   www.audit-commission.gov.uk.

74   The Community Care Services to Carers and Children's Services (Direct Payments (England)) Regulations 2003 SI 762.

75   The Community Care, Services for Carers and Children's Services (Direct Payments) (England) Regulations 2009 SI 2009/1887.

76   Department of Health (2008) LAC (DH) 2008/1 *Transforming Social Care* January 2008.

77   Department of Health (2008) A guide to receiving direct payments from your local council DH.

78   Logan PA, Murphy A, Drummond AER, Bailey S, et al. (2007) An investigation of the number and cost of assistive devices used by older people who had fallen and called a 999 ambulance. *British Journal of Occupational Therapy,* **70**(11), 475–8.

79   The Community Care, Services for Carers and Children's Services (Direct Payments) (England) Regulations 2009 SI 2009/1887.

80   Department of Health (2009) *A Guide to Receiving Direct Payments from your Local Council – a Route to Independent Living*. DH, London.

81   *Morgan v Phillips* [2006] All ER (D) 189 March.

82   Department of Health (2005) *Green Paper; Independence, Well-being and Choice*. DH, London.

83   Department of Health (2005) *Responses to the Consultation on adult social care in England: analysis of feedback from the Green paper Independence, Well-being and Choice*. DH, London.

84   Department of Health (2005) *Green Paper; Independence, Well-being and Choice*. DH, London.

85   Department of Health (2006) *Our health, our care, our say: A new direction for community services*. DH, London.

86   Department of Health (2008) LAC (DH) 2008/1 Transforming Social Care January 2008.

87   www.dh.gov.uk/en/SocialCare/Socialcarereform

88   www.csed.csip.org.uk/

89   www.dh.gov.uk/en/SocialCare/Socialcarereform/Personalisation

90   Department of Health (2009) Shaping the Future of Care together Cm 7673 Stationery Office.

91   Disability Discrimination (Meaning of Disability) Regulations 1996 SI 1996/1455.

92   Disability Discrimination (Blind and Partially Sighted Persons) Regulations 2003 SI 2003/712.

93   Doyle, B.J. (1996) *Disability Discrimination: the New Law*. Jordans, Bristol.

94   Cooper, J. (ed) (2000) *Law, Rights and Disability*. Jessica Kingsley, London.

95   Thurgood, J. (1999) The employment implications of the Disability Discrimination Act 1995 and a suggested format for developing reasonable adjustments. *British Journal of Occupational Therapy*, **62**(7), 290–94.

96   Disability Discrimination (Providers of Services) (Adjustment of Premises) Regulations 2001 SI 2001/3253.

97   Disability Rights Commission (2002) 2004 – what it means for disabled people; www.drcgb.org/rights/newsdetails.

98   The Disability Discrimination Act 1995 (Taxis)(Carrying of Guide Dogs etc.) (England and Wales) Regulations 2000 SI 2000/7559.

99   Frean, A. (2000) Disabled rights group launched. *The Times*, 20 April.

100   White Paper Fairness For All: A New Commission for Equality and Human Rights. DTI and DCA, May 2004.

101   www.equalityhumanrights.com

102   OJ 2000 I 303 p. 16.

103   Coleman (Social Policy) [2008] EUECJ C-303/06 31 January 2008.

104   Coleman (Social Policy) [2008] EUECJ C-303/06 17 July 2008.

105   Council Directive 2000/78 ([2000] OJL303/16).

106   Employment Equality (Age) Regulations 2006 SI 2006/1031.

107   *Richmond Court (Swansea) Ltd v Williams* [2006] EWCA Civ 1719 (14 December 2006).

19 Employment Law

This chapter sets out the basic principles of employment law and how they relate to the practitioner. The law relating to contract for services and the self-employed practitioner is considered in Chapter 28. The following topics are covered in this chapter:

- The employment contract
- Statutory rights
- Termination of contract
- Protection against unfair dismissal
- Local bargaining
- Agenda for change
- Rights of the pregnant employee
- Other rights relating to family responsibilities
- Rights in relation to sickness
- Minimum Wage
- Working time directive
- Protection against discrimination: race, sex, age and disability
- Rehabilitation of Offenders Act 1974
- Part-time workers
- Trade Unions
- Whistle blowing
- Grievance procedures
- Pre-employment checks
- Future changes in employment law

The employment contract

As soon as an unconditional offer of employment (by the employer) or to be employed (by the employee) has been accepted by the other party, a contract of employment comes into existence. The contract may be subject to conditions, e.g. receipt of satisfactory references or satisfactory medical examinations. If these prove not to be satisfactory, then the contract will either not come into existence or will cease to exist.

Legal Aspects of Occupational Therapy, Third Edition By Bridgit Dimond
© 2010 Bridgit Dimond

As a result of the contract of employment both employer and employee have duties and rights. These terms can be either express terms, agreed by the parties individually or resulting from collective bargaining procedures; or implied terms; or terms set by statute.

Express terms

Some duties arise by express agreement between the parties. These would include the basic terms of the contract: title of the post, starting date, salary, holidays, sickness, pensions, etc. Some of these terms may have already been part of collective bargaining within the work place either at national or at local level.

The employee might also agree specific terms with the employer when commencing: e.g. that a previously booked holiday can be taken, or that she can start the day an hour later than usual because of child commitments. Such terms are enforceable, but written evidence of the agreement that the term is to be part of the contract of employment would be of considerable assistance to an employee who claimed that these terms were not being upheld.

Implied terms

The law implies into a contract of employment certain terms which are binding on both parties even though such terms were never expressly raised by the parties. Figure 19.1 lists the terms which would be implied by law as obligations upon the employer, and Figure 19.2 lists the terms which would be implied by law as obligations upon the employee.

The basic principle is that where express terms cover the issue, terms will not have to be implied.

Figure 19.1   Implied terms binding upon the employer.

(1)   A duty to take reasonable care for the health and safety of the employee, including the duty to ensure that the premises, plant and equipment are safe, that there is a safe system of work and that the staff are competent
(2)   A duty to co-operate with the employee to enable him to fulfil his contract of employment
(3)   To pay the employee

Figure 19.2   Implied terms binding upon the employee.

(1)   A duty to obey the reasonable instructions of the employer
(2)   A duty to act with reasonable care and safety
(3)   A duty to co-operate with the employer. This would include the duty to account for profits, to disclose misdeeds, not to compete with the employer
(4)   A duty to maintain the confidentiality of information learnt during employment

In the case of a junior hospital doctor it was argued that there was an implied term that an employer would take care of his employees and not ask them to work an excessive amount of overtime.[1] In this case the junior doctor became ill as a result of the excessive amount of overtime he was asked to work. The Court of Appeal held that the employer's right under the contract to ask the doctor to work up to 84 hours a week had to be exercised in the light of their implied duty of care to the employee. The Unfair Contracts Terms Act 1977 could apply to terms set out in the contract of employment (see Chapter 10). However, it considered that such matters were more properly negotiated by the professional bodies concerned or resolved by Parliament rather than the courts.

Human Rights

The Human Rights Act 1998 raises new issues in the employment field, since in certain circumstances an employee of a public authority or of an organisation exercising functions of a public nature may be able to argue that he is being treated in an inhuman or degrading way contrary to Article 3. In addition, where civil rights and obligations are in dispute, a person is entitled to have a hearing by an independent and impartial tribunal under Article 6 (see Appendix and Chapter 6). The Working Time Directive now applies to hours of work (see later). Cases where human rights breaches have been alleged include: an employee of a school facing a disciplinary hearing for allegations of sexual misconduct was entitled to an enhanced measure of procedural protection afforded by Article 6.1 of the ECHR guaranteeing the right to a fair hearing, which included the right to legal representation at the disciplinary hearing;[2] the procedure of effectively banning care workers from working with vulnerable people without giving them an opportunity to answer any allegations of unsuitability, was incompatible with the right to a fair hearing under Article 6 of the ECHR.[3] Issues of discrimination have also given rise to allegations of breach of the ECHR. For example the House of Lords held that the policy of disentitling persons without accommodation from receiving the disability premium to which they would otherwise be entitled in their income support amounted to discrimination within article 14 of the ECHR but was lawful as it could be justified on policy grounds.[4] The High Court held that placing an offender on the sex offenders indefinitely was a disproportionate interference with the right to respect for private and family life.[5]

Performance of the contract

Both parties under the contract of employment have a duty to fulfil the express, implied and statutory requirements in the contract of employment. Failure by the employee to fulfil the contractual requirements could result in her facing disciplinary proceedings. Failure by the employer to fulfil his contractual obligations could result in the employee claiming that she has been constructively dismissed by the employer; i.e. the employer has shown an intention of no longer abiding by the contract of employment and this therefore gives the employee the right either to see the contract as ended by this breach of contract or of seeing the contract as continuing. If the employee elects to see the contract as continuing then the employee has the right to claim damages or compensation for this breach of contract. Rights in a constructive dismissal are considered below.

It is a basic principle of contract law that one party to a contract cannot unilaterally change the terms of the contract without the consent of the other person. Thus an employer who required an employee to work in a different capacity or in a different location could be seen as being in breach of the contract if the capacity and the location were express terms in the contract.

Situation: Change of location

An occupational therapist who has worked at Roger Park Hospital for five years is asked by the trust to work at another location. She is unwilling to change her location since this would be inconvenient for home and schools.

In the above situation the OT might find that her contract does not actually give her a right to work at Roger Park Hospital, in which case her employer could change the location without being in breach of contract. On the other hand, if it was agreed in her contract that she would work at Roger Park Hospital, the employer can only change the location by agreement with her. She may be able to negotiate some benefits for changing the location. However, if there is any danger that she may be in a redundancy situation if she fails to move, she could be asked by the employer to accept suitable alternative employment, i.e. in a different location as an alternative to redundancy.

Statutory rights

The employer does not have complete discretion over what terms he can negotiate with the employee. Acts of Parliament require the employer to recognise certain rights, known as statutory rights, to which the employee is entitled. The employer could offer terms which improve upon these rights, but not reduce the benefits under the rights. Certain qualifying conditions stipulate which employees are entitled to benefit from these statutory rights. Figure 19.3 sets out the principle rights given by statute. Many statutory rights have given rise to judicial decisions on their interpretation. For example the Court of Appeal has held that the basic salary fixes holiday pay and therefore an airline which based its paid annual leave rate for pilots on their basic salary rather than on what they might

---

Figure 19.3   Statutory rights.

- Written statement of particulars
- Itemised statement of pay
- Time off provisions:
  - to take part in trade union duties and training,
  - to take part in trade union activities,
  - to look for a job or undergo training, in a redundancy situation
  - to attend ante-natal clinics
  - to act as a JP and undertake certain public service duties
- Provisions relating to pregnancy and maternity including pay
- Sickness pay
- Health and safety rights
- Rights relating to trade union membership and activities
- Bank holidays
- Guarantee payments
- Redundancy payment
- Medical suspension payment
- Rights under the Working Time Directive
- Rights under the Parental Leave Directive
- Part-time workers' right not to be treated less favourably
- Right to request flexible working

be expected actually to earn was not in breach of the statutory holiday pay requirements.[6] The House of Lords has held that employees who were entitled to statutory holiday pay were also entitled to claim its non-payment as an unlawful deduction from wages.[7] ACAS has provided guidance on some of the statutory rights such as a Code of Practice for time off for trade union duties and activities.

Health professionals employed within the NHS or by local authorities, and health professionals employed by contractors to the NHS and local authorities, are required to be registered with the Health Professions Council or another relevant registration body (see Chapter 3).

Termination of the contract

A contract of employment can come to an end in the following ways:

- by performance
- by the expiry of a fixed term contract
- by giving notice
- by a breach of contract by one or other party
- by frustration.

Ending by performance

A contract which identifies specific services to be provided will come to an end when these services have been given.

Ending of a fixed term contract

A fixed term contract will come to an end at the passing of the specified time unless the contract is renewed. Failure to renew a fixed term contract is seen in law as a dismissal.

Ending by notice

Under the employment protection legislation the employee is entitled to a minimum length of notice terminating the job, the period depending on the length of continuous service. However, notice provisions in excess of the statutory lengths will usually be agreed in the contract of employment. Where the employer dismisses an employee without regard to the length of notice, this constitutes a wrongful dismissal. Even when the correct length of notice is given to end a contract, there may still be an unfair dismissal by the employer (see below).

Ending by breach of contract

Breach of contract by the employer – If the employer is in fundamental breach of the contract of employment, the employee might see herself as being constructively dismissed and bring an application for unfair dismissal (see below).

Breach of contract by the employee – Where an employee is in breach of contract the employer can, if the circumstances justify it, see the contract of employment as at an end and dismiss the employee. The employee does, however, have the right to claim that the dismissal is unfair (see below).

Ending by frustration

Where an event occurs that was not in the contemplation of the parties at the time the contract was agreed, and it makes the performance of the contract impossible, then the contract will end by law without any requirement for the employer to terminate it, i.e. the performance of the contract is 'frustrated'. The following events have been seen as frustrating and therefore bringing to an end a contract of employment: death, imprisonment, and blindness (in a pilot).

Protection against unfair dismissal

One of the most important statutory rights has been the right not to be unfairly dismissed. There was a requirement that employees had to have worked continuously for the same employer for two years for at least 16 hours a week or for five years for at least eight hours a week. This requirement of 2 years' continuous service was challenged and the Court of Appeal[8] ruled that it was incompatible with the equal treatment enshrined in the Equal Treatment Directive of the European Community.[9] The qualifying period for bringing an unfair dismissal application has since been reduced from two years to one year of continuous service.[10]

No continuous service requirement

There are certain dismissal situations where no continuous service requirement exists. These are shown in Figure 19.4.

Application for unfair dismissal

If an allegation of unfair dismissal arises, and the employee has failed to win an internal appeal, an application to an employment tribunal can be made. The time limit for making such an application is three months from the date of dismissal, but the tribunal has the power to extend this if it is reasonable to do so.

The Advisory, Conciliation and Arbitration Service (ACAS) will contact the employee in an attempt to conciliate between the parties, so that a hearing of the case is unnecessary. From 1 April 2009 this is no longer a statutory duty but a discretionary power of ACAS. ACAS has prepared a note, 'Conciliation and tribunals', that describes the criteria, agreed by the ACAS Council, that its

---

Figure 19.4   Unfair dismissal with no continuous service requirement.

- Dismissal in connection with trade union activity and membership
- Dismissal in connection with pregnancy, childbirth maternity or parental leave
- Dismissal in connection with discrimination
- Dismissal in connection with health and safety
- Dismissal for asserting a statutory right
- Dismissal for exercising a right under the Working Time Regulations, or the Part-time Workers Regulations
- Dismissal for making a protected disclosure

conciliators use when deciding whether they can exercise the power to conciliate in these case. ACAS has a general duty of promoting the improvement of industrial relations. It can provide advice on employment legislation and industrial relations and can also assist in the settling of disputes. ACAS is able to offer an arbitration scheme for unfair dismissal disputes which is a voluntary alternative to the tribunal. Information is available on the ACAS website[11] and it also provides free advice on employment matters on a national helpline.[12] Information can also be obtained on the website for the Department for Business Innovation and skills (replacing the Department for Business, Enterprise and Regulatory Reform (which replaced the DTI)) on its website.[13] Dispute resolution procedures which set a three stage process for handling disputes and grievances were repealed by the Employment Act 2008 (but still apply to those cases which commenced before 6 April 2009) which gave powers to employment tribunals to amend awards if parties have failed to comply with a relevant statutory code. In April 2009 a revised ACAS Code of Practice on disciplinary and grievance issues, incorporating the new rules on employment dispute resolution, came into force. The new procedure is a less formal process, with lower penalties for those failing to follow the letter of the rules and a greater emphasis on resolving disputes quickly. The revised ACAS Code of Practice on disciplinary and grievance procedures explains what's fair and 'reasonable' behaviour when tackling problems at work.[14] There is a fear that ambiguities over the new procedures could lead to an increase in tribunal claims.[15] The new code does not apply to non-renewal of fixed term contracts or redundancies. Employers are expected to deal with issues promptly and without reasonable delay. Failure by the employer to follow fair procedures could lead to a 25% increase in compensation (in contrast to the 50% under the old statutory dispute resolution procedures). ACAS has also produced as a supplement to the Code of Practice a revised non-statutory guide which provides more information on handling discipline and grievance solutions in the workplace.[16]

Employment Rights (Dispute Resolution) Act 1998

This Act substituted the name 'employment tribunal' for 'industrial tribunal' and introduced provisions designed to speed up the hearing of complaints. These include: cases which can be heard by a chairman alone; certain matters being dealt with by a legal officer alone; non-lawyers being able to enter into compromise agreements; and an alternative method for resolving disputes about employment rights by means of a new voluntary arbitration scheme.

Unfair dismissal – the hearing

If the dispute resolution fails and a hearing is held, then the employee must show that there has been a dismissal and not a resignation. A dismissal may be:

- an ending of the contract of employment by the employer
- a constructive dismissal where the employee is able to regard the contract as ended by the employer's fundamental breach of contract
- the failure to renew a fixed term contract.

Defence to an unfair dismissal application

The employer must show the reason for the dismissal and the fact that the reason is recognised in law as capable of being a reason for dismissal. He must also show that he acted reasonably in

Figure 19.5 Statutory reasons for a fair dismissal.

- Conduct
- Capability
- Redundancy
- Going on strike
- Legal impossibility
- Other substantial reason

Figure 19.6 Elements in the reasonableness of the employer's action.

- Consistency
- Following the code of practice
- Clarity
- Hearing the employee's case
- Allowing the employee to be represented
- Giving a warning
- Making a fair investigation of the facts

treating this statutory reason as justifying the dismissal. The statutory reasons are set out in Figure 19.5 and the factors which are taken into account in determining the reasonableness of the dismissal are shown in Figure 19.6.

An example of a fair dismissal is a case where an occupational therapist in the NHS was doing private work in working hours.

Case: private work in working hours[17]

An OT was warned not to engage in private work during his working week. He was seen by a manager seeing a private client during his lunch break and was dismissed for gross misconduct. He had ignored the warning and continued seeing private clients. He was dismissed from his post and he applied to an industrial tribunal.

His dismissal was held by the tribunal to have been fair and he also failed in his appeal to the employment appeal tribunal. His defence that he was doing no more than taking an early lunch was rejected on the grounds that lunch hours are for lunch and not for seeing private patients. The employment appeal tribunal was satisfied that the employer had conducted a reasonable and fair enquiry into what had happened and that the decision of the industrial tribunal was beyond any sensible criticism.

Dismissal and pornography

A local authority[18] which had dismissed an employee for gross misconduct for using an office computer during office hours to access hard core pornography, appealed to an employment appeal tribunal against a finding that the dismissal was unfair. The EAT held that the employment tribunal had correctly asked itself whether the dismissal for gross misconduct fell within the band of reasonable response by the employer, but it had then gone on to consider its own view on the seriousness of the breach of contract and categorised it as no more than misconduct. The EAT held that no reasonable tribunal could have reached a conclusion other than that dismissal for gross misconduct was a reasonable response. A finding that the dismissal was anything other than fair was perverse.

Sanctions of employment tribunal

If an employee wins the case for unfair dismissal, the tribunal has the following options:

- Compensation – basic award; compensatory award; special award
- Reinstatement or Re-engagement

Further information on these remedies can be obtained from the Department for Business Innovation and skills (replacing the Department for Business, Enterprise and Regulatory Reform (which replaced the DTI)) on its website.[19]

Employee protection and health and safety

The Trade Union Reform and Employment Rights Act 1993 (now consolidated into the Employment Rights Act 1996) has given the employee considerable protection against dismissal where the employee is taking action on grounds of health and safety. There is no continuous service requirement placed upon the employee to obtain protection against dismissal or any other action short of dismissal.

The criteria for judging the appropriateness of the employee's actions are 'all the circumstances including, in particular, his knowledge and the facilities and advice available to him at the time'.

A defence is available to the employer if the employee's actions were so negligent that a reasonable employer might have dismissed him as the employer did (section 100(3)).

These provisions should give the employee much greater protection against unfair dismissal when bringing issues of health and safety hazards to the attention of the employer. These provisions have been strengthened by the insertion of new sections (43A–43L) into the Employment Rights Act 1996 as enacted by the Public Interest Disclosure Act 1998 which is considered later under whistle blowing.

The ambit of section 100 was considered in a case brought against St George's Hospital[20] where it was held that S 100 was not confined to the health and safety of the employees, but the employee's dismissal could relate to his or her fears about the health and safety of others.

Local bargaining

Most practitioners are employed by NHS trusts. A minority are employed in the independent sector. Within the NHS the framework of collective bargaining is provided by the Whitley Councils. Foundation hospitals may have greater powers of local bargaining than other NHS trusts (see Chapter 17). The practitioner needs to ensure that she understands the principles of contract law and employment law in order to make maximum use of any system of local bargaining.

Agenda for Change (AfC)

In 1999 the Government published a paper Agenda for Change: Modernising the NHS pay system. This included

- a single job evaluation scheme to cover all posts in the NHS to support a review of pay and all other terms and conditions for health service employees;
- three pay spines for doctors and dentists; for other professional groups covered by the Pay Review Body and for remaining non-Pay Review Body staff; and
- A wider remit for the Pay Review Body.

The Agenda for Change introduced a national modernised pay and grading framework into the NHS which required a specially designed NHS job evaluation scheme to be used as the basis for deciding the appropriate AfC grade for NHS posts. A second edition of the NHS Job Evaluation Handbook was published in 2004.[21] The COT has provided several briefing notes on agenda for change including OT titles, job clustering, preceptorships, job descriptions and how to challenge the outcome. [22]

The National Audit Office in a report in 2009[23] stated that the agenda for change scheme had not delivered noticeable improvements in staff morale, many trusts had failed to improve training and there was no evidence of better working. The Knowledge and Skills Framework had not been fully implemented with many managers perceiving it as complex and burdensome. Far from leading to an increase in productivity across the NHS, the NAO said that the Agenda for change had led to a fall in productivity of 2.5% a year. (The National Audit Office (which is totally independent of Government) scrutinises public spending on behalf of Parliament. The Comptroller and Auditor General is an Officer of the House of Commons.) A COT/BAOT briefing note no 31 provides guidance on the Knowledge and Skills framework for OT staff (February 2006) and briefing note no 108.[24] The Knowledge and Skills framework is considered in Chapter 5.

Situation

An OT takes on additional duties which under the Agenda for Change and the Knowledge and skills framework should have been preceded by an appraisal and re-evaluation of pay. Her job description is unilaterally changed by her employer. Where does she stand? A job description is not seen as part of the contract of employment and can be changed by the employer without the agreement of the employee provided the agreed contractual terms are not breached. Failure of the employer to act within the spirit of the Agenda for Change and Knowledge and Skills framework should lead to discussion between the employee and the human resources department. However as can be seen above from the National Audit Office report, such a situation is not uncommon. Collective action from a whole department may be necessary.

Rights of the pregnant employee

Statutory rights given to the pregnant employee are shown in Figure 19.7. The rights shown in Figure 19.7 are the rights given by statute. Many employers, however, give far more generous benefits than those given as a statutory right. The employee cannot have both. The Whitley Council conditions are in many ways superior to the statutory rights for those who have been in employment for more than two years. The rights of the pregnant woman are contained in the Employment

Figure 19.7 Statutory rights in pregnancy.

- Time off to attend for ante-natal care
- Maternity leave
- Maternity pay
- Right to return after confinement
- Protection against dismissal on grounds of pregnancy or childbirth
- Right to receive pay during suspension on grounds of pregnancy, recently given birth or breastfeeding
- Health in Pregnancy Grant

Rights Act 1996, the Employment Relations Act 1999, the Employment Act 2002 and the Work and Families Act 2006. Full details of all the entitlements are available on the Department for Business Innovation and skills (replacing the Department for Business, Enterprise and Regulatory Reform (which replaced the DTI)) on its website.[25] All employed women whose babies were due on or after 1 April 2007 are now entitled to additional maternity leave: 39 weeks for statutory maternity pay and maternity allowance; 8 weeks (instead of 28 days) notice must be given if she wishes to change the date of her return from maternity leave. All women have the right to return to work after maternity leave regardless of the size of the employer. Under the Health and Social Care Act 2008 section 131 a pregnant women is entitled to the payment of a lump sum (known as a health in pregnancy grant) if she meets certain conditions (including that she has received advice on matters relating to maternal health from a health professional and is in Great Britain at the time she makes a claim for the grant).

The Court of Justice of the European Communities held that the dismissal of a woman when her ova had been fertilised in an in vitro procedure, but had not been transferred to her uterus was not prohibited by the Community directive on the safety and health of pregnant workers but was prohibited by the equal treatment directive if it was established that the dismissal was based on the fact that she had undergone in vitro fertilisation.[26]

Other rights relating to family responsibilities

Parental leave[27]

A right is given by the Employment Relations Act 1999 to enable either parent to be absent from work for the purpose of caring for a child or making arrangements for the child's welfare.[28] The right can be claimed by an employee who has a baby or adopts a child after 15 December 1999 and who has completed one year's continuous service with their employer by the time they wish to take leave. Anyone satisfying the conditions could have leave of up to 13 weeks per child. Parental leave can be taken any time up to the child's fifth birthday, or five years after the adoption takes place, or in the case of a child with a disability, living with the parent, up to the child's 18th birthday.

The parent is entitled to return to the same job if the leave is for less than four weeks, or a similar job if the leave was for longer than four weeks. Procedures can be agreed between employer and employees for the details of parental leave. An employee who has been refused parental leave can take a case to the employment tribunal.

Time off for dependants[29]

From 15 December 1999, reasonable time off is permitted for an employee to deal with a domestic incident. This includes: when a dependant is ill, gives birth, is injured or dies; unexpected disruption of arrangements for the care of the dependant; an incident at a child's school. The employee must notify the employer of the reason for his absence as soon as is reasonably practicable, and of how long he is likely to be off. 'Dependant' includes a spouse, a child, a parent, a person who lives in the same household as the employee (other than a tenant or lodger) and includes any person who reasonably relies on the employee for assistance when ill or injured. An employer's refusal to give time off for dependants could be followed by an application by the employee to an employment tribunal.

Neither the parental leave nor time off for dependants give a right to paid leave.

Flexible working

Section 47 of the Employment Act 2002 introduced a new statutory right from April 2003 for an employee to request a variation in her contract. The right only arises for the purposes of the care of a child below 6 years or a disabled person below 18 years (This was extended under the Work and Families Act 2006 to carers of adults from April 2007 – see below). The employer has a statutory duty to consider the request and can refuse the request if one of the following grounds exist:

- the burden of additional costs
- detrimental effect on ability to meet customer demand
- inability to re-organise work among existing staff
- inability to recruit additional staff
- detrimental impact on quality
- detrimental impact on performance
- insufficiency of work during the periods the employee proposes to work
- planned structural changes
- such other grounds as the Secretary of State may specify by regulations.

Clear procedures for dealing with requests by employees for changes in their contracts are essential.

Work and Families Act 2006

The Work and Families Act 2006 followed a consultation on Work and Families: Choice and Consultation published in October 2005. As well as enhancing the rights of the pregnant employee, the Act:

- extended the right to request flexible working to carers of adults from April 2007
- gave employed fathers a new right to up to 26 weeks Additional Paternity Leave
- introduced measures to assist employers manage the administration of leave and pay
- introduced measures to improve communications during maternity leave.

Information on adoption leave and pay, flexible working and work life balance, paternity leave and pay, additional paternity leave and pay, parental leave, part-time work and time off for dependants can be obtained from the website of the Department for Business Innovation and skills (replacing the Department for Business, Enterprise and Regulatory Reform (which replaced the DTI)) on its website.[30]

Rights in relation to sickness

Employees are entitled to receive statutory sick pay from their employer when they are sick. Those who are not in work or are self-employed may be able to claim a state incapacity benefit instead. These include sickness benefit, invalidity benefit, and severe disablement allowance.

Statutory sick pay is payable for up to 28 weeks' incapacity. Many employees receive superior sickness benefits under their contracts of employment: in the NHS most employees with the necessary continuous service have, under Whitley Council conditions, received six months' full pay and six months' half pay to cover sickness. Details of the conditions and actions to be taken by the employee and employer are set out on the website for the Department for Works and Pensions.[31]

The European Court of Justice has held that a worker can defer his holiday entitlement arising when he is off work ill or to compensation in lieu.[32] The ruling was a victory for Revenue and Customs staff and reverses a Court of Appeal decision in 2005.

Minimum wage

The National Minimum Wage Act 1998 aims to combat poverty pay. Subject to certain exceptions the national minimum wage will apply at the same rate to all workers, regardless of the sector in which they work. The Act creates a framework for the minimum wage to be implemented and enforced and the details are contained in regulations issued by the Secretary of State. The Act refers to workers, including agency workers and homeworkers, and created the Low Pay Commission (LPC) which works with the Secretary of State in creating the minimum wage and advising on policy matters. The Low Pay Commission is an independent statutory non-departmental public body set up to advise the Government about the National Minimum Wage. Its permanent status was confirmed in 2001. Its most recent report in 2008[33] assessed the impact of the 2007 increase and recommended a minimum of £5.73 an hour from October 2008. Further information on the LPC can be found on its website.[34]

Working Time Regulations

Working Time Regulations were introduced following EC Directives.[35] Employers are subject[36] to restraint on the maximum average weekly working time, the average normal hours of night workers, the provision of health assessments for night workers, rest breaks and entitlement to annual leave.[37] There was criticism that the Directive was not fully implemented in the regulations and in February 2001 the Advocate General of the European Community ruled that the UK's requirement of a 13-week period of continuous service before there was an entitlement to annual leave was unlawful. The regulations were revised in 2002[38] to give enhanced rights to young workers. Obligations are imposed on employers concerning:

- a limit of an average weekly working time of workers of 48 hours
- the average normal hours of night workers of 8 hours in any 24-hour period
- the provision of health assessments for night workers

- workers have a right to 11 hours rest in any 24-hour period
- workers have a right to a day off each week
- workers have a right to an in-work rest break if the working day is longer than 6 hours
- Workers have a right to 5.6 weeks paid leave a year (from 1 April 2009 – increased from 4.8 weeks)
- the keeping of records of workers' hours of work.

The right of employees to opt-out of the regulations is being examined by the European Commission and is being negotiated through out the EU. The rights to time limits and health assessments are enforced through the Health and Safety Executive and local authority environmental health departments. Entitlements to rest and leave are enforced by individuals through the employment tribunals. Further information is available from the Department for Business Innovation and skills (replacing the Department for Business, Enterprise and Regulatory Reform (which replaced the DTI)) on its website[39] and also from the Employments Tribunal Service. The NHS Employers (see below) (which represents trusts in England on workforce issues) also provide information on the working time regulations in their applicability to the NHS including the significance of on call times and the prevention of abuse of the ability to opt out.[40]

The House of Lords held in *HM Revenue & Customs v Stringer and others*[41] that a worker:

- can take paid annual leave under the Working Time Directive during a period of sick leave. However, if a worker is on sick leave for part of their leave year and then returns to work before the end of their leave year, they should be able to take their annual leave then
- may be able to make a holiday pay claim under the deduction from wages provisions of the Employment Rights Act 1996, not just under the Working Time Regulations 1998.

The working time directive of a 48 hour week applies to junior doctors from August 2009, despite considerable opposition from surgeons amongst others. Deborah Kendall and others describe how the NHS North West recruited a team of junior doctors to implement the directive one year ahead.[42]

NHS employers

NHS Employers act on behalf of NHS Trusts in four priority areas:

- pay and negotiations
- recruitment and planning the workforce
- healthy and productive workplaces
- employment policy and practice.

It aims to keep employers up to date with the latest workforce thinking; provide practical advice and information; and help them to network and share knowledge. NHS Employers have agreed with the NHS Unions and Department of Health a partnership agreement[43] which covers roles and responsibilities principles for effective working, benefits and working arrangements at national, regional and local level.

Protection against discrimination: race, sex, age and disability

The main legislation protecting persons against discrimination over race and sex are the Race Relations Act 1976 and the Sex Discrimination Act 1975 and subsequent amendments. The Sex Discrimination Act 1986 equalised the position of men and women in relation to retiring age following the decision of the European Court in *Marshall v Southampton AHA*.[44] The Equal Pay Act 1970 implies an equality clause into an employment contract, that a woman employed on like work to a man is entitled to have similar terms and conditions. The Race Relations (Amendment) Act 2000 and Regulations 2003 place a duty on public authorities to eliminate unlawful discrimination and promote equality.

The basic principles under the race and sex discrimination laws, and these apply both within and outside the employment field, are shown in Figures 19.8 and 19.9.

A test case[45] on the Equal Pay Act 1970 was brought by speech therapists who claimed that they were employed on work of equal value with male principal grade pharmacists and clinical psychologists employed in the NHS whose salaries exceeded theirs by about 60%. The Court of Appeal referred the case to the European Court of Justice.[46] This decided that the fact that differences in pay were mainly arrived at through collective bargaining is not sufficient objective justification for the difference in pay between the two jobs. It is for the national court to determine, whether and to what extent the shortage of candidates for a job and the need to attract them by higher pay constitutes an objectively justified economic ground for the difference in pay between the jobs in question. Subsequently, the Court of Appeal held that the speech therapist was entitled to receive the same pay as a male comparator was currently earning[47] The Court of Appeal held that it was sufficient notice of an equal pay claim for an employee to send a written statement of grievance to the employer identifying the issue as an equal pay claim.[48]

Figure 19.8   Principles of protection from discrimination on grounds of race.

Basic principle
Discrimination on grounds of colour, race, nationality or ethnic or national origins is unlawful.

Direct discrimination
This occurs where one person treats another less favourably on racial grounds than he would treat a person of another race.

Indirect discrimination
This exists when an employer applies a requirement or condition which, although applicable to all people, is such that a proportion of people of one race who can comply with it is smaller that the proportion in another, or where the employer cannot show that the requirement is justifiable on other than racial grounds and it is to the detriment of the complainant because he or she cannot comply with it.
   It is also unlawful to victimise or segregate on grounds of race.

Exempt areas
● Genuine occupational grounds (e.g. the essential nature of the job requires a particular physique and authenticity (like playing the Moor in Othello))
● National security
● Charitable trusts

Other provisions
The Act does not apply to immigration rules or civil service regulations.

Enforcement
This is through an application to an employment tribunal.
   Assistance can be provided by the Equality and Human Rights Commission

> **Figure 19.9**   Principles of protection from discrimination on grounds of sex.
>
> **Basic principle**
> To treat a person less favourably on the grounds of sex than a person of the other sex
> would be treated is unlawful. It is also unlawful for an employer to discriminate against a
> person on grounds of marital status.
>
> **Indirect discrimination**
> This occurs where an employer applies a requirement or condition which, even though
> it applies equally to all persons, is such that a proportion of people of one sex who can
> comply with it is considerably smaller that the proportion in the other, and where the
> employer cannot show justification on other than sexual grounds and it is to the detriment
> of the complainant. It is also unlawful to victimise or segregate on grounds of sex.
>
> **Exempt areas**
> - Genuine occupational qualification:
>   - essential nature of the job requires a person of a different sex
>   - authenticity, decency and privacy, personal services
>   - work abroad which can only be done by a man
>   - the job is one of two held by a married couple
> - National security
> - Work in private households
> - Charitable trusts
> - Ministers of religion
> - Sports and sports facilities
> - Police and police cadets in respect of certain terms only
>
> **Enforcement**
> This is through an application to an employment tribunal.
>   The Equality and Human Rights Commission has a duty to work towards the elimination
> of discrimination, promoting the equality of opportunities and keeping under review the Sex
> Discrimination Act.

A Code of Practice on Equal Pay came into force on 1 December 2003, replacing the 1997 edition.[49] The Equal Pay Directive 1975 and the Equal Pay Treatment Directive 1976 were brought together in the Consolidated Equal Treatment Directive 2006.[50] Member states must implement it by 15 August 2009.

The Sex Discrimination Act 1975 (Amendment) Regulations 2008[51] implements the 2002 Directive[52] which applies the principle of equal treatment of men and women to access to employment, vocational training and promotion and working conditions. The Regulations amend the 1975 Act amending the definition of harassment and discrimination on grounds of pregnancy or maternity leave.

The Equality Act 2010 is discussed in Chapter 18.

Discrimination on grounds of religion or belief or sexual orientation

New regulations came into force in December 2003 as a result of employment directives from the European Community. The Employment Equality (Religion or Belief) Regulations[53]) and the Employment Equality (Sexual Orientation) Regulations[54]) protect employees and applicants and those in vocational training against discrimination, victimisation or harassment on the grounds of religion or belief or sexual orientation. Exceptions to equality in respect of religion or belief are recognised for national security, positive action and the protection of Sikhs from discrimination in connection with requirements as to wearing of safety helmets. Exceptions to equality in respect of sexual orientation are recognised for national security and positive action and also for benefits that are dependent on marital status. Enforcement in respect of both sets of regulations is through the employment tribunal.

Respect for religious diversity can cause issues within the NHS and the DH has said that it is reviewing the state provision of hospital chaplains. A guide on Religion or Belief: A practical guide for the NHS states that practicing or attempting to convert people at work can cause many problems as non-religious people and those from other religions or beliefs could feel harassed and intimidated by this behaviour. A nurse who offered to pray for a patient was suspended without pay by North Somerset Primary Care Trust. She was eventually reinstated following protests by the Christian Legal Centre amongst others.[55] It was stated that the patient had made no complaint.

The first successful case under the Sexual Orientation regulations was the case of *Whitfield v Cleanaway UK*[56] where a manager won £35,000 for constructive dismissal as a result of suffering sustained abuse including references to 'queer', 'queen' and 'dear' from senior management. The Court of Appeal held that a straight man who was the victim of gay gibes could bring an action for sexual harassment. The case brought by Stephen English against his employers Thomas Sanderson Blinds had been turned down by the employment tribunal and the employment appeal tribunal but Court of Appeal in a majority judgment ruled that he could be harassed by homophobic banter even though he was not gay and remitted the case to the EAT for the assessment of compensation.[57]

Employment Equality Regulations[58] came into force on 1 October 2005 which brought sexual indirect discrimination in line with racial discrimination. Article 9 of the European Convention on Human Rights gives a qualified right in respect of freedom of thought, conscience and religion.

Age discrimination

Protection from discrimination on grounds of age came into force in October 2006 as a result of a European Directive[59] which was implemented by the Employment Equality (Age) Regulations 2006.[60] The Regulations only apply to employment and vocational training and only protect employees up to 65 years who can be dismissed after that age provided the employer satisfies the specified procedure set out in the regulations. If the employer agrees to keep the employee on after that age, the employee is protected against other forms of discrimination in relation to discipline, pay, harassment and job classification. Employees have the right to request working beyond 65 years and in such a case employers have a duty to consider the request according to Schedule 6. In a case on 16 October 2007[61] involving a Spanish worker who challenged his forced retirement, the European Court of Justice said that the EU states can introduce and enforce mandatory retirement ages as long as they are justified. Heyday, an offshoot of the charity Age Concern, had awaited this ruling before pursuing its own case (see below). One possible distinction between the UK and the ruling in the Spanish case is that in the UK retirement ages are fixed by collective bargaining with individual employers and not by the Government. Subsequently Age Concern challenged the right of employers to impose retirement at the age of 65 years. The Court of Justice of the European Communities ruled that member states had to justify age discrimination[62] but the burden of proof was on the member state to establish that the discrimination was objectively and reasonably justified. The case then had to return to the High Court where the Government had to justify Britain's compulsory retirement age as having a legitimate aim linked to social or employment policy.

The Age Discrimination Regulations do not only protect the older worker: in March 2008 a teenager won an age discrimination claim.[63] Leanne Wilkinson who worked as an administrative assistant in Springwell Engineering was sacked and told that she was too young for the job. She obtained £16,000 compensation, the tribunal concluding that she had been discriminated against on grounds of age. Provisions in the new Equality Act 2010 prohibit age discrimination beyond the work place (see Chapter 18).

Disability discrimination

The Disability Discrimination Act was passed in 1995 and gives the disabled person certain rights in relation to employment, pensions and insurance, the provision of goods and services, access to premises, education and public transport. The main provisions of the Act are considered in Chapter 18. Part II of the Act covers discrimination in relation to employment and a summary of the provisions of Part II are shown in Figure 19.10. A Code of Practice for the elimination of discrimination in the field of employment has been published and this sets out guidance on the status and use of the Code, the main employment provisions of the Act, recruitment, and employment and particular provisions. Appendices to the Code of Practice cover what is meant by discrimination, and how to get further information, help and advice.

Part II of the Act, which covers discrimination in employment, makes it unlawful for an employer to discriminate against a disabled person (i.e. unjustifiably treat the disabled person less favourably) in arrangements for recruitment, and also in the terms of employment which are offered, including opportunities for promotion and training and other benefits. The disabled employee is also protected against dismissal or other detriment. Regulations have been made to cover these provisions and also to define further the duties of the employer in relation to physical arrangements.[64]

The disabled person has the right to apply to an Employment Tribunal over any discrimination. The Department for Education and Employment (DEE) has issued guidance for employers.[65] Annex B gives practical suggestions for avoiding discrimination in recruitment and employment. They include:

- Do not make assumptions
- Consider whether you need expert advice
- Plan ahead
- Consult

Figure 19.10   Part II Disability Discrimination Act 1995.

- Discrimination against applicants and employees
- Meaning of discrimination
- Duty of employer to make adjustments
- Exemption for small businesses
- Enforcement, remedies and procedure
- Discrimination by other persons
- Premises occupied under leases
- Occupational pension schemes
- Insurance services

- Specify the job carefully
- Be able to justify any health requirement
- Think ahead for interviews
- Only ask about a disability if it is relevant
- Be fair
- Review recruitment, promotion and career development arrangements.

The House of Lords has held that an employer can allow a disabled employee to be treated more favourably.[66] An employee who had become disabled could be transferred to a more suitable post without being required to compete with other applicants. The House of Lords has also held that in determining whether a person was disabled under the DDA 1975 by reason of having an impairment which, although capable of being controlled by measures taken to treat it, would be likely to have substantial adverse effects but for those measures, the word 'likely' did not mean 'probably' but 'could well happen'. The employee whose propensity to develop vocal nodules was controlled by a strict management regime based on avoiding raising her voice, was a disabled person for the purposes of the Act. The employers who placed her in a noisier work environment in spite of her claim that it would require her to speak louder and jeopardise her voice management regime, had to answer her claim that they had failed to make reasonable adjustments for her disability.[67] Further guidance is available in the statutory code of practice. This Code, which covers the duty to promote disability equality and clarifies the statutory duties, was published by the Disability Rights Commission in 2005.[68] (The Codes of Practice on Gender equality duty, race equality duty and disability equality duty are available from the new Equality and Human Rights Commission website.[69]) A chief inspector of police claimed that he had been unfairly discriminated against on account of his dyslexia. The tribunal found that the dyslexia did not have a substantial adverse effect on his ability to carry out normal day-to-day activities and therefore he was not disabled within the meaning of S 1 of the DDA 1995. The employee's appeal to the Employment Appeal Tribunal succeeded.[70] It held that once the tribunal had accepted that the employee was disadvantaged to the extent of requiring 25% extra time to do an assessment, it inevitably followed that there was a substantial adverse effect on normal day-to-day activities. He was therefore a disabled person within the meaning of the Act. Further consideration of the Disability Discrimination Act 1995 is provided in Chapter 18.

The Disability Discrimination Act 2005

This Act puts into law some of the recommendations of the Disability Rights Task Force which was set up by the Government in 1997. Section 18 of the Act extends the definition of disability in respect of those with a mental illness (It is no longer a requirement that mental illness must be clinically well-recognised if it is to be the basis of 'mental impairment') and includes those diagnosed with cancer, multiple sclerosis and HIV infection from the point at which the disease was diagnosed rather than from the point at which their illness had an adverse effect on them. Its other provisions are considered in Chapter 18.

The Court of Appeal has held that the rights recognised in the Disability Discrimination legislation applied to the services provided in prisons, police custody and detention centres for failed asylum seekers.[71] Whether an adverse effect on a person's ability to carry out normal day-to-day activities was likely to recur should be determined by an employment tribunal on the basis of evidence available at the time of the alleged disability discrimination.[72]

Clients and employments

The OT is not only concerned with employment law in respect of her own situation, but also with the problems of ensuring employment for her disabled clients. For example OTs working in the field of mental health may be concerned about how much information should be disclosed to other services or organisations about known risks to and from clients who are moving into vocational, community or educational settings, and who may have a forensic or complex history. They need to balance disclosure of information which may hinder the client being employed with the attempt to secure the social integration of the client into the work force. The OT has a responsibility to notify a prospective employer about any reasonable risks of harm as a result of a client being taken on, but the employer also has a responsibility under the Disability Discrimination laws not to discriminate against such clients. The definition of discrimination now includes 'mental illness'.

The Equality and Human Rights Commission

In October 2003 the Government announced plans for a single equality body for Great Britain: the Commission for Equality and Human Rights (CEHR). Under the proposals the CEHR was to take responsibility for new laws on age, religion and belief and sexual orientation and would replace the Commission for Racial Equality (CRE), the Equal Opportunities Commission (EOC) and the Disability Rights Commission (DRC). Following consultation on the proposals, a task force was set up to explore and develop ways in which the new body would work and it published its draft paper, *A Vision for the Commission for Equality and Human Rights*, in December 2003. A White Paper was published in May 2004. The Equality and Human Rights Commission was established on 1 October 2007 under the Equality Act 2006 replacing the Equal Opportunities, the Disabilities Rights Commission and the Commission for Racial Equality. See Chapter 18 for further details on the Equality and Human Rights Commission role. The provisions of the Equality legislation of 2008 and 2009 are also considered in that chapter. ACAS has published a guide on delivering equality and diversity for employers (March 2009) which can be down loaded from the ACAS website. NHS Employers has also provided guidance on diversity[73] which is available on its website.[74]

The Coleman Case

Ms Coleman worked for her former employer as a legal secretary from January 2001. In 2002, she gave birth to a son who suffered from apnoeic attacks and congenital laryngomalacia and bronchomalacia. Her son's condition required specialised and particular care. The claimant in the main proceedings was his primary carer. On 4 March 2005, Ms Coleman accepted voluntary redundancy, which brought her contract of employment with her former employer to an end. On 30 August 2005, she lodged a claim with the Employment Tribunal alleging that she had been subject to unfair constructive dismissal and had been treated less favourably than other employees because she was the primary carer of a disabled child. She claimed that that treatment caused her to stop working for her former employer. The Tribunal referred the case to the European Court of Justice to determine whether there could be discrimination where the employee herself was not the disabled person, but was the mother of the disabled person. The European Court of Justice held that the interpretation of the Directive[75] should not be limited in its application only to people who are themselves disabled since that would deprive the directive of an important element of its effectiveness and reduce the protection which it is intended to guarantee.[76]

The decision is an extremely important one for carers of those with disabilities.

Rehabilitation of Offenders Act 1974

The aim of this Act is to prevent discrimination against those who have had criminal convictions. It works by regarding certain offences as 'spent' after a certain length of time. This means that the person does not have to disclose the offence, and to dismiss an employee on grounds that she failed to disclose a spent offence is automatically unfair. However, the Act does not apply to serious crimes and many occupations are excluded from its effect, including health service employment. Under Schedule 1 to the Statutory Instrument,[77] all members of any profession coming under the aegis of the Professions Supplementary to Medicine Act 1960 (and now the Health Professions Council) are excepted from the provisions of the 1974 Act and no convictions are considered spent. All convictions will remain on the record. All registered OTs are therefore excluded from the provisions of the 1974 Act.

Part-time workers

On 1 July 2000 regulations came into force to prevent part-time workers being treated less favourably than full-time workers,[78] implementing the European Directive.[79] Paragraph 5 of these regulations gives the part-time worker

the right not to be treated by his employer less favourably than the employer treats a comparable full-time worker:

- As regards the terms of his contract, or
- By being subjected to any other detriment by any act, or deliberate failure to act, of his employer.

The right applies only if the treatment is on the ground that the worker is a part-time worker and the treatment is not justified on objective grounds. The part-time worker has to compare himself with full-time workers working for the same employer. The right also applies to workers who become part-time or, having been full-time, return part-time after absence, to be treated not less favourably than they were before going part-time. It does not give an employee the right to insist on having part-time work.

The Regulations (Para. 6) also entitle a worker, who considers that he has been treated in a manner which infringes this right, to request from this employer a written statement giving particulars of the reasons for the treatment. The worker must be provided with a statement within 21 days of his request. Failure to provide a statement at all or only in an evasive or equivocal way will enable the tribunal to draw any inference which it considers just and equitable, including an inference that the employer has infringed the right in question. The regulations also enable a part-time worker who is dismissed to be regarded as unfairly dismissed if he has taken advantage of the Regulations. The part-time worker is also given a right not to be subjected to any detriment (Para. 7).

Any worker who considers that his rights have been infringed can present a complaint to an employment tribunal within three months of the day of less favourable treatment or detriment taking place. This is subject to the right of the tribunal to consider out of time cases if in all the circumstances it is just and equitable to do so.

At present employees do not have a right to insist on working part-time but this is being considered.

Trade unions

The protection and immunities which trade unions and their members enjoyed in the 1970s and 1980s have been eroded until they have very few rights in relation to protection as a result of industrial action. Industrial action itself is defined in narrow terms if it is to be construed as 'lawful'. Rules are laid down in relation to the holding of elections, and secret ballots before a strike can commence. Secondary industrial action is prohibited, so that trade unions are not immune from liability for the effects of any secondary action. The individual citizen has been given a right to prevent disruption to his supply of any goods or services because of unlawful industrial action. If he can show that he has been or will be deprived of goods or services and that the industrial action is unlawful, then he can apply to the court for an order to restrain the action.

Employment Relations Act 1999

This Act introduced a number of reforms to employment and trade union law as a result of the White Paper *Fairness at Work*. There are new procedures for the recognition and derecognition of trade unions as being entitled to conduct collective bargaining on behalf of groups of workers. The Act has also introduced new maternity rights and a right to leave for domestic and paternity leave (see above).

The reader is referred to one of the specialist books on employment in the Further Reading list for further information on trade union rights and duties.

Whistle blowing: Public Interest Disclosure Act 1998

Whistle blowing is the term which refers to a person (usually an employee) who draws attention to concerns which have health and safety implications. The Public Interest Disclosure Act 1998 provides protection from victimisation for an employee who brings to the attention of specified persons certain information which is considered 'protected' under the legislation. The Public Interest Disclosure Act 1998 came into force on 2 July 1999 and introduces amendments to the Employment Rights Act 1996. The explanatory memorandum envisages that the Act will protect workers, who disclose information about certain types of matters, from being dismissed or penalised by their employers as a result. The Act applies to specific disclosures:

- that a criminal offence has been committed, is being committed or is likely to be committed
- that a person has failed, is failing or is likely to fail to comply with any legal obligation to which he is subject
- that a miscarriage of justice has occurred, is occurring or is likely to occur
- that the health or safety of any individual has been, is being or is likely to be endangered
- that the environment has been, is being or is likely to be damaged
- that information tending to show any matter falling within any one of the preceding paragraphs has been, is being or is likely to be deliberately concealed.

To qualify for protection, the worker making the disclosure must:

- make the disclosure to his employer or to another person to whom the failure relates or who has legal responsibility
- be acting in good faith.

Protected disclosures include:

- disclosures made to obtain legal advice
- disclosures to a Minister of the Crown if the employee's employer is appointed by the Crown.

The Secretary of State has the power to make an order identifying other organisations or persons to whom a protected disclosure could be made, provided that the employee makes it in good faith and reasonably believes that any allegations are substantially true.

Other disclosures are protected subject to specified conditions. These disclosures would include disclosures to the press, police, media and MPs. The specified conditions are that the worker:

- makes the disclosure in good faith
- reasonably believes that the information disclosed, and any allegation contained in it, are substantially true
- does not make it for personal gain
- satisfies one of the conditions set out in 43G(2)
- and in all the circumstances of the case, it is reasonable for him to make the disclosure.

The conditions in 43G(2) include the belief by the worker that he would be subjected to a detriment by his employer if he were to make the disclosure to him or the Secretary of State; that he fears that evidence will be concealed or destroyed; or that he has previously made a disclosure of substantially the same information to his employer. The reasonableness of the employee's actions are judged in relation to:

- the person to whom the disclosure was made
- the seriousness of the relevant failure
- whether the disclosure was made in breach of a duty of confidentiality
- any action which the employer or other person could have taken when first notified
- whether the worker followed the procedure.

When the failure being reported is of an exceptionally serious nature, it will be a protected disclosure if the worker makes the disclosure in good faith, believes it to be substantially true, does not make it for personal gain, and in all the circumstances it is reasonable for him to make the disclosure.

Any provision in an agreement between employer and worker is void if it purports to preclude the worker from making a protected disclosure.

Guidance has been issued by the Department of Health[80] which requires every NHS trust and health authority to have in place local policies and procedures which comply with the provisions of the Act. Further details of the legislation can be obtained from the website of the Department for Business Innovation and skills (replacing the Department for Business, Enterprise and Regulatory Reform (which replaced the DTI)) on its website.[81]

Implementation of the Public Interest Disclosure Act

In one of the first cases to be reported after the coming into force of the Act, compensation of more than a quarter of a million pounds was awarded.[82] A consultant in obstetrics and gynaecology who was sacked after highlighting the high infant death rate and appalling treatment of patients at a Tyneside hospital won her case for unfair dismissal and racial discrimination.[83] The Bristol Inquiry,[84] which is considered in Chapter 17, recommended an open honest partnership between the patient and the health professional. It stated that a duty of candour, i.e. a duty to tell a patient if adverse events have occurred, must be recognised as owed by all those working in the NHS to patients. When things go wrong, patients are entitled to receive an acknowledgement, an explanation and an apology. Concerns of patients should be addressed in a one-stop shop and complaints dealt with swiftly and thoroughly. If this recommendation were fully implemented, there would be less need for whistle blowers within the NHS. Consultation on a new scheme for compensation for clinical negligence[85] considered the possibility of a statutory duty of candour, accompanied by an exemption from disciplinary or professional conduct proceedings (unless the health professional has committed a criminal offence or it would not be safe for the professional to continue to treat patients). However, such provisions were not contained in the NHS Redress Act. (See Chapter 10 for further details of the consultation paper.) Concern was expressed about the striking off from the nursing and mid-wifery register of Margaret Haywood following her actions in reporting on TV abuses of elderly patients. The Council for Healthcare Regulatory Excellence (see Chapter 3) issued a statement saying that it acknowledged public concern around the case, explaining its function but noting that it had no powers in relation to decisions which result in removal from the register. In these cases, the registrant has the right to appeal against such a decision.

It had requested a copy of the transcript of this case from the NMC and would review it and would publish a report on the conduct and outcome of the case when all legal processes had been concluded. Subsequently the NMC replaced the striking off with a 12 month caution. The British Medical Association has set up a whistleblower helpline because of growing evidence of staff reluctance to speak out for fear of recrimination. The helpline is part of new guidelines[86] In 2008 the British Standards Institute published standards for whistle blowing which can be down loaded free of charge[87] from its website.[88]

Criminal actions by health staff

Following the offences by Beverly Allit (who killed or harmed several children when working as a nurse), the Clothier Inquiry made several recommendations for detecting the possibility of personal disorder in applicants for nursing posts, to set up procedures for management referrals to occupa-tional health staff and to clarify the criteria for triggering such referrals. There would therefore be a duty on any employee who suspects that a colleague is acting suspiciously to advise the appropri-ate manager.

The Clothier recommendations were reinforced by an inquiry chaired by Richard Bullock follow-ing the case of Amanda Jenkinson, a Nottinghamshire nurse who was jailed for harming a patient. The Government has accepted the recommendations that all NHS staff will have a pre-employment health assessment. Information provided to occupational health staff will remain confidential unless disclosure is necessary because a member of staff is considered to be a danger to patients, other staff or themselves. In these circumstances there should be disclosure to the appropriate person or authority.

The Shipman case

An inquiry was established following the conviction of Dr Shipman for 15 murders of patients (The Inquiry considered him to have probably been responsible for over 200 deaths). Six reports followed the conviction of Dr Harold Shipman.[89] The first report of the inquiry identified the victims of Dr Shipman. The second report of the inquiry examined how such events could be prevented in the future and reported in July 2003. Significant changes were recommended to professional regulation, certification of death and the coronial system. These are considered in chapters 4 and 25.

Grievance procedures

As stated above, the Department of Health has recommended that each trust should provide a procedure to ensure that an employee can bring any concerns to the awareness of senior management without suffering victimisation. The jurisdiction of the Health Service Commissioner does not extend to complaints and grievances of staff (see Chapter 14) but the Care Quality Commission (see Chapter 17) would be receptive to complaints from staff where these relate to deficiencies in the standards of care available to patients.

Pre-employment checks

In addition to the checks on the sex offenders' register, employers are required to carry out checks on illegal working. As a result of section 8 of the Asylum and Immigration Act 1996 it is a criminal offence to employ someone aged 16 or over who has no right to work in the UK. Employers have a statutory defence against conviction if they have checked and copied certain original documents. From 1 May 2004 there were changes to the type of document which must be checked and copied. Further information can be obtained from the Home Office.[90]

The Protection of Children Act 1999

The Protection of Children Act 1999 makes statutory the Department of Health's Consultancy Service Index list and it requires childcare organisations to refer the names of individuals considered unsuitable to work with children for inclusion on the list. It also provides rights of appeal against inclusion and requires regulated childcare organisations to check the names of anyone they propose to employ in posts involving regular contact with children, with the list, and not to employ them if they are listed. Finally, it amends Part V of the Police Act 1997 to allow the Criminal Records Bureau to act as a central access point for criminal records information, List 99[91] and the new Department of Health list. In other words, the Criminal Records Bureau will act as a one-stop shop in the carrying out of checks.

The effect of the legislation is that organisations such as health trusts who work with children have a statutory duty from October 2000 to vet prospective employees, paid or unpaid, for work involving contact with children. From October 2000 organisations who have registered with the DH are able to check names from their own computers via the internet. In October 2000 there were about 1000 names on the DH Consultancy Service Index,[92] who had been notified to the DH because they had been dismissed from childcare posts or who had left such a post in circumstances where the employer considered that a child would be at risk of harm from them. The Protection of Children and Vulnerable Adults and Care Standards Tribunal Regulations were passed in 2002 and amended in 2003.[93]

The Sexual Offenders Act 1997

The Sexual Offenders Act 1997 was passed in order to ensure that once a sex offender had served his sentence and was about to be released, he would still be subject to some form of supervision to protect persons against the risk of his re-offending. Part 1 of the Act requires the notification of information to the police by persons who have committed certain sexual offences. Guidance on the Act was provided by the Department of Health in 1997.[94]

Sexual Offences (Amendment) Act 2000

Under this Act the age at which certain sexual acts (for example, homosexual acts in private) are lawful is reduced to 16 years and a new defence is available so that when one party to homosexual activity is below the age of 16 and the other over 16, the younger one does not commit any offence. However, a new offence is introduced for a person, A, over 18 years to have sexual intercourse with a person or engage in any other sexual activity with another person, B, if A is in a position of trust in relation to B. 'Position of trust' is defined in section 4 as where B is detained in an institution or is resident in a home, or cared for in a hospital, residential care home or nursing home, where A is looking after such persons, or A looks after persons under 18 who are receiving full-time education at an educational institution and B is receiving such education.

   Local authorities may be liable for employees who fail to take action when children are subjected to abuse (see Chapter 23).

The Safeguarding Vulnerable Groups Act 2006

This Act aimed at strengthening current safeguarding arrangements for individuals in the workplace and reducing the risk of individuals suffering harm at the hands of those employed in either paid or voluntary capacity to work with them. The Independent Barring Board (IBB) was set up on 2 January 2008 and people included in lists maintained under the Protection of Children Act 1999 or the Care Standards Act 2000 or who are subject to a direction under the Education Act 2002 section 142 will be included or considered for inclusion by the IBB in the children's barred list of the adults' barred lists.

   The IBB was renamed the Independent Safeguarding Authority (ISA) which was established to support the implementation of the Safeguarding Vulnerable Groups Act and bring together the existing barring schemes, Protection of Vulnerable Adults (POVA), Protection of Children Act and List 99. From the autumn of 2008 ISA covered the following areas:

- coverage of all workforce areas where children or vulnerable adults may be exposed to abuse or exploited instead of just regulated social care settings.
- pre-employment vetting
- independent and consistent decision-making by employers
- continuous monitoring: ISA can review decision not to bar on receipt of new information
- reduction in bureaucracy: online and free of charge checking system, once people have joined the scheme
- wide range of sources of information: duty of employers and service providers to give information to the scheme
- coverage across the UK

ISA issued a consultation paper on the barring process in June 2007 covering the time period for making representations; the minimum no-review period; the age boundary in relation to the minimum barred period and automatic barring offences. It is estimated that 11 million individuals will have to be passed through the ISA's checking process in the first five years of its operations.

From October 12th 2009 the ISA responsibilities for barring individuals who pose a known risk from working or volunteering with children and vulnerable adults were further strengthened as more sectors such as the NHS and the Prison Service came under the Scheme and new criminal offences came into force. Further details on the Vetting and Barring Scheme Programme can be found on the Home Office website.[95]

The Department for Children, Schools and Families (DCSF) has also developed a cross-Government strategy for children and young people called 'Staying Safe' which can be accessed on the DCSF website and the police website.[96]

Future changes in employment law

Major changes have taken place in the law relating to employment as the result of the European Directives. The White Paper Fairness at Work.[97] set out proposals for significant changes in employment law, most of which have now been implemented. The ten years following the White Paper were reviewed in a speech in May 2008 by the Secretary of State for Business, Enterprise and Regulatory Reform.[98] He envisaged that the UK had reached the end of any new regulations and believed that in future there would be a changing balance of rights and responsibilities; business success would be boosted by investing in employees; a need to ensure more effective enforcement of existing laws; recognising that consumers can drive up standards at work. Some of these ideas are contained in the Employment Act 2008. The Act aims to:

- Improve the effectiveness of employment law to the benefit of employers, trade unions, individuals and the public sector;
- Bring together both elements of the government's employment relations strategy increasing protection for vulnerable workers and lightening the load for law-abiding businesses
- Promoting compliance and help to ensure a level playing field for law-abiding businesses.

The Act's provisions were:

- to repeal the Employment Act 2002 and the Dispute Resolution Regulations 2004 and thus abolish the existing statutory dispute resolution procedures and related provisions about procedural unfairness
- to establish a new non-regulatory scheme for dispute resolution
- to clarify and strengthen the enforcement framework for the National Minimum Wage
- to implement the changes required following the ECHR decision in *Aslef v UK*[99] which ruled that clearer rights for TUs to determine their membership
- employment tribunals are given discretionary powers to amend awards if parties have failed to comply with a relevant statutory code. Tribunals are able to reach a determination without a hearing. Tribunals will also be able to award compensation for financial loss, in certain cases. The law relating to conciliation by ACAS is also amended.

Section 78 of the Equalities Act 2010 will require companies to carry out gender pay audits to identify employers who routinely pay women less.[100] Section 77 also bans secrecy clauses that prevent colleagues comparing their salaries. Employment tribunals will also be given new powers to make recommendations to companies on equal pay if a company is taken to court by an employee (see Chapter 18).

NHS Professionals

In implementing the NHS Plan,[101] NHS Professionals[102] was introduced by the Department of Health in November 2000. It is a national scheme for managing and providing temporary staffing services. The key characteristics of NHS Professionals are set out in a circular.[103] The initiative has been implemented and is likely to have an impact on more flexible working and lead to greater uniformity in the payment of bank and agency staff. NHS Professionals is seen by the Government as being part of a whole systems approach modernising human resource systems in the NHS. It will link into the new NHS HR/Payroll system, and with NHS Careers (a national service to provide information about careers in the NHS) and a new e-pensions service being developed by the NHS Pensions Agency. Such developments are likely to have a major impact on the human resource function of individual NHS trusts and health authorities. NHS Professionals was established as a special health authority on 1 April 2004 and is accountable for the effective management of the NHS temporary labour market.

Conclusions

There is pressure on the UK Government to implement the wider employment rights which are set out in the European Community's Charter of Fundamental Social Rights. It is likely therefore that over the next few years there will continue to be significant changes in the laws relating to employment as workers' rights are expanded across the European Community, and the remainder of the Government's White Paper *Fairness at Work* is implemented.

The now proactive role of ACAS in unfair dismissal cases has made it more likely that a dispute will be resolved internally and made it less likely that a case will go to the employment tribunal. The tighter laws on discrimination and in particular the Equality Act 2006, have still to be embedded within the NHS which still remains an organisation where racism and other blatant forms of discrimination abound. OTs are concerned with employment laws both for themselves and for their clients and the constant changes and new regulations present considerable challenges for them.

 Questions and exercises

1   What rights do part-time employees have?
2   Look at the letter setting out your contract conditions and identify the source of each term of employment, i.e. statutory, expressed as a result of personal agreement or as a result of collective bargaining. What terms would be implied?
3   There are very few men employed as OTs or OT assistants. What action do you consider your NHS trust or social services employer could take to encourage the recruitment of more men, without breaking the law on sex discrimination?
4   Consider the issues relating to finding employment or vocational training for your clients in the context of the laws preventing discrimination in employment and education.

References

1   *Johnstone v Bloomsbury Health Authority* [1991] ICR 269.
2   *R v Governors of X School* The Times Law Report 24 April 2009 QBD.
3   *R (Wright and Others) v Secretary of State for Health and Another* The Times Law Report 23 January 2009 HL.
4   *R (RJM) v Secretary of State for Work and Pensions* The Times Law Report 27 October 2008 HL.
5   *R (F) v Secretary of State for Justice; R (Thompson) v Secretary of State for the Home Department* The Times Law Report 23 January 2009 QBD.
6   *British Airways plc v Williams and Others* The Times Law Report 28 April 2009 CA.
7   *Ainsworth and others v Inland Revenue Commissioners* HL Times Law Report 15 June 2009.
8   *R v Secretary of State for Employment, ex parte Seymour-Smith and Perez* [1995] IRLR 464.
9   EEC Equal Treatment Directive 76/207: Articles 1(1), 2(1) and 5(1) 1976.
10 Unfair Dismissal and Statement of Reasons for Dismissal (Variation of Qualifying Period) Order 1999 SI 1999/1436.
11 www.acas.org.uk
12 Acas Helpline – 08457 47 47 47- open from 8am–8pm Monday to Friday and 9am–1pm on Saturdays.
13 www.bis.gov.uk (information is still available on the www.berr.gov.uk/employment site).
14 www.acas.org.uk/dgcode2009
15 Tynan Roger Will reform fuel workplace disputes The Times 26 March 2009.
16 ACAS (2009) Discipline and grievances at work – an Acas guide ACAS.
17 *Watling v Gloucestershire County Council Employment Tribunal*, EAT/868/94, 17 March 1995, 23 November 1994, Lexis transcript.
18 *Thomas v Hillingdon LBC*, The Times, 4 October 2002.
19 www.bis.gov.uk (information is still available on the www.berr.gov.uk/employment site).
20 *Von Goetz v St George's Hospital Employment Appeal Tribunal* EAT/1395/97 18 October 2001.
21 Department of Health (2004) *NHS Job Evaluation Handbook*. DH, London.
22 College of Occupational Therapists (2008) Agenda for Change OT job titles Briefing note no 106; Briefing note no 107: Job clustering; Briefing note no 109: Preceptorship for OTs; Briefing note no 110: Reviewing job descriptions; Briefing note no 114: how to challenge your outcome. COT, London.
23 National Audit Office NHS Pay Modernisation in England: Agenda for Change Report by the Comptroller and Auditor General HC 125 Session 2008–2009 (29 January 2009).
24 College of Occupational Therapists (2008) Knowledge and Skills Framework for OT staff in the NHS Briefing note no 108. COT, London.
25 www.bis.gov.uk (information is still available on the www.berr.gov.uk/employment site).
26 *Mayr v Backerel und Konditorei Gerhard Flockner OHG* The Times Law Report 12 March 2008 Case C-506/06.
27 Paragraphs 76–80, Part I, Schedule 4 of Employment Relations Act 1999.
28 Maternity and Parental Leave Regulations 1999 SI No. 3312.
29 Part II, Schedule 4, Employment Relations Act 1999.
30 www.bis.gov.uk (information is still available on the www.berr.gov.uk/employment site).
31 www.dwp.gov.uk/lifeevent/benefits/statutory_sick_pay.asp.
32 *Stringer and others v HM Revenue and Customs* Court of Justice of the European Communities Cases no C-520/06 and C-350/06 The Times Law Report 28 January 2009.
33 Secretary of State for Business, Enterprise and Regulatory Reform (2008) National Minimum Wage Low Pay Commission Report Cm 7333 Stationery Office.
34 www.lowpay.gov.uk/
35 Council Directive 93/104/EC; and Council Directive 94/33/EC.
36 *Broadcasting, Entertainment, Cinematographic and Theatre Union (BECTU) v Secretary of State for Trade and Industry*, Case C-173/99, Opinion of Advocate General.
37 Dimond, B. (1999) Working Time Regulations and the midwife. *British Journal of Midwifery*, **7**(4), 232–1.
38 Working Time (Amendment) Regulations 2002 SI 3128.
39 www.bis.gov.uk (information is still available on the www.berr.gov.uk/employment site).

40   www.nhsemployers.org/
41   *HM Revenue & Customs v Stringer and others* [2009] UKHL 31.
42   Kendall Deborah, Ahmed-Little Yasmin, Cousins Darren, Sunderland Howard, Johnston Mark and Najim Omar (2009) Achieving the 48 hour week for junior doctors. *British Journal of Healthcare Management*, **15**(3), 127–31.
43   NHS Employers (2007) Partnership Agreement DH.
44   *Marshall v Southampton and SW Hampshire AHA* [1986] 2 All ER 584.
45   *Enderby v Frenchay Health Authority and the Secretary of State for Health* [1991] IRLR 44.
46   *Enderby v Frenchay Health Authority and Health Secretary* (C-127/92) October 1993 ECJ Current Law (1994) 4813.
47   *Enderby v Frenchay HA and the Secretary of State for Health (No 2)* [2000] IRLR 257, CA.
48   *Suffolk Mental Health Partnership NHS Trust v Hurst and Others; Sandwell Metropolitan Borough Council v Arnold and Others* The Times Law Report 28 April 2009 CA.
49   Code of Practice on Equal Pay Order 2003 SI 2003/2865.
50   Directive 2006/54/EC.
51   The Sex Discrimination Act 1975 (Amendment) Regulations 2008 SI 656.
52   Directive 2002/73 (2002) OJ L269/16.
53   The Employment Equality (Religion or Belief) Regulations SI 2003/1660.
54   The Employment Equality (Sexual Orientation) Regulations SI 2003/1661.
55   Gledhill Ruth Victory for nurse suspended in prayer dispute The Times 7 February 2009.
56   Martin Wainwright Landmark ruling on homophobic taunts The Guardian 29 January 2005.
57   *English v Thomas Sanderson Ltd* The Times Law Report 5 January 2009 CA.
58   Employment Equality (Sex Discrimination) Regulations SI 2005/2467.
59   Council Directive 2000/78 ([2000] OJL303/16).
60   Employment Equality (Age) Regulations 2006 SI 2006/1031.
61   *Felix Palacios de la Villa v Cortefiel Servicios SA* ECJ [2007] 16 October Case C-411/05; [2008] All ER (EC) 249; The Times Law Report 23 October 2007.
62   *R (Incorporated Trustees of the National Council on Ageing (Age Concern England)) v Secretary of State for Business, Enterprise and Regulatory Reform* Case C-388/07 The Times Law Report 8 March 2009.
63   Frances Gibb Teenager wins age discrimination claim The Times 4 March 2008 page 27.
64   See Department for Education and Employment Code of Practice for the elimination of discrimination in the field of employment against disabled people or persons who have had a disability. Stationery Office, London.
65   DEE (1999) Disability Discrimination Act 1995: What employers need to know. Stationery Office, London.
66   *Archibold v Fife Council* Times Law Report, 5 July 2004, HL.
67   *Boyle v SCA Packaging Ltd, Equality and Human Rights Commission Intervening* The Times Law Report 6 July 2009 HL.
68   Disability Rights Commission (2005) The Duty to promote disability equality Stationery Office.
69   www.equalityhumanrights.com
70   *Paterson v Metropolitan Police Commissioner* [2007] All ER (D) 346 July.
71   *Gichura v Home Office* The Times Law Report 4 June 2008.
72   *McDougall v Richmond Adult Community College* The Times Law Report 22 February 2008.
73   NHS Employers (2009) Managing Diversity: making it core business Briefing note no 60.
74   www.nhsemployers
75   Council Directive 2000/78/EC of 27 November 2000.
76   Coleman (Social policy) [2008] EUECJ C-303/06.
77   Rehabilitation of Offenders Act 1974 (Exceptions) Order 1975 SI 1975/1023.
78   The Part-time Workers (Prevention of Less Favourable Treatment) Regulations 2000 SI 2000/1551.
79   Directive 97/81/EC Part-time Work Directive as extended to the UK by Directive 98/23/EC.
80   DoH. Public Interest Disclosure Act, HSC(99)198.
81   www.bis.gov.uk (information is still available on the www.berr.gov.uk/employment site).

82 Booth, J. (2000) Man who shopped boss wins £290 000. *The Times*, 11 July.

83 Bate, J. (2002) Whistle blowing doctor wins dismissal claim. *The Times*, 14 May, p. 5.

84 Bristol Royal Infirmary. *Learning from Bristol: the report of the public inquiry into children's heart surgery at the Bristol Royal Infirmary 1984–1995*. Command paper CM 5207.

85 DoH (2003) *Making Amends*. A consultation paper setting out proposals for reforming the approach to clinical negligence in the NHS. CMO.

86 Lister Sam Doctors set up whistleblower helpline as concerns grow for patient safety in NHS The Times 27 June 2009.

87 British Standard Institute (2008) PAS (i.e. Publicly available specification) 1998 *Whistleblowing Arrangements Code of Practice*. BSI, London.

88 www.bsigroup.co.uk.

89 Shipman Inquiry First Report Death Disguised published 19 July 2002; www.the-shipman-inquiry.org.uk/reports.asp; Shipman Inquiry Second Report The Police Investigation of March 1998 published 14 July 2003; www.the-shipman-inquiry.org.uk/reports.asp; Shipman Inquiry Third Report Death and Cremation Certification published 14 July 2003; www.the-shipman-inquiry.org.uk/reports.asp; Shipman Inquiry Fourth Report the Regulation of Controlled Drugs in the Community published 15 July 2004 Cm 6249 Stationery Office; www.the-shipman-inquiry.org.uk/reports.asp; The Shipman Inquiry Fifth report Safeguarding Patients: Lessons from the Past – Proposals for the Future. Command Paper CM 6394 December 2004 Stationery Office. Online. Available: www.the-shipman-inquiry.org.uk/reports.asp; The Shipman Inquiry Sixth Shipman: The Final Report January 2005 Stationery Office. Online. Available: www.the-shipman-inquiry.org.uk/reports.asp.

90 www.ind.homeoffice.gov.uk Helpline: 0845 010 6000.

91 List 99 is a list held by the Department for Education and Employment of those considered unsuitable to work with children. It has always been a statutory list.

92 Department of Health Press Notice, 2 October 2000.

93 Protection of Children and Vulnerable Adults and Care Standards Tribunal Regulations 2002 SI 2002/816; SI 2003/626.

94 HDG(97)37; LASSL (97)17 Guidance of Hospital Managers and local authority social services departments on the Sex Offenders Act 1997.

95 http://police.homeoffice.gov.uk/about-us/police-policy-operations/vettingandbarringscheme/.

96 http://police.homeoffice.gov.uk/operational-policing/bichard-implementation.

97 Department of Trade and Industry (1998) White Paper *Fairness at Work* CM 3968. Stationery Office, London.

98 www.berr.gov.uk/pressroom/Speeches/page46408.html

99 *Associated Society of Locomotive Engineers and Firemen (ASLEF) v The United Kingdom* 11002/05 [2007] ECHR 184 (27 February 2007).

100 Bennett Rosemary Wage bill spot checks to force bosses to pay women more The Times 24 April 2009.

101 DoH (2000) *The NHS Plan*. Stationery Office, London.

102 www.nhsprofessionals.nhs.uk/aboutnhspro/index.asp

103 NHS Executive (2001) HSC 2001/02 NHS Professionals Flexible organisations, Flexible staff. DoH, London.

20 Physical Disabilities

This chapter considers legal issues which mainly arise in the course of caring for those with physical disabilities, but there are, of course, many clients with multi-handicaps and who therefore also come under other client groupings (such as mental disorder (Chapter 21), learning disabilities (Chapter 22), children (Chapter 23) and older people (Chapter 24)) Reference should also be made to Chapters 3–9 which cover issues arising across all client groups. Of particular relevance to the care of those with physical disabilities are the laws on health and safety, especially manual handling (see Chapter 11); confidentiality (see Chapter 8); access to records (see Chapter 9); record keeping (see Chapter 12) and community care laws (see Chapter 18). Possible situations of negligence in relation to this group and in relation to equipment and adaptations are considered in Chapters 10 and 15 respectively; and complaints from this client group are discussed in Chapter 14.

A comprehensive textbook[1] on occupational therapy and physical dysfunction is edited by Turner and others. Occupational therapists should also find a book by Sally French and John Swain of assistance in understanding disability[2] and a Textbook of Rehabilitation Medicine by Michael Barnes and Anthony Ward.[3] The COT has published several works on vocational rehabilitation including a guide to current practice in the UK (2007).[4] It is important for the OT to be able to access information about the services and organisations available and works such as those published by the Disabled Living Centres and Independent Living Centre, and Michael Mandelstam's compilation on how to get equipment for disability[5] are invaluable. The Department of Health also publishes a practical guide for disabled people or carers, which provides information on services and equipment available.[6] The College of Occupational Therapy also publishes many guides to different aspects of the OT role including Occupational Therapy in vocational rehabilitation.[7]

The following topics are covered in this chapter:

Legal Aspects of Occupational Therapy, Third Edition By Bridgit Dimond
© 2010 Bridgit Dimond

- Guidance from the College of Occupational Therapists
- Chronically Sick and Disabled Persons Act and related legislation
- Social security provision for the disabled
- Accommodation
- Disabled Facilities Grants

- Education and training and employment facilities
- Inter-agency co-operation
- Use of volunteer agencies and other non-statutory bodies
- Limitations on resources and priority setting
- Role of the OT and the physically disabled

Guidance from the College of Occupational Therapists

The College of Occupational Therapists (COT) prepared a Standards, Policies and Proceedings (SPP) document on Services for Consumers with Physical Disabilities in 1995.[8] which has now been replaced by the professional standards and statements set out in initially in 2003 and revised in 2007.[9] They cover the following topics:

- referral
- consent
- assessment and goal planning
- intervention and evaluation
- discharge, closure or transfer of care
- record keeping
- service quality and governance
- professional development/lifelong learning
- practice placements
- safe working practice
- research ethics.

The *Professional standards for occupational therapy practice* are those expected by the professional body. They have been written to be attainable, with practice improvements if necessary. They are not considered to be minimum standards, but neither are they purely aspirational.

It should be noted, however, that these standards are not in themselves legally enforceable. They could, nevertheless, be used in evidence if negligence were alleged. They do not detract from the duty of each OT to use her professional discretion as to what and how services should be supplied to each client. The introduction points out that:

> However, in some circumstances, local organisations or services may have their own specific requirements to ensure the quality of service provision. In such a case, occupational therapists must, first and foremost, follow local policy. Where this differs significantly from these standards, the occupational therapist or occupational therapy service should attempt to uphold the principles of the particular professional standard and should seek advice.

The Chronically Sick and Disabled Persons Act 1970 and related legislation

The general duties placed upon local authorities in respect of the needs of disabled persons are set out in the Chronically Sick and Disabled Persons Act 1970. The principal duties are shown in Figure 20.1, with the detailed arrangements to be made shown in Figure 20.2. It should be noted that the

---

Figure 20.1   Duties under the Chronically Sick and Disabled Persons Act 1970 – section 1.

(1)   It shall be the duty of every local authority having functions under section 29 of the National Assistance Act 1948 to inform themselves of the number of persons to whom that section applies within their area and of the need for the making by the authority of arrangements under that section for such persons.

(2)   Every such local authority—

(a)   shall cause to be published from time to time at such times and in such manner as they consider appropriate general information as to the services provided under arrangements made by the authority under the said section 29 which are for the time being available in their area; and

(b)   shall ensure that any such person as aforesaid who uses any of those services is informed of any other *service provided by the authority (whether under any such arrangements or not)* which in the opinion of the authority is relevant to his needs *and of any service provided by any other authority or organisation which in the opinion of the authority is so relevant and of which particulars are in the authority's possession.*

[words in italics introduced by the 1986 Act.]

Figure 20.2   Arrangements which the LA has a duty to make – section 2.

(a)   the provisions of practical assistance for that person in his home;

(b)   the provision for that person of, or assistance to that person in obtaining, wireless, television, library or similar recreational facilities;

(c)   the provision for that person of lectures, games, outings or other recreational facilities outside his home or assistance to that person in taking advantage of educational facilities available to him;

(d)   the provision for that person of facilities for, or assistance in, travelling to and from his home for the purpose of participating in any services provided under arrangements made by the authority ... or in any services provided otherwise than as aforesaid which are similar to services which could be provided under such arrangements;

(e)   the provision of assistance for that person in arranging for the carrying out of any works of adaptation in his home or the provision of any additional facilities designed to secure his greater safety, comfort or convenience;

(f)   facilitating the taking of holidays by that person, whether at holiday homes or otherwise and whether provided under arrangements made by the authority or otherwise;

(g)   the provision of meals for that person in his home or elsewhere;

(h)   the provision for that person of, or assistance to that person in obtaining, a telephone and any special equipment necessary to enable him to use a telephone.

---

provisions apply to those suffering from mental disabilities as well as those with physical disabilities, but for convenience are dealt with here and not repeated in Chapters 21, 22 or 24.

Section 2 of the 1970 Act lists the provisions that the local authority has a duty to make in the following circumstances:

- The local authority has the functions under section 29 of the National Assistance Act (NAA) 1948.
- It is satisfied that the section applies to an individual.

- The person is ordinarily resident in its area.
- It is necessary, in order to meet the needs of that person, to make arrangements for all or any of the matters set out in Figure 20.2.

(The duties referred to in section 29 of the NAA are that the LA may make arrangements for promoting the welfare of persons over 18 who are blind, deaf, dumb, or who suffer from mental disorder, and other persons who are substantially and permanently handicapped by illness, injury or congenital deformity or such other disabilities.)

The right to enforce provision under section 2 was considered by the House of Lords in a case[10] where disabled persons applied for judicial review of the decision by Gloucester County Council to cut social services for the disabled (see the section on limitations on resources and priority setting later in this chapter).

In a case involving the closure of a day centre, J a person with learning disabilities applied for permission to seek judicial review of the action taken by the local authority alleging that he was ordinarily resident within the catchment area of the local authority and entitled to receive services under section 2 of the Chronic Sick and Disabled Persons Act 1970. It was also alleged that the closure was an infringement of article 8(2) of the European Convention on Human Rights. Permission to seek judicial review was granted on the grounds that J came within S 2 of the 1970 Act and the LA's approach to those for whom the service was a central part of their life was unnecessary or disproportionate or both.[11]

A novel way to avoid paying the accumulated fees in respect of a person's residential care after their death was attempted in vain in the following case.

Sandford and another v London Borough of Waltham Forest[12]

The claimants were executors of the deceased's estate. In an assessment of the deceased's home based needs, an occupational therapist recommended the provision of cot-sides for her bed. In April 2003 the deceased fell whilst getting out of bed and fractured her right femur. Following her recovery she was admitted to a nursing home where she died in October 2006. She was required to contribute to the fees for her accommodation. The claimants brought proceedings, claiming that the failure to fit cot-sides was a breach of the defendants statutory duty for which they could recover damages in respect of the costs of her accommodation in the nursing home and damages in respect of the pain, suffering and loss of amenity caused to the deceased by the injuries she had suffered as a result of her fall.

The claim failed. The authority had not owed the deceased a common law duty of care arising out of the statutory duty. The duty was not actionable at the suit of a private individual, and, in any event, in performing its duties, the authority had not voluntarily assumed any responsibility but was doing that which was required of it by statute. Further on the evidence the claimants had failed to make out that, on the balance of probabilities, if the cot-sides had been fitted then the deceased would not have suffered her injury.

It is inevitable, given the range of services required and the limited resources of local and health authorities, that services for individual patient groups will vary. Unfortunately, the scope of this book is not such as to enable a thorough review of the services provided for each individual patient group. The importance of occupational therapy intervention in wide-ranging physical conditions can also be seen from OTs' work in pain relief and pain management.[13] Reference could also be made to all the specialist groups who operate under the aegis of the College of Occupational Therapists, many of which have drafted guidance material for OTs working in those specialist areas.

Health and Social Care (Independent Living) Bill

A Health and Social Care (Independent Living) Bill was debated in Parliament but failed to be passed before the 2010 general election. If enacted the following provisions would have been introduced:

- each disabled person to make decisions about their own independent living arrangements by choosing whether allocated resources are provided in cash, services or a combination of both;
- advocacy to be provided where there are disputes between careers and disabled persons;
- new rights to ensure a disabled person is not placed in care against their wishes;
- amend the Mental Health Act 1983 to ensure independent living options are investigated before authorities decide to section or provide compulsory treatment;
- care homes will come within the definition of public authority for the purposes of the Human Rights Act 1998 (see Chapter 6 for the significance of this);
- the Care Standards Act 2000 is to be amended to ensure that disabled people in residential care have an individual living agreement;
- a duty would be placed on local housing authorities to provide disabled people with accessible and affordable homes.

Social security provision for the disabled

It is impossible to cover in detail the benefits available to those suffering from mental and physical disabilities; reference must be made to the publications of the Royal Association for Disability and Rehabilitation (RADAR) and others, included in the bibliography, which are updated on an annual basis. An excellent guide to the rights and benefits available is also provided by the *Disability Rights Handbook* (published by Disability Rights Group, London). This provides far more detail than can be given in this chapter. Information is also available from the direct government website.[14]

The OT should be careful to ensure that she knows the limitations of her knowledge in this very complex area that is constantly changing. She could be liable for giving negligent advice if clients relied on her advice to their financial loss. It is preferable for her to ensure that she knows how to guide the client to the best sources of advice available.

Accommodation

Local authorities have a duty to provide accommodation for those suffering from physical and mental disabilities under the provisions of the NAA 1948 and other legislation. Figure 20.3 sets out the basic provisions of section 21(1) of the 1948 Act as amended by the NHS and Community Care Act 1990.

Residential accommodation

Directions issued under the amended section 21[15] cover:

- Residential accommodation for persons aged 18 or over who by reason of age, illness, disability or any other circumstances are in need of care and attention not otherwise available to them.

Figure 20.3   National Assistance Act 1948 – section 21(1) (as amended).

[A] local authority may with the approval of the Secretary of State, and to such extent as he may direct, shall, make arrangements for providing—

(a)   residential accommodation for persons aged eighteen or over who by reason of age, *illness, disability*, or any other circumstances are in need of care and attention which is not otherwise available to them and

(aa) *residential accommodation for expectant and nursing mothers who are in need of care and attention which is not otherwise available to them.*

[words in italics added by 1990 Act.]

- Temporary accommodation for persons in urgent need where the need for that accommodation could not reasonably have been foreseen.
- Accommodation:
  - for persons who are or have been suffering from mental disorder, or
  - (to prevent mental disorder) for persons who are ordinarily resident in the LA area or have no settled residence.
- Accommodation in order to:
  - prevent illness
  - care for those suffering from illness
  - provide the after care for those so suffering.
- Arrangements specifically for persons who are alcoholic or drug-dependent.
- Residential accommodation for expectant and nursing mothers (of any age) who are in need of care and attention not otherwise available to them.

Services for residents

Further arrangements (in relation to persons provided with accommodation) cover all or any of the following purposes:

- the welfare of all such persons
- supervising the hygiene of the accommodation so provided
- enabling such persons to obtain:
  - medical attention
  - nursing attention
  - services provided by the NHS.

The LA is also required to review the accommodation and the arrangements. However, it is not required to provide any accommodation which is the duty of the NHS to provide.

Conveyance of residents and provision of accommodation

LAs may make such arrangements as they consider appropriate to provide for transport of residents to and from premises in which accommodation is provided. The statutory duties set out in the 1948

Figure 20.4   Provisions of the 1990 Act relating to accommodation and charging.

Section 42

Amends section 21 of the NAA 1948 in the definition of those for whom local authorities have a duty to provide accommodation and makes changes to the agency arrangements which LAs can make. Additional amendments are made in Schedule 9.

Amends section 30 of the NAA 1948 and extends the nature of the organisations with which the LA may make arrangements for accommodation to private sector and voluntary organisations.

Amends section 45(3) of the Health Services and Public Health Act 1968 and extends the organisations and persons with which the LA can make arrangements for promoting the welfare of old people.

Section 43

Amends section 26 of the NAA 1948, excluding certain persons (generally those who were already in homes on 31 March 1993) from the powers of local authorities to provide accommodation.

Section 44

Amends the provisions of section 22 of the NAA 1948 under which local authorities can charge for the accommodation provided.

Amends section 29 of the NAA 1948 under which arrangements can be made for the provision of hostel accommodation for those in receipt of welfare services.

Section 45

Amends sections 21, 22 23 and 24 of the Health and Social Services and Social Security Adjudication Act 1983 under which the local authority can recover sums due to it where persons in residential accommodation have disposed of assets and gives powers to the Secretary of State to make directions.

Act were amended by the NHS and Community Care Act 1990 to implement the recommendations of the Griffiths Report[16] and the White Paper.[17] The main changes brought about by the 1990 Act are shown in Figure 20.4.

The result of these changes is that, whilst the basic duties of the local authority to provide accommodation to specific categories of people have been slightly modified, the range of organisations with whom they can contract has increased.

In addition, since 1 April 1993 the purchasing of the accommodation for persons is the responsibility of the local social services authorities, who can recover fees from residents on a means tested basis, rather than the department of social security. Reference should also be made to Chapter 18 on community care. Details of how these provisions can be applied can be seen from the example of a case brought on assessment set out below; although this case is concerned with the needs of a person with learning disabilities, the principles apply to those with physical disabilities.

Case: *R v Avon County Council ex parte M*[18]

The applicant was 22 and suffered from Down's syndrome. By section 21 of the NAA 1948, the local authority was required to make arrangements for providing residential accommodation for him as a person who by reason of infirmity was in need of care and attention not otherwise available to him. In 1989 the local authority began an assessment of the applicant's needs. At first he lived in a training unit, where he remained. In 1991 he was offered a place at Milton Heights. He spent three weeks there, and he and his family were set on his going there. However, the local authority proposed various alternatives which were not acceptable. In January 1992 a review panel recommended that he should be placed at Milton Heights. The social services committee rejected the recommendation. In March 1992 the applicant commenced judicial review proceedings.

The judicial review proceedings were provisionally compromised on the basis that the local authority's social worker and the applicant's psychologist would prepare a joint assessment of the applicant's needs and the matter would be reconsidered by the review panel. This was done. In a decision in January 1993 the review panel found that the applicant had formed an entrenched wish to go to Milton Heights and recommended that he should be placed there. The social services committee declined to accept this recommendation and decided to place the applicant elsewhere. As a result the applicant revived his application for judicial review to challenge the local authority's decision.

The High Court held (quashing the local authority's decision):

1. Residential accommodation which the local authority was obliged to provide should be appropriate to the needs of the individual applicant – by virtue of section 47 of the NHS and Community Care Act 1990 (see Figure 18.4). The applicant's needs properly included his psychological needs and, in the present case, his entrenched wish to go to Milton Heights was not mere personal preference but part of his psychological needs.
2. The social services committee could not overrule the recommendation of the review panel without a substantial reason and without having given it the weight it required. The review panel had properly arrived at its decision on the evidence before it. The strength, coherence and apparent persuasiveness of that decision had to be addressed head on if it were to be set aside and not followed. Anybody required, at law, to give reasons for reconsidering and changing such a decision must have a good reason for doing so and must show that they had given the decision sufficient weight. The local social services committee had failed to do so and its decision must be quashed.

A dispute arose over the accommodation which should be provided to a disabled person arose in the following case.

R (on the application of A) v London Borough of Bromley[19]

A, a young man of 19 years, profoundly autistic with severe learning disabilities and petit mal epilepsy had been in a boarding school run by the Hesley group in Purbeck in Dorset. His time there had come to an end and all agreed that he needed a placement on a 52 week basis. His parents wished him to go to Hesley Village and College in Yorkshire but the LA disagreed and wished him to go to Robinia Care in Horndean. The LA also had suggested a home in Lee on Solent. Judge Crane found the decision making of the LA to be flawed: Hesley was ruled out as too expensive before any alternatives had been considered. He stated his role was not to substitute his decision for that of the LA, but to determine the lawfulness of the LA's actions and if he made a positive order to send the claimant to Hesley Village in Yorkshire the court would be substituting its decision for that of the LA. He therefore quashed the LA's decision and left his judgment to speak rather than grant declarations. Discussions then took place between the barristers and the judge in order to reach agreement over the immediate care of A whose condition would deteriorate unless he was immediately placed in the appropriate accommodation.

Health or social services responsibility?

A National Framework for NHS Continuing Healthcare was published in October 2007 which was designed to resolve the disputes over whether it was an NHS or social services duty to provide care (this is considered in Chapter 24).

Disabled facilities grants

Under section 1 of the Housing Grants, Construction and Regeneration Act 1996 grants are available for the provision of facilities for disabled persons in dwellings, and in the common parts of buildings containing one or more flats. These are known as disabled facility grants (DFGs). The application must be made in writing to the local housing authority and must contain: particulars of the works for which the grant is sought; two estimates from different contractors of the costs of carrying out the works (unless this is dispensed with); particulars of any preliminary or ancillary services and charges; and any other prescribed particulars. Either an owner's or tenant's certificate must accompany the application, containing the information specified in sections 21 and 22.

An application for a disabled facilities grant *must* be approved (subject to the stated conditions) if it is an application for the purposes set out in Figure 20.5.

Guidance is provided by the Department of the Environment.[20] However, the duty is subject to certain conditions which must be present and these are set out in Figure 20.6.

Even where the purpose of the grant does not come within those set out in Figure 20.5, a local housing authority *may* approve a disabled facility grant:

> for the purpose of making the dwelling or building suitable for the accommodation, welfare or employment of the disabled occupant in any other respect. (section 23(2))

This is also, however, subject to the conditions set out in Figure 20.6.

For the purposes of DFGs a person is disabled (section 100(1)) if:

(a) his sight, hearing or speech is substantially impaired
(b) he has a mental disorder or impairment of any kind, or
(c) he is physically substantially disabled by illness, injury, impairment present since birth, or otherwise.

Section 100(2) A person, aged 18 or over shall be taken for the purposes of the Part of the Act to be disabled if:

(a) he is registered in pursuance of any arrangements made under section 29(1) of the NAA 1948, (disabled persons' welfare) or
(b) he is a person whose welfare arrangements have been made under that provision or, in the opinion of the social services authority, might be made under it.

Section 100(3) A person under 18 years shall be taken for the purposes of the Part of the Act to be disabled if:

(a) he is registered in a register of disabled children maintained under paragraph 2 of Schedule 2 to the Children Act 1989, or
(b) he is in the opinion of the social services authority a disabled child as defined for the purposes of Part III of the Children Act 1989 (local authority support for children and their families).

The social services authority means the council which is the LA for the purposes of the Local Authority Social Services Act 1970 for the area in which the dwelling or building is situated (section

Figure 20.5 Section 23 Housing Grants, Construction and Housing Act 1996.

(1) The purposes for which an application for a disabled facilities grant must be approved, subject to the provisions of this chapter, are:

(a) facilitating access by the disabled occupant to and from the dwelling or the building in which the dwelling or, as the case may be, flat is situated;

(b) making the dwelling or building safe for the disabled occupant and other persons residing with him;

(c) facilitating access by the disabled occupant to a room used or usable as the principal family room;

(d) facilitating access by the disabled occupant to, or providing for the disabled occupant, a room used or usable for sleeping;

(e) facilitating access by the disabled occupant to, or providing for the disabled occupant, a room in which there is a lavatory, or facilitating the use by the disabled occupant of such a facility;

(f) facilitating access by the disabled occupant to, or providing for the disabled occupant, a room in which there is a bath or shower (or both), or facilitating the use by the disabled occupant of such a facility;

(g) facilitating access by the disabled occupant to, or providing for the disabled occupant, a room in which there is a wash hand basin, or facilitating the use by the disabled occupant of such a facility;

(h) facilitating the preparation and cooking of food by the disabled occupant;

(i) improving any heating system in the dwelling to meet the needs of the disabled occupant or, if there is no existing heating system in the dwelling or any such system is unsuitable for use by the disabled occupant, providing a heating system suitable to meet his needs;

(j) facilitating the use by the disabled occupant of a source of powers, light or heat by altering the position of one of more means of access to or control of that source or by providing additional means of control;

(k) facilitating access and movement by the disabled occupant around the dwelling in order to enable him to care for a person who is normally resident in the dwelling and is in need of such care;

(l) such other purposes as may be specified by order of the Secretary of State.

100(4)). The maximum amount of mandatory (for specified purposes) disabled facilities grant which a housing authority can be required to pay under the Housing Grants, Construction and Regeneration Act 1996 has been increased from £20 000 to £25 000 for dwellings and buildings in England.[21] However, where the cost of the eligible work is more than the grant limit, the council may use its discretionary powers under the Regulatory Reform (Housing Assistance)(England and Wales) Order 2002 to bridge the part or all of the gap between what they are required to pay and the full cost of the works. Social services can also provide community care equipment and minor adaptations which a person has been assessed to need and for which he is eligible, free of charge, provided the cost, including fittings, is less than £1,000.

For further information on disability facilities grants, see the works by Michael Mandelstam.[22] Further information on DFGs is available on the website for communities and local government[23] and a booklet has been published.[24] See also Housing and Children published by the Joseph Rowntree Foundation.[25]

It was held by the High Court in the case of *R v Birmingham City Council*[26] that financial resources are not relevant when a local authority is deciding whether to provide someone with a disabled

Figure 20.6 Conditions which must be present for a Disability Facilities Grant (section 24 Housing Grants, Construction and Regeneration Act 1996).

(3)   A local housing authority shall not approve an application for a disabled facilities grant unless they are satisfied:
   (a)   that the relevant works are necessary and appropriate to meet the needs of the disabled occupant; and
   (b)   that it is reasonable and practicable to carry out the relevant works, having regard to the age and condition of the dwelling or building;
   In considering the matters specified in paragraph (a) above, a local housing authority which is not itself a social services authority shall consult the welfare authority.
(4)   An authority proposing to approve an application for a disabled facilities grant shall consider:
   (a)   in the case of an application in respect of works to a dwelling, whether the dwelling is fit for human habitation;
   (b)   in the case of a common parts application, whether the building meets the requirements in section 604(2) of the Housing Act 1985;
(5)   A local housing authority shall not approve a common parts application for a disabled facilities grant unless they are satisfied that the applicant has a power or is under a duty to carry out the relevant works.

facilities grant under section 23(1) of the Housing, Grants, Construction and Regeneration Act 1996. The judge allowed an application for judicial review of a decision of Birmingham City Council which took account of financial resources when deciding whether to offer the applicant a disabled facilities grant. However entitlement to receive a disabled facilities grant is means tested, and this fact may dampen demand. The decision in the Birmingham case was considered together with the nature and ambit of section 23 of the 1996 in the following case:

Case: *B v Calderdale Metropolitan Council*[27]

The claimant was the father of four children, the eldest of whom, D, was autistic and thought to suffer from Asperger's syndrome. The family lived in a rented three-bedroom house in which D shared a bedroom with his brothers. D was uncontrollably aggressive towards S, frightening him while he slept and attacking him when they were in the bedroom together. The family wanted a grant to build an additional bedroom in which D could sleep on his own. The Council refused a grant and B's application was rejected in the High Court. The Court of Appeal allowed the appeal, quashing the decision to refuse a DFG and ordering the Council to reconsider the application in the light of the judgment of the Court. Lord Justice Sedley stated that whilst the additional bedroom would not completely remove the risk of harm to the brother, it would obviate the risk caused by their sharing a bedroom. He considered the facts fell within section 23(1)(b) of the 1996 Act (see Figure 20.5).

Disabled facility grants and OTs

These statutory provisions can give rise to many difficulties for OTs. Although the local housing authority should ensure that the welfare authority is consulted over the decision to give a grant, this is not always implemented. It may happen that applications go straight to the housing authority, which places them on a waiting list without first obtaining the advice and assessment of a registered OT.

It is inevitable that priorities have to be established to meet the demand for DFGs, and OTs may be encouraged to make an assessment in the light of the available resources rather than in the light of the needs of the disabled person. OTs must consider priorities in the light of the eligibility criteria published by the local authority and must ensure that they fulfil their professional responsibilities by identifying that any proposed adaptation is necessary and appropriate to meet the needs of the person with disabilities. It is essential that reference should be made to the guidance from the COT on carrying out assessments to ensure that professional standards of probity are maintained. The COT standards for practice in home assessment with hospital inpatients were published in September 2000.[28] (see Chapter 18). OTs involved in housing issues will find a book by Sylvia Clutton and others published in 2006 of value[29] in unravelling the maze of legislation and complexities in this field. See also the OT briefing note on housing in an ageing society.[30] See also a work on Occupational Therapists and housing.[31] The COT and the Housing Corporation have jointly published a book on securing minor adapations without delay.[32]

Other aspects of DFGs

Entitlement to receive a DFG is means tested, and this may limit demand. It should also be remembered that, in addition to its powers under section 1, the local housing authority has the power to make grants in respect of improvements and repairs under sections 7–18 of the Housing Grants, Construction and Regeneration Act 1996. These depend on the age of the property, its condition and the nature of the applicant's interest in the property. It is possible that where parents are separated, a dispute could arise between them over which house should be adapted to meet the disability needs of a child. The situation of a dispute between parents is considered in Chapter 23 on children.

Education and training and employment facilities

Duties are placed upon local authorities under the NAA 1948, the Chronically Sick and Disabled Persons Act 1970 and the Disabled Persons (Employment) Acts 1944 and 1958 (as amended by subsequent legislation) to provide education and training and employment facilities for those with physical and mental disabilities.

Sheltered employment for the seriously physically or mentally disabled must therefore be established by LAs and it is likely that the OT employed by the social services authority will be significantly involved both in the assessment of clients for this sheltered employment and in the management and choice of activities undertaken. The LA's duty extends to those disabled people who are ordinarily resident within its catchment area. The National Network of Assessment Centres[33] is a UK wide network of specialist services that work together to facilitate access for disabled people to education, training, employment and personal development. Assessment Centre Services include quality assessment and support in the use of assistive technology and/or specialised learning strategies. Students in higher education in the UK claiming the Disabled Students Allowance are often referred to an Assessment Centre for DSA-funded Study Aids and Strategies Assessment on behalf of higher education students.

OTs also have a role in the planning of such facilities and in bringing to the attention of the social services authority deficiencies and shortcomings in the arrangements. The COT published *Work matters: vocational navigation for OT staff* in 2007[34] and a *Vocational Rehabilitation strategy* in 2008.

Duty of care and the local authority

In Chapter 22 a case is discussed where it was held that the local authority owed a duty of care towards a husband and wife with learning disabilities who were being victimised and assaulted by a gang of youths.[35] The Court of Appeal allowed the appeal by the defendant holding that no duty of care was owed.[36]

Inter-agency co-operation

Local authorities have a statutory duty to co-operate with other statutory authorities and the voluntary sector in the provision of services (section 26 of the Health Act 1999 (see Chapter 17)). There is a statutory duty under section 72 of the NHS Act 2006 for NHS bodies to co-operate with each other in exercising their functions and under section 82 for NHS Trusts and local authorities to co-operate with one another in order to secure and advance the health and welfare of the people of England and Wales. Under the NHS and Community Care Act 1990 local authorities also have the responsibility of preparing and each year revising a community care plan, in conjunction with health authorities and voluntary agencies, setting out the provision for those receiving community care services (see Chapter 18). In practical terms the cooperation between health staff and LA staff is vital to the interests of the client and its lack can cause the OT considerable problems. The establishment of care trusts should, in theory, ensure greater co-ordination in the planning and provision of services across the NHS/social services divide.

Use of volunteer agencies and other non-statutory bodies

LAs are increasingly using non-direct labour for the provision of services and entering into contracts with other organisations, usually of a non-profit making kind, to provide the services which the LA has a statutory duty to ensure exist. Such arrangements can create complex issues relating to responsibility and accountability, as can be seen from Chapter 15 on equipment issues. It is advisable for the OT who may have to deal with complaints about the services provided by these non-statutory organisations to have sight of the agreements drawn up with the LA in order to be certain of the terms on which their services are given and to be aware of which duties are enforceable. The use of such organisations and agencies does not, however, remove the statutory responsibility from the LA to ensure that the services are available. The same principles apply to health services and the use of volunteers and voluntary or charitable organisations within the NHS.

Limitations on resources and priority setting

In 1995 certain disabled people in Gloucestershire challenged, by judicial review, the decision by Gloucestershire County Council to reduce or withdraw certain welfare assistance provided to them under section 2 of the Chronically Sick and Disabled Persons Act 1970. The court had to decide the issue of resources and statutory duties.

Case: *R v Gloucester County Council, ex parte Barry and ex parte Mahfood*[37]

Disabled persons complained when services were curtailed following withdrawal of a government grant upon which the County Council's plans had been based and the Council gave greater priority to the more seriously disabled. The Council had not reassessed in the light of the cut-backs but had simply sent out a standard letter withdrawing services.

The Queen's Bench Division at first instance held that an LA was right to take account of resources both when assessing needs and when deciding whether it was necessary to make arrangements to meet those needs:

> A balancing exercise had to be carried out assessing the particular needs of that person in the context of the needs of others and the resources available but, if no reasonable authority could conclude other than that some practical help was necessary, that would have to be its decision. Furthermore, once it had decided that it was necessary to make the arrangements, it was under an absolute duty to make them. That was a duty owed to a specific individual and not a target duty. No term was to be implied that the LA was obliged to comply with the duty only if it had the revenue to do so. Once under that duty resources did not come into it.

It was acknowledged that an LA faced an impossible task unless it could have regard to the size of the cake of resources so that it could know how fairest and best to cut it. However, the failure of Gloucester County Council to reassess once the cuts became known amounted to treating the cut in resources as the sole factor to be taken into account and that was unlawful.

Mr Barry took the case to the Court of Appeal,[38] which allowed the appeal and held:

> A local authority was not entitled to take into account the availability or otherwise of resources when carrying out its duty under section 2 of the 1970 Act in assessing the needs of any disabled person for those services. However, where a local authority had identified such needs of a disabled person, resources might be relevant in considering how the needs might be met.

Once Gloucestershire CC had identified Mr Barry's need for cleaning and laundry service, the manner in which that need was met, for example by someone doing his laundry at home in a washing machine or by it being taken away, was within the discretion of the authority and costs would be a relevant consideration. Any reassessment of the disabled person's needs could not be based solely on the absence of resources to meet the person's needs.

Leave was given for an appeal to be made to the House of Lords,[39] where the appeal was upheld in a majority decision.

Case (cont): Decision of the House of Lords in the *Gloucester* case

> For the purposes of section 2(1) of the 1970 Act a chronically sick and disabled person's needs were to be assessed in the context of, and by reference to, the provision of certain types of assistance for promoting the welfare of disabled persons using eligibility criteria decided upon by a local authority as to whether the disability of a particular person dictated a need for assistance and, if so, at what level. Those criteria had to be set taking into account current acceptable standards of living, the nature and extent of disability and the relative cost balanced against the relative benefit and the relative need for that benefit. In deciding how much weight was to be attached to the cost of providing the benefit, the authority had to make an evaluation about the impact which the cost would have on its resources, which in turn would depend on the authority's financial position. It followed that a chronically sick or disabled person's need for services could not sensibly be assessed without having some regard to the cost of providing them, since his need for a particular type or level of service could not be provided in a vacuum from which all considerations of cost were expelled.'

Comment on *Gloucester* case

It is to be noted that this case related to section 2 of the Chronically Sick and Disabled Persons Act 1970. The ruling would not necessarily apply to other community care assessments under section

47(1) of the NHS and Community Care Act 1990. Reference should be made to Chapter 18 on community care for the statutory duties placed upon the local and health authorities under the 1990 Act.

The final outcome of the *Gloucester* case, though disappointing for the disabled and chronic sick, is a sensible one for local authorities (and in fact represents Department of Health policy since 1970) in that resources are relevant to both the assessment and the provision of services under the 1970 Act. This does not mean that authorities can take decisions on the basis of resources alone; the authority must still take into account all other relevant factors. Pressure on resources cannot be used as an excuse for taking arbitrary or unreasonable decisions.[40] Failure to provide services can be challenged under the complaints and representation procedures of the local authority. It is essential, therefore, that all those involved in the assessment and allocation of resources have clear documentation of the decisions which have been made and the factors which have been taken into account in making those decisions. Failure to assess priorities in a reasonable way according to reasonable standards of professional practice could be grounds for complaint by a client.

The House of Lords ruling in the Gloucester case was applied in *R v E Sussex CC ex p Tandy*,[41] which is considered in Chapter 23. In the following case the High Court held that it was lawful for the local authority to charge for services provided under the Chronic Sick and Disabled Persons Act 1970.

Case: *R v Powys County Council ex parte Hambridge*[42]

> The applicant who was disabled received care services provided by the local authority for which she paid £10 per week. She applied for judicial review arguing that the LA had not power to demand payment for services provided under the 1990 Act. Her application was dismissed. S 17 of the Health and Social Services and Social Security Adjudications Act 1983 enabled a local authority to charge for services provided under S 29 of the National Assistance Act 1948. The Local authority was not providing services under section 2 of the 1990 Act; they were making arrangements under the 1948 NA Act for the provision of their services. The charges for welfare services was lawful.

At the same time as the Gloucester case, the court heard an application by Mr McMillan[43] for judicial review of the decision of Islington Borough Council not to provide him with home help cover, when his carers were ill or away. This application failed on the grounds that the Council had conducted a proper balancing exercise taking into account resources and the comparative needs of the disabled in its area. The court held that the Council was not in breach of the duty which it owed to the applicant.

The Gloucester case was followed in a case[44] involving adaptions and aids for two severely disabled children of 17 and 13. The LA asked for details of the parents' means. The parents said they could not afford to pay for the alterations but refused to provide information about their means and sought judicial review of the authority's action. The High Court held that the authority was entitled to take into account the parents' financial resources when deciding whether or not to provide and pay for alterations. The claimants appealed, arguing that section 2 of the 1970 Act created a free-standing duty on the authority to provide services without any right to charge. The Court of Appeal dismissed the appeal holding that the local authority could charge for the provision of services provided under S 2 of the 1970 Act and section 17 of the Children Act 1989 and could reasonably expect that parents who could afford the expense, would make any alterations to their home, that were necessary for the care of their disabled children. The LA was entitled to decline to provide services to meet the needs of disabled children until it was demonstrated that having regard to their means, it was not reasonable to expect their parents to provide them.

In the case of *R (on the application of Hefferman) v Sheffield City Council*,[45] the claimant, who suffered from Still's disease and was almost totally blind and had both hips and knees replaced, argued that the amount he was paid to enable him to obtain care was insufficient and that he required 27–30 hours per week as opposed to the 24 ½ provided. The court held that it could not be said that the allocation of care was perverse. It was not at all generous but it did not have to be: it had to be adequate to meet the proper needs. The claimant's condition was deteriorating and there had to be regular reviews of his care, but such a reconsideration would not inevitably result in more hours of care.

In 2005 the Department of Health published a Green paper on Independence, Well-being and Choice[46] which placed considerable emphasis on users of social care and LA services having individual budgets to buy in the care services they require. This is considered in Chapter 18. Reference should also be made to Chapter 24 and the care of the elderly.

Priority setting in hospital care

Similar problems exist in determining priorities in hospital care, where OTs might find that they cannot see all patients referred to their care and some patients may be discharged before the OT can arrange a home assessment.

Situation: no pre-discharge assessment

Nora, an OT, is attached to the orthopaedic department. She is very short staffed and has advised her manager that she is not able to arrange pre-discharge visits for all the patients. Before she can assess one patient, she discovers that the doctor has discharged the patient assuming that the patient was able to manage at home. She subsequently hears that the patient has been severely hurt in a fall at home. Who, if anyone, is liable? Would it make any difference if Nora had assessed the patient and recommended that discharge should be delayed, but the doctor decided to discharge the patient immediately because of a shortage of beds?

An OT must make decisions on priorities on a reasonable basis according to the Bolam test (see Chapter 10), which means that she must have adequate information on which to prioritise. If harm occurs to a patient who is being cared for in hospital, the argument that there is a lack of resources will not be a defence when there is negligence. Reasonable standards of care must be provided. The OT should ensure that her senior manager is aware of the situation. Clinical governance and quality standards (see Chapter 17) should ensure that action is taken to provide a reasonable standard of care to patients, including the provision of OT services. The responsibility for discharging a patient contrary to OT advice is that of the doctor. The OT must ensure that her records clearly show evidence of her assessment and her recommendations and that these were drawn to the attention of those having clinical responsibility for discharge. She should still, if possible, follow up the patient in the community to ensure that the appropriate equipment is made available or contact her colleagues in social services so that they can provide a service to the patient.

Where there is a serious OT shortage or inadequate resources to provide a full OT service, it may have to be accepted that the OT will not be able to see all patients referred to the service and will have to decide according to agreed criteria those patients who have priority. The clinical consequences of such a situation would have to be discussed at the highest level of management.

Scope of professional practice of the OT and the physically disabled

The opportunities for constructive intervention in the care of the physically disabled and others with short-term disabilities are extensive and varied and continuously developing. For example, Gill Carlill, Elizabeth Gash and Glenis Hawkins[47] discuss the role of OTs in A&E in preventing unnecessary admissions. Following an audit the OT service in A&E was made available 7 days a week between 11.00 and 19.00 hours with extended hours from 08.00 to 19.00 on three days when two OTs worked. Such work is an exciting development in the expanded role of the OT, and the principles considered in Chapter 10 in relation to the standard of care need to be followed. Where an OT takes on responsibilities which might have been carried out by another health professional, she must ensure that there is no lowering in the standard of care provided.

Conclusions

It is not possible in a book of this kind to consider every possible type of physical disability and the legal implications of each. Emphasis has to be placed on the general principles. The Disability Discrimination Act 1995 (see Chapter 18) has already led to considerable improvements in the quality of life and environments of those with physical disabilities but much still needs to be done. In 1992 the National Audit Office[48] reported on health services for physically disabled people aged 16 to 64 and concluded that more action needed to be taken to provide more rehabilitation services generally and in particular the treatment of incontinence and prevention of pressure sores. Specific recommendations were made for health authorities to ensure that rehabilitation services were provided to meet identified needs, including services for brain damaged people. Gaps in the provision of respite care should be identified and action taken to fill them. In addition, there should be improvements in the timeliness, quality and availability of information on services provided for physically disabled people. The picture however does not seem to have improved greatly since 1992. A CSCI report on the state of social care in England 2006–7[49] describes a gloomy picture of the social care for the elderly and disabled. This is discussed in Chapter 24. Occupational therapists have a key role to play in identifying the gaps in service provision and in ensuring that the appropriate services are provided and monitored. In spite of the legislative changes and the recognition of the rights of those with disabilities many challenges still remain.

 Questions and exercises

1   A client suffering from multiple sclerosis who lives on her own complains to you that her home help visits have been reduced to three a week. What advice do you give her and what action do you take?

2   Your assessment of the physical needs of a person suffering from arthritis is overruled by the disability officer (who is not a registered OT), who decides that your recommendations for specific adaptations in the home need not be carried out. What is the legal situation if the client is subsequently harmed as a result of a failure to provide her with the necessary equipment and adaptations?

3   Draw up a protocol which identifies the role and function of the occupational therapy assistant in the care of those suffering from physical impairment.

References

1   Turner, A., Foster, M. & Johnson, S.E. (2002) *Occupational Therapy and Physical Dysfunction: Principles, Skills and Practice*, 5th edn. Churchill Livingstone, Edinburgh.

2   French Sally and Swain John (2008) *Understanding Disability*. Churchill Livingstone/Elsevier, Edinburgh.

3   Barnes Michael P and Ward Anthony B (2000) *Textbook of Rehabilitation Medicine*. Oxford University Press, Oxford.

4   College of Occupational Therapy (2007) *Occupational Therapy in Vocational Rehabilitation*. COT, London.

5   Mandelstam, M. (1993) *How to Get Equipment for Disability*, 3rd edn. Jessica Kingsley Publishers for the Disabled Living Foundation.

6   DoH (2003) *A Practical Guide for Disabled People or Carers*; www.doh.gov.uk/disabledguide/index.htm

7   Tim Barnes, Jain Holmes and College of Occupational Therapists (2007) *Occupational Therapy in Vocational Rehabilitation*. COT, London.

8   College of Occupational Therapists (1995) *Statement on Occupational Therapy Services for Consumers with Physical Disabilities*, SPP 105B. COT, London.

9   College of Occupational Therapists (2007) *Professional Standards*. COT, London.

10 *R v Gloucester County Council, ex parte Barry* [1997] 2 All ER 1 HL; (QBD) Times Law Report, 21 June 1995; (CA) Times Law Report, 12 July 1996.

11 *R (on the application of Jones) v Southend-on-Sea BC* [2005] EWHC 1439 (admin), (2007)10 C.C.L. Rep 428.

12 *Sandford and another v London Borough of Waltham Forest* [2008] EWHC 1106 (QB).

13 Contact: Input, St Thomas's Hospital, London, 0171 922 8107 (Jackie Adams) or The Old Police Station, High Street, Newnham, Gloucester, 01594 516450 (Pat O'Hara) for information on the OT and pain management. See also Dimond, B. (2002) *Legal Aspects of Pain Management*. Quay Books, Dinton, Wiltshire.

14 www.direct.gov.uk/en/DisabledPeople/FinancialSupport/index.htm

15 LAC(93)10 (consolidating).

16 Sir Roy Griffiths (1988) *Community Care: Agenda for Action*. HMSO, London.

17 Secretary of State for Health (1989) *Caring for People: Community care in the next decade and beyond*. Cm 849. HMSO, London.

18 *R v Avon County Council, ex parte M* [1994] 2 FLR 1006.

19 *R (on the application of A) v London Borough of Bromley* [2004] EWHC 2108 (Admin).

20 Department of the Environment 17/96 Disabled Facilities Grants; SI 1996/2888; Disabled Facilities Grants and Home Repair Assistance (Maximum Amounts) Order 1996.

21 Disabled Facilities Grants and Home Repair Assistance (Maximum Amounts) (Amendment No 2) (England) Order 2001 SI 2001/4036.

22 Mandelstam, M. (1997) *Equipment for Older or Disabled People and the Law*. Jessica Kingsley Publishers, London.

23 www.communities.gov.uk/publications/housing/disabledfacilitiesgrant/

24 Department for Communities and Local Government and Welsh Assembly Government (2007) *Disabled Facilities Grants*. Stationery Office, London.

25 Beresford Bryony and Rhodes Dave (2008) *Housing and Disabled Children*. Joseph Rowntree Foundation, York.

26 *R v Birmingham City Council, ex parte Mohammed* [1998] 3 All ER 788; The Times Law Report, 14 July 1998.

27 *B v Calderdale Metropolitan Council* [2004] EWCA Civ 134.

28 College of Occupational Therapists (2000) *Standards for Practice: Home assessment with hospital in-patients*. COT, London.

29 Clutton Sylvia, Grisbrooke Jani and Pengelly Sue (2006) *Occupational Therapy in Housing: Building on firm foundations*. Whurr, London.

30 College of Occupational Therapists (2008) National Strategy for housing in an ageing society Briefing note no 103. COT, London.

31 Clutton Sylvia, Grisbrook Jane and Sue Pengelly (2006) *Occupational Therapy in Housing: Building on firm foundations*. Whurr, London.

32 College of Occupational Therapists and Housing Corporation (2006) *Minor adaptations without delay*. COT and Housing Corporation, London.

33 www.nnac.org/

34 College of Occupational Therapists (2007) *Work Matters: vocational navigation for OT staff*. COT and National Social Inclusion Programme, London.

35 *X and Y v London Borough of Hounslow* [2008] EWHC 1168 (QB) 23 June 2008.

36 *X and Y v London Borough of Hounslow* [2009] EWCA Civ 286.

37 *R v Gloucester County Council, ex parte Mahfood et al.* (QBD) Times Law Report, 21 June 1995; (1995) 30 BMLR 20.

38 *R v Gloucester County Council, ex parte Barry* (CA) Times Law Report, 12 July 1996; [1996] 4 All ER 421.

39 *R v Gloucester County Council, ex parte Barry* [1997] 2 All ER 1 HL.

40 LASSL(97)13 Responsibilities of Local Authority Social Services Departments: Implications of recent legal judgments.

41 *R v E Sussex CC ex p Tandy* (1995) 95 LGR 745.

42 *R v Powys County Council ex parte Hambridge* [1998] 1 FLR 643; 7 October 1997.

43 *R v Gloucestershire County Council* [1997] AC 584 HL [1997] 2 All ER 1.

44 *R (on the application of Spink and another) v Wandsworth London Borough Council* [2005] EWCA Civ 302.

45 *R (on the application of Hefferman) v Sheffield City Council* [2004] All ER (D) 158 June.

46 Department of Health (2005) *Green Paper; Independence, Well-being and Choice*. DH, London.

47 Carlill, G., Gash, E. & Hawkins, G. (2002) Preventing unnecessary hospital admissions: an occupational therapy and social work service in an accident and emergency department. *British Journal of Occupational Therapy*, **65**(10), 440–46.

48 National Audit Office (1992) *Report on Health Services for Physically Disabled People aged 16 to 64*. HMSO, London. See also NAHAT Briefing Summary, September 1992.

49 Commission for Social Care Inspection (2008) *The state of social care in England 2006–7*. CSCI.

21 Mental Disorder

This chapter covers the legal issues arising in the care of the mentally ill. The issues arising in the care of those with learning disabilities are considered in Chapter 22, and of older people in Chapter 24.[1] The intention is to deal with some of the more common dilemmas faced by OTs in the care and treatment of the mentally ill. Figures will provide a summary of some of the main points of the Mental Health Act 1983 as amended by the Mental Health Act 2007. This Act as amended is the main legislation covering the detention of the mentally disordered and for the most part replaces the Act of 1959 which by the end of the 1970s was seen as failing to protect the rights of the mentally disordered.

The following topics are covered in this chapter:

- Informal patients
- The Mental Health Act 1983
- Definition of mental disorder
- Holding power
- Compulsory admission
- Role of the nearest relative
- Role of the approved mental health professional
- Informing the patient
- Informing the relative
- Provisions for the mentally disordered offenders
- Consent to treatment provisions
- Long-term detentions
- Role of OT

- Physical illness
- Short-term detention and informal patients
- Community Provisions
- Guardianship
- Section 17
- Section 117 after care
- Supervised community treatment
- Mental Health Review Tribunal
- Mental Health Managers
- Care Quality Commission (replacing the Mental Health Act Commission)
- Mentally ill and the European Convention of Human Rights
- National Service Frameworks

Legal Aspects of Occupational Therapy, Third Edition By Bridgit Dimond
© 2010 Bridgit Dimond

Emphasis will be placed on those areas where the OT can have a significant input into the legal process; for example, the provision of advice to a second opinion appointed doctor, the provision of a report for a mental health tribunal or managers' hearing, or for the renewal of a section. Reference should be made to the Department of Health's Code of Practice on the Mental Health Act which was revised in 2008[2] guidance on the new Code was provided by the Mental Health Act Commission in October 2008.[3] The MHAC was incorporated into the Care Quality Commission in April 2009 and the guidance can be downloaded from the CQC website. A useful textbook on occupational therapy and mental health is edited by Jennifer Creek.[4] Chapter 8 on record keeping, by Mary Booth, gives guidance on the content of patient records which OTs working in this field should keep, and the requirements of record keeping under the care programme approach, the supervision register and after care under section 117. In Chapter 9 of the same book, Sarah Cook and Penny Spreadbury outline the implications of clinical governance and clinical audit on mental health services. Chapter 11 by Ian E. Thompson considers ethics and looks at issues relating to the client's rights to privacy, and the client's right to know and to receive care and treatment. Unfortunately there is no comparable chapter on the legal rights of the client in mental health care, nor is there any chapter on mental health law. An overview of the appraisal and implementation process of clinical guidelines within mental health services is considered by Edward Duncan and colleagues[5] and they urge for quality research to underpin the development of guidelines which can be used as the basis of clinical interventions. Jennifer Creek and Lesley Lougher have edited a textbook on occupational therapy and mental health[6] and a handbook on mental health is available edited by Catherine Jackson and Kathryn Hill.[7] A book on women in secure units is edited by Nikki Jeffcote,[8] a book on evidence in mental health by C Lond[9] and advance OT in mental health by Elizabeth McKay and colleagues[10] See also the publication by the Mental Health Act Commission on Women detained in Hospitals.[11]

The College of Occupational Therapists has published Standards for Practice in forensic residential settings[12] (see later in this chapter) and a research and development vision and action plan for forensic occupational therapy (2000). OTs may well be working with many support staff in the field of mental health and the COT has published a briefing note in the light of the NSF on Mental Health which recommended Support, Time and Recovery Workers in mental health.[13] This discusses the role and management of such workers and their pay, education and training. The COT published a 10 year strategy for Occupational Therapy in Mental health covering the years 2007–2017 in 2006.[14] At the same time it published a literary review and the results from service user and carer focus groups.

Informal patients

The vast majority (well over 90%) of patients who are cared for in psychiatric hospitals are not detained. They have either given consent to admission or, if they lack the mental capacity to consent to admission, they were being treated by common law powers recognised by the House of Lords in the *Re F* case[15] (see Chapter 7), which have now been replaced by the Mental Capacity Act 2005. The House of Lords in the *Bournewood*[16] case considered the question of whether a mentally incapacitated person, incapable of giving consent to admission, could be held at common law in a psychiatric hospital and not placed under the Mental Health Act 1983. It decided that section 131 of the Mental Health Act 1983 did not require a mentally ill person to have the capacity to consent to admission as an informal patient.

Case: lack of capacity to consent to admission: the Bournewood case

An adult with learning disabilities was informally admitted to a mental health unit. He was not detained under the Mental Health Act 1983. His carers asked for his discharge but his psychiatrist considered that it was not in his best interests to be discharged and that he should remain in hospital. The carers challenged the legality of this decision. They lost in the High Court, but the Court of Appeal held that section 131 of the Mental Health Act required a person to have the mental capacity to agree to admission; a person lacking the requisite capacity should be examined for compulsory admission under the Act. The House of Lords upheld the appeal of the NHS trust, holding that an adult lacking mental capacity could be cared for and detained in a psychiatric hospital, using common law powers.

Grave concern was expressed in the House of Lords at the absence of statutory protection for such patients and the Department of Health stated that the legislative provisions were being reviewed. Such revision was necessary to ensure compliance with the Human Rights Act 1998 (see Chapter 1). Article 5 of the European Convention of Human Rights which is set out in Schedule 1 in the Human Rights Act 1998 states:

(1) Everyone has the right to liberty and security of person. No one shall be deprived of his liberty save in the following cases and in accordance with a procedure prescribed by law.

Included in the 'following cases' under (e) are 'persons of unsound mind'.

An application was then made to the European Court of Human Rights which held that on the facts of the Bournewood case there was a breach of Article 5 of the Convention (see Appendix 1) The UK Government was therefore required to ensure the legislative changes necessary to provide protection for those people lacking the mental capacity to agree to admission. Safeguards which are known as the Bournewood Safeguards or Deprivation of Liberty Safeguards were enacted by means of amendments to the Mental Capacity Act 2005. They are considered in detail in Chapter 22.

Other rights of the informal patient

As well as being entitled to the rights as set out in the Articles of the European Convention on Human Rights, a patient who has mental health difficulties may also come under the provisions of the Chronic Sick and Disabled Persons legislation and may also be entitled to community care assessments and provisions under the NHS and Community Care Act 1990. The care programme approach ensures that each person with mental health needs is assessed and the appropriate services made available for him or her. The Chronic Sick and Disabled Persons Act 1970 and subsequent provisions are considered in Chapter 20.

Mental Health Act 1983 as amended by the 2007 Act

As stated above, only about 10% of psychiatric patients are at any one time detained under the Mental Health legislation. The next section gives an account of the main statutory provisions which apply to the detention and treatment of such patients. The 1983 Act was amended by the Mental Health Act 2007, but the changes are less radical than those originally envisaged in the Report of the Expert Committee chaired by Professor Richardson. Its terms of reference included the degree to which the current legislation needed updating and to ensure that there was a proper balance between safety (both of individuals and the wider community) and the rights of individual patients.

It was required to advise the Government on how mental health legislation should be shaped to reflect contemporary patterns of care and treatment and to support its policy as set out in *Modernising Mental Health Services*.[17] The Expert Committee presented its preliminary proposals, which set out the principles on which any future legislation should be based, in April 1999 and its full report was published in November 1999.[18] The Government presented its proposals for reform in 1999 with a final date for response by 31 March 2000.[19] Subsequently significant debates took place in Parliament but eventually new legislation replacing the 1983 Act was abandoned and the 1983 Act was amended to incorporate changes enacted by the 2007 Act.

Julie Carr provided an analysis of the proposed reforms of the Mental Health Act 1983 for the occupational therapist.[20] She concluded that:

> occupational therapists will need to reflect upon how the philosophy of empowerment held at the core of their interventions will balance with a legal framework based in compulsion.

This is a concern which is shared across many health professionals.

Principles to be included in the Code of Practice

The guiding principles that the consultation paper suggested should be contained in a new Mental Health Act are set out in Figure 21.1. Other principles, recommended by the Review Committee and which the Government considered should be included in a Code of Practice on the new Act, were:

- non-discrimination
- patient autonomy
- consensual care
- reciprocity
- respect for diversity
- equality
- respect for carers
- effective communication
- provision of information
- evidence-based practice.

Figure 21.1 Guiding principles recommended by Review Committee to be included in a new Mental Health Act.

- Informal care and treatment should always be considered before recourse to compulsory powers
- Patients should be involved as far as possible in the process of developing and reviewing their own care and treatment plans
- The safety of both the individual patient and the public are of key importance in determining the question of whether compulsory powers should be imposed
- Where compulsory powers are used, care and treatment should be located in the least restrictive setting consistent with the patient's best interests and safety and the safety of the public

> **Figure 21.2**   Statement of Fundamental Principles in Code of Practice to cover following matters.
>
> (a)   respect for patients' past and present wishes and feelings,
> (b)   respect for diversity generally including, in particular, diversity of religion, culture and sexual orientation (within the meaning of section 35 of the Equality Act 2006),
> (c)   minimising restrictions on liberty,
> (d)   involvement of patients in planning, developing and delivering care and treatment appropriate to them,
> (e)   avoidance of unlawful discrimination,
> (f)   effectiveness of treatment,
> (g)   views of carers and other interested parties,
> (h)   patient wellbeing and safety, and
> (i)   public safety.

Ultimately the Mental Health Act 2007 required the Secretary of State to include in the Code of Practice a statement of principles which included reference to the matters set out in Figure 21.2. A much reduced list than those contained in the Review Report. The Secretary of State is also required to have regard to the desirability of ensuring:

(a)   the efficient use of resources, and
(b)   the equitable distribution of services.

The Mental Health Act 2007 requires those referred to in section 118(1)(a) and (b) of the 1983 Act to have regard to the Code in performing their functions under the Act. These include registered medical practitioners, managers and staff of hospitals and mental nursing homes, approved mental health professionals and members of other professions in relation to the medical treatment of patients suffering from mental disorder.

Children may be detained under the provisions of the Mental Health Act, but there are different time limits over the application to mental health review tribunals. Concern was expressed in a report *Out of the Shadows* published by the charity Young Minds in 2008 which found that only 15% of health trusts have complied with the Government's commitment that all young people would be treated in special units, and not with adults by November 2008. Half of the trusts make no special provision for the children detained on adult wards. The Children's Commissioner for England published an account of young people's experience of adult mental health facilities in 2007.[21]

Definition of mental disorder

No person can be compulsorily detained under the Mental Health Act 1983 unless they are suffering from mental disorder as defined in the Act. The definition as amended by the 2007 Act is as follows:

'mental disorder' means any disorder or disability of the mind;
and
'mentally disordered' shall be construed accordingly;".
A person with learning disability shall not be considered by reason of that disability to be—

(a)   suffering from mental disorder for the purposes of the provisions mentioned in subsection (2B) below; or
(b)   requiring treatment in hospital for mental disorder for the purposes of sections 17E and 50 to 53 below,

unless that disability is associated with abnormally aggressive or seriously irresponsible conduct on his part. Learning disability is defined as: a state of arrested or incomplete development of the mind which includes significant impairment of intelligence and social functioning.

The 1983 Act stated that a person could not be dealt with under the Act as suffering from mental disorder 'by reason only of promiscuity or other immoral conduct, sexual deviancy or dependence on alcohol or drugs'. However this was replaced by the 2007 Act with the words:

dependence on alcohol or drugs is not considered to be a disorder or disability of the mind for the purposes of the definition of mental disorder.

This means that if a patient is abusing drugs he cannot be detained under the Mental Health Act 1983 unless he is shown to be suffering from mental disorder apart from the drug abuse.

The holding power

Situation: The holding power of the nurse

Harold Graves, an informal patient admitted to a psychiatric hospital three weeks ago, is attending the industrial therapy department which is managed by Gill Evans, an occupational therapist, when he becomes very aggressive and starts abusing an occupational therapy assistant.

Since Gill Evans is not a nurse or a doctor she does not have any statutory powers to detain Harold. In the past she would have been able to use common law powers to restrain him so that help could be summoned. Common law powers have been replaced by the Mental Capacity Act 2005 for those who lack the mental capacity to make decisions and action must be taken in their best interests. Restraint can be used in the circumstances described in Chapter 7. Gill also has the powers of the citizen to effect an arrest on the limited occasions set out in the Police and Criminal Evidence Act. If she feared for the life of Harold were he to be allowed to leave hospital immediately, or for the life of anyone else, she could legally prevent his leaving the industrial therapy unit in an emergency. Since Harold is an in-patient, a nurse who is qualified in mental health care and therefore recognised for the purposes of section 5(4) of the Mental Health Act could detain Harold.

Figure 21.3 sets out the main points of the holding power of the nurse laid down by section 5(4) of the Act. The only nurses designated as prescribed nurses under the Act are those who are registered nurses with an entry in the register indicating that the nurse's field of practice is either mental health nursing, or learning disabilities nursing.[22]

Figure 21.3   The holding power: Mental Health Act 1983 section 5(4).

(1)   The patient is receiving treatment for mental disorder
(2)   The patient is an in-patient
(3)   It appears to the prescribed nurse that the patient is suffering from mental disorder to such a degree that it is necessary for his health or safety or for the protection of others for him to be immediately restrained from leaving the hospital
(4)   It is not practicable to secure the immediate attendance of a practitioner who could exercise the powers under section 5(2)

If all the requirements set out in Figure 21.3 are present, then a prescribed nurse has the power to detain Harold for up to six hours. As soon as the appropriate medical practitioner or approved clinician arrives, however, the holding power will cease. The nurse must fill in the appropriate forms and ensure that these are taken to the managers of the hospital immediately. Procedures vary; in some hospitals it is the practice for the hospital manager to be on call for such purposes; in others this duty is delegated to the nurse manager on duty at night and weekends. If the doctor or approved clinician arrives and decides that Harold should be detained under section 5(2) then whatever part of the holding power has elapsed before his arrival will become part of the 72 hours' detention. Unlike section 5(4), section 5(2) can be used for any in-patient, even one admitted for a physical disorder. Section 5(4), in contrast, can only be used when the patient is being treated for mental disorder.

If the appropriate doctor or approved clinician is not able to arrive within the six hours, it is essential for the doctor or approved clinician to exercise his powers of nomination under section 5(3) so that another medical practitioner or approved clinician can act as nominee and see Harold at the earliest possibility.

In this situation it is stated that Harold is an in-patient and therefore Harold is attending the industrial therapy unit in his capacity as an in-patient. If Harold were not an in-patient, then he could not be detained under either sections 5(4) or 5(2) and in an emergency situation professionals would have to consider section 4 if only one doctor could be obtained, or section 2 (see Table 21.1).

Compulsory admission

There are three main sections for the compulsory admission of the mentally disordered person other than through the courts: sections 3, 2 and 4. (For the admission of the mentally disordered offender see later in the chapter. Section 37 is the main section for detention by the courts and this can be linked with a restriction order under section 41.) These are shown in full in Table 21.1, which sets out the section numbers and requirements for each section that enables compulsory admission to take place, and the maximum length of detention (unless there is a renewal). The requirements in relation to the two medical recommendations are set out in Figure 21.4. Mutual recognition of section 12 approved status has been agreed between England and Wales.[23] Regulations relating to the documents which must be kept and providing further details of the statutory provisions were replaced in 2008.[24]

Renewal

Section 4, section 2, section 5(4) or section 5(2) are not renewable. A patient on section 2 who needs to be detained for longer can be further detained on section 3. Section 3 can be renewed for a further six months and then for one year at a time. The procedure for the renewal is that the responsible clinician in charge of the patient's care examines the patient, within the period of two months ending with the date the section is due to end and, if it appears to him that the specific condition of mental disorder is present and the other conditions required by section 20 are present, he must furnish to the managers a report to that effect, and the patient's detention is then renewed. The managers in their review can decide that the patient should be discharged. An OT may be asked by the responsible clinician about the possibility of a section being renewed. She should be able to justify her opinion with evidence and should record the discussion in her documentation.

Table 21.1 Compulsory admission provisions.

Section	Duration (up to)	Applicant	Medical requirements	Other requirements
4 Emergency admission for assessment	72 hours	Approved mental health professional or nearest relative	1 Recommendation only stating that patient is suffering from mental disorder and stating the provisions of section 2 exist (see below)	Applicant must have personally seen patient within 24 hours before the application. Admission must be of urgent necessity
2 Admission for assessment	28 days	Approved mental health professional or nearest relative	2 Medical recommendations (a) patient is suffering from mental disorder of a nature or degree which warrants detention in hospital for assessment and (b) he/she ought to be so detained in the interests of his/her own health or safety or with a view to the protection of others and (c) appropriate medical treatment is available	Applicant must personally have seen patient within the period of 14 days ending with the date of the application
3 Admission for treatment	6 months, renewable for a further 6 months, then for a period of 1 year	Approved mental health professional or nearest relative	2 Medical recommendations that: (a) The patient is suffering from mental disorder (b) deleted (c) It is necessary for the health or safety of the patient or for the protection of others that he should receive such treatment, and it cannot be provided unless he is detained under this section and (d) appropriate medical treatment is available for him	As above under section 2. Approved mental health professional must consult with nearest relative before making an application unless this would not be reasonably practicable or would involve unreasonable delay. The application cannot be made if the nearest relative objects

continued

Table 21.1 Continued

Section	Duration (up to)	Applicant	Medical requirements	Other requirements
37 Hospital order without restrictions	6 months, renewable for a further 6 months, then for a period of 1 year	Order can be made by Crown Court in case of person convicted of an offence punishable by imprisonment or by magistrates (a) if convicted of offence punishable on summary conviction with imprisonment or (b) if person is suffering from mental illness or severe mental impairment and magistrates are satisfied that he committed the crime	2 Doctors required to give oral or written evidence that (a) offender is suffering from mental disorder of a degree which makes it appropriate for him/her to be detained for medical treatment and (b) the court is of the opinion, having regard to all the circumstances, that the most suitable method of disposing of the case is by means of a hospital order	
41 Restriction order (imposed in conjunction with hospital order section 37)	For a specified period or without limit of time	Crown Court which has made a hospital order can impose a restriction order. Magistrates Court cannot make a restriction order but can send offender over 14 to Crown Court for a restriction to be made	As for section 37; at least one of the two doctors must give evidence orally before the court.	

The Approved Clinician

The 2007 Act enables other professional groups to have powers which were formally restricted to the responsible medical officer. Directions[25] which have been issued on the requirements for becoming an approved clinician are that the person:

(a) fulfils at least one of the professional requirements (a registered medical practitioner; a Registered psychologist; a first level nurse with the inclusion of an entry indicating their field of practice is mental health or learning disabilities nursing; an occupational therapist; a social worker)

Figure 21.4   Requirements for the two medical recommendation.

(1)   Practitioners must have personally examined the patient either together or separately, but where they have examined the patient separately not more than 5 days must have elapsed between the days on which the separate examinations took place.

(2)   One of the medical recommendations must be from a practitioner approved by the Secretary of State for such purposes as having experience in the diagnosis or treatment of mental disorder and unless that practitioner has previous acquaintance with the patient, the other practitioner should have, if practicable.

(2A)   A registered medical practitioner who is an approved clinician shall be treated as also approved for the purposes of this section under subsection (2) above as having special experience as mentioned there (added by 2007 Act).

(3)   One (but not more than one) of the medical recommendations should be given by a practitioner on the staff of the hospital to which the patient is to be admitted.

(4)   Point (3) above does not apply, i.e. both medical recommendations can be given by staff of the hospital in question, if
   (a)   compliance with (3) above would result in delay involving serious risk to the health and safety of the patient; and
   (b)   one of the practitioners works at the hospital for less than half of the time which he is bound by contract to devote to work in the health service; and
   (c)   where one of the practitioners is a consultant, the other does not work in a grade in which he is under that consultant's directives.

(5)   A medical recommendation cannot be given by
   (a)   the applicant;
   (b)   a partner of the applicant or of a practitioner by whom another medical recommendation is given for admission;
   (c)   a person employed as an assistant by the applicant or by any such practitioner;
   (d)   a person who receives or has an interest in the receipt of any payments made on account of the maintenance of the patient;
   (e)   except as set out in (3) and (4) above a practitioner on the staff of the hospital to which the patient is admitted or by specified relatives of the other practitioner giving the medical recommendation.

(6)   A general practitioner who is employed part-time in a hospital shall not be regarded as a practitioner on its staff.

These provisions also apply to the two medical recommendations for guardianship.

(b)   possesses the relevant competencies (set out in Schedule 2 of the Directions) and
(c)   has:
   (i)   completed a course for the initial training of approved clinicians within the previous two years or
   (ii)   been approved, or been treated as approved, to act as an approved clinician in England or Wales within the previous five years

Role of the nearest relative

The nearest relative has an important role to play and has to be given specific information. The definition of nearest relative and the hierarchy is given in Figure 21.5. This figure also illustrates the powers of the nearest relative.

Figure 21.5　Definition and powers of the nearest relative.

Definition: the highest in the following hierarchy, section 26(i):

- relative who ordinarily resides with or cares for the patient
- husband or wife or civil partner
- son or daughter
- father or mother
- brother or sister
- grandparent
- grandchild
- uncle or aunt
- nephew or niece

Preference is given in relatives of the same description to the whole blood relation over the half-blood relation and the elder or eldest regardless of sex. Husband and wife include a person who is living with the patient as the patient's husband or wife and has been so living for not less than six months. A person other than a relative with whom the patient ordinarily resides for a period of not less than 5 years shall be treated as if he were a relative. However, such a person is at the bottom of the above hierarchy.

Power of nearest relative

(1)　To apply for the admission of the patient for assessment, for assessment in an emergency, for treatment and for guardianship.

(2)　To be informed about the approved mental health professional's application to admit the patient for assessment.

(3)　To be consulted about the approved mental health professional's proposed application for treatment and to object to it.

(4)　To be given information about the details of the patient's detention, consent to treatment, rights to apply for discharge, etc. (but subject to the patient's right to object to this information being given).

(5)　To discharge the patient after giving 72 hours' notice in writing to the managers.

(6)　To apply to a Mental Health Review Tribunal under sections 16, 25 and 29.

Role of the approved mental health professional

Table 21.2 sets out the main tasks of the approved mental health professional who, as a result of the changes of the 2007 Act, replaces the approved social worker. Only health professionals who have completed the specified training can be recognised as approved for the purposes of the Act.[26] Whilst the Act allows the nearest relative to be an applicant for compulsory admission under sections 2, 3, 4, and 7, in practice the applicant will usually be the approved mental health professional and this is the preferred procedure.

Informing the patient

The task of explaining his legal rights to the patient once a detention order has been imposed may fall upon the OT (see Figure 21.6), who must ensure that she is conversant with the conditions of the different sections and can explain these to the patient by word of mouth as well as handing out the appropriate leaflet. If the patient is too ill to understand what is being said, this fact should be

Table 21.2   Role of the approved mental health professional and of any social worker.

Duty	Details
Duties of the approved mental health professional	
Section 11 (3)	
Inform nearest relative of admission of patient and of nearest relative's right to discharge	1. In admission for assessment (sections 2 and 4) 2. Before or within a reasonable time after an application for admission for assessment is made 3. Such steps as are practicable to inform the person appearing to be the nearest relative
Section 11 (4)	
Consult nearest relative on admission for treatment or guardianship and discontinue application if nearest relative notifies objection	1. Consultation with person appearing to be the nearest relative of the patient 2. Unless it appears that in the circumstances such consultation is not reasonably practicable or would involve unreasonable delay
Section 13 (1)	
To apply for admission or guardianship order if satisfied application ought to be made and is of the opinion that it is necessary or proper for application to be made by him	1. In respect of patient within the area of local social services authority by whom he is appointed 2. Must have regard to wishes expressed by relatives of patient or any other relevant circumstances that are necessary or proper for application to be made by him
Section 13 (2)	
To interview patient in suitable manner and satisfy himself that detention in a hospital is in all the circumstances of the case the most appropriate way of providing the care and medical treatment of which the patient stands in need	1. Before making application for admission to hospital
Section 13 (4)	
To take patient's case into consideration with a view to making an application for admission. If decides *not* to make an application he will inform the nearest relative in writing of his reasons	1. If nearest relative requires local social services authority of area in which patient resides, authority must direct approved mental health professional as soon as practicable
Duties of any social worker	
Section 14	
To provide report on social circumstances	1. Where patient admitted to hospital an application by nearest relative other than section 4 2. Managers must as soon as practicable give notice of that fact to local social services authority for area in which patient resided immediately before his admission

continued

Table 21.1   Continued

Duty	Details
Duties of any social worker Section 117 Duty of district health authority and of local social services authority to provide after-care services	1. Applies to patients detained under section 3 or admitted under hospital order (section 37) or transferred under transfer direction (sections 47 or 48) who cease to be detailed and leave hospital 2. Authorities must co-operate with relevant voluntary agencies 3. After-care services to be provided until such time as the authorities are satisfied that the person concerned is no longer in need of such services (they shall not be so satisfied if the person is subject to after-care under supervision)

Figure 21.6   Informing the patient: Mental Health Act 1983 section 132.

The managers of the hospital in which a patient is detained under the Act must:

(1) Take such steps as are practicable to ensure the patient understands:
   (a)   under which provisions of the Act he is for the time being detained and the effect of that provision; and
   (b)   what rights of applying to a Mental Health Review Tribunal are available to him in respect of his detention under that provision;
   (c)   the effect of certain provisions of the Mental Health Act including the consent to treatment provisions, the role of the Mental Health Act Commission (now the CQC) and other provisions relating to the protection of the patient.
(2) The steps to inform the patient must be taken as soon as practicable after the commencement of the patient's detention under the provision in question.
(3) The requisite information must be given to the patient in writing and also by word of mouth.

recorded and an attempt made later to give the information to the patient. The leaflets have been translated into many different languages and an interpreter should be used to assist in the provision of the information by word of mouth.

Informing the relatives

Where the patient is too disturbed to take in the information, the statutory duty to inform the nearest relative assumes even greater importance. Section 132(4) requires the managers to furnish the person appearing to them to be the patient's nearest relative with a copy of any information given to the patient, in writing, under the duty outlined above. The steps for this must be taken when the information is given to the patient or within a reasonable time thereafter. The patient has the right of veto and can request that this information is not given.

Provisions for mentally disordered offenders

In addition to section 37 (and 41) (see Table 21.1) the courts can order the patient to be detained for specific purposes:

- Section 35 – remand for 28 days (renewable) for reports
- Section 36 – remand for 28 days (renewable) for treatment
- Section 38 – interim hospital order up to twelve weeks (renewable)
- Section 47 – transfer direction for those under sentence
- Section 48 – transfer direction for other prisoners

The College of Occupational Therapists has published Standards for Practice in forensic residential settings.[27] This guide contains seven standards with the evidence of criteria to be met, which can be audited on a regular basis. The standards cover:

- safe and therapeutic environment
- framework for practice
- assessment
- intervention
- evaluation
- transfer and discharge
- accommodating the legal status of the patient.

Consent to treatment provisions

See Figures 21.7 and 21.8.

Long-term detained patients

Under the provision of Part IV of the Mental Health Act 1983, those patients who are detained under long-term detention provisions (e.g. sections 2, 3, 37 and 41) can in certain circumstances be given compulsory treatment. For these patients the Act covers all possible treatments for mental disorder, both in emergency and nonemergency situations. The provisions are set out in Figures 21.7 and 21.8. Treatment is defined in the amended Act:

> 'Medical treatment' includes 'nursing, psychological intervention and specialist mental heath habilitation, rehabilitation and care (section 145(1)). Any reference to medical treatment, in relation to mental disorder shall be construed as a reference to medical treatment the purpose of which is to alleviate, or prevent a worsening of the disorder or one or more of the symptoms or manifestations. (S.145(3)).

It has been held[28] that preliminary care given to enable the treatment for mental disorder to be given was within the original definition and so covered by section 63. Thus a detained patient who was anorexic could be given tube-feeding, even though that was not the treatment that justified admission under section 3. The Court of Appeal held that compulsory feeding by tube came under section 63.

Figure 21.7   Consent to treatment: Mental Health Act 1983 sections 57, 58 and 63.

(1)   Treatments involving brain surgery or hormonal implants can only be given with the patient's consent, which must be certified, and only after independent certification of the consent and of the fact that the treatment should proceed (section 57).

(2)   Treatments involving electroconvulsive therapy, or medication where 3 months or more have elapsed since medication was first given during that period of detention, can only be given either (a) with the consent of the patient and it is certified by the patient's own registered medical practitioner or another registered medical practitioner appointed specifically for that purpose that he is capable of understanding its nature, purpose and likely effects, or (b) the registered medical practitioner appointed specifically certifies that the patient has refused or is incapable of consenting but agrees that the treatment should proceed (section 58). Subject to 58A

(3)   **S. 58A ECT and other specified treatments**
A person shall not be given such treatments unless he or she falls within certain specified conditions:
These conditions include

1.   where the patient is at least 18 years, has consented to the treatment and his capacity to consent has been certified by the approved clinician in charge of it or by the appointed registered medical practitioner

2.   The patient is below 18 years, has consented to the treatment and an appointed registered medical practitioner (not being the approved clinician in charge of the treatment) has certified in writing the patient's capacity to consent and that it is appropriate for the treatment to be given or

3.   an appointed registered medical practitioner (not being the responsible clinician/ approved clinician in charge of the treatment) has certified in writing:
   a.   that the patient is not capable of understanding the nature, purpose and likely effects of the treatment; but
   b.   that it is appropriate for the treatment to be given and
   c.   that giving him the treatment would not conflict with:
      i.   an advance decision which the registered medical practitioner concerned is satisfied is valid and applicable or
      ii.   a decision made by a donee or deputy or by the Court of Protection.

Before a certificate is given in circumstances 3, the appointed registered medical practitioner must consult two person who have been professional concerned with the patient's medical treatment, one must be a nurse and the other neither nurse nor a registered medical practitioner. In addition neither shall be the responsible clinician (if there is one) or the approved clinician in charge of the treatment in question.

(4)   All other treatments: these can be given without the consent of the patient provided they are for mental disorder and are given by or under the direction of the responsible medical officer (section 63).

Seclusion

There is no provision in the Mental Health Act 1983 in relation to seclusion, but the Code of Practice of the Mental Health Act Commission has given guidance on the use and monitoring of seclusion. The House of Lords[29] reviewed the policy on seclusion at Ashworth Hospital which had been developed at variance from the Code of Practice. It held that the Code of Practice is guidance and not law and that all hospitals should observe the Code unless they had good reason for departing from it

Figure 21.8   Consent to treatment: urgent treatments.

Urgent treatments can be given according to the degree of urgency and whether they are irreversible or hazardous:

a	Any treatment	which is immediately necessary	to save the patient's life
b	Treatment which is not irreversible	if it is immediately necessary	to prevent serious deterioration
c	Treatment which is not irreversible or hazardous	if it is immediately necessary	to alleviate serious suffering
d	Treatment which is not irreversible or hazardous	if it is immediately necessary and represents the minimum interference necessary	to prevent the patient from behaving violently or being a danger to himself or others

Irreversible is defined as 'if it has unfavourable irreversible physical or psychological consequences' and hazardous is defined as 'if it entails significant physical hazard'.

As a result of changes by the 2007 Act, ECT cannot be given under a or b, and other specified treatment cannot be given under any subsection of a to d if so specified in the directions.

in an individual case. Unjustifiable failure to follow the guidance in the code could mean that seclusion was in breach of Article 3, Article 5 and/or Article 8 of the European Convention of Human Rights. However on the particular facts before it, the House of Lords held, in a majority judgment that it was lawful for Ashworth to have developed its own seclusion policy at variance to the Code and that there was no breach of articles 3, 5 or 8.

Role of the occupational therapist

What is the role of the OT in consent to treatment provisions? Under the provisions of sections 57 and 58, the independent registered medical practitioner, in determining whether the treatment should proceed, must consult with a nurse and another professional who have been professionally concerned with the patient's medical treatment. An occupational therapist may be called upon as that second professional, to provide an opinion. The independent doctor must record the fact that he has consulted these two persons. Interestingly, however, there is no requirement on the form that he should actually record their opinions, so it could well happen that both the nurse and the other professional counselled against certain medication but the doctor still recommended it. A disagreement is unusual but it is advisable for the OT, whether there is agreement or not with her views, to ensure that the advice she gave is recorded clearly and comprehensively.

Situation: consulting an OT

Brian Evans, an older severely depressed man, was admitted to hospital under section 3 and the responsible medical officer decided that ECT would be beneficial for him. Brian refused to give consent for ECT and a second opinion appointed doctor (SOAD) was requested as required under section 58. It was clear that the SOAD would not be able to see Brian for two days and section 62 was used to give Brian the first treatment.

The SOAD consulted Brian's named nurse over the treatment and then asked for the name of another professional whom he could consult who was neither nurse nor doctor. It was suggested that Meryl Jenkins, an occupational therapist, should talk to the SOAD. Meryl, however, had only met Brian once shortly after his admission, when he was too disturbed to communicate with her and was reluctant to provide any opinion to the SOAD. What is the law?

Clearly the OT cannot provide an opinion of a patient with whom she has had barely any contact. She should inquire whether there is any other health professional who has been concerned in Brian's treatment who would have more information than she had, possibly a clinical psychologist or social worker. If there is no such person, then she could ask to be given time to interview Brian so that she can give an informed opinion to the SOAD. As a consequence of the amendments introduced by the Mental Health Act 2007 in adding a new section 58A (see Figure 21.7), ECT cannot be forced upon a patient who has the mental capacity to refuse to give consent. Where a patient is incapable of giving consent to ECT, then the independent doctor must decide that it is appropriate for the treatment to be given. He or she must also check that there is no valid advance decision under which the patient is refusing ECT.

Unfortunately, pressure is sometimes placed on OTs to provide a speedy opinion, when they have had very little or even no contact with the patient. After the OT has been consulted by the SOAD she should ensure that she records information relating to the consultation in her records of the patient. The COT has published a briefing on occupational therapy staff involved in the second opinion process under the Mental Health Act 1983.[30] It advises that the interview with the SOAD gives the OT the opportunity to advise on:

- the nature of her contact with the client
- a description of the client's history and mental state as seen by the OT
- the impact of OT interventions on the progress of treatment
- her professional opinion of the proposed medical interventions, on the basis of her knowledge of the client and the client's response to treatment.

In providing advice to the SOAD, the OT should remember that she is a member of a mental health team which should share concerns about the patient's treatment. In law the team has no legal entity, each individual takes personal and professional responsibility for what she does or advises (see Chapter 10). A guide to current practices for community mental health teams is provided by Tom Burns.[31]

Physical illness

These provisions on consent to treatment for mental disorder would thus appear to cover all eventualities concerning the long-term detained patient. However, there is a gap in relation to treatment for physical illness. Sections 57, 58, 58A and 63 only apply to the treatment of mental disorder. Where a patient detained under the Act refuses treatment for a physical illness, then Part IV of the Act does not cover the situation and the Mental Capacity Act 2005 would apply where the patient lacked the requisite mental capacity to give consent. This would mean that treatment could be given to a person who lacks the mental capacity to give consent, provided that it was given in the best interests of the patient and in the absence of any advance decision by which such treatment was refused. The common law power to act out of necessity in the best interests of the patient was replaced by the powers and duties set out in the Mental Capacity Act 2005 which only apply when the patient lacks the capacity to give a valid consent. In the case of *Re C* (discussed in Chapter 7 under 'Determination of competence') a Broadmoor patient's refusal to have an amputation was upheld by the court. The court held that he had the mental capacity to be able to refuse an amputation. This right of the mental capacitated adult to refuse even life saving treatment is now underwritten by the Mental Capacity Act 2005.

Courts have in the past interpreted 'treatment for mental disorder' in a wide way. Thus, in the case of *B v Croydon Health Authority*, the Court of Appeal held that compulsory feeding by tube came under section 63.[32] There have also been several cases where a pregnant woman detained under the Mental Health Act 1983 has been compelled to undergo a caesarean section under section 63 of the Act.[33] This has been overruled by the Court of Appeal in *Re MB*[34] (see Chapter 7 under 'Determination of competence'). It is clear that if a detained patient, suffering from mental disorder, has the mental capacity to understand the proposed treatment and the implications of his or her refusal, then the court would not order the treatment to proceed unless it could clearly be seen to be treatment for the mental disorder and therefore comes within section 63. If, however, the patient lacks the mental capacity to refuse treatment in his or her best interests, treatment for physical conditions could lawfully be given in his best interests under the provisions of the Mental Capacity Act 2005. There are considerable advantages in securing a declaration of the court that it is lawful to provide the treatment. The Court of Appeal has recently ruled that where a patient is detained under the Mental Health Act 1983, he can only be treated for the specified form of mental disorder for which he was detained.[35] In the actual case, the patient had been detained under section 37/41 and the specified form of mental disorder was mental illness. He could not therefore be compulsorily treated under section 63 for a personality disorder in a ward for those suffering from personality disorder. As a result of the changes to the Mental Health Act 1983 by the Act of 2007 there are no separate specified forms of mental disorder.

Multiple disabilities

Patients who are detained under Mental Health legislation may have physical disabilities which gives rise to additional issues as the following situation illustrates.

Situation: Equipment needs in a forensic setting

Mary a patient in a High Secure Psychiatric Hospital requires a physical functional assessment and the OT, Ted Jones is asked to provide one. One of his conclusions is that equipment must be prescribed. Ted prepares a care plan and writes a risk assessment on the correct use of the equipment. The equipment is provided to the unit through 2 sources: the on-site medical centre but more usually through the short loans department of the local social services. Ted is concerned about who is liable for the maintenance and servicing of this equipment especially if the patient is not on the OT caseload.

It would be the responsibility of Ted as the prescriber of the equipment to ensure that issues relating to the responsibility for monitoring and maintenance of the equipment and the relevant time scales were identified when the equipment was first issued. Any failure on his part to ensure that there was a safe system of equipment issue, installation and maintenance which resulted in harm could lead to the vicarious liability of the NHS Trust (see Chapter 15 on equipment).

Short-term detained patients and informal patients

Short-term detained patients and informal patients are not covered by the Part IV treatment provisions of the Mental Health Act. There is only one exception to this: informal patients are specifically covered by the provisions of section 57 relating to brain surgery and hormonal implants, and by the relevant provisions of sections 62, 59 and 60. The basic principles of consent, discussed in Chapter 7, apply to the short-term detained patients and informal patients; if they have the necessary mental capacity, they can refuse even life-saving treatment for a good reason, a bad reason or no reason at all; if they lack the necessary mental capacity then treatment out of necessity can be given to them in their best interests in accordance with the Mental Capacity Act 2005.

A useful insight into the making of informed choices in the context of mental health services and the Mental Capacity Act 2005 is provided by Tish O'Brien and Katrina Bannigan.[36] The importance of empowering the individual to make his or her own decisions in occupational therapy practice is emphasised. See Chapter 7 and the principles set down under the Mental Capacity Act.

Community provisions

The philosophy behind the Mental Health Act 1983 is that a patient should only be compulsorily detained in hospital if informal admission is not an option and if alternative services in the community cannot be provided. There are very few community provisions in the 1983 Act except for section 7 guardianship, section 17 leave, section 117 after care and after care under supervision. The 2007 Act repealed the Mental Health (Patients in the Community) Act 1995 and the concept of after-care under supervision or supervised discharge, and introduced a community treatment order. This is discussed below. The occupational therapist has a significant role to play in multi-disciplinary planning and care and should ensure that her involvement is weighty and meaningful. She should also ensure that her input and the team's decisions are recorded. She has an important role in ensuring the involvement of the patient in after care planning and discussing with him long-term plans for rehabilitation, employment and accommodation. She should also refer to the standards set by the National Service Framework for Mental Health, which are referred to later in this chapter.

Guardianship

Situation

David has been under a guardianship order for three months. He lives with his mother, the guardian, and attends a day centre three times each week, where he receives occupational therapy. One day he decides that he does not wish to attend the day centre. His mother pleads with him but is unable to persuade him to go. She informs the OT that he will not be attending. What action can the OT take?

There are three statutory powers in relation to guardianship and these are set out in Figure 21.9.

In the situation above, in theory the OT could ask for David to be brought to the day centre since this is a condition of his guardianship. However, this is unlikely to be a practical suggestion, since he may be extremely disturbed and aggressive towards other patients/clients. It would probably be preferable to advise David's mother that his refusal to attend the centre would suggest that the guardianship order should be reviewed and for her to report the situation to the appropriate social worker and David's responsible medical officer. This situation should be compared to the situation on a community treatment order discussed below.

One of the weaknesses in the provision of guardianship is that whilst the patient can be required to attend a specified place for treatment, there are no means of enforcing the guardianship powers

> **Figure 21.9**   Statutory powers of the guardian.
>
> (1)   The power to require the patient to reside at a place specified by the guardian;
> (2)   The power to require the patient to attend at places and times specified for the purpose of medical treatment, occupation, education and training; and
> (3)   The power to require access to the patient to be given at any place where the patient is residing to any registered medical practitioner, approved mental health professional or any person specified.

over the patient other than the right of returning the patient to the specified place if he absconds. The ultimate sanction is possibly the knowledge that if the patient does not fare well in the community, then he is likely to be admitted to hospital. It is not, however, good professional practice to use this as a threat. Apart from gentle professional persuasion, there is no way to force a patient to undertake occupational therapy. As a result of the new supervised community treatment order, it may be that less use is made of guardianship orders.

Section 17 leave

A detained patient can be given leave of absence by the responsible clinician in charge of the patient. The leave does not have to be in writing but good practice, as recommended by the Code of Practice of the Department of Health,[37] suggests that there should be a written record of the leave granted and the terms on which it is granted. Section 17 leave can be used as part of the care plan of the patient towards ultimate discharge from the section and from the hospital. Thus a patient on section 17 leave can be required to stay in residential accommodation. (The patient cannot be charged for residential accommodation he is required to stay in as a condition of section 17; see later text regarding section 117). Section 17 leave can be withdrawn at any time on the written instructions of the responsible clinician. Any OT who is responsible for a patient would have to assess the patient prior to leave commencing to establish that there were no grounds for preventing the leave taking place.

Situation

Avril, an OT, is due to take Bob on a shopping trip one afternoon. He is detained under section 3 but has been granted section 17 leave by the responsible clinician. Avril sees Bob at an OT session in the morning when he appears to be extremely disturbed. In the afternoon, she considers that he has not improved and it would be unwise to continue with the shopping trip. Bob becomes extremely aggressive and says that the consultant had said that he could go out three afternoons a week and only the consultant could stop him going. What is the law?

Where section 17 leave has been granted and the patient has left hospital, then the responsible clinician has the power to withdraw the leave at any time in writing. Where, as in the circumstances of the situation above, the patient has not yet left the hospital, it is open to any member of the multi-disciplinary team to advise the responsible clinician that it would be unwise for the patient to leave the hospital, and prevent the patient going. The OT should have easy access to a copy of the section 17 leave approval and conditions and should have an input into the multi-disciplinary discussions which precede the granting of section 17 leave. Leave can be agreed on the basis of a treatment plan, e.g. two weeks escorted ground parole, followed by three afternoons of escorted community visits, followed by overnight leave one night per week. The responsible clinician does not have to agree to each individual leave, provided that it is within the overall agreed plan. The OT should ensure that she documents any outings under section 17 leave. Where she finds the patient too disturbed to take his outing under section 17, she should ensure that the responsible clinician is consulted and the withdrawal of the leave put in writing.

Sections 17A, 17B, 17C 17 D, 17E , 17 F and 17G were added to the Mental Health Act 1983 by the Mental Health Act 2007 and relate to supervised community treatment order (see below).

Section 117 After care services

A statutory duty is placed upon the health authority and local authority, in conjunction with the voluntary sector, to arrange for the provision of after care services for the patient. This duty continues until such time as the health and local authority consider that the patient is no longer in need of the services they can provide. (The duty cannot end if the patient is under a supervised community treatment order; see next section.) The section applies to patients who have been detained under sections 3, 37, 47 and 48. However, the duty to provide a community care assessment under section 47 of the National Health Service and Community Care Act 1990 applies to these patients and also to patients detained under other sections of the Act (e.g. sections 2, 4, 5(2) and 5(4)) and also to informal patients. As a consequence patients who come under the care programme approach and those who are owed section 117 duties may in practice not be kept separate.

However, there are advantages in ensuring that section 117 patients are clearly identified, since a House of Lords decision has made it clear that they cannot be compelled to pay for the treatment which is provided under the after care plans. Some local authorities had been charging patients on a means tested basis for residential accommodation provided under section 117. The House of Lords[38] dismissed an appeal from the judgment of the Court of Appeal and held that where accommodation is provided under section 117 for a patient, then a local authority may not provide it under section 21 nor charge for it under section 22 of the National Assistance Act 1948. Where patients are required to live in residential accommodation under section 17, they are entitled to this accommodation as an after-care service under section 117 when discharged from detention under the Act. Further guidance on the implications of the House of Lords judgment is provided by the Department of Health.[39] The Court of Appeal[40] clarified that the appropriate health and social services authorities for the purpose of section 117 were those where the patient was resident at the time of admission to hospital, but if the patient had no current residence on admission, the authorities for the area where the patient must reside as part of his or her conditional discharge had responsibility for providing after-care under section 117.

Delays in discharging a patient who had been placed under conditional discharge because the responsible social authority had been unable to implement the conditions set by the MHRT were held to be a breach of Article 5 of the European Convention on Human Rights by the European Court of Human Rights in Strasbourg.[41]

Supervised community treatment and community treatment order (CTO)

The Mental Health Act 2007 replaced after care under supervision or supervised discharge with supervised community treatment and a community treatment order. The details are shown in Figure 21.10. Sections 17A to 17G which make provision for a community treatment order (CTO) to be

Figure 21.10 Community treatment order under supervision.

Under 17A(4) the responsible clinician may not make a community treatment order unless—

    (a)   in his opinion, the relevant criteria are met; and

    (b)   an approved mental health professional states in writing—

        (i)   that he agrees with that opinion; and

        (ii)   that it is appropriate to make the order.

(5)   The relevant criteria are—

    (a)   the patient is suffering from mental disorder of a nature or degree which makes it appropriate for him to receive medical treatment;

    (b)   it is necessary for his health or safety or for the protection of other persons that he should receive such treatment;

    (c)   subject to his being liable to be recalled as mentioned in paragraph (d) below, such treatment can be provided without his continuing to be detained in a hospital;

    (d)   it is necessary that the responsible clinician should be able to exercise the power under section 17E(1) below to recall the patient to hospital; and

    (e)   appropriate medical treatment is available for him.

(6)   In determining whether the criterion in subsection (5)(d) above is met, the responsible clinician shall, in particular, consider, having regard to the patient's history of mental disorder and any other relevant factors, what risk there would be of a deterioration of the patient's condition if he were not detained in a hospital (as a result, for example, of his refusing or neglecting to receive the medical treatment he requires for his mental disorder).

17B Conditions for a community treatment order

(1)   A community treatment order shall specify conditions to which the patient is to be subject while the order remains in force.

(2)   But, subject to subsection (3) below, the order may specify conditions only if the responsible clinician, with the agreement of the approved mental health professional mentioned in section 17A(4)(b) above, thinks them necessary or appropriate for one or more of the following purposes—

    (a)   ensuring that the patient receives medical treatment;

    (b)   preventing risk of harm to the patient's health or safety;

    (c)   protecting other persons.

(3)   The order shall specify—

    (a)   a condition that the patient make himself available for examination under section 20A below; and

    (b)   a condition that, if it is proposed to give a certificate under Part 4A of this Act in his case, he make himself available for examination so as to enable the certificate to be given.

(4)   The responsible clinician may from time to time by order in writing vary the conditions specified in a community treatment order.

(5)   He may also suspend any conditions specified in a community treatment order.

(6)   If a community patient fails to comply with a condition specified in the community treatment order by virtue of subsection (2) above, that fact may be taken into account for the purposes of exercising the power of recall under section 17E(1) below.

(7)   But nothing in this section restricts the exercise of that power to cases where there is such a failure.

continued

Figure 21.10 Continued.

17C Duration of community treatment order

A community treatment order shall remain in force until—

(a) the period mentioned in section 20A(1) below (as extended under any provision of this Act) expires, but this is subject to sections 21 and 22 below;

(b) the patient is discharged in pursuance of an order under section 23 below or a direction under section 72 below;

(c) the application for admission for treatment in respect of the patient otherwise ceases to have effect; or

(d) the order is revoked under section 17F below,

whichever occurs first.

17D Effect of community treatment order

(1) The application for admission for treatment in respect of a patient shall not cease to have effect by virtue of his becoming a community patient.

(2) But while he remains a community patient—

(a) the authority of the managers to detain him under section 6(2) above in pursuance of that application shall be suspended; and

(b) reference (however expressed) in this or any other Act, or in any subordinate legislation (within the meaning of the Interpretation Act 1978), to patients liable to be detained, or detained, under this Act shall not include him.

(3) And section 20 below shall not apply to him while he remains a community patient.

(4) Accordingly, authority for his detention shall not expire during any period in which that authority is suspended by virtue of subsection (2)(a) above.

17E Power to recall to hospital

(1) The responsible clinician may recall a community patient to hospital if in his opinion—

(a) the patient requires medical treatment in hospital for his mental disorder; and

(b) there would be a risk of harm to the health or safety of the patient or to other persons if the patient were not recalled to hospital for that purpose.

(2) The responsible clinician may also recall a community patient to hospital if the patient fails to comply with a condition specified under section 17B(3) above.

(3) The hospital to which a patient is recalled need not be the responsible hospital.

(4) Nothing in this section prevents a patient from being recalled to a hospital even though he is already in the hospital at the time when the power of recall is exercised; references to recalling him shall be construed accordingly.

(5) The power of recall under subsections (1) and (2) above shall be exercisable by notice in writing to the patient.

(6) A notice under this section recalling a patient to hospital shall be sufficient authority for the managers of that hospital to detain the patient there in accordance with the provisions of this Act.

17F Powers in respect of recalled patients

(1) This section applies to a community patient who is detained in a hospital by virtue of a notice recalling him there under section 17E above.

(2) The patient may be transferred to another hospital in such circumstances and subject to such conditions as may be prescribed in regulations made by the Secretary of State (if the hospital in which the patient is detained is in England) or the Welsh Ministers (if that hospital is in Wales).

continued

Figure 21.10 Continued.

(3) If he is so transferred to another hospital, he shall be treated for the purposes of this section (and section 17E above) as if the notice under that section were a notice recalling him to that other hospital and as if he had been detained there from the time when his detention in hospital by virtue of the notice first began.

(4) The responsible clinician may by order in writing revoke the community treatment order if—

   (a) in his opinion, the conditions mentioned in section 3(2) above are satisfied in respect of the patient; and
   (b) an approved mental health professional states in writing—
      (i)   that he agrees with that opinion; and
      (ii) that it is appropriate to revoke the order.

(5) The responsible clinician may at any time release the patient under this section, but not after the community treatment order has been revoked.

(6) If the patient has not been released, nor the community treatment order revoked, by the end of the period of 72 hours, he shall then be released.

(7) But a patient who is released under this section remains subject to the community treatment order.

(8) In this section—

   (a) "the period of 72 hours" means the period of 72 hours beginning with the time when the patient's detention in hospital by virtue of the notice under section 17E above begins; and
   (b) references to being released shall be construed as references to being released from that detention (and accordingly from being recalled to hospital).

Section 20A Community treatment period

A community treatment order shall cease to be in force on expiry of the period of six months beginning with the day on which it was made and this period is referred to in this Act as "the community treatment period". The community treatment period may be extended for a period of six months and then on for further periods of up to one year at a time. Section 20A subsections 4–10 set out the conditions for renewal and the procedure to be followed.

20B Effect of expiry of community treatment order

When the community treatment order expires, the community patient shall be deemed to be discharged absolutely from liability to recall under this Part of this Act, and the application for admission for treatment ceases to have effect.

Treatment provisions for those on a community treatment order

The Mental Health Act 2007 inserts into the Mental Health Act 1983 a new Part 4A which sets out the provisions for the treatment of community patients who are not recalled to hospital.

imposed in certain circumstances (section 17A(1)) and define a person subject to a CTO as a 'community patient' (section 17(7)). An application will be made to the hospital managers by the responsible clinician with a supporting recommendation by an AMHP. The relevant criteria for the use of a CTO are set out in the section 17A(5). Section 17B provides that a CTO shall specify conditions to which the patient is to be subject under the order. Section 17E provides a power for a responsible clinician to recall a community patient to hospital where the patient fails to comply with a condition or make himself available for examination.

OT and a supervised community treatment order

The occupational therapist may be involved a patient who is on a supervised community treatment order in several ways:

- She may be involved in the discussions which precede an application for the patient to be placed under a supervised community treatment order and therefore contribute to the formulation of the decisions on the required after care services.
- She may be one of the persons specifically consulted in respect of her professional involvement with the patient or as an approved mental health professional, before the responsible clinician makes an application for a supervised community treatment order.
- She may be identified as the person who is to supervise the patient who is subject to a supervised community treatment order.
- She may be a member of the team which is responsible for the after care of the patient in the community.

She needs to be familiar with the implications of the statutory framework on the rights of the patient and her own legal duties and powers.

Situation: community treatment order (CTO)

> After having been detained under section 3, Harold Graves is placed under supervised community treatment and one of the conditions of the order is that he tries to engage with the Occupational Therapist. She is concerned as to whether this constitutes a referral and as to whether a client can be ordered to undertake occupational therapy. What are the legal implications for the occupational therapist?

It would have been hoped that the conditions of the CTO would have been discussed on a multi-disciplinary basis prior to the CTO being put in place, and that the OT would have had a significant part in these discussions. If so, she would have been already aware of the "tries to engage with OT" condition. Clearly if a client is not prepared to take part in OT activity, it cannot be undertaken without his consent (as Chapter 7 discusses). Failure by Harold to comply with the conditions of his community treatment order gives the responsible clinician the power to recall him to hospital. It would be reasonable to discuss this refusal to engage in OT with Harold since ultimately failure to comply with the requirements could lead to a review by the responsible clinician and ultimately to readmission to hospital. Occupational Therapy performed under duress is probably of little thera-peutic value. However that does not mean that there is not some value in including occupational therapy in the conditions of a CTO.

Removal to place of safety, section 135

Figure 21.11 sets out the basic provisions of this power of the approved mental health professional. The section was amended by the Police and Criminal Evidence Act 1984 so it does not now have to be a named constable who accompanies the approved mental health professional to the house. The House of Lords held that S 135 did not give the magistrate the power to identify the health profes-sionals who were to accompany the police officer in execution of the warrant.[42]

Figure 21.11   Mental Health Act 1983 section 135.

(1)   If it appears to a justice of the peace, on information on oath laid by an approved
mental health professional, that there is a reasonable cause to suspect that a person
believed to be suffering from mental disorder
(a)   has been, or is being, ill-treated, neglected or kept otherwise than under proper
control, in any place within the jurisdiction of the justice; or
(b)   being unable to care for himself, is living alone in any such place the justice
may issue a warrant authorising any constable to enter, if need be by force, any
premises specified in the warrant in which that person is believed to be, and, if
thought fit, to remove him to a place of safety with a view to the making of an
application in respect of him under Part II of this Act, or of other arrangements for
his treatment or care (section 135(4)). In the execution of a warrant issued under
section 135(1) a constable shall be accompanied by an approved mental health
professional and by a registered medical practitioner (as amended by Police and
Criminal Evidence Act 1984 Schedule 6 para 26).

Figure 21.12   Police powers section 136.

(1)   If a constable finds in a place to which the public have access a person who appears
to him to be suffering from mental disorder and to be in immediate need of care or
control, the constable may, if he thinks it necessary to do so in the interests of that
person or for the protection of other persons, remove that person to a place of safety
within the meaning of section 135.
(2)   A person removed to a place of safety under this section may be detained there for a
period not exceeding 72 hours for the purpose of enabling him to be examined by a
registered medical practitioner and to be interviewed by an approved mental health
professional and of making any necessary arrangements for his treatment or care.

Removal from a public place by police, section 136

The basic provisions of this section are set out in Figure 21.12. There has been considerable concern
over the use of the section since the documentation has been inadequate; the police have not always
recorded the details as to when they have used this section, and when the patient has been brought
to hospital the details have not always been recorded by the hospital staff and managers. Many
hospitals have now designed their own forms for this purpose which record the date and time the
patient arrives and the number and name of the constable who brings in the patient.

The Mental Health Review Tribunal

Table 21.3 illustrates the time limits for applying to the Mental Health Review Tribunal, the powers
of the tribunal, and the applicants. A major innovation of the 1983 Act was that the managers must

Table 21.3 Applications to Mental Health Review Tribunals.

Section	Patient	Nearest relative	Manager
2	Applications by patients within first 14 days of detention	No application by nearest relative	No application by manager (Unless patient still under S2 whilst nearest relative is being displaced, when managers have a duty to refer at 6 months)
3	Application by patient within first 6 months of detention, once within second 6 months, then annually	Yes, within 28 days of being informed that responsible medical officer has issued report barring discharge of patient When an order is made appointing a nearest relative under section 29 On reclassification of patient under section 16	Automatic referral if tribunal has not considered case within first 6 months of detention, thereafter if tribunal has not considered case within previous 3 years* (1 year if patient is under 18) *Power for S of S to reduce length of time.
37	Yes, once within second 6 months of detention, then annually	Yes, once within second 6 months of detention, then annually	Automatic if the case has not been considered by tribunal within previous 3 years (1 year if patient is under 18)
41	Yes, once within second 6 months of detention, then annually	No application by nearest relative	Automatic referral by Home Secretary if tribunal has not considered case within the preceding 3 years

automatically refer a patient to the tribunal if he has failed to apply himself. There must be a tribunal hearing at least once every three years Every child under 18 must be referred by the managers every year if he has not himself applied.

An occupational therapist may be asked to provide a report for a Mental Health Review Tribunal or for a Managers' Hearing. She should ensure that she follows the guidance for report writing (see Chapter 13) and that her conclusions are drawn from the evidence she cites in the report. She should also ensure that she would be able to substantiate her report by oral evidence to the hearing. It is important that she makes a decision as to whether any information should be withheld from the patient (see below).

Mental health managers

The managers are given certain statutory duties under the Act. These are set out in Figure 21.13. Of these all can be delegated by the NHS trust board to officers except the duty to hear an application from a patient for discharge. In this case the NHS trust is empowered to appoint a subcommittee, which can include co-opted members provided they are not officers of the NHS trust, for hearing such applications. A decision of the court has stated that in a decision to discharge a patient at least three of the managers should be in agreement.[43]

Figure 21.13   Role of the managers.

1. To accept a patient and record admission (section 140).
2. To give information to detained patient (section 132).
3. To give information to nearest relative (section 132(4)) and inform him of discharge (section 133(1)) or of detention (section 25(2)).
4. To discharge patient (section 23(2)(b)). Powers may be exercised by any three or more members of the authority (section 23 (4)).
5. To refer patient to Mental Health Review Tribunal (section 63(1)(2)).
6. To transfer patient (section 19(3), section 19(la) Reg. 7(2) and Reg. 7(3)).
7. To give notice to local social services authority specifying hospitals in which arrangements are made for reception in case of special urgency of patients requiring treatment for mental disorder (section 140).

Definition of managers: The Primary Care Trust, Health Authority or Special Health Authority responsible for the administration of the hospital, the Trust or the person(s) registered in respect of a registered establishment (section 145).
● All powers can be delegated by managers to the officers except for (4) above: discharging the patient.

Role of the OT and appeals against detention

Often OTs are asked to provide reports for appeals to Mental Health Review Tribunals or to Managers' Hearings. They should follow the principles for report writing which are considered in Chapter 13. They should ensure that they are able to justify every point they make in the report, since they will be expected to give evidence at the hearing. They should also be aware that the patient would be entitled to see any reports, unless the health professional has appended a note setting out information which she would not wish to be shared with the patient. For Managers' Hearings the criteria for withholding information from the patient should be the same as that of the data protection provisions (see Chapter 8), i.e. information can be withheld if serious harm would be caused to the physical or mental health or condition of the patient or any other person, or if a third person has asked not to be identified. Criteria for withholding information from the patient who is appealing to a Mental Health Review Tribunal are not set out in the regulations, but are within the discretion of the Tribunal. However, the Tribunal is required to show the withheld information to the representative of the patient, if the latter is within the specified categories. The information which the OT has decided should not be disclosed should be kept separate from the rest of the report which may be disclosed to the patient.

Danger to OT from aggressive patients

The tragic death of an occupational therapist who worked at the Edith Morgan Unit in Torbay is a sad reminder of the fact that working with the mentally disordered can be dangerous. Those OTs working in acute and specialist units should be aware of the recommendations of the Blom-Cooper report.[44] The employers have a duty to ensure that reasonable care is taken of the health and safety of each employee and also of the general public; this is discussed in Chapter 11. Occupational therapists should be involved in the risk assessment of any unit for the care of the mentally ill and should take active steps to ensure that recommendations for improving health and safety and preventing accidents are implemented.

The Care Quality Commission (CQC)

Figure 21.14 illustrates the powers and constitution of the Mental Health Act Commission. On 1 April 2009 the powers formerly held by the Mental Health Act Commission were transferred to the CQC. These included powers in relation to the special hospitals to review decisions to (a) withhold an item brought to a patient in a High Secure Hospital; (b) withhold internal post sent by a patient in a High Secure Hospital to another patient in the same hospital; or (c) monitor and record a telephone conversation made by a patient in such a hospital.[45] The CQC has the responsibility of updating the Code of Practice on the Mental Health Act and of ensuring that SOADs are appointed and arranging visits to detained patients.

Mentally disordered patients and the European Convention on Human Rights

Several patients have won cases in Strasbourg for breach of their rights as set out in the European Convention on Human Rights. Thus in one case[46] the European Court of Human Rights held that the UK was in breach of Article 5 of the European Convention on Human Rights because for a considerable time the patient was not lawfully detained. Several Mental Health Review Tribunals had given the patient a deferred conditional discharge under section 73 of the Act, but discharge had been delayed because the local authority had been unable to find suitable supervised hostel accommodation. Since 2 October 2000 those who allege that their human rights have been infringed are able to bring action in the courts of the UK instead of going to Strasbourg (see Chapter 6). The Bournewood case (see above) is another example of the ECHR upholding the rights of a patient suffering from mental disorder.

Patients in the secure hospital at Rampton unsuccessfully relied on a human rights argument when they contested the smoking ban imposed on hospital premises. They argued that the policy of prohibiting smoking in the premises of an NHS trust was a violation of their human rights as set out under articles 8 and 14. The Court of Appeal in a majority judgement held that whilst Rampton

---

Figure 21.14 Powers and constitution of the Mental Health Act Commission.

(1) Composition: chairman and about 90 members (doctors, nurses, lawyers, social workers, academics, psychologists, other specialists and lay members)
(2) Headquarters in Nottingham
(3) National Standing Committees
(4) Duty to draft and monitor Code of Practice
(5) Prepare a biennial report to Parliament
(6) Review any decision at a special hospital to withhold a postal packet or its content
(7) Carry out on behalf of the Secretary of State duties in relation to the review of the exercise of powers and discharge of duties under the Act, visiting and interviewing detained patients, and hearing complaints from detained patients
(8) Exercise duties and appointment of second-opinion doctors in relation to Part IV. Consent to treatment provisions

was the claimants' home, it was not a private home but a public institution operated as a hospital under Section 4 of the 2006 Health Act which required all premises used by the public to be smoke free by 1 July 2007.[47] Article 8 did not protect the right to smoke at Rampton. The dissenting judge Lord Keene held that the concept of personal autonomy which the Strasbourg court had adopted in *Pretty v United Kingdom*[48] was wide enough to incorporate a right to choose to smoke.

National Service Frameworks

As envisaged in the White Paper on the NHS,[49] the Government has published National Service Frameworks for different specialties to ensure that there is a minimum standard of provision across the country. The National Service Frameworks for Mental Health were published in 1999 and set seven standards in five areas:

(1)   Mental Health promotion
(2) and (3) Primary care and access to services
(4) and (5) Effective services for people with severe mental illness
(6)   Caring about carers
(7)   Preventing suicide.

The Frameworks document describes the standards as 'realistic, challenging and measurable, and are based on the best evidence available. They will help to reduce variations in practice and deliver improvements for patients, service users and their carers, and for local health and social care communities – health authorities, local authorities, NHS trusts, primary care groups and trusts, and the independent sector.'

OTs working in mental health services should ensure that they obtain a copy of these standards, and their updates, in order that they can ensure that the services they are providing are comparable with these national standards. Unfortunately there is little specific mention in these service frameworks of the OT contribution to mental health standards, and it is hoped that in future years the OT interventions and benefits could be specified. The DH published a review of the NSF on mental health on its 5th birthday in 2004.

Guidance on standards in mental health care have also been published by NICE (see Chapters 10 and 17). The guidance includes post traumatic stress disorder (2005), self harm (2004), treating and managing schizophrenia (2002), schizophrenic core interventions (2009), eating disorder (2004), obsessive compulsive disorder (2005), depression in primary and secondary care (2004 revised 2007), depression in children and young people (2005), antenatal and post natal mental health (2007) attention deficit hyperactive disorder (2008), mental well-being in older people (2008) and OT interventions and physical activity to promote the mental well-being of older people in primary care and residential care (2008). All these guidelines can be downloaded from the NICE website.[50]

The Mental Health Act 2007 did not contain the radical proposals contained in the Expert Report, but it has introduced supervised community treatment, independent mental health advocates and made other changes to the 1983 Act already noted in this chapter. It also amended the Mental Capacity Act 2005 to provide Deprivation of Liberty Safeguards.

Conclusions

There have been considerable delays in reforming both the law on decision making by mentally incapacitated adults and also the Mental Health Act 1983. Both provisions now they are in force should have profound implications for the care of those with mental health problems and also for those adults who lack mental capacity. There is evidence that both sets of legislation will be closely monitored and it is hoped that any necessary revisions will be enacted speedily. The College of Occupational Therapists drafted a strategy for mental health from 2007 to 2017 Recovering Ordinary Lives (December 2006). Its stated vision for OT in mental health services was:

> By 2017 mental health service provision in the UK will be better for the active role and inspirational leadership provided by the cultural heritage and identity of occupational therapy, which at its core is social in nature and belief and, therefore, will deliver the kind of care that service users want, need and deserve.

The strategy set out the guiding principles for mental health occupational therapy practice and identified key messages for OT practitioners, managers, the COT, OT educators, OT researchers and commissioners of mental health services.

The literary review which accompanied the strategy concluded that:

> However, there are also opportunities to move into new areas of practice where the values and skills of the occupational therapist could make an effective contribution. Occupational therapists have the knowledge, skills and attitudes that will enable them to work effectively in three main areas of practice:
>
> - institutional services and settings (including community-based work), providing individualised care for people receiving primary, secondary and tertiary services;
> - public health, including the primary promotion and maintenance of health and disease prevention;
> - community development, working with communities to build capacity and resources to support health and quality of life.

A National Director of Mental Health has been appointed. Consultation on the future of mental health care known as 'New Horizons' was launched in 2009. The New Horizons consultation aims to help come up with an approach to make services for adults with mental health problems better in the future, and to help everyone have better mental health. Occupational Therapists should ensure that they have an input into any subsequent developments.

 Questions and exercises

1   A day patient comes to the industrial therapy centre and is clearly highly disturbed and may need to be detained. What is the legal situation?

2   An occupational therapist is asked by the second opinion appointed doctor for her views on the giving of electro convulsive therapy to an older patient who is extremely depressed, has been starving herself and appears incapable of giving consent. What information should she obtain and what principles should she follow in providing her recommendation?

3   A patient asks an occupational therapist to accompany her to a Manager's Hearing on her application for discharge. What action should the OT take?

4   The occupational therapist is a member of a community mental health team which is caring for a former detained patient who has been placed under a supervised community treatment order. She has been asked to be the patient's community supervisor. What are the implications of this for the work of the occupational therapist?

5   What are the implications for the OT of the new role of approved mental health professional?

References

1 See Dimond, B. & Barker, F. (1996) *Mental Health Law for Nurses*. Blackwell Publishing, Oxford.
2 Mental Health Act Commission (2008) *Code of Practice on the Mental Health Act 1983*. DH, London.
3 Mental Health Act Commission (2008) *Guidance for Commissioners: The Revised Code of Practice*. Care Quality Commission, London.
4 Creek, J. (ed) (2008) *Occupational Therapy and Mental Health*, 4th edn. Churchill Livingstone, Edinburgh.
5 Duncan, E., Thomson, L. & Short, A. (2000) Clinical guidelines within mental health services: an overview of the appraisal and implementation process. *British Journal of Occupational Therapy*, **63**(11), 557–60.
6 Creek Jennifer and Lougher Lesley (eds) (2008) *Occupational Therapy and Mental Health*, 4th edn. Churchill Livingston, Edinburgh.
7 Jackson, Catherine and Hill Kathryn (2006) *Mental Health Today: a Handbook*. Pavilion Brighton.
8 Jeffcote Nikki (ed) (2005) *Working Therapeutically with Women in Secure Mental Health Settings*. Jessica Kingsley. London.
9 Long C, Cronin-Davis J (eds) (2006) *Occupational Therapy Evidence in Practice for Mental Health*. Blackwell, Oxford.
10 McKay Elizabeth Anne, Craik Christine, Lim Kee Hean and Richards Gabrielle (eds) (2008) *Advancing Occupational Therapy in Mental Health Practice*. Blackwell, Oxford.
11 Mental Health Act Commission (2009) *Women detained in hospital*. MHAC now available from CQC, London.
12 College of Occupational Therapists (2002) *Standards for Practice Occupational Therapy in forensic residential settings*. COT, London.
13 College of Occupational Therapy (2003) Mental Health Policy Implementation Guidance: Support, Time and Recovery Workers Briefing No 6. COT, London.
14 College of Occupational Therapy (2006) *Recovering ordinary lives: The strategy for occupational therapy in mental health services in 2007–2017, a vision for the next 10 years*. COT, London.
15 *F v West Berkshire Health Authority* [1989] 2 All ER 545.
16 *R v Bournewood Community and Mental Health NHS Trust ex parte L* [1998] 3 All ER 289; [1999] AC 458.
17 Department of Health (1998) *Modernising Mental Health Services*. DH, London.
18 Department of Health (1998) *Review of Expert Committee Review of the Mental Health Act 1983*. DH, London.
19 Department of Health (1999) Reform of the Mental Health Act 1983 Proposals for Consultation Cm 4480 Stationery Office, London.
20 Carr, J. (2001) Reform of the Mental Health Act 1983: Implications of safety, capacity and compulsion. *British Journal of Occupational Therapy*, **64**(12), 590–4.
21 Aynesely-Green Al (2007) *Pushed into the shadows – young people's experience of adult mental heath facilities*. Office of Children's Commissioner, London.
22 The Mental Health (Nurses) (England) Order 2008 SI 2008/1207.
23 The Mental Health (Mutual Recognition) Regulations 2008 SI 2008/1204.
24 Mental Health (Hospital, Guardianship and Treatment) (England) Regulations 2008 No.1184.
25 Mental Health Act 1983 Approved Clinician (General) Directions 2008 (amended in 2009).
26 The Mental Health (Approved Mental Health Professionals) (Approval). (England) Regulations 2008 SI 2008/1206.
27 College of Occupational Therapists (2002) Standards for Practice Occupational Therapy in forensic residential settings. COT, London.
28 *B v Croydon Health Authority* [1994] The Times Law Report, 1 December 1994, [1995] 1 All ER 683.
29 *Munjaz, R (on the application of) v Ashworth Hospital Authority* [2005] UKHL 58.
30 College of Occupational Therapy (2003 revised in 2006) *Briefings: Occupational therapy staff involved in the second opinion process under the Mental Health Act 1983*. COT/BAOT, London.
31 Burns Tom (2004) *Community Mental Health Teams – a guide to current practice*. Blackwell, Oxford.
32 *B v Croydon Health Authority*. Times Law Report, 1 December 1994 [1995] 1 FLR 470.
33 *Tameside and Glossop Acute Services Trust v CH* [1996] 1 FLR 762; *Norfolk & Norwich (NHS) Trust v W* [1996] 2 FLR 613.

34   *Re MB (An Adult: Medical Treatment)* [1997] 2 FLR 426.

35   *R v Ashworth Hospital Authority*, Times law Report, 24 April 2003.

36   O'Brien Tish and Bannigan Katrina (2008) Making informed choices in the context of service user empowerment and the Mental Capacity Act 2005. *British Journal of Occupational Therapy*, **71**(7), 305–7.

37   Department of Health (2008) *Code of Practice of the Mental Health Act 1983*. Stationery Office, London.

38   *R v London Borough of Richmond ex parte Wilson; R v Redcar and Cleveland Borough Council ex parte Armstrong; R v Manchester City Council ex parte Stennett; R v London Borough of Harrow ex parte Cobham* [2002] UKHL 34; [2002] 4 All ER 124.

39   HSC 2000/003; LAC(2000)3 After-Care under the Mental Health Act 1983.

40   *R v Mental Health Review Tribunal, ex parte Hall* [1999] 3 All ER 131.

41   *Stanley Johnson v The United Kingdom* [1997] series A 1991 VII 2391.

42   *Ward v Commissioner of Police for the Metropolis & Ors* [2005] UKHL 32.

43   *R (Tagoe-Thompson) v Central & North West London Mental Health NHS Trust*. Times Law Report, 18 April 2003.

44   Blom-Cooper L. Hally, H. & Murphy E. (1995) *The Falling Shadow – One patient's mental health care 1978–1993*. Duckworth, London.

45   The Care Quality Commission (Additional Functions) Regulations SI 2009/410.

46   *R v Mental Health Review Tribunal, ex parte Hall* [1999] 3 All ER 131.

47   *R (E) v Nottinghamshire Healthcare NHS Trust* and *R (N) v Secretary of State for Health* The Times Law Report 10 August 2009.

48   *Pretty v United Kingdom* (2002) 35 EHRR 1.

49   White Paper *The New NHS Modern Dependable*, 1997. Stationery Office, London.

50   www.nice.org.uk

22 Learning Disabilities

This chapter considers the law relating to the care of those with learning disabilities. However, it should be pointed out that, whilst for convenience the different client groups (those suffering from mental illness, children, older people, the physically disabled) are considered in separate chapters, many clients may come in more than one category and reference should be made to the other relevant chapters. Some clients with learning disabilities for example also suffer from a mental illness, and these can present some of the most challenging behaviours for occupational therapists (OTs) to deal with – a challenge which is made more difficult because the health and social services organisations may classify the client groups differently so that the OT could be having to deal with different teams and even different NHS trusts, primary care or care trusts.

The OT should also be aware of the provisions of the Mental Health Act 1983 and subsequent legislation which may become relevant in the situation where compulsory powers are needed. The definition of mental disorder includes those who suffer from mental impairment with associated specified conditions (see Chapter 21 on mental disorder). It should also be noted that the statutory duties placed on local and health authorities in respect of those with disabilities apply to both physical and learning disabilities. To avoid repetition, an account of these and the financial benefits available is included in Chapter 20 on Physical Disabilities and reference must be made to that chapter for the information which also relates to those with learning disabilities. See also Chapter 18 for details of the community care legislation and disability discrimination. Chapter 23 includes information on the assessment and statementing of children with special educational needs. Reference should also be made to the general chapters covering areas such as professional accountability, health and safety and the different rights of the client, and to the more specialist works included in the further reading section.

Those OTs caring for clients with learning disabilities will also find it helpful to refer to such works as the textbook *Learning Disabilities* edited by Bob Gates[1] which was written in the light of the White Paper[2] on learning disabilities (see below) and aims to provide all those health and social professionals who work in, or are interested in this area, with a sufficient knowledge base concerning people with learning disabilities. Chapter 13 of *A Handbook of Care* edited by S. Eamon & S. Thomas[3] considers the ethical issues which arise and the principles which can be applied in the resolution of moral problems in decision making. Some of the situations discussed can also be related to the legal principles considered here. A practical guide on OT for those with learning disabilities is provided by Jane Goodman and colleagues[4] and a book on risk assessment for those with LD has been written by Carol Sellers.[5] The specialist section of the COT has also published guidance on the principles of education and practice in OT services for adults with learning disabilities (2003) based on the OT standards as set out in 2003? Four principles are set out for OT services for those with learning disabilities:

Principle 1: Occupational therapists working in learning disability services provide a service for people whose primary reason for referral relates to the effect of their learning disability upon their occupational performance.

Principle 2: People with learning disabilities need to be enabled to have choice and influence over their occupational therapy intervention.

Principle 3: People with learning disabilities have the right to access generic health and social care.

Principle 4: Occupational therapy services should be provided in partnership with the person with learning disabilities, his or her carers and all relevant agencies.

These should now be read in the light of the OT professional standards of practice published in 2007.

The COT/BAOT has also published a position statement on supporting people with long term conditions (2005) which responded to the DH's Supporting people with long term conditions and stated that community matron posts should not be taken by OTs.

The effect of the community care initiative has meant that fewer clients with learning disabilities are cared for in institutions administered under health service organisations and more are cared for either within the family setting or in community homes specially built or adapted for their needs. Some of this accommodation has been provided by housing associations who may work in conjunction with care organisations which undertake the day-to-day management of the home. Many such clients are therefore under the care of OTs employed by the social services departments (SSDs) rather than NHS trusts. Some may come under the newly formed care trusts (see Chapter 18).

The following topics are covered in this chapter:

• Duty of care owed by local authorities	• Sheltered housing and workshops
• Learning disabilities, mental capacity and mental disorder	• Risk assessment and risk taking
• Strategic planning for those with learning disabilities	• Rights of the client and incapacity
	• Law Commission and decision making
• Philosophy behind the care of those with learning disabilities	• Mental Capacity Act 2005
	• Rights of relatives
• Community homes for those with learning disabilities	• Sexual relations, sterilisation, abortion
	• Refusal to partake in activities
	• Property and exploitation

Duty of care owed by Local Authorities

The High Court[6] has recently held that a duty of care is owed by a local authority.

Case: *X(1) and Y(2) v London Borough of Hounslow*

The claimants had learning disabilities and lived in a Council house with their 2 children, one of whom had learning difficulties. They were assaulted and abused by a group of youths who virtually imprisoned them in their home. The claimants brought an action against the Council on the grounds that the Council was negligent and in breach of the claimants rights under Articles 3 and 8 of the European Convention for the Protection of Human Rights (see Appendix 1) The Council defended on the grounds that no duty of care was owed to the claimants. The Judge held that the injury and loss suffered was reasonably foreseeable and the relationship between defendants and claimants was sufficiently proximate to warrant the imposition of the duty of care. The Council which was well aware of the circumstances (two independent reports had been commissioned on the situation) should have invoked the emergency transfer scheme to move the claimants to alternative accommodation. The judge found it unnecessary and too complex because of the timings to determine whether in fact there was a breach under the Human Rights Act 1998.

The implications of this decision would have been considerable for local social services authorities who may in future have to give evidence of the steps which they have taken to fulfil the duty of care they owe, and also the steps which they have taken to fulfil any statutory duties they may have.

The case which was heard in June 2008 went to the Court of Appeal which allowed the defendant's appeal.[7] The Court of Appeal concluded:

> While this has been a very troubling case and we have every sympathy for the respondents in being subjected to an appalling ordeal, and while we fully appreciate the careful way the judge approached the evidence and the issues, we have reached a different conclusion from him. Our conclusion is that the Council did not assume a responsibility to the respondents at common law, that neither it nor its employees owed them a duty of care at common law and, in any event, that neither it nor its employees was in breach of a duty to take reasonable care to remove them from the flat into emergency accommodation as found by the judge. It follows that the appeal must be allowed.

Criminal offence of ill-treatment or wilful neglect

Section 44 of the Mental Capacity Act 2005 creates a new statutory offence of ill treatment or wilful neglect. It can arise where a person (D) has the care of a person (P) who lacks, or whom D reasonably believes to lack, capacity, or is the donee of a lasting power of attorney, or an enduring power of attorney created by P, or is a deputy appointed by the court for P.

Learning disabilities, mental capacity and mental disorder

Mental capacity

Mental capacity is now statutorily defined in the Mental Capacity Act 2005. This is explained in Chapter 7 the two stages of defining capacity: (a) is there an impairment in the functioning of brain or mind and (b) if so, does this cause an inability to make decisions?

A person is unable to make decisions if he or she is unable:

(a) to understand the information relevant to the decision,
(b) to retain that information,
(c) to use or weigh that information as part of the process of making the decision, or
(d) to communicate his decision (whether by talking, using sign language or any other means). (S.3(1))

It should be noted however that under section 3(2) a person is not to be regarded as unable to understand the information relevant to a decision if he is able to understand an explanation of it given to him in a way that is appropriate to his circumstances (using simple language, visual aids or any other means). This means that when attempting to assess the capacity of someone with learning disabilities and assisting them in communicating their wishes, every practicable means must be used to assist. This might include using the services of a speech therapist, obtaining specialist equipment, speaking to those who can communicate with that person and generally using any available means of communicating with the client.

Mental disorder

The provisions of the Mental Health Act 1983 (as amended by the Mental Health Act 2007) may become relevant in the situation where compulsory powers are being considered. The amended definition of mental disorder is "any disorder or disability of the mind" and would therefore include those who suffer from mental impairment with associated specified conditions. Learning disability (which is defined as "a state of arrested or incomplete development of the mind which includes significant impairment of intelligence and social functioning") is not considered to come under the definition of mental disorder unless the disability is associated with abnormally aggressive or seriously irresponsible conduct on the person's part (Section 2 of 2007 Mental Health Act) (see Chapter 21 on mental illness).

Strategic planning for those with learning disabilities

In 1992 guidance on the development of health services for people with learning disabilities was published.[8] Both the White Paper on the NHS[9] and the White Paper for Social Services[10] envisaged that improved service provision for those with learning disabilities would be made. The Green Paper[11] *Our Healthier Nation* was concerned that vulnerable and disadvantaged people should have the best possible health. *Signposts for Success* was issued in 1998 by the Department of Health to provide good practice guidance for planners, commissioners and providers of health services.[12] Further advice was provided for those working in primary care to enhance their understanding, improve their practice and promote their partnerships with other agencies and NHS services in provision for those with learning disabilities.[13] A White Paper setting out a new strategy for learning disability for the twenty-first century was published by the Department of Health in March 2001.[14] This White Paper set out a new vision based on the key principles of rights, independence, choice and inclusion.

The strategy covers the problems and challenges relating to children and young people and their transition into adult life, providing more choice and control, supporting carers, improving health for people with learning disabilities, housing, fulfilling lives and employment, quality services and partnership working and bringing about the changes. An annex sets out objectives and sub-objectives, targets and performance indicators. Implementation guidance was published in August 2001.[15]

White Paper: *Valuing People*

The White Paper *Valuing People – a new Strategy for Learning Disability for the 21st Century*[16] (which held that long-term hospitals were not an appropriate home environment for people with learning disabilities) recognised 4 key principles: Rights, Independence, Choice and Inclusion as lying at the heart of the Government's proposals. The White paper is described by the Government as taking a life-long approach, beginning with an integrated approach to services for disabled children and their families and then providing new opportunities for a full and purposeful adult life. The proposals should result in improvements in education, social services, health, employment, housing and support for people with learning disabilities and their families and carers. The White Paper estimates that there are about 210,000 people with severe learning disabilities and about 1.2 million with a mild or moderate disability. It sets out the following proposals:

- new national objectives for services for those with learning disabilities
- a new Learning Disability Development fund
- a new central implementation support fund
- disabled children and their families to be an integral part of the Quality Protects programme, the Special Educational Needs Programme of Action and the Connexions Service
- development of advocacy services to assist them in having as much choice and control over their lives as possible
- supporting carers by implementing the Carers and Disabled Children Act 2000 (see Chapter 18) and by funding the development of a national learning disability information centre and helpline in partnership with Mencap.
- improving health of those with learning disabilities by providing the same rights of access to mainstream health services as the rest of the population by appointing health facilitators, ensuring registration with a GP and a health action plan for each client
- giving greater choice over where they live with more appropriate accommodation
- more local day services to assist them in leading a full and purposeful life.
- new targets for increasing numbers of people with learning disabilities in work
- raising of standards and quality of services provided for those with learning disabilities including training and qualifications for care staff through a learning disability awards framework
- effective partnership working through Learning Disability Partnership Boards

To implement these changes a Learning Disability Task Force was set up to advise the Government, supported by an Implementation Support Team to promote change at regional and local level.

In December 2007 the Department of Health published a consultation document *Valuing People now*[17] which set out the next steps on the Valuing People policy and its delivery. It saw the main priorities for 2008–2011 to be personalisation; what people do during the day; better health; access to housing and making sure that change happened. The wider agenda would include an emphasis on advocacy and human rights; partnership with families; ensuring all those with learning disabilities were included; working with the criminal justice system and the department of transport and local groups to ensure those with learning disabilities can become full members of their local communities; providing the same opportunities as others in the transition from childhood to adulthood and supporting those who work with those with learning disabilities. The consultation ended in March 2008 and a summary of the responses was published by the Government in 2009.[18] One of the conclusions was that:

> There were consistent worries about whether *Valuing People Now* will make a real difference to people's lives, particularly in terms of funding and legislative 'teeth'. Many respondents felt that *Valuing People Now* was strong on vision but short on the detailed implementation plans to make the vision a reality, particularly compared to the 'view from the ground' that many respondents were experiencing.

In Chapter 24 the Green Paper on Independence, Well-being and Choice[19] and the White Paper on Our Health, our care, our say[20] published in 2006 are discussed in relation to risk management, together with the subsequent guidance published by the DH on a guide to independence, choice and risk[21] which provides a risk management framework for use by everyone involved in supporting adults using social care within any setting, including NHS staff working in multi-disciplinary or joint teams. A report published in 2008 which gave stark evidence of the discrimination suffered by those with learning disabilities in accessing healthcare[22] shows the extent of the challenge in ensuring equality of healthcare provision for those with learning disabilities. See also Jo Corbett's work on health provision for people with learning disabilities.[23] The following situation is probably not unusual

Situation: Not worth bothering about

> Stan had fallen from a first floor window in his community home and was taken to A&E by his carer. He had very limited speech and was unable to explain where he hurt and screamed when the doctor tried to examine him. The doctor suggested that the carer should take him home and give him paracetamol and a hot drink and return to the A&E department if it looked as though he had a fracture or any other serious problems.

Clearly the carer should try to ensure that Stan receives the reasonable standard of care which any person is entitled to in the A&E department and if the approved practice would have been to take X-Rays and even admit over night, then Stan is entitled to that standard. His difficulties in speaking, should not be used by clinicians as a reason to provide a lower standard of care.

Other examples can be given where because of a failure to X-Ray, fractures are not diagnosed, or there is a failure to offer screening (e.g. cervical, breast etc.) facilities which would be available to those with mental capacity. A situation may be that of a client with LD, who was non-verbal and autistic and whose fingers in her hand curled tightly into her palm, getting tighter over recent few years. Her fingernails were growing into her palm and causing her a lot of pain. She was referred to a plastic surgeon who suggested that the tendons in her fingers should be cut, rather than opening up her hand gradually using a splint. The OT protested pointing out that she still used her hands, and made good use of her thumb and little finger to manipulate objects. In such conflicts where an OT is aware that a client with LD is not receiving an acceptable standard of care an application can be made to the Court of Protection which has the power to appoint a Deputy (see below).

Crossing service provision boundaries

Individuals do not of course fit into neat categories and all health professionals must be aware of the dangers of failing to treat the whole person and ignoring problems which do not fit into a specific form of service provision. These individuals are often vulnerable but can be excluded from support mechanisms due to having the "wrong" diagnosis to access services. For example teenagers who have a dual diagnosis of learning disability and mental health may not come within any particular service. The Child and Adolescent Mental Health Service may not see a child with an IQ of 60 or less, the paediatric services may not work with major mental health issues. Pressure is often put on "adult" learning disability services to pick such individuals up when therapists do not have the skill set for working with children with mental health problems. Any health professional, including the OT, who is involved in the care of the child would have a legal responsibility to ensure that all the appropriate services from other agencies and departments were involved and may herself become the co-ordinator of care for that client. The law requires that a reasonable standard of care is provided for the client, irrespective of the different service providers he or she may come under. Failures to co-operate across service boundaries was evident in the Baby P case discussed in Chapter 23.

Philosophy behind the care of those with learning disabilities

The White Paper recognized four key principles: Rights, Independence, Choice and Inclusion as being central to government in the provision of services for those with learning disabilities. These implicitly include: autonomy, normalisation and maximum potential of each individual.

Autonomy

A basic principle accepted by most twentieth century western philosophers is that the autonomy of the adult person should be respected and enhanced. Autonomy or self-rule or self-determination is based on the principle of respect for the person. It does not follow that, because a person has learning disabilities, he or she is unable to act autonomously. There may be some decisions which are within the person's competence, and the aim of any carer – informal or professional – should be to maximise the person's ability to enjoy his or her autonomy. It therefore follows that the rights of the person with learning disabilities should be protected. The Mental Capacity Act 2005 sets out a general principle that a person must be assumed to have capacity unless it is established that he lacks capacity (see Chapter 7). Any rebuttal of the presumption of capacity is on a balance of probabilities.

The rights shown in Figure 22.1 were identified by Knapp and Slade[24] in relation to a socio-sexual developmentally disabled person. Those with learning disabilities are also entitled to the human rights as set out in the European Convention of Human Rights (see Chapter 6 and Appendix 1) and discrimination against such persons would be unlawful under Article 14.

The Joint Committee on Human Rights (the Committee) published its report *A Life like Any Other? Human Rights of Adults with Learning Disabilities* on 6 March 2008.[25] The Joint Committee put forward 81 conclusions and recommendations for the Government and other organisations on ensuring that the human rights of those with adults with learning disabilities were respected. The Government

Figure 22.1   Rights of the socio-sexual developmentally disabled person.

- The right to equal educational opportunity
- The right to education and habilitation which includes the right to receive information about sex and contraception
- The right to be free unless proven dangerous
- The right to privacy, especially concerning one's intimate bodily functions, including the right to sexual expression
- The right to equal access to medical services
- The right to have relationships with one's peers, including the members of the opposite sex – this right includes the right to sexual expression
- The right to equal opportunities for housing
- The right to equal and fair treatment by public agencies and officials

responded to the report in May 2008[26] outlying the action it intended taking in relation to each recommendation, including the review of Valuing People and the importance of the role of the Equality and Human Rights Commission in safeguarding the human rights of those with learning disabilities. Both the Joint Committee's Report and the Government Response can be accessed on the parliamentary website.[27] See also the DH publication on a review of human rights and equality of opportunity in mental health and learning disabilities.[28]

Empowerment

It follows from the principle that the autonomy of an individual should be respected that, as far as possible, those with learning disabilities should be supported in enjoying as 'normal' a life as possible.

Figure 22.2 shows the rights that these same authors considered essential to implement this principle of normalisation.

Empowerment has as its aim to ensure the full potential of such clients and attempt to prevent any restriction on their life and opportunities which is not an inevitable consequence of their condition. In this work the OT has a key role to play. The College of Occupational Therapy (COT) prepared guidelines in 1995[29] covering topics which are now included in the Professional Practice Standards set out in 2007.[30] In 2003 the COT published guidance on OT services for adults with learning disabilities[31] and in 2004 published guidance on disability and learning. This latter publication explained and clarified the Disability laws in relation to this particular client group setting out the principles which apply to disability and learning and looking at practice placements.[32] Empowerment means taking all reasonable steps to ensure that those with learning disabilities can as far as is practicable make decisions for themselves and look after themselves and thus such practical handbooks as the Travel Training Resource Pack (2004) published jointly by West Sussex Health and Social Care NHS Trust and the National Association of OTs working with people with learning disabilities are invaluable resources.

Services for those with learning disabilities should no longer be seen as the 'Cinderella service' and it is clear that in the setting of priorities considerable sums should be available for staffing and equipment. (Refer also to Chapter 15 on equipment issues.) Quality care for those with learning disabilities may require considerable expenditure in both staffing and equipment and other facilities.

Figure 22.2   Rights to implement the normalisation principle.

- The right to a normal rhythm to the day (regular mealtimes, work and leisure time)
- The right to experience the normal life cycle
- The right to grow up, to leave parents and to move into the community
- The right to live in and experience male/female relationships
- The right to the same economic standards
- The right to make choices
- The right to fail – if developmentally disabled persons are offered as much autonomy as they are capable of, this necessarily will include the possibility of failing, just as everyone enjoys this possibility

Maximum development of potential

The principles which govern the care of those with learning disabilities include not only that of empowerment but also the aim of ensuring the maximum development of the potential of each individual. This requires individual assessment and the preparation of an individual care plan covering all aspects of life – education, health and social and economic development. In this strategic planning for each individual the OT has a major role to play. Activities in which OTs may be involved include horse riding[33] and similar therapeutic pastimes. It is essential that the OT ensures that she obtains the necessary training, works within her field of competence and has her employer's agreement to taking on expanded role activities.

Community homes for those with learning disabilities

More and more persons with learning disabilities now live in community homes. The activities of housing associations supported by funds from housing corporations have enabled many clients with special needs to live in such homes. Sometimes the administration of the homes is under a separate care organisation. These organisations often provide a code of practice covering the rights which the client/tenant/resident should enjoy, and setting quality standards.

The OT should have a major role to play in these community homes, not only in the selection of clients for each home but also in providing support and guidance on the activities and lives of the clients.

Sheltered workshops

Clients, whether living in their family homes or in community homes, should have the facility of attending sheltered workshops and other forms of industrial therapy. However, provision is patchy across the country.

Risk assessment and risk taking

The philosophy of normalisation requires that health and social services professionals working with those with learning disabilities should be acquainted with and implement a risk assessment strategy in relation to each individual client. It would be possible to prevent any harm arising by keeping the client indoors under close supervision and denying him or her opportunities to go shopping, go to work or undertake everyday tasks. However, quality of life would be severely reduced if opportunities were not taken for holidays, trips and other activities. The law requires that reasonable precautions are taken to prevent reasonably foreseeable risks of harm. Thus a risk assessment of each individual client is needed to identify the potential risks of possible harm to that client or to other people and to determine what action would be reasonable to prevent such risks occurring.

It is essential that records should be kept of this risk assessment so that, should the client's condition deteriorate, it is possible to identify the significance of these changes to the proposed participation in the activities and so that other healthcare workers can identify, through the treatment plan, what a client should or should not be encouraged to do. Risk assessment in people with learning disabilities is considered by Carol Sellars[34] in her book which covers the problems in predicting risks and linking risks with care planning. She also considers the issues arising with parents with learning disabilities, violence and offenders with learning disabilities and sex offenders who have learning disabilities.

Records are also extremely important if harm arises to the client or another person and the professional is required to justify her action before the civil or criminal courts, or in disciplinary or professional conduct proceedings. If the professional can establish that her actions were reasonable in relation to reasonably foreseeable risks, then civil liability should not exist.

In Chapter 11 the use of a risk assessment strategy is considered in the context of health and safety and this strategy could also be used in relation to individual care planning.

Restraint

Under the Mental Capacity Act 2005 restraint can only be used where a person reasonably believes that it is necessary to do the act in order to prevent harm to the person who lacks the requisite mental capacity and where the act of restraint is a proportionate response to (a) the likelihood of P's suffering harm, and (b) the seriousness of that harm. As a consequence of amendments to the Mental Capacity Act 2005 introduced by the Mental Health Act 2007 safeguards have been introduced where a person lacking the requisite mental capacity is deprived of his or her liberty. This topic is further considered in Chapter 7.

Deprivation of Liberty Safeguards (DOLS) (The Bournewood Safeguards)

In the Bournewood case the European Court of Human Rights[35] declared that the detention of a patient under common law powers was contrary to his article 5 rights. As a consequence of this decision the Government, introduced amendments to the Mental Capacity Act 2005 to enable restrictions of patients to be lawfully made. These amendments were originally known as the Bournewood safeguards and are now referred to as deprivation of liberty safeguards. The Mental Health Act 2007 amended the Mental Capacity Act 2005 to introduce the safeguards necessary to justify loss of liberty of residents in hospitals and care homes. They are set out in the new Schedule A1 to the MCA as introduced by the Mental Health Act 2007 and can be found in a briefing paper available from the Department of Health.[36] They came into force in April 2009 and a Code of Practice to supplement the existing Code of Practice on the Mental Capacity Act 2005 was issued by the Lord Chancellor in 2008.

The use of the deprivation of liberty safeguards may be indicated in the following circumstances:

- where restraint is used to admit a person or to prevent their leaving
- where movement is controlled for a significant period
- where a request for discharge by relatives is refused
- where an individual is prevented from having social contact because of restrictions placed on access by others
- where continuous supervision and control has led to a loss of autonomy by an individual.[37]

Who is covered by the deprivation of liberty safeguards?:

- Those over 18 years
- Who suffer from a disorder or disability of mind

- Who lack the capacity to give consent to the arrangements made for their care and
- For whom such care (in circumstances that amount to a deprivation of liberty within the meaning of article 5 of the European Convention on Human Rights) is considered after an independent assessment to be a necessary and proportionate response in their best interests to protect them from harm

What procedures are required?

1. *Application for authorisation:* The hospital or care home, i.e. the managing authority, must identify a client/patient as lacking capacity and who risks being deprived of his/her liberty. It must apply for the authorisation of deprivation of liberty to the supervisory body i.e. where the person is in hospital, the Primary Care Trust (PCT) or for Wales, a Local Health Board or the National Assembly; where the person is in a care home, the local authority for the area in which the person is ordinarily resident or, if the person is not ordinarily resident in the area of a local authority, the area in which the care home is situated. A third party, who is concerned that there is an unauthorised deprivation of liberty taking place can apply to the supervisory body to assess whether the person is deprived of liberty.
2. *Assessments required:*
   Age assessment – client/patient must be over 18 years
   Mental Health Assessment – client/patient must be suffering a mental disorder
   Mental Capacity Assessment – client/patient must lack the capacity to decide whether to be admitted to or remain in the hospital or care home
   Eligibility assessment- the client/patient must:
   - Not be detained under the Mental Health Act
   - Not be subject to a conflicting requirement under the Mental Health Act
   - Not be subject to powers of recall under the Mental Health Act nor to a treatment order in hospital to which the client/patient objects

   Best interests assessment - the authorisation would be in the client/patient's best interests, that it is necessary that the person be a patient in the hospital or care home in order to prevent harm to him or her and is a proportionate response to the likelihood of suffering harm and the seriousness of that harm. A registered occupational therapist could provide a best interests assessment provided that she has at least two years post-registration experience and has successfully completed training to be a best interests assessor.
   There must be no conflict between the authorisation sought and a valid decision by a donee of a lasting power of attorney or a deputy and the authorisation does not conflict with a valid and applicable advance decision made by the client/patient.
3. *Appointment of representative for the client/patient:* If the best assessor concludes that the client/patient has the capacity to appoint her own representative, then he/she can do this. Otherwise the best interests assessor can appoint a representative. If the assessor notifies the supervisory body that a representative has not been appointed for him/her, then it can appoint a representative who can be paid to act as the client/patient's representative. Regulations came into force in November 2008 on the appointment of the representatives.[38]
4. *Authorisation granted:* If all the assessments are satisfactory then authorisation by the supervisory body can be granted for the deprivation of the client/patient's liberty for up to 12 months.
5. *Review and monitoring:* The supervisory authority should keep under review the client/patient's deprivation of liberty and the whole process of the assessments and authorisation will be monitored to ensure that all the required procedures were followed.

A standard authorisation is requested by a managing authority when it appears likely that a person will be accommodated in circumstances amounting to a deprivation of liberty. If the criteria are met the authorisation can be for up to 12 months duration. An urgent authorisation is possible where a standard authorisation cannot be made in advance and it is necessary in the best interests of the person to deprive him or her of liberty. A managing authority can issue an urgent authorisation for a maximum of 7 days. Further information on DOLS is available on the DH website and from MIND.

Carers

The implementation of the Mental Capacity Act 2005 has major implications for carers of those with learning disabilities. Their role in the decision making process where a person lacks the mental capacity to make a specific decision has been clarified. Information which they can give about the mentally incapacitated person includes his or her passed wishes and feelings, views, beliefs and any other relevant information. Whilst the Act does not stipulate that informal (i.e. unpaid) carers are required to follow the guidance in the Code of Practice, they would find the advice of considerable help.[39]

Independent Mental Capacity Advocates (IMCA)

Where a relative or friend is not available to be consulted in the process of determining the best interests of a person lacking the requisite mental capacity, the Mental Capacity Act 2005 requires the appointment of an independent mental capacity advocate in specified circumstances. These include: where serious medical treatment is being considered and where accommodation is being arranged by the NHS or social services. Under the regulations[40] under the Mental Capacity Act 2005 an Independent Mental Capacity Advocate should be appointed in an adult protection case even though relatives or informal carers are available.

Further information on the independent mental capacity advocate can be found in the author's work.[41]

Refusal to grant accommodation

The rights of relatives to refuse to take back a client who has been in respite care also need to be considered. In the case of an adult person suffering from mental impairment, if the relatives refuse to take the person back home this is their right and they cannot be compelled to look after him or her. Health and social services professionals would have to look for other accommodation for the client. Reference should be made to the discussion in Chapter 18 on the guidelines for the division between health services' and social services' respective responsibilities on continuing care.

Protection of the autonomy of the client

Conversely it may happen that an extremely diligent parent/carer is unwilling to allow a son or daughter with learning disabilities to leave home and enter sheltered accommodation. In a recent case a mother had been placed under an injunction not to visit her son who had been moved to alternative accommodation. The Court of Appeal ruled that the injunction should be lifted as it was not appropriate to threaten her with imprisonment but the case illustrates the difficulties of 'letting go'.

The role of the OT

If OTs are aware of a conflict between the rights (as shown in Figure 22.1) of the person with learning disabilities and the wishes of the carer, they should take action to protect the client and endeavour to secure a harmonious outcome, bearing in mind the rights of the client. Again, this is another area where, the Mental Capacity Act protects the client who lacks the mental capacity to make his own decisions. Reference should also be made to Chapter 20 on physical disabilities, where rights to accommodation are considered.

Decision making and incapacity

Many clients with learning disabilities may still have the capacity to make decisions on their own account. The client's capacity must be related to the nature of the decision to be made. The client may be able to choose what clothes to wear or buy but may not have the capacity to decide whether or not to undergo an operation to be sterilised. Decisions for a person under 18 years can be made by the parents (or local authority if the child is in care) provided that it is in the best interests of the child. The Mental Capacity Act 2005 has since October 2007 filled the gap which existed in statutory provision in decision making on behalf of the mentally incapacitated adult. It thus provides statutory provision for decisions to be made in the best interests of the mentally incapacitated adult, replacing the common law principles established by the House of Lords in the case of Re F.[42]

Mental Capacity Act 2005

The Law Commission, following an extended period of consultation on the issue of decision making and mental incapacity, prepared draft legislation in 1995.[43] The Lord Chancellor issued a consultation document in December 1997[44] *Who Decides*. Following this consultation a Bill was introduced into Parliament to enact the Law Commission's recommendations. The Mental Capacity Act 2005 received royal assent in 2005 and was brought into force in October 2007. The Act is discussed in full in Chapter 7. The Act sets out statutory principles which should apply and can be found in Box 7.1. The Act defines mental capacity and also sets out the steps to be taken to determine the best interests of those lacking the requisite mental capacity. Independent mental capacity advocates are to be appointed in specific circumstances to provide information on the best interests of the patient. The Act recognises the power to appoint a lasting power of attorney (discussed in Chapter 24) and sets up a new Court of Protection with jurisdiction over personal welfare decisions as well as matters relating to property and affairs. The Court of Protection can appoint deputies to make decisions who come under the supervision of a new Office of Public Guardian. Further information can be found in the author's work.[41]

The Bournewood case

A House of Lords decision in 1998[45] held that the power of acting out of necessity in the best interests of a person who lacks mental capacity can also apply to the admission of such patients to psychiatric care. The House of Lords had overruled a Court of Appeal decision which had held that any adult who lacked the mental capacity to give consent to voluntary admission to psychiatric care had to be examined with a view to detention under the provisions of the Mental Health Act 1983 (see Chapter

21). The carers applied to the European Court of Human Rights holding that its decision was contrary to article 5 in the European Convention. The European Court of Human Rights held that there had been a breach of Article 5 of the European Convention on Human Rights.[46] The Bournewood case is considered in Chapter 21 and the Bournewood safeguards are considered on pages 440–2.

The issue of capacity arose in the following case.

Local Authority X v MM 2007[47]

The Local Authority brought the case seeking orders that M lacked capacity to conduct litigation, make decisions as to where she should reside, determine with whom she should have contact, manager her own affairs or enter into marriage. It also wanted a declaration that it was in M's best interests to reside in supported accommodation and had limited contact with K, her partner. M was a vulnerable adult who suffered paranoid schizophrenia and learning disabilities. She had been with K for 15 years. The LA received information that K was intending to move M from her supported accommodation and disengage from psychiatric services. They therefore applied for an interim injunction to prevent M being moved from her supported accommodation or have unsupervised contact with K.

The judge held that the test of mental capacity to consent to medical treatment was also applicable to decisions over residency and with whom the person was to have contact. There was no relevant distinction between the test in Re MB[48] and the statutory definition in the Mental Capacity Act 2005 (see Chapter 7); The capacity to consent to sexual intercourse depended on a person having sufficient knowledge and understanding of the sexual nature and character of the act of sexual intercourse and of the reasonably foreseeable consequences of sexual intercourse, to have the capacity to choose whether or not to engage in it. It was issue specific not partner specific. M had the capacity to consent to sexual intercourse, but lacked the capacity to litigate; to manage her finances; to decide where and with whom she should live, to marry and to decide with whom she should have contact. M's human rights had to be taken into account and her wishes and feelings should be considered and the court had to pay regard to M's wishes to have an ongoing sexual relationship with K. The judge made the order required by the LA subject to the qualification that her contact with K did not have to be supervised. The LA was directed to file a care plan setting out its final proposals.

Court of Protection and Code of Practice

Appointment of Deputy

The Court of Protection can make a single order or appoint a deputy in relation to a matter within its jurisdiction which includes personal welfare as well as finance and property. Section 16 makes provision for the Court of Protection to make decisions and for the appointment of deputies. The deputy must act on behalf of the patient in accordance with the principles set out in the Mental Capacity Act 2005, in the best interests of the patient (see Chapter 7) and within the powers granted him by the Court of Protection. The deputies can be given powers (with specified limitations) over matters of personal welfare which extend in particular to:

- deciding where P is to live (where a deputy makes a decision on this, it is subject to the restrictions on deputies)

- deciding what contact, if any, P is to have with any specified persons (the deputy has no power to make an order prohibiting a named person from having contact with P)
- giving or refusing consent to the carrying out or continuation of a treatment by a person providing healthcare for P.

A deputy cannot give a direction that a person responsible for P's health care allows a different person to take over that responsibility: Only the Court of Protection has that power.

Where the deputy is given powers over a person's property and affairs, they could include the following:

- the control and management of P's property
- the sale, exchange, charging gift or other disposition of P's property
- the acquisition of property in P's name or on P's behalf
- the carrying on, on P's behalf, of any profession, trade or business
- the taking of a decision which will have the effect of dissolving a partnership of which P is a member
- the carrying out of any contract entered into by P
- the discharge of P's debts and of any of P's obligations, whether legally enforceable or not
- the settlement of any of P's property, whether for P's benefit or for the benefit of others
- the execution for P of a will (unless P is under 18 years old) (subject to restriction on deputies)
- the exercise of any power (including a power to consent) vested in P whether beneficially or as trustee or otherwise
- the conduct of legal proceedings in P's name or on P's behalf.

The Code of Practice identifies the following list as duties to be followed by the court appointed deputy.[49] It notes that when agreeing to act as deputy whether in relation to welfare or financial affairs, the deputy is taking on a role which carries powers that s/he must use carefully and responsibly. The standard of conduct expected of deputies involves compliance with the following duties as an agent and with the statutory requirements:

- to comply with the principles of the Act
- to act in the best interests of the client
- to follow the Code of Practice
- to act within the scope of their authority given by the Court of Protection
- to act with due care and skill (duty of care)
- not to take advantage of their situation (fiduciary duty)
- to indemnify the person against liability to third parties caused by the deputy's negligence
- not to delegate duties unless authorised to do so
- to act in good faith
- to respect the person's confidentiality, and
- to comply with the directions of the Court of Protection.

To be appointed as a deputy an individual must be 18 years or over. An individual of at least 18 years or a trust corporation can be appointed as a deputy in respect of powers relating to property and affairs. The deputy must give consent to the appointment. The holder of a specified office or position may be appointed as deputy. Two or more deputies could be appointed to act jointly or jointly and severally. (Jointly means that they act together in making decisions and exercising the powers; severally means that they act as individuals separately).

The deputy is entitled to be reimbursed out of P's property for his reasonable expenses in discharging his functions. In addition, if the court so directs when appointing the deputy, the deputy can receive remuneration out of P's property for discharging his functions. The court can give the deputy powers to take possession or control of all or any specified part of P's property and to exercise all or any specified powers in respect or it, including such powers of investment as the court decides.

The Office of Public Guardian acts as supervisor of the deputy and any complaints about the conduct of a deputy can be made to that Office. Further information on the role of the deputy, the Office of Public Guardian and the Court of Protection can be obtained from the Ministry of Justice website.[50] See also the author's work.[41]

Safeguarding vulnerable adults

A new Safeguarding Vulnerable Adults Policy and a protocol for joint working between the Office of the Public Guardian and Local Authorities was launched in December 2008.[51] This policy provides a framework for delivering the OPG's role in safeguarding vulnerable adults, as the Mental Capacity Act 2005 introduced a statutory duty for the Public Guardian to supervise, investigate concerns and regulate Court appointed Deputies. The policy is supported by the OPG's Safeguarding Vulnerable Adults Procedures and Guidance document. The protocol for joint working outlines the respective roles that the OPG, the Court of Protection and local authorities play in adult protection, ensuring that areas of overlap can be harmonised. The agencies will work together to help prevent and respond to abuse, by sharing information and following principles laid down in the guidelines. To view the policy, protocol and guidelines see the OPG website.[52]

Sexual relations and related issues

Implicit in the concept of normalisation is the view that those suffering from learning disabilities should be able to participate in sexual activity according to their mental understanding. See the case of *Local Authority X v MM*[53] discussed above in relation to the mental capacity to consent to having sexual relations.

Protection by the criminal code

The law protects those who do not have the capacity to give consent to sexual intercourse. It was an offence for a man to have unlawful sexual intercourse with a woman who is a defective under the Sexual Offences Act 1956, section 7. This has now been repealed and replaced by the criminal offences under the Sexual Offences Act 2003. It was a defence if a man is able to prove that he did not know and had no reason to suspect that the woman was defective. In the case of *R v Hudson*,[54] the Court of Criminal Appeal allowed the appeal of the defendant against conviction on the grounds that a subjective test should have been applied to determine whether he had reason to suspect this.

The Sexual Offences Act 2003 repealed the provisions of section 128 of the Mental Health Act 1959 which made it an offence for a man on the staff of or employed by a hospital or mental nursing home to have extra-marital sexual intercourse with a woman who is receiving treatment for mental disorder in that hospital or home either as an out-patient or an in-patient.

Under the Sexual Offences Act 2003 the following offences are created in relation to carers:

- Section 38 Care worker: sexual activity with a person with mental disorder
- Section 39 Care worker: causing or inciting sexual activity
- Section 40 Care worker: sexual activity in the presence of a person with mental disorder
- Section 41 Care worker: causing a person with a mental disorder to watch a sexual act.

Section 42 includes in the definition of care worker a person who has functions in a home in the course of employment which have brought him or likely to bring him into regular face to face contact with the person with mental disorder. The definition also covers the situation where the patient is receiving NHS independent hospital or clinic services and the person has functions to perform in the course of employment. Those who have regular face to face contact with B as a result of providing care, assistance or services to him in connection with his mental disorder, whether or not in the course of employment also come within the definition.

Sexuality training

The practical problem for carers is on the one hand protecting a person with learning disabilities from abuse and exploitation, and on the other hand ensuring that where the capabilities exist the client should enjoy the rights set out in Figure 22.2. Thompson has looked at the issue of sexuality training in occupational therapy for people with a learning disability[55] and followed up the draft policy which was started four years before for use in sexuality training in occupational therapy. He also provides a useful summary of the law relating to sexual relations. OTs should be aware of the importance of protecting vulnerable people who may not have the capacity to consent and who may be exploited in sexual relationships. It is also important to ensure that they are protected against the risk of AIDS/HIV or other infections.[56] Preventing pregnancy is only one aspect of safe sex.

Emily White and Rosemary Barnitt[57] undertook a collaborative study on intimate relationships of eight adults with learning disabilities. They concluded that seven of the eight interviewed had a positive attitude towards intimate relationships and anticipated that their current partner would stay with them forever. Whilst they felt supported by family members, sexual activity was not discussed between the interviewees and their parents and sex education was provided through education sources for four subjects. (See Chapter 26 for research involving adults with mental incapacity.)

The right to procreate

The rights set out in Figures 22.1 and 22.2 relate only to the client; no other person's rights are affected. However, the right to procreate involves the rights of the future child. There is considerable debate as to whether a person with severe learning disabilities has a right to procreate.[58]

Sterilisation

As the result of the case of *Re D* in 1976[59] (where a mother sought a declaration that her daughter, a sufferer of Sotos Syndrome, could be sterilised), it became a requirement that those seeking a non-therapeutic sterilisation (i.e. one which was not required for the physical health of the patient) should first obtain a declaration of the court. In this case the judge refused to permit the sterilisation of a girl of 11 years since it was not established that the child would not have the ability to make a decision for herself at a later date. On the other hand, in Jeanette's case[60] the House of Lords gave its approval to the sterilisation of a girl of 17 years who suffered from learning disabilities and her parents consented to the sterilisation. In the case of *Re F*[61] (see earlier), the House of Lords declared that it would be lawful to sterilise a woman who lacked the capacity to consent if it were in her best interests and the doctors acted according to the Bolam test.

The situation is now covered by either the Children Act 1989 or the Mental Capacity Act 2005. Where the person is under 16 years an application for sterilisation would be made to the Family Division of the High Court. Where the person is over 18 years an application could be made to the Court of Protection. A young person or 16 or 17 could be referred to either court as appropriate. If there is a request from a relative that the client be sterilised then the professional should raise this issue with the multi-disciplinary team and ensure that, if necessary, an application is made to the appropriate court. The decision to sterilise an individual is one of the most significant which can be taken and it is essential that any health professional who is involved in the court proceedings and the evidence which is required should follow the principles considered in Chapter 13. The Code of Practice on the Mental Capacity Act (issued by the Department of Constitutional Affairs and now available from the website of the DCA's successor, the Ministry of Justice[62]) notes in paragraph 8.22:

> that cases involving non-therapeutic sterilisation will require a careful assessment of whether such sterilisation would be in the best interests of the person who lacks capacity and such cases should continue to be referred to the court.

In the case of *Re A* a mother applied for a declaration that a vasectomy was in the best interests of A, her son, (who had Down's syndrome and was borderline between significant and severe impairment of intelligence), in the absence of his consent. After balancing the burdens and benefits of the proposed vasectomy to A, the Court of Appeal held that the vasectomy would not be in A's best interests.[63]

Abortion

A person with learning disabilities who has the capacity to give a valid consent could sign the form for an abortion to be carried out provided that the requirements of the Abortion Act 1967 (as amended by the Human Fertilisation and Embryology Act 1990) are met. Where the adult with learning disabilities lacks competence, then the Mental Capacity Act 2005 would now apply. The Code of Practice paragraphs 6.18–6.19 points out that some treatment decisions are so serious that they must be made by the Court and it includes within this category termination of pregnancy in certain circumstances. The court has also given guidance on when certain termination of pregnancy cases should be brought before the court.[64]

Refusal to partake in activities

The care of those with learning disabilities should be aimed at ensuring the maximum autonomy and decision making by the clients. However, difficulties have arisen over the refusal of the client to take part in work and industrial therapy activities. The situation has been made more difficult, since the payment of Disability Living Allowance reduces the incentive which the small payment for taking part in these activities might have played in the past. There is no power to compel clients to take part in any activities arranged for them. It may be possible as part of a treatment plan to build in incentives for the client to be involved and thus encourage participation.

Property and exploitation

The duty of care owed by the health professional to care for a client would also include a duty of care in relation to any property of the client. Where the client has the capacity to look after his own property, then the health professional does not become responsible for that property unless it has been specifically entrusted to her care or unless the client has become incapacitated and cannot care for the property herself.

However, special precautions have to be taken in the care of those with learning disabilities who may be vulnerable to exploitation and who may not have the capacity to care for their own property. Any moneys belonging to the client and handled by staff must be strictly accounted for and records kept. Facilities should be provided for cash or other valuables to be safely stored, and care should also be taken to prevent one client misappropriating property belonging to another. (See further discussion on liability for property in Chapter 10.)

The new Court of Protection set up in October 2007 has a remit to make decisions on behalf of mentally incapacitated adults in respect of personal welfare and property and financial decisions. A deputy could be appointed to make decisions in relation to any property or financial interests of an adult lacking mental capacity. The jurisdiction of the Court of Protection is normally restricted to those over 16 years but where it is anticipated that the lack of the requisite mental capacity could continue beyond 16 years then it can hear cases involving persons who are younger than 16 years. For example if a child was severely injured in a road accident which led to serious brain damage and received a payment for several million pounds as a consequence the Court of Protection could hear an application relating to his case since the disability will persist beyond 16 years.

Direct payments

Those with learning disabilities may be entitled to receive direct payments to purchase services for their care and support their independent living. Direct payments are considered in detail in Chapter 18.

Future Strategy

The White Paper *Valuing People* in 2001[65] set out the aim of investing at least £1.3 million a year for the next three years to develop advocacy services for people with learning disabilities in partnership with the voluntary sector in order to enable people with learning disabilities to have as much choice and control as possible over their lives and the services and support they receive. The eligibility for direct payments was to be extended through legislation. In addition a national forum for people with learning disabilities was to be set up to enable them to benefit from the improvement and expansion of community equipment services now under way. New guidance on person-centred planning was to be issued with resources for implementation through the Learning Disability Development Fund.

In spite of the White Paper, a scandal was reported in Cornwall where significant failings were found at Buddock Hospital (a unit for 14 patients with severe disabilities). The Healthcare

Commission carried out a national audit of learning disability services and then consulted on a 3 year plan.[66] The 3 year plan envisaged:

- audit of all inpatient care being provide for learning disability service users across the NHS and independent sector, including commissioning arrangements
- investigation into long-stay hospitals to ensure that they are providing a safe and acceptable service
- review of the care of people with LD who are placed outside their local area away from family and friends
- increasing the accessibility of the Commission's services so that people with a learning disability can better raise complaints and concerns about their care
- establishing champions at the regional offices of the Healthcare Commission responsible for monitoring services for people with a disability.

In December 2006 as a result of the Equality Act, public bodies were placed under a new disability equality duty to ensure that their organisations had a policy to identify and eradicate discrimination against disabled people. Public authorities are required to carry out six duties:

- to promote equality of opportunity between disabled and other persons
- to eliminate discrimination that is unlawful under the DDA 1995
- to eliminate harassment related to their disabilities
- to promote positive attitudes
- to encourage participation in public life and
- to take account of their disabilities, even where that involves them more favourably than other persons.

It remains to be seen how effective this duty is in relation to those with learning disabilities.

Conclusions

The implementation of the Mental Capacity Act 2005 and the changes to the Mental Health Act 1983 made by the Mental Health Act 2007 should provide greater clarity for those caring for persons with learning disabilities. Undoubtedly questions and uncertainties are likely to emerge as the new legislation is implemented and it is hoped that the Court of Protection will provide ongoing review of the workings of the MCA. The Care Quality Commission replacing the Mental Health Act Commission should also monitor the effects of the amended Mental Health Act.

The strategy set out in the White Paper Valuing People should in theory lead to the appropriate resources being made available for this client group. The follow up consultation document, Valuing People Now should result in the implementation of the policy remaining a high priority for the Department of Health. The consultation recognised that strong local and national leadership would be required over the next three years to ensure the vision became a reality. In addition the establishment of a new multi-inspection agency in the form of the Care Quality Commission (see Chapter 17) should reinforce appropriate standards of care in health and social care settings. MENCAP[67] is a useful source for further information on good practice, standards of care and many other aspects in the care of those with learning disabilities. The regulation of children's services moved from CSCI to the Office for Standards in Education, Children's Services and Skills (Ofsted) in 2007 (see Chapter 23).

Questions and exercises

1 It is suggested that one of your clients with learning disabilities should go for a week's holiday at the sea-side. In carrying out a risk assessment for this client, what aspects would you take into account?

2 The mother of a girl with severe learning disabilities who is now 13 years old has asked you to assist in ensuring that she will be sterilised as soon as possible. What action would you take and what advice would you give the mother?

3 You are aware that one of your clients with learning disabilities, who lives in a community home and who has a private income from a family trust fund, is extremely generous with his money and is being exploited by the other residents. What action would you take and what is the law?

4 What are the implications of the Mental Capacity Act 2005 for the making of decisions on behalf of those who have severe learning disabilities? (See Chapter 7.)

References

1   Gates, B. (2003) *Learning Disabilities: Towards Inclusion*, 4th edn. Churchill Livingstone, Edinburgh.
2   Department of Health (2001) *Valuing People: A new strategy for learning disability for the 21st century*. White Paper CM 5086. DH, London.
3   Hessler, I. & Kay, B. (1993) Chapter 13. In: *Learning Disabilities: A Handbook of Care* (eds S. Eamon & S. Thomas) 2nd edn. Churchill Livingstone, Edinburgh.
4   Goodman Jane, Hurst Jenni Locke Christopher (2009) *Occupational Therapy for People with Learning Disabilities*. Churchill Livingston, Edinburgh.
5   Sellers Carol (2002) *Risk Assessment in people with learning disabilities*. Blackwell, Oxford.
6   *X and Y v London Borough of Hounslow* [2008] EWHC 1168 (QB) 23 June 2008.
7   *X and Y v London Borough of Hounslow* [2009] EWCA Civ 286.
8   HSG(92)42 Development of health services for people with learning disabilities.
9   Department of Health (1997) *The New NHS – Modern Dependable*. DH, London.
10 Department of Health (1998) *Modernising Social Services*. DH, London.
11 Department of Health (1999) *Saving Lives: Our Healthier Nation*. DH, London.
12 Department of Health (1998) *Signposts for Success*. DH, London.
13 HSC 1999/103; LAC (99)17 *Once a Day: A Primary Care Handbook for People with Learning Disabilities* (1999) DH, London.
14 Department of Health (2001) *Valuing People: A new strategy for learning disability for the 21st century*. White Paper CM 5086. DH, London.
15 HSC 2001/016; LAC (2001)23 *Valuing People: a New Strategy for Learning Disability for the 21st Century: implementation*.
16 Department of Health (2001) *White Paper: Valuing People A New Strategy for Learning Disability for the 21st Century*. CM 5086. The Stationery Office, London.
17 Department of Health (2007) White Paper *Valuing People now – from progress to transformation – a consultation on the new three years of learning disability policy*. DH, London.
18 HM Government (2009) Summary of Responses to the Consultation on Valuing People Now: from progress to transformation.
19 Department of Health (2005) *Green Paper; Independence, Well-being and Choice*. DH, London.
20 Department of Health (2006) *Our Health, Our Care, Our Say: A New Direction for Community Services*. DH, London.
21 Department of Health (2007) *Independence, Choice and Risk: a Guide to Best Practice in Supported Decision Making*. DH, London.

22   Michael, Jonathan (2008) Healthcare for all: report of the independent inquiry into access to healthcare for people with learning disabilities. DH, London. iahpld.org/uk/healthcare.final.

23   Corbett Jo (2007) *Health provision for people with learning disabilities – a guide for health professionals*. Wiley, Chichester.

24   Knapp, M.B. & Slade, C.L. (1984) Sexuality and the developmentally delayed teenager. In: N. Fulgate-Woods (ed) *Human Sexuality*. Mosby, London.

25   Joint Committee on Human Rights *A Life like Any Other? Human Rights of Adults with Learning Disabilities* Seventh Report of session 2007–8 HL Paper 40-1/HC73-1; www.publications.parliament.uk

26   Government Response to the Joint Committee on Human Rights: A Life Like Any Other? Human Rights of Adults with Learning Disabilities Cm 7378 The Stationery Office.

27   www.publications.parliament.uk

28   Department of Health (2006) *Human Rights and equality of opportunity Bamford Review of Mental Health and Learning Disabilities*. DH, London.

29   College of Occupational Therapists (1995) *Statement on Occupational Therapy Services for Clients with Learning Disabilities*, SPP 115A. COT, London.

30   College of Occupational Therapists (2007) *Professional Standards for Occupational Therapy Practice*. COT, London.

31   College of Occupational Therapy (2003) *Occupational Therapy services for adults with learning disabilities*. COT, London.

32   College of Occupational Therapy (2004) *Guidance on Learning and Disability*. COT, London.

33   Bracher, M. (2000) Therapeutic horse riding: What has this to do with occupational therapists? *British Journal of Occupational Therapy*, **63**(6), 277–82.

34   Sellars, C. (2002) *Risk Assessment with People with Learning Disabilities*. Blackwell, Oxford.

35   *HL v United Kingdom* [2004] ECHR 720 Application No 45508/99 5 October 2004; Times Law Report 19 October 2004.

36   Department of Health (2006) Briefing Sheet Bourne wood November 2006 Gateway Reference 6794.

37   Ministry of Justice and Department of Health (2008) *Impact assessment of the Mental Capacity Act 2005 – deprivation of liberty safeguards to accompany the code of practice and regulations*. Ministry of Justice, London.

38   The Mental Capacity (Deprivation of Liberty: Appointment of Relevant Person's Representative) Regulations 2008 SI No 1315.

39   Code of Practice Mental Capacity Act 2005 Department of Constitutional Affairs February 2007 available on the website of the Ministry of Justice www.justice.gov.uk.

40   The Mental Capacity Act 2005 (Independent Mental Capacity Advocates)(Expansion of Role) Regulations 2006 SI 2006/2883.

41   Dimond, B. (2008) *Legal Aspects of Mental Capacity*. Blackwell, Oxford.

42   *F v West Berkshire Health Authority and another* [1989] 2 All ER 545; also reported as Re F.

43   Law Commission (1995) Report No. 231 *Mental Incapacity*. HMSO, London.

44   Lord Chancellor's Office (1997) *Who Decides?* HMSO, London.

45   *R v Bournewood Community and Mental Health NHS Trust, ex parte L.* (HL) reported in *The Times* 30 June 1998, [1998] 3 All ER 289.

46   *HL v United Kingdom* [2004] ECHR 720 Application No 45508/99 5 October 2004; Times Law Report 19 October 2004.

47   *Local Authority X v MM* [2007] EWHC 2003 Fam.

48   *Re M B (Caesarian Section)* [1997] 2 FLR 426; [1997] 2 FCR 541; The Times Law Report, 18 April 1997.

49   Code of Practice Mental Capacity Act 2005 Department of Constitutional Affairs February 2007 Paragraph 8.56.

50   www.justice.gov.uk.

51   Department of Health and Welsh Assembly Government Mental Capacity Act Update Edition 20 February 2009.

52   www.publicguardian.gov.uk/about/843.htm

53   *Local Authority X v MM* [2007] EWHC 2003 Fam.

54   *R v Hudson* [1965] 1 All ER 721 (CCA).

55   Thompson, S.B.N. (1994) Sexuality training in occupational therapy for people with a learning disability, four years on, policy guidelines. *British Journal of Occupational Therapy*, **57**(7), 255–8.

56   Royal College of Nursing/Society of Mental Handicap Nursing (1991) *AIDS – a proactive approach to mental handicap*. Scutari Press, Harrow.

57   White, E. & Barnitt, R. (2000) Empowered or discouraged? A study of people with learning disabilities and their experience of engaging in intimate relationships. *British Journal of Occupational Therapy*, **63**(6), 270–76.

58   Dimond, B.C. (1988) Ethical and legal issues raised by the sterilisation of the mentally handicapped. MA thesis. University College Swansea.

59   *Re D (a minor) (wardship: sterilisation)* [1976] 1 All ER 326.

60   *Re B (a minor) (wardship: sterilisation)* [1987] 2 WLR 1213.

61   *F v West Berkshire Health Authority and another* [1989] 2 All ER 545; also reported as Re F.

62   www.justice.gov.uk

63   *Re A (medical treatment: male sterilisation)* (1999) 53 BMLR 66.

64   *D v An NHS Trust (Medical Treatment: Consent: Termination)* [2004] 1 FLR 1110.

65   Department of Health (2001) *White Paper: Valuing People A New Strategy for Learning Disability for the 21st Century*. CM 5086. The Stationery Office, London.

66   Healthcare Commission (2005) *Three year plan for adults with learning disabilities*. Stationery Office, London.

67   www.mencap.org.uk/

23 Care of Babies, Children and Young Persons

This chapter sets out the law relating to the care and rights of children, considers some situations which could arise and identifies some of the special situations which arise when OTs are caring for children. The BMA has published guidance on the rights of the child and young person, which considers both the legal and ethical issues.[1] A book edited by Chia Swee Hong and Lynne Howard[2] considers occupational therapy in childhood and includes a chapter on bereavement and ME. A book edited by Sylvia Rodger and Jenny Ziviani considers the roles, occupations and participation of children in order to enhance the purpose and value of OT.[3] An edited work explores the more specialist area of children with rheumatic disease.[4] An explanation of the Children Act 1989 is provided by Caroline Gibson et al.[5]

The following topics are covered in this chapter:

- Rights of the child
- Children Act 1989
- Child protection
- Children and Family Court Advisory and Support Service (CAFCASS)
- Protection of vulnerable adults and children
- Corporal Punishment
- Carers and Disabled Children Act 2000

- Discrimination in Education
- Consent by child: child/parent disputes
- Confidentiality of child information
- Access of the child to health records
- Standards in the care of children
- National Service Frameworks
- Health and safety and the child
- Research using children

Rights of the child

Like any other person a child could bring an action against a public authority alleging violation of his human rights as set out in the European Convention of Human Rights (see Appendix 1). Article

Legal Aspects of Occupational Therapy, Third Edition By Bridgit Dimond
© 2010 Bridgit Dimond

14 gives a right not to be discriminated against in the implementation of the rights set out in other Articles, and whilst age is not specifically mentioned this could be a reason for discrimination and therefore unlawful under Article 14. In addition, a child can draw on the United Nations Convention on the Rights of the Child. Whilst this has not been incorporated into UK law and is not therefore directly enforceable in the UK, compliance by the signatories is monitored by the United Nations on a biennial basis and the UK is warned about any failures of compliance. (See the report by the Joint Committee of the House of Lords and House of Commons on the UK observation of the Convention which was published in June 2003.[6]) In addition, there are many other charters which have been drawn up by charities and organisations caring for children and these would have persuasive force in that they indicate good practice, while they do not in themselves set down laws which can be enforced.

Children Act 1989

The Children Act 1989 set up a new framework for the protection and care of children and established clear principles to guide decision making in relation to their care. The principles that the court should take into account are shown in Figure 23.1. The overriding principle is that:

> The child's welfare shall be the court's paramount consideration.

The involvement of the child in the decision making is also a major principle and Figure 23.2 sets out the considerations that the court should take into account in making certain orders. Finally, in deciding whether or not to make an order, the court

> shall not make the order or any of the orders unless it considers that doing so would be better for the child than making no order at all.

Whilst the considerations set out in Figure 23.2 apply to specific decisions to be made under the Children Act 1989, there is good reason for the practitioner to follow these same considerations in the general care of the child.

Figure 23.1   Principles of the Children Act 1989.

(1) The welfare of the child is the paramount consideration in court proceedings.
(2) Wherever possible children should be brought up and cared for in their own families.
(3) Courts should ensure that delay is avoided, and may only make an order if to do so is better than making no order at all.
(4) Children should be kept informed about what happens to them, and should participate when decisions are made about their future.
(5) Parents continue to have parental responsibility for their children, even when their children are no longer living with them. They should be kept informed about their children and participate when decisions are made about their children's future.
(6) Parents with children in need should be helped to bring up their children themselves.
(7) This help should be provided as a service to the child and his family, and should:
    (a) be provided in partnership with parents;
    (b) meet each child's identified needs;
    (c) be appropriate to the child's race, culture, religion, and language;
    (d) be open to effective independent representations and complaints procedures; and
    (e) draw upon effective partnership between the local authority and other agencies including voluntary agencies.

Figure 23.2   Circumstances to be taken into account by the court under the Children Act 1989 – section 1(3).

(a)   the ascertainable wishes and feelings of the child concerned (considered in the light of his age and understanding);

(b)   his physical, emotional and educational needs;

(c)   the likely effect on him of any change in his circumstances;

(d)   his age, sex, background and any characteristics of his which the court considers relevant;

(e)   any harm which he has suffered or is at risk of suffering;

(f)   how capable each of his parents, and any other person in relation to whom the court considers the question to be relevant, is of meeting his needs;

(g)   the range of powers available to the court under this Act in the proceedings in question.

The National Association of Paediatric Occupational Therapists (NAPOT) (now the special section of children, families and young people) of the COT published a guide to the Children Act 1989.[7] It sets out simply and clearly the main principles of the Act and the key issues including a welfare checklist, parental responsibility and the court system, and discusses possible implications of the Act for occupational therapists. There is also a useful glossary. The COT in conjunction with its specialist section for children, families and young people has also published guidance and briefing notes on the National Service Framework and on Every Child Matters[8] and other topics of concern. They can all be down loaded from the COT website.

The House of Lords held that where care proceedings under the Children Act 1989 were being held, the test to be used was the civil test of the balance of probabilities. Care proceedings were there to protect the child from harm. The consequences for the child of getting it wrong were equally serious either way.[9]

The duties and powers of the local authority under the Chronically Sick and Disabled Persons Act 1970 (see Chapter 20) can be combined with those under the Children Act 1989. For example in the case of *R (on the application of BG) v Medway Council*,[10] the Court held that the funding by the local authority to provide adaptations to the family home to provide for a disabled child was reasonable. The boy was three years old with severe mental and physical disabilities, including 4 limb cerebral palsy, epilepsy, asthma, and sleep problems. He needed assistance with all aspects of daily living and mobility. The family was suffering from sleep deprivation because there was insufficient space to cater for his needs. Adaptations were required to create more space , so that he could have his own room, and for more storage space for his equipment and to provide room for his treatment such as daily physiotherapy. The adaptations would cost £65,000. The LA planned to meet the shortfall in the costs of the works remaining after the maximum available disability facility grant (DFG) by a loan secured on the home, which would be discharged after 20 years without any requirement for repayment. The loan was subject to conditions, so that the authority would not seek repayment unless the claimant ceased to live at the home during these 20 years. The father sought judicial review of the conditions on the loan. The court held that the relevant conditions were not unreasonable.

Resources are relevant in any question relating to the statutory duties of the LA. For example in the Tandy case parents brought an application to review a reduction in the hours of home tuition from 5 to 3 hours per week. They won in the High Court but the local authority's appeal succeeded. The Court of Appeal applied the ruling in the Gloucester case[11] (see Chapter 20) where the House of Lords accepted that resources were relevant in fulfilling a statutory duty. The Court of Appeal held that the authority was justified in balancing the individual's requirements against the cost of making arrangements.[12]

Specific issue order

This is the procedure where action is to be taken rather than prevented, for example in a dispute between parents over adaptations for a disabled child. A situation could arise where adaptations are required for a child under the Housing Acts (see Chapter 20); the parents live in different houses but the local authority is only prepared to pay for adaptations to one house. How is such a dispute resolved?

Either parent could take the case to court for a specific issue order and for a declaration from the court as to which parent was entitled to have the adaptations in his or her house. Obviously account would be taken of where the child was likely to want to spend most time and which parent, if any, had a residence order. (It would of course be possible, funds permitting, for an individual parent to pay for the second house to be adapted as well.)

In the following case,[13] the father applied to the local authority for assistance as a homeless person, but the LA decided that he was not in priority need of housing and that it was only in very exceptional cases that a child might be considered to reside with both parents.

Case: *Holmes-Moorhouse v Richmond upon Thames London Borough Council* [2007]

The father and mother had separated and a consent order was made by the family court that the father would leave the property of which the mother was the sole tenant. Both parents were to have a shared residence with the 3 younger children who would spend alternate weeks with the parents and half of each school holiday. The Court of Appeal held that once the court had made a residence order, it was not open to the local housing authority to take the view that the child was only staying with the father (as opposed to residing with him), even though the order was obtained by consent. The Court quashed the authority's decision and the father's application was to be reconsidered in the light of the court's decision.

A useful book on Housing and Disabled Children has been published by the Joseph Rowntree Foundation[14]

Children in need

Section 17 of the Children Act 1989 places a general duty on the local authority in relation to children in need.

It shall be the duty of every local authority (in addition to the other duties imposed on them by this Part):

a. to safeguard and promote the welfare of children within their area who are in need; and
b. so far as is consistent with that duty, to promote the upbringing of such children by their families,

by providing a range and level of services appropriate to those children's needs.

This section was considered by the House of Lords in three appeals[15] over the responsibilities of local authorities for the accommodation of children who were in need.

Cases: *R (on the application of A) v Lambeth London Borough Council; R (on the application of G) v Barnet London Borough Council* and *R (on the application of W) v Lambeth Borough Council* [2003]

The claimants' case was that S.17(1) required a local social services authority to assess the needs of a child who was in need, and to meet his needs when they had been assessed. They also considered whether a local authority might insist on providing accommodation for a child alone, as distinct from a child and his mother, when a child was in need of accommodation and it would cost no more to provide accommodation for both of them. The first appeal concerned two children who were in need because they were disabled, in the other two appeals, the children were in need because their mothers, with whom they were living, were homeless. The House of Lords held in a majority judgment that Section 17(1) did not impose on local social services a duty to meet the assessed needs of a child. The section set out duties of a general character which were intended to be for the benefit of children in need in the local social services authority's area in general. Although the services under S 17 could include the provision of accommodation, the provision of residential accommodation to re-house a child in need so that he could live with his family was not the principal or primary purpose of the legislation. Housing was the function of the local housing authority, for the acquisition and management of whose housing stock detailed provisions were contained in the Housing Acts. The LA could insist on providing accommodation for a child alone. A LA is entitled to adopt a general policy under which it is made clear that it will make accommodation available to the children of the family in order to prevent the children becoming homeless, but will not permit parents to use the children as stepping stones by means of which to obtain a greater priority to be re-housed than that to which they would otherwise be entitled.

In another dispute over section 17 of the Children Act 1989 and section 2 of the Chronically Sick and Disabled Persons Act 1970 and the provision of services to a child in need, the claimant argued that the local authority had failed to act reasonably and infringed the article 8 rights of the child Z.[16] Z suffered from Sanfilippo a disease like juvenile dementia which was degenerative and life limiting. Her mother was her sole carer and an independent review recommended a care plan which suggested that the mother should no longer remain the primary carer and that there should be 2 carers around the clock. The plan was rejected by the Council and the mother on behalf of the child claimed that this action amounted to Wednesbury unreasonableness (the Wednesbury[17] case laid down the principle that the court will intervene to prevent or remedy abuses of power by public authorities if there is evidence of unreasonableness or perversity.) The High Court judge analysed the independent review and concluded that the Council had not acted unreasonably in deciding that the current care plan was adequate nor did he find any breach of article 8 in that there was no evidence that the disabled person was not so circumscribed and so isolated as to be deprived of the possibility of developing his personality.

Child protection

The key statute is the Children Act 1989 and Department of Health guidance on the Act is available from the DH website.[18] Reference could also be made to a book about occupational therapy for child and adolescent mental health.[19] Chapter 15 in that book covers child protection legislation. The Audit commission has published guidance on preventing unintentional injury to children[20]

The importance of a knowledge of child protection principles and practice by the OT cannot be overstated. Where a practitioner is concerned that a child, or the sibling or child of one of her patients, is being abused, whether physically, sexually or mentally, she should take immediate action to ensure that this is drawn to the attention of the appropriate persons. For example, the practitioner may notice bruising, signs suggesting cigarette burns or other scars. She may also see a parent inflicting severe corporal punishment on a child and consider that action should be taken. This means that she must be familiar with the provisions for child protection and who are the persons to be contacted. It is not always easy to decide if action is necessary, and the practitioner should see as her main priority the safety of the child. As the guidelines on inter-agency co-operation state:[21]

> The difficulties of assessing the risk of harm to a child should not be underestimated. It is imperative that everyone who deals with allegations and suspicions of abuse maintains an open and inquiring mind. (Paragraph 1.13)

Should the practitioner be wrong in her fears, and it appears that there is no abuse, her name could not be divulged to the parents[22] (see below). Nor, if her actions were reasonably taken in the best interests of the child, would a parent have a right of action against her.[23] (See below). Abuse may include an over zealous dietary or religious regime. For example a 12-year-old girl was brought up on a strict vegan diet and was admitted to hospital with a degenerative bone condition said to have left her with the spine of an 80-year-old woman.[24]

Procedure for the management of child abuse

In May 2003 the Department of Health launched a single source document for safeguarding children, with the aim that all agencies would be working from the same succinct set of advice.[25] The publication was the result of one of the recommendations of the Laming Inquiry which investigated the circumstances surrounding the death of Victoria Climbié.[26] The Inquiry made over 100 recommendations for future practice by health and social services. A Green Paper *Every Child Matters* was published by the Department of Health in September 2003 (see the COT Guide[27]). The Green Paper focused on four main areas:

- supporting parents and carers
- early intervention and effective protection
- accountability and integration – locally, regionally and nationally
- workforce reform.

The new single source booklet set out:

- What people should do if they have concerns about children.
- What will happen once they have informed someone about those concerns.
- What further contribution they may be asked or expected to make to the process of assessment, planning and working with children, reviewing that work and how they should share that information.
- Some basic information and background about the legislative framework within which children's welfare is promoted and safeguarded.

There should be in existence an agreed procedure for the management of child abuse cases in accordance with the national guidelines, and the practitioner should be acquainted with this. The procedure should specifically refer to the role of the department if child abuse is suspected. This would require any professional staff working in the department who suspect that there is a possibility of ill-treatment, serious neglect, sexual or emotional abuse of a child, to inform the senior practitioner in charge of the department who should then contact a consultant paediatrician. If the paediatrician confirms the possibility of abuse, then the paediatrician should inform the Social Services Department immediately.

Inter-agency co-operation

There used to be in each local authority area a forum to ensure co-operation between all the agencies involved in the protection of children at risk. This forum was known as the Area Child Protection Committee (ACPC). On this forum there would be representatives of the medical and nursing services. There were also advantages in having representatives from professions allied to medicine. This representation would be at a senior level and there would be a designated senior professional for child protection within the hospital or community unit. Subsequently significant changes were made to Child Protection Provisions as a result of the Green Paper *Every Child Matters* and the enactment of the Children Act 2004. A Children's Commissioner was appointed and each local authority was required to appoint a Director of Children's Services, covering education and child welfare. Information is available from the website of the Department for Children, Schools and Families[28] and from the specific website set up by the Department of Health for child protection.[29]

Children Act 2004

The Children Act 2004 provides the legal underpinning for *Every Child Matters* and its provisions are shown in Figure 23.3 and was followed by the publication Working together to safeguard Children.[30] Significant features of the Children Act 2004 include the new Local Safeguarding Children's Boards (which each local authority is required to set up under section 13), and the duty on local authorities to appoint a director of children's services and a lead member for children's services. The Local Safeguarding Children Boards, (LSCB) which came into being on 1 April 2006, are designed to ensure that the agencies work effectively together to protect children. The old area child protection committees which they replace are in effect placed on a statutory footing. The core

---

Figure 23.3   Main Provisions of Children Act 2004.

Part 1 Children's Commissioner

Part 2 Children's services in England: Co-operation to improve well-being
Arrangements to safeguard and promote welfare
Information databases
Local Safeguarding Children Boards:
establishment, functions, procedure and funding;
Children and young people's plans
Director of children's services
Lead member for children's services
Inspections of children's services

Part 3 Children's Services in Wales

Part 4 Advisory and support services for family proceedings

membership includes local authorities, health boards, the police and others. Guidance on the functioning of the LSCBs is obtainable on the Every Child Matters website.[31] The guidance is incorporated as chapter 3 of Working Together to Safeguard Children which was published in 2006. The guidance describes the LSCB as "the key statutory mechanism for agreeing how the relevant organisations in each local area agree to co-operate to safeguard and promote the welfare of children in the locality and for ensuring the effectiveness of what they do".

Advice for LSCBs on safeguards for protecting disabled children was published in February 2006.[32] Disabled children are more vulnerable to abuse or neglect than non-disabled children. The resource is intended to help those with a strategic or planning responsibility for children understand their particular needs and consider how best to safeguard and promote their welfare. Supplementary guidance has also been published for LSCBs on safeguarding children in whom illness is fabricated or induced.[33]

Following the Lord Laming inquiry into the death of Victoria Climbié the Joint Chief Inspectors reported on safeguarding arrangements for children and young people in England. The regulation of children's services moved from CSCI to the Office for Standards in Education, Childrens Services and Skills (Ofsted) in 2007. This Office reviews the work of local safeguarding children boards.

Failures since the Children Act 2004

In spite of the changes following the Children Act 2004 serious failings in protecting children have still arisen, of which the most infamous Baby P is considered below. A baby girl died at 54 days old after she was abused and then murdered by her father. She may have been saved had 30 health and social services staff not missed vital signs that she was being ill-treated.[34] In May 2008 Khyra Ishaq, 7 years old, apparently starved to death, despite an initial welfare check on the family in January 2008. Her mother and her partner were accused of causing or allowing her death contrary to section 5 of the Domestic Violence, Crime and Victims Act 2004. The House of Lords criticised the fact that the Housing Services and the Children's services did not communicate with each other in a case brought by a girl of 18 who was held not to be entitled to further council support in her own right. She had been provided with accommodation by the LA's housing department but had not come to the attention of the children's services department and so was not entitled to further support.[35] The Housing Department should have referred her to the children's services so that she would have become a relevant child for the purposes of the duties of the children's department. The Court of Appeal held that there was no breach of the mother's right to a fair hearing under article 6 of the European Convention on Human Rights when she was represented by the Official Solicitor in a case concerning a care order for her child. The Court of Appeal held that the Official Solicitor was right to concede that the threshold criteria under section 31 of the Children Act 1989 were satisfied and that a care order was in the child's best interests.[36] The employment checks required for those who work with children and vulnerable persons are considered in Chapter 19.

Baby P

Baby P died in Haringey as a result of appalling abuse, despite being seen on over 60 occasions by health professionals, social services staff, police and others. He was known to be at risk. The Director of Children's Services was dismissed. Lord Laming was invited to report on the failings which had led to Baby P's death. Lord Laming's report[37] published on 12 March 2009 put forward 52

Figure 23.4   Recommendations from Lord Laming's Report in March 2009.

National agency to oversee reform implementation. Cabinet minister responsible for
    success;
Social work students must get child protection training and work experience before starting
    their job;
Increased quality of degrees; introduction of a children's social worker postgraduate
    qualification;
Court fees for applying to take children into care should be scrapped if they affect
    decisions;
Ofsted inspectors examining children's social services to have child protection experience;
A national strategy to address recruitment problems;
Guidelines on case-loads;
Directors with no child protection experience should appoint an experienced social work
    manager to support them.

---

recommendations for improving child protection services, some of which are shown in Figure 23.4.
It was also hoped that the £4,000 court fee (a rise from £125) introduced in May 2008 for taking a
child into care would be scrapped. In February 2009 it was reported that two thirds of hospitals fail
to conduct routine checks on injured children suspected of being at risk, despite warnings after the
death of Baby P.[38] The Healthcare Commission was expected to publish a review of the situation
shortly.

There have been many official reports into the circumstances surrounding the death of Baby P.
Two have been carried out by Haringey Council itself; the Audit Commission on children's services
reported on 4 March 2009 and Laming report on Baby P was published on 12 March 2009.

The Healthcare Commission investigation on the NHS care surrounding Baby P was published
by the Care Quality Commission in May 2009.[39] This report found systematic errors in how the NHS
Trusts dealt with the case of Baby P and made recommendations to the Trusts involved. These
included:

● The NHS Trusts should ensure that their staff are clear about child protection procedures and
  have received safeguarding training to an appropriate level.
● A sufficient number of appropriately qualified paediatric staff should be available when required,
  in line with established guidelines.
● The adequacy of consultant cover should be reviewed at one hospital.
● All 4 NHS Trusts need to establish clear communication and working arrangements with relevant social services departments and, in particular, ensure that there is no delay in establishing
  contact between agencies once a safeguarding referral has been made to social services.
● The trusts must ensure that appropriate arrangements are in place to enable:
  ○ safeguarding supervision
  ○ staff to attend multi-agency child protection case conferences
  ○ appropriate training to be undertaken
  ○ signing off the trusts' own declarations against core standards, assuring themselves that they
    can do so and do so adequately.

The Baby P case shows that co-ordination between the various services involved meant no-one
took control and that there were serious failures by doctors and health visitors to detect evidence

of non-accidental injuries. There were also poor links between health and social services. As a consequence of Government action all children's services directors will be sent for compulsory training in the realities of frontline social work under plans to drive up standards in child protection announced on 13 March 2009.[40] A course will be created at the National College for School Leadership.

Criticism of the care system was made by the cross party Children, Schools and Families Select Committee on 20 April 2009. The Committee called for a new national framework of fees and allowances for foster parents who look after about two thirds of the 60,000 children in the care system, in order to attract and retain better families. Other criticisms related to the fact that many children left care at 16 years, encouraged by local authorities on financial grounds yet this was the time when they could go off the rails, and of the lack of training of staff in care homes. Care should become a positive experience for the child.

ContactPoint has a database of 11 million children in England see Chapter 12.

If the doctor disagrees with the practitioner

The practitioner should ensure that any concerns are made known to a senior member of the department who should decide whether it is appropriate to bring a consultant paediatrician in to see the child. It is important to ensure that the practitioner records in writing all the facts which have given rise to the suspicions and fears, and keeps a copy of this document. If the consultant subsequently takes the view that there is no abuse, the practitioner has to accept this but should remain vigilant about the safety of the child and continue to report any further concerns. Unfortunately, insufficient attention is often given to the views and evidence of non-medical staff and particularly non-registered staff. Louis Blom-Cooper pointed out in his Report on the Investigation of Jason Mitchell,[41] that vital information about the patient's mental condition was ignored by the multi-disciplinary team because it was reported by an occupational therapy assistant (see Chapter 10). Assertion skills and determination are obviously essential if there is a conflict over suspected abuse.

The practitioner's duty of confidentiality

Certain apparent breaches of confidentiality are justified by most health professional organisations where it is necessary to protect the welfare of the patient or to prevent harm, or it is justified in the public interest. If the practitioner is in doubt, then advice should be sought. The Caldicott Guardian and the lawyers to the NHS trust would be able to advise on the legality of breaching confidentiality in exceptional circumstances (see Chapter 8). Any reasonable suspicion of child abuse should be notified to the appropriate agencies without fear of a successful action for breach of confidentiality by the parents. If a suspected case is reported to the police, social services or NSPCC and it turns out that the suspicions are unfounded, the parents have no right to be given the name of the person reporting them. The House of Lords has held that it is not in the public interest for such information to be disclosed to the parents.[42]

Errors in suspecting child abuse

The local authority has a duty of care to ensure that children are protected and if necessary taken into care. This is considered in Chapter 10. However the House of Lords has held that there is no right of action by parents, where children have been taken into care as a result of suspected child abuse, which has subsequently been shown not to exist.[43] In this case in East Berkshire, a mother was suspected of Munchausen's syndrome by proxy when her son suffered from allergic reactions following birth and he was placed on the 'at risk' register. However, it was subsequently discovered that he did have allergy problems. The mother claimed compensation on the grounds that the original diagnosis was made negligently. The House of Lords held that it would not be fair, just or reasonable to impose a duty of care on a doctor in respect of a negligent clinical diagnosis where there was a concurrent and potentially conflicting duty of care towards a child patient. No duty of care was owed to the parents. The East Berkshire case was followed where a father of a child, who had been suspected of sexual abuse, brought a claim against the local authority. It was held that a duty of care was not owed by the social workers to the parents where the children were the subject of an investigation, whether the social workers were carrying out operational functions such as interviewing or relaying the results of the interview, or evaluating evidence and deciding whether intervention was necessary.[44] These rulings must however be reviewed in the light of the decision of the European Court of Human Rights that parents could win damages when the baby was taken into care following medical diagnosis.[45] The facts of the case were that the baby aged two months was taken into hospital with a fractured femur. The doctors considered that it was a non-accidental injury and she was placed in the care of her aunt. Following another fracture, the doctors diagnosed brittle bone disease. The ECHR held that there was no breach of the parents Article 8 rights, since the doctors had acted reasonably in concluding that it was a non-accidental injury and took the appropriate action following the second fracture. However the ECHR held that there had been a violation of Article 13, which guaranteed an effective remedy before a national authority. The applicants should have had available to them a means of claiming that the local authority's handling of the procedures was responsible for any damage which they suffered and of obtaining compensation for that damage. Compensation of £8,000 was ordered. In December 2008 a couple, whose 3 children spent two years in care, received an undisclosed six figure sum in compensation.[46] The couple were completely exonerated of any abuse in October 2006 and subsequently Newport City Council agreed to give a full written apology and pay compensation.

In April 2009 the family courts were opened to the media, though the courts would still have the power to impose reporting restrictions. The onus was on the judge to restrict the press only if absolutely necessary.

The Integrated Children's System (ICS) (replacing child protection registers)

In Working Together to Safeguard Children the Government stated that child protection registers would be phased out by 1 April 2008 and replaced by the Integrated Children's System (ICS) Each local authority is required to ensure that its local ICS is able to use data from the ICS child protection plans. The ICS has been developed to improve outcomes for children defined as being in need, under the Children Act 1989. It provides a conceptual framework, a method of practice and a business process to support practitioners and managers in undertaking the key tasks of assessment, planning, intervention and review. It is based on an understanding of children's developmental needs in the context of parental capacity and wider family and environmental factors. It is supported by an electronic case record system. A key aim of ICS is to provide frontline staff and their managers with the necessary help, through information communication technology, to record, collate, analyse and output the information required. Further information on the ICS and the technical details are available from the website of every child matters.[47] The aims of ICS are set out in Figure 23.5. All authorities were required to have the ICT support for all new referrals in place by 1 January 2006 and to be fully operational by 1 January 2007.

> **Figure 23.5** Aims of the Integrated Children's System (ICS).
>
> - All practitioners and managers, responsible for children in need, should work in accordance with the ICS conceptual framework, from case referral to case closure
> - Assessments of children in need should be completed with the necessary detail and within the required timescales
> - Case-based information should be aggregated through computer systems into management information, required for day-to-day service planning
> - All practitioners should feel they are supported in their work by working directly with Information Communication Technology (ICT) systems that support ICS

If the abuse is not confirmed by the consultant

If the consultant is not able to confirm that a child who was of concern to an OT has been subjected to abuse, and there were no medical grounds for requiring the child to be detained in hospital, then the parent could not be stopped from taking the child home. However, there should be arrangements in place for all such concerns to be notified to the appropriate health visitor or school nurse and also to the appropriate general practitioner and for ongoing monitoring of the child.

If a suspected child abuse is confirmed by the consultant paediatrician

The agreed procedures and the inter-agency arrangements should be followed immediately. The provisions of the Children Act 1989 enable the following orders to be made: section 43 (child assessment order); section 44 (Emergency protection order); and section 46 (Removal and accommodation of children by police in cases of emergency).

For further details of these sections and the other provisions of the Children Act 1989, reference should be made to the Department of Health guides to the Children Act 1989.[48]

Removal and accommodation of children by police in cases of emergency – section 46

This section enables the child to be taken in to police protection. Where a constable believes that a child would be likely to suffer significant harm he may remove the child to suitable accommodation and keep him there. He may also take reasonable steps to ensure that the child's removal from hospital, or any other place in which he is being accommodated, is prevented. The section, once invoked, lasts a maximum of 72 hours.

A new scheme is being piloted by Community Service Volunteers in Bromley and Sunderland with volunteers who do not have a social work background working with the families of children on the at-risk register.[49]

Working together to safeguard children[50]

This publication is a guide to inter-agency working to safeguard and promote the welfare of children. It replaces the publication *Working Together under the Children Act 1989* published in 1991. It highlights the duties in the Children Act 1989 which require inter-agency co-operation:

Section 27 enables a local authority to request help from any local authority; any local education authority; any local housing authority; any health authority; and any person authorised by the Secretary of State or in Wales, the National Assembly.

Children and Family Court Advisory and Support Service (CAFCASS)

In April 2001 as a result of the Criminal Justice and Court Services Act 2000, the Children and Family Court Advisory and Support Service (CAFCASS) was established as a non-departmental public body responsible to the Lord Chancellor to look after the interests of children involved in family court proceedings. The new service combines the Family Court Welfare Service, the Children's Branch of the Official Solicitor's Department, and Guardian ad Litem and Reporting Officer services previously provided by local authorities. Guidance[51] by the Department of Health emphasises that CAFCASS should be included as a core member of each Area Child Protection Committee. Annex B to the circular provides revised guidance on complaints about the functioning of child protection conferences and amends paragraphs 5.71–5.73 of *Working Together to Safeguard Children*.[52]

The Children and Family Court Advisory Support Service (Cafcass) has been criticised in Ofsted inspection reports. In the first Ofsted inspection of Cafcass in the East Midlands, Ofsted held that the Cafcass operation was inadequate and child safety was compromised on numerous occasions[53] and it had failed to protect children who are involved in divorce and separation cases.[54] Criticism was also made about a new protocol for managing child-care cases which has onerous requirements and the new court fee of £4,000 (from £150) for taking children into care, which appears to have led to a fall in care order applications by a third[55] and was criticised in the Laming Inquiry of 2009 (see above).

Protection of vulnerable adults and children

Various measures have been taken in law to prevent those who are likely to abuse children from having contact with them. The Protection of Children Act 1999, the Sexual Offenders Act 1997 and the Care Standards Act 2000 enable employers to establish if there are grounds for not employing prospective employees. These are considered in Chapter 19.

Corporal punishment

A case heard by the European Court of Human Rights ruled that severe corporal punishment by a stepfather to discipline his stepson was a breach of Article 3 of the European Convention on Human Rights.[56] The stepfather had on several occasions beaten a 9-year-old boy with a garden cane. The stepfather had been prosecuted for assault occasioning actual bodily harm, but had been acquitted by the jury who had accepted his defence that the caning had been necessary and reasonable to discipline the boy. The European Court of Human Rights held that ill-treatment must attain a minimum level of severity if it is to fall within the scope of Article 3. It depended on all the circumstances of the case, such as the nature and context of the treatment, its duration, its physical and mental effects and in some instances, the sex, age and state of health of the victim (these factors are known as the reasonable chastisement test). In finding that there had been a breach of Article 3 in this case, it awarded the boy £10 000 against the UK Government, and costs. The UK Government acknowledged that the UK law failed to provide adequate protection to children. Subsequently a consultation document[57] was issued by the Government on a range of proposals relating to the physical punishment of children. The analysis of the responses was published in November 2001.[58] The Government's policy was against any change of law at that time and favoured a common sense approach, in 'the need to balance the needs of children with the reality of the difficulties of parenting'.[59] The use of the reasonable chastisement test would be kept under review by the Department of Health. The Joint Committee of House of Lords and House of Commons,[60] in monitoring the UK compliance with the UN Convention on the Rights of the Child, considered that the retention in the UK of the defence of 'reasonable chastisement' is incompatible with the provisions of Article 19 of the Convention.

Subsequently the Children Act 2004 was enacted. Section 58 states that battery of a child cannot be justified on the ground that it constituted reasonable punishment.

S.58(1) In relation to any offence specified in subsection (2) below, battery of a child cannot be justified on the ground that it constituted reasonable punishment.

(2) The offences referred to in subsection (1) are:

a. an offence under section 18 or 20 of the Offences against the Person Act 1861 (wounding and causing grievous bodily harm)

b. an offence under section 47 of that Act (assault occasioning actual bodily harm)

c. an offence under section 1 of the Children and Young Persons Act 1933 (cruelty to persons under 16).

(3) Battery of a child causing actual bodily harm to a child cannot be justified in any civil proceedings on the ground that it constituted reasonable punishment.

(4) For the purposes of subsection (3) "actual bodily harm" has the same meaning as it has for the purposes of section 47 of the Offences against the Person Act 1861.

(5) In section 1 of the Children and Young Persons Act 1933, omit subsection (7).

(section 1(7) made any parent or person having lawful control or charge of a child to administer punishment an exception of the offence of assaulting or wilfully ill treating a child.)

The effect of this section is that a parent who causes harm to her or his child and is prosecuted under the Offences Against the Person Act sections 18, 20 or 47 or under the Children and Young Persons Act 1933 section 1 cannot use as a defence that the battery constituted reasonable punishment. The same applies in civil proceedings where actual bodily harm is caused.

In 2007 the Children's Commissioner for England called for a complete ban on smacking children[61] as a consultation on the effect of the change in the law was initiated. As a result of the review the Children's Minister ruled out a total ban on smacking children in 26 October 2007.[62] In April 2009 a boy of 8 years was taken into care after his mother admitted that she had hit him with a hairbrush.[63]

Carer's (Recognition and Services) Act 1995

This Act placed a duty upon a local authority to respond to a request for a carer assessment, when undertaking an assessment of the child.

Section 1(2) states that in any case where a local authority assesses the needs of a disabled child for the purposes of Part III of the Children Act 1989 or section 2 of the Chronic Sick and Disabled Persons Act 1970, and the carer provides or intends to provide a substantial amount of care on a regular basis for the disabled child the carer may request the local authority, before they make their decision as to whether the needs of the relevant person call for the provision of any services, to carry out an assessment of his ability to provide and to continue to provide care for the disabled child. If such a request is made, the local authority shall carry out such an assessment and shall take into account the results of that assessment in making that decision.

This does not apply where the carer provides services under a contract of employment or as a volunteer for a voluntary organisation.

Carers and Disabled Children Act 2000

This Act gives a right to carers to be assessed and enables the local authority to provide services to carers following such an assessment. Under the Act, vouchers can be issued by local authorities for short-term breaks and direct payments to carers in lieu of services which they have been assessed as needing. A person with parental responsibilities for a disabled child has the right to an assessment, from a local authority under section 6, of his ability to provide care for the child. The local authority must take that assessment into account in deciding what services to provide under section 17 of the Children Act 1989. Vouchers and direct payments to disabled children and to persons with parental responsibility for disabled children can be made under section 7 of the Carers and Disabled Children Act. Regulations relating to the vouchers came into force on 29 May 2003.[64] These state that the value of a voucher may be expressed in terms of money or the delivery of a service for a period of time (time vouchers) but not both. Rules are laid down on the issue and redemption of vouchers. In an early decision on the Act, a judge stated that on the facts of the case an assessment should be carried out within 35 days.[65] (See below.) (See Chapter 18 for further discussion on the rights of the carer and on direct payments.)

Case: assessment of needs of a child

J, a 7-year-old boy with autism and challenging behaviour, sought judicial review of the local authority's refusal to carry out an assessment of his needs. He had been accepted as homeless and placed in temporary accommodation together with his family. There was no indication of when the family might be moved to permanent accommodation. J's mother had difficulties in coping with his care. The local authority took the view that an assessment should not be carried out as the family could be moved to permanent accommodation, with the result that an assessment at the present time would be an inappropriate use of its resources.

The judge allowed the application and said that the assessment should be carried out within 35 days. J's mother could not be expected to cope without support other than for a short period. As there was no likely date for J's move to permanent accommodation, there was no basis for delaying the assessment required by section 6 of the Carers and Disabled Children Act 2000.

Action by victim of child abuse

The European Court of Human Rights recently held that where the local authority failed to protect children from sexual abuse by the stepfather, the local authority was in violation of Article 3 and Article 13 and was held liable to pay damages.[66] In another case, the European Court of Human Rights held that there was no violation of Article 3 by the local authority, but there was a failure to provide an appropriate means of obtaining a determination of their allegations and therefore a breach of Article 13.[67] (Article 13 is not included in Schedule 1 of the Human Rights Act 1998 (see

Appendix 1).) The court has a discretion to dispense with the time limits set by the Limitation Act 1980 and this discretion can be used in determining the date of knowledge test (see Chapter 10) under section 14 of the Limitation Act 1980 in cases of sexual abuse. In another case against a local authority, this time by a couple who adopted a violent child, the couple won their case that they should have been notified by the LA of the boy's serious and emotional behavioural difficulties.[68] The court held that the local authority could be held vicariously liable for negligence by its employees in failing to fulfil their duty of care owed to those who might foreseeably be injured if the duty was carelessly exercised.

Discrimination in education

Part IV of the Disability Discrimination Act 1995 covers discrimination in education and has been amended by the Special Educational Needs and Disability Act 2001. (For other provisions of the Disability Discrimination Act, see Chapters 18 and 19.) Annual school reports are required to include information as to:

(a)   the arrangements for the admission of disabled pupils
(b)   the steps taken to prevent disabled pupils from being treated less favourably than other pupils
(c)   the facilities provided to assist access to the school by disabled pupils (section 29(2)).

Under section 30 of the Disability Discrimination Act 1995, the conditions under which financial support is given to further and higher education institutions:

(a)   shall require the governing body to publish disability statements at such intervals as may be prescribed, and
(b)   may include conditions relating to the provision made, or to be made, by the institution with respect to disabled persons.

A disability statement means a statement containing information or a prescribed description about the provision of facilities for education of disabled persons by the institution (section 30(3)).

Codes of Practice have been published covering discrimination in education, one for schools and for the over 16-year-olds. The Code of Practice for schools[69] covers the following areas:

- The duties: who is covered, who is responsible, what activities are covered
- What is discrimination? Less favourable treatment
- What is discrimination? A failure to make reasonable adjustments
- Lack of knowledge defence and confidentiality
- Redress and conciliation in Scotland, England and Wales
- Other duties under the Disability Discrimination Act 1995
- Relationship with other legislation and responsibilities
- Appendix One The meaning of disability
- Appendix Two Definitions of disability under other legislation
- Appendix Three Publications and useful addresses.

There are two key duties involved in ensuring that schools do not discriminate against disabled pupils:

- not to treat disabled pupils less favourably
- to take reasonable steps to avoid putting disabled pupils at a substantial disadvantage.

This latter duty is known as the 'reasonable adjustments' duty.

The Code of Practice states that the duties in the Disability Discrimination Act are designed to dovetail with existing duties under the Special Educational Needs (SEN) framework. The main purpose of the SEN duties is to make provision to meet the special educational needs of individual children. A child has special educational needs if he or she has a learning difficulty which calls for special educational provision (section 312 of the Education Act 1996). A child has a learning difficulty if he or she:

- has a significantly greater difficulty in learning than the majority of children of the same age or
- has a disability which prevents or hinders the child from making use of educational facilities of a kind generally provided for children of the same age in schools within the area of the LEA or
- is under five and falls within either of the two above definitions or would do so if SEN provision was not made for the child.

Special education provision means:

- for a child of two or over, educational provision which is additional to, or otherwise different from, the educational provision made generally for children of the child's age in maintained schools (other than special schools) in the area
- for a child under two, educational provision of any kind.

The SEN framework consists of the primary legislation, the regulations, and the guidance. The statutory duties that form the core of the SEN framework in England and Wales are set out in Part 4 of the Education Act 1996, as amended by the SEN and Disability Act 2001. The rest of the framework is provided by the Education (Special Educational Needs) (England) (Consolidation) Regulations 2001, the Education (Special Educational Needs) (Wales) Regulations 2002, the Education (Special Educational Needs) (Information) (England) Regulations 1999, the Education (Special Educational Needs) (Information) (Wales) Regulations 1999, the Special Educational Needs (Provision of Information by Local Education Authorities) (England) Regulations 2001, the Special Educational Needs (Provision of Information by Local Education Authorities) (Wales) Regulations 2002, and guidance, including the Special Educational Needs Code of Practice and Inclusive Schooling – Children with Special Educational Needs 2001. In Wales, regulations and guidance, including the SEN Code of Practice for Wales, are provided separately by the National Assembly for Wales.

The SEN framework makes an increasing assumption that children with special educational needs will be educated in mainstream schools. Amendments to section 316 of the Education Act 1996 (by section 1 of the SEN and Disability Act 2001) strengthen the general duty to provide a mainstream school place for a child with special educational needs where their parents want that, and so long as that is compatible with the efficient education of other children. The Secretary of State, in England, and the National Assembly for Wales, provide guidance on the operation of the amended section 316 and new section 316A.

Within this framework, which increasingly emphasises inclusion and parental participation, the SEN duties require local education authorities, maintained schools and others to identify, assess and make provision for children's special educational needs. The SEN Codes of Practice in England and the SEN Code of Practice for Wales support schools and local education authorities in interpreting their duties under the SEN framework.

The disability duties in Part 4 of the Disability Discrimination Act are designed to dovetail with existing duties under the SEN framework.

Special Educational Needs and Disability Act 2001

As mentioned above, this Act makes significant changes to the rights of the disabled child within the context of education. Its contents are shown in Figure 23.6.

Schedules to the Special Educational Needs and Disability Act cover Amendments to Statement of Special Educational Needs: the Procedure and Appeals; definitions of the responsible bodies for schools and educational institutions; and amendments and modifications to the Disability Discrimination Act 1995, the Disability Rights Commission Act 1999 and other legislation.

The occupational therapist may be involved in assessments and preparing reports for the Special Educational Needs Tribunals. She should follow the principles of report writing set out in Chapter 13 and ensure that she is able to support her written report if called upon to be a witness at the tribunal. The OT may be concerned as to whether the statement should include what the child would need in an ideal world in contrast to what therapies could realistically be provided by the OT service. If only the latter are included in the statement, then there would be no recognition of the opportunities which additional resources could provide for the child. Resources are relevant to the provision of appropriate services, but it may be helpful to identify the further services which would be of value to the child. It may be that services which one OT department finds to be beyond its resources, are provided as basic in another part of the country. Figures 23.7–14 set out the provisions of the Education Act and Code of Practice in relation to Special Educational Needs.

Figure 23.6   Special Educational Needs and Disability Act 2001.

Part 1 Special educational needs: mainstream education, general duties of Local Education Authorities, appeals, identification and assessment of educational needs

Part 2 Disability Discrimination in Education: Chapter 1 Schools; Chapter 2 Further and Higher Education

Part 3 Supplementary

Figure 23.7   S. 19(1) Education Act 1996.

Each local education authority shall make arrangements for the provision of suitable full time or part time education at school or otherwise than at school for those children of compulsory school age who, by reason of illness, exclusion from school or otherwise, may not for any period receive suitable education unless such arrangements are made for them.

Figure 23.8   S.19(4) Education Act 1996.

The local education authority may make arrangements for the provision of suitable full time or part time education otherwise than at school for those young persons who, by reason of illness, exclusion from school of otherwise, may not for any period receive suitable education unless such arrangements are made for them.

Figure 23.9   Children with special educational needs.

- Meaning of 'special educational needs' and 'special educational provision' etc. – section 312 Education Act 1996
- Code of Practice – sections 313 to 314
- Special educational provision – sections 315 to 320
- Identification and Assessment of children with special educational needs – sections 321 to 332
- Special Educational Needs Tribunal (SENT) – sections 333 to 336 (now SENDIST)
- Special Schools and Independent Schools – sections 337 to 348
- Variation of deeds (changing a school's constitution) – section 349

Figure 23.10   Definition of special educational needs – section 312 Education Act 1996.

(1) For the purposes of the Education Acts, a child has 'special educational needs' if he has a learning difficulty which calls for special educational provision to be made for him.
(2) For the purposes of this Act, subject to subsection (3) below, a child has a 'learning difficulty' if—
    (a) he has a significantly greater difficulty in learning than the majority of children of his age;
    (b) he has a disability which either prevents or hinders him from making use of educational facilities of a kind generally provided for children of his age in schools within the area of the local education authority; or
    (c) he is under compulsory school age and is, or would be if special educational provision were not made for him, likely to fall within paragraph (a) or (b) when over that age.

[The definition of child includes any person who has not attained the age of nineteen years and is a registered pupil at a school]

Figure 23.11   Code of Practice on special educational needs and assessment.

(1) Principles and Policies
(2) Working in partnership with parents
(3) Pupil participation
(4) Identification, assessment and provision in early education settings
(5) Identification, assessment and provision in the primary phase
(6) Identification, assessment and provision in the secondary sector
(7) Statutory Assessment of Special Educational Needs
(8) Statements of special educational needs
(9) Annual Review
(10) Working in partnership with other agencies

Annex A   The Education (Special Education Needs) Regulations 2001
           The Education (SEN)(Provision of Information by Local Education Authorities)
           Regulations 2001
           The Education (SEN) Regulations 1999
Glossary

Figure 23.12   Fundamental principles in the Code of Practice.

- A child with special educational needs should have their needs met
- The special educational needs of children will normally be met in mainstream schools or settings
- The views of the child should be sought and taken into account
- Parents' have a vital role to play in supporting their child's education
- Children with special educational needs should be offered full access to a broad, balanced, and relevant education, including an appropriate curriculum for the foundation stage and the National Curriculum

Figure 23.13   Critical success factors in the Code of Practice.

- **The culture, practice, management and deployment of resources in a school or setting are designed to ensure** all children's needs are met
- **LEAs, schools and settings work together to ensure that any child's special educational needs are** identified early
- **LEAs, schools and settings exploit** best practice **when devising interventions**
- **Those responsible for special educational provision take into account** the wishes of the child **concerned, in the light of their age and understanding**
- **Special education professionals and** parents **work in** partnership
- **Special education professionals take into account the** views of individual parents **in respect of** their child's particular needs
- **Interventions for each child are** reviewed regularly **to assess their impact, the child's progress and the views of the child, their teachers and their parents**
- **There is close co-operation between all the agencies concerned and a** multi-disciplinary approach **to the resolution of issues**
- **LEAs make assessments in accordance with the** prescribed time limits
- **Where an LEA determines a child's special educational needs, statements are** clear and detailed, **made within** prescribed time limits, specify monitoring arrangements, **and are** reviewed annually.

(Bold as in the Code of Practice)

Consent by child: child/parent disputes

Chapter 7 covers the basic principles relating to trespass to the person and the importance of obtaining the consent of the patient. This section deals with the specific laws relating to consent by or on behalf of the child or young person (i.e. a person under 18 years of age).

The child of 16 and 17

A child of 16 or 17 has a statutory right to give consent to treatment under section 8(1) of the Family Law Reform Act 1969. This is shown in Figure 23.15, together with the definition of treatment under

Figure 23.14   Exceptions to disclosure of statements of special educational needs requiring the consent of the child under the SEN Regulations 2001 Regulation 24.

The consent of the child is required to disclosure of the statement except:

- To persons to whom, in the opinion of the authority concerned, the statement should be disclosed in the interests of the child.
- For the purposes of any appeal under the Act.
- For the purposes of educational research which, in the opinion of the authority, may advance the education of children with special educational needs. This may be done if, but only if, the person engaged in the research undertakes not to publish anything contained in or derived from, a statement otherwise that in a form which does not identify any individual concerned, including in particular the child concerned and his or her parents.
- On the order of any court or for the purpose of any criminal proceedings.
- For the purposes of any investigation under the Local Government Act 1974 Part III (investigation of maladministration).
- To the Secretary of State when he requests disclosure to decide whether to give directions or make an order under Section 496, 497 or 497A of the Education Act 1996.
- For the purposes of an assessment of the needs of the child with respect to the provision of any statutory services for him being carried out by officers of a social services authority under section 5(5) of the Disabled Persons (Services, Consultation and Representation) Act 1986.
- For the purposes of a local authority performing its duties under the Children Act 1989.
- To Her Majesty's Inspectors.
- To the Connexions Service for the purposes of writing or amending a transition plan
- To a Young Offender institution for the purposes of the performance of its duties under rule 38 of the Young Offender Institution Rules 2001

Figure 23.15   The Family Law Reform Act 1969 – section 8.

(1)   The consent of a minor who has attained the age of 16 years, to any surgical, medical or dental treatment, which in the absence of consent, would constitute a trespass to the person, shall be as effective as it would be if he were of full age; and where a minor has by virtue of this section given an effective consent to any treatment it shall not be necessary to obtain any consent for it from his parent or guardian.
(2)   In this section 'surgical, medical or dental treatment' includes any procedure undertaken for the purposes of diagnosis and this section applies to any procedure (including, in particular, the administration of an anaesthetic) which is ancillary to any treatment as it applies to that treatment.
(3)   Nothing in this section shall be construed as making ineffective any consent which would have been effective if this section had not been enacted.

section 8(2). The definition of treatment under section 8(2) would probably cover most treatments given by a health practitioner where these are under the aegis of a doctor. Care provided by an occupational therapist would be included in this definition.

Section 8(3) (see Figure 23.15) covers two situations: the giving of consent by a parent on behalf of a child of 16 or 17 years and the giving of consent by a child below 16 years.

Overruling a young person's refusal

The fact that a young person of 16 or 17 has a statutory right to give consent to treatment does not mean that they cannot be compelled to have treatment or that their refusal cannot be overruled. The Court of Appeal in the case of *Re W*[70] upheld the decision of the High Court judge to order a child of 16 years who was suffering from anorexia nervosa to undergo medical treatment against her will. Clearly, overruling a child or young person's refusal is an extremely significant step and would only occur in very serious circumstances of a life-saving kind.

The child under 16

The parent has a right at common law to give consent on behalf of the child. In addition, as a result of the House of Lords ruling in the Gillick case,[71] a child under 16 years who has sufficient under-standing and intelligence to be capable of making up his own mind could give a valid consent to treatment. As a result of this case we have the term 'Gillick competent' which signifies a child who has the maturity and competence to make a decision in the specific circumstances arising. (The term 'Competent according to Lord Fraser's guidelines' is occasionally used instead of 'Gillick compe-tent'.) The Court of Appeal applied the Gillick principle to a case where parents were not informed that an abortion was to be carried out on a competent girl under 16 years.[72] The COT has prepared a briefing note on Gillick competence and consent.[73]

In life-saving situations, however, it is unlikely that the child under 16 years would be able to make a decision contrary to his or her best interests. In the case of *Re M*[74] a girl of 15 years refused to have a heart transplant which was essential for her survival. The parents sought an injunction from the court that the transplant operation could proceed and this was granted in the best interests of the child. In contrast when Hannah Jones, who was terminally ill with leukaemia, refused a heart transplant on the grounds that she would prefer to die with dignity, her parents respected her wishes and despite doctors reporting the case to the child protection officers, no application was made to court to enforce a transplant. After interviewing the child the child protection officer accepted that her wishes should prevail.[75] (Several months later it was reported that she had changed her mind and agreed to the transplant)

Even where the child and parents both agree that treatment should not be given, as in the case of a Jehovah's Witness family, the court can order treatment to proceed if it is considered to be in the best interests of the child (case of *Re E* (1993)).[76]

Situation: referral by paediatrician

> A child of 12 years is referred by the paediatrician for occupational therapy. She is being looked after by a relative as her parents were abroad. Is consent necessary and if so who gives it?

Only in extreme emergencies would a clinician act without consent from those with parental respon-sibilities or from a competent child in order to take life saving action on behalf of a child. In this situ-ation the 12-year-old child may have the mental capacity as defined in the Gillick case to give consent to the therapy. Alternatively the relative who brings the child to the clinic can give consent under the provisions of section 3(5) of the Children Act 1989. This states that a person who (a) does not have parental responsibility for a particular child, but (b) has care of the child, may (subject to the provision of this Act), do what is reasonable in all the circumstances of the case for the purpose of safeguarding or promoting the child's welfare.

Giving information to children and young persons

As can be seen from the discussion in Chapter 7, information giving is part of the duty of care and therefore in order that both the child/young person or the parent can understand the implications of giving consent to treatment, they need to be told the significant risks of substantial harm which could occur and also the existence of alternative treatments or even of no treatments. The British Medical Association publication,[77] which considers the rights of the child, emphasises the importance of ensuring that appropriate information is given to the child or young person. For example, in a study of families experienced in caring for children with chronic arthritis, Carrie Britton[78] shows that there was a wide variation in the understanding about the aims and methods of exercise and splinting programmes. She concludes that improvements in compliance could arise from greater *mutual* understanding and shared information between therapist and family.

Disputes between parents

Those who have parental responsibilities are the married parents of the child, the unmarried mother, or the father of the child who has not married the mother (or married her after the birth of the child), but only where he has assumed the rights of a parent by ensuring that the necessary papers were completed. Even when parents are divorced or separated, under the Children Act 1989 section 2(1), both parents retain parental responsibility for their children. Under section 2(7), where more than one person has parental responsibility for a child, each of them may act alone and without the other (or others) in meeting that responsibility. Even where one parent has a residence order in his or her favour, the other still retains parental responsibilities and can exercise these to the full. It also follows that one parent does not have the right of veto over the other's actions. If, however, there has been a specific order by the court relating to a decision affecting the care or treatment of the child, then a single parent cannot change this or take any action which is incompatible with this order unless the approval of the court is obtained.

It therefore follows that if there is a dispute between parents over treatment decisions in respect of the child, either can go to court for a specific issue or prohibited steps order to be made.

Prohibited steps order

Where one parent wishes to prevent the other taking action which he or she does not consider is in the interests of the child, he or she may seek a prohibited steps order. This can be ordered under section 8 of the Children Act 1989 and means that no step which could be taken by a parent in meeting his parental responsibility for a child, and which is of a kind specified in the order, shall be taken without the consent of the court. Thus if one parent feared that the other was likely to agree to a daughter with learning disabilities being sterilised, then that parent could obtain a prohibited steps order preventing consent being given without the consent of the court.

If the child is considered to be 'Gillick competent' and disagreed with actions which the parents were intending, the child could seek the leave of the court to obtain a prohibited steps order. The child would have to apply to the Family Court.[79] The court must be satisfied that the child has sufficient understanding to make the proposed application (section 10(8)).

In a recent case[80] the Court of Appeal declared that it was lawful for Siamese twins to be separated, even though the operation would necessarily involve the death of the twin who was dependent on the heart and the lungs of the other for survival. The Court of Appeal held it was lawful for doctors to carry out the operation to separate the twins. The court concluded that the operation would give J the prospects of a normal expectation of relatively normal life. The operation would shorten M's life but she remained doomed for death. M was alive because she sucked the life blood out of J. She would survive only as long as J survived. The operation could be carried out under the doctrine of necessity. The essential elements of that doctrine were all satisfied: (1) the act was needed to avoid inevitable and irreparable evil; (2) no more should be done than was reasonably necessary for the purpose to be achieved; and (3) the evil inflicted must not be disproportionate to the evil avoided. The court held that its decision was not in conflict with Article 2 of the European Convention on Human Rights.

The parents were given leave to appeal to the House of Lords but decided not to do so. The operation was carried out: M died and J survived.

Parents' refusal

In what circumstances could parental refusal to consent to occupational therapy be overruled? For example, an OT might consider it vital for the social and intellectual development of a child that he should participate in play therapy. In such a situation, parental refusal to allow the child to participate might not be considered so harmful to the child that the Children Act should be invoked. However, where there are fears of serious harm to the best interests of the child because of parental refusal, it is probable that the local authority would be involved and an application could be made to court under the Children Act 1989 for the necessary therapy to be carried out. The parents' refusal could therefore be overruled if the refusal was considered to be contrary to the best interests of the child. Evidence would be required on what was in the child's best interests.

It may be that some therapies are desirable but not absolutely essential and the parents' refusal can be accepted. If this is not so and the therapy is necessary in the best interests of the child, then an application would be made to court for a declaration that it can be lawfully carried out. In such situations there will be examples where it is of life-saving necessity that certain treatments are carried out (for example, failure of parents to give a diabetic child insulin), in which case the appropriate action will be taken and court authorisation obtained. At the other extreme there will be treatments which would have been helpful, but can be omitted without serious harm to the child, and between these two extremes there will be very difficult decisions to make.

Parents' refusal upheld by the courts

In the case of *Re T*[81] the court unusually upheld the parents' refusal to consent to a liver transplant for their baby. The facts were unusual in that the parents lived outside the country and were health professionals. The Court of Appeal upheld the appeal of the parents against the High Court judge's order that the transplant should proceed. The paramount consideration was the welfare of the child and not the reasonableness of the parents' refusal of consent. It must be stressed that *Re T* is a very unusual case and there were very special circumstances which led to the court upholding the wishes of the parents over those of the doctors. OTs should, however, be aware that there may be circumstances where the courts uphold the wishes of parents even when these are contrary to medical opinion. The paramount consideration in all cases will be the welfare of the child. However, any overruling on parental wishes should be subjected to the consideration of the court, as the *Glass* case, discussed below illustrates.

Right to insist on treatment

Parents do not have the right to insist upon care or treatment which the doctors consider is not in the best interests of the child. The court would not order the doctors to carry out treatment on a child which the doctors considered was not in the best interests of the child. See the case of Jamie Bowen discussed in Chapter 6.

Case: A dispute between parents and clinicians: the case of *Glass*[82]

A boy of 12 was severely disabled and the relatives fought with staff to try and prevent morphine being given to him. The relatives resuscitated the boy and the mother sought an application for judicial review from the court, and a declaration on the action that the doctors should take in the future. She appealed to the Court of Appeal against the decision of the High Court refusing judicial review.

The Court of Appeal turned down her appeal and held that it would be inappropriate for the court to grant a declaration to act in anticipation and indicate to doctors at a hospital what treatment they should or should not give in circumstances which had not yet arisen. The best course of action was for the parents and doctors to agree on the course of treatment, but if this were not possible, then the actual circumstances must be brought before the court so that the court could resolve what was in the best interests of the child in the light of the facts existing at that time. There were a number of principles in conflict:

- sanctity of life
- the non-interference by the courts in areas of clinical judgement
- the refusal of the courts to dictate appropriate treatment to a medical practitioner, subject to the powers of the court to act in the best interests of the child
- treatment without consent save in an emergency was a trespass to the person
- the court would interfere to protect the interests of a minor or person under a disability.

How these principles would be applied to particular facts was very difficult to answer and would depend on the actual circumstances of the case, which could not be anticipated. The relatives were subsequently prosecuted for assaulting staff.

Mrs Glass subsequently took her case to the European Court of Human Rights where it was held that the failure of the NHS trust to seek a declaration from the court before administering diamorphine to her son without her consent, and in writing him up for DNR instructions without her knowledge, was a breach of her Article 8 rights.[83]

Confidentiality of child information

The same principles apply in relation to maintaining the confidentiality of information provided by the child patient, as apply to information provided by the adult patient (see Chapter 8). However, there may be situations where the interests of the child require confidential information to be passed on to an appropriate authority. If possible, the consent of the child should be obtained to the disclosure. However, where the child refuses consent, or where the child lacks the capacity to give consent, the practitioner should notify the child of her view that the information should be passed on in the best interests of the child. She should not make a commitment to the child that the confidential information will never be passed on. She should also ensure that she takes advice before breaching confidentiality. She should record the action she has taken and the reasons for it, and be prepared to justify her actions if subsequently challenged.

Access to child health records: by the child

Chapter 9 covers the basic principles which apply to access to records. Here we are concerned with access to records about children. The Data Protection Act 1998 applies to both computerised and manually held records and the provisions of the Access to Health Records Act 1990 are repealed except in relation to the records of dead people. The Data Protection Act 1998 does not make express provision for access by a child, but such an application would come under section 7. Where the child has the capacity, he can apply for access to his personal health data kept in both computerised form and held manually under the Data Protection Act 1998. The Department of Health recommended under the provisions covering the 1984 Data Protection Act[84] that a certificate should be signed in which a responsible adult certifies that the child understands the nature of the application, and this procedure could be followed in implementing provisions of access under the 1998 Act. No definition of the capability of the child is given in the Act but it is submitted that the Gillick test of competence adapted to the specific conditions of access to records would be applied. (This test of competence is discussed above.) Access can be refused if serious harm to the physical or mental health or condition of the patient or another person would be caused, or where a third person (not being a health professional involved in the treatment) who has asked not to be identified would be identified by the disclosure (see Chapter 9).

Access to child health records: by the parent

Under the Data Protection Act 1998, a parent or other relative could apply for access to data and the data controller can comply with the request under section 7(4) if:

(a) The patient has consented to the disclosure of the information to the person making the request, or
(b) it is reasonable in all the circumstances to comply with the request without the consent of the other individual, or
(c) the information is contained in a health record and the other individual is a health professional who has compiled or contributed to the health record or has been involved in the care of the data subject in his capacity as a health professional.

Whether the records are held in computerised or manual form, the application for access can be refused if serious harm would be caused to the physical or mental health or condition of the patient or another person or would identify a third person (not being a health professional involved in the care of the child) who did not wish to be identified.

The Data Protection (Subject Access Modification) (Health) Order 2000[85] prevents the disclosure of information to a person other than the data subject if:

(a) the information was provided in the expectation that it would not be disclosed to the person making the request, or
(b) obtained as a result of any examination or investigation to which the data subject consented in the expectation that the information would not be so disclosed, or
(c) which the data subject has expressly indicated should not be so disclosed.

These provisions apply where the applicant has parental responsibility for the data subject or has been appointed by a court to manage the affairs of a data subject who is incapable of managing his own affairs.

Standards in the care of children

Chapter 10 sets out the principles of law which apply in ensuring that reasonable standards of professional care are provided. This will include multi-disciplinary team working and the rational determination of priorities. Practitioners must ensure that they maintain their competence and that they keep up to date with developments in their field of specialisation. Multi-disciplinary care of the child may involve the use of unorthodox treatments and investigations. However, the practitioner must be aware that there is no legal concept of team liability, and if she acts contrary to the standards of professional competence of a reasonable practitioner, she could not use as a defence that she was carrying out the instructions of the team. If, therefore, a team member proposes an unorthodox treatment or investigation in the care of a child, she must be assured that this complies with the reasonable standards of care and that the parents and/or the child have given consent to the treatment, in the full knowledge that the proposed treatment is not of the usual kind but is in the circumstances justifiable.

Karen Stagnitti and Carolyn Unsworth[86] consider the use of pretend play in child development as an effective means of reducing the participation restrictions that some children experience in learning and social situations. There may be professional differences of opinion over the most appropriate procedure in a given set of circumstances. National criteria based on research of clinically effective practice will always have to be updated in the light of changing developments. The Department of Health has issued guidance for professionals working with disabled children (birth to third birthday) and their families.[87] The guidance is aimed at ensuring a more co-ordinated, family-centred approach to multi-agency working. Twenty-eight pilot projects have been set up as part of the DfES-funded Early Support Pilot Programme. Key themes explored include:

- effective multi-agency family support
- involvement of parents in planning and delivery of services
- better information to parents
- better training to improve professional knowledge and skills
- agreed joint family support plans
- better co-operation between agencies and knowledge of what works well, and where.

Following a consultation exercise, guidance was issued in 2001 to local social services authorities on the social care of deafblind children and adults.[88] Authorities are required to identify, make contact with and keep a record of deafblind people in their catchment area, ensure that assessments are carried out by specifically trained persons, appropriate services are provided, access to specifically trained one-to-one support is ensured and that one member of senior management includes overall responsibility for deafblind services.

National Service Frameworks (NSFs)

The NHS Plan[89] envisaged that National Service Frameworks would be established to improve services through setting national standards to drive up quality and tackle existing variations in care.

The Children's NSF was published in September 2004.[90] Five core standards are set in Part one for the NHS, local authorities and partner agencies to achieve high quality service provision for all children and young people and their parents or carers.

Standard 1: Promoting Health and Well-being, Identifying Needs and Intervening Early

The health and well-being of all children and young people is promoted and delivered through a co-ordinated programme of action, including prevention and early intervention wherever possible, to ensure long term gain, led by the NHS in partnership with local authorities.

Standard 2: Supporting Parenting

Parents or carers are enabled to receive the information, services and support which will help them to care for their children and equip them with the skills they need to ensure that their children have optimum life chances and are healthy and safe.

Standard 3: Child, Young Person and Family-Centred Services

Children and young people and families receive high quality services which are coordinated around their individual and family needs and take account of their views.

Standard 4: Growing Up into Adulthood

All young people have access to age-appropriate services which are responsive to their specific needs as they grow into adulthood.

Standard 5: Safeguarding and Promoting the Welfare of Children and Young People

All agencies work to prevent children suffering harm and to promote their welfare, provide them with the services they require to address their identified needs and safeguard children who are being or who are likely to be harmed.

Part two sets standards for the following areas:

- Children and young people who are ill
- Children in hospital
- Disabled children and young people and those with complex health needs
- The mental health and psychological well-being of children and young people
- Medicines for children and young people

Part three relating to maternity services
Part 3 of the NSF is concerned with Midwifery standards and Standard 11 is as follows:

Women have easy access to supportive, high quality maternity services, designed around their individual needs and those of their babies.

The expansion of that standard identifies:

- woman-centred care services;
- care pathways and managed care networks;
- improved pre-conception care;
- the identifying and addressing of mental health problems;
- choice of options in relation to place of birth;
- professional skilled in neonatal resuscitation at every birth; and
- post-birth care based on a structured assessment provided by a multi-disciplinary team
- breastfeeding information and support for mothers.

The NSF should have a major impact on children's and maternity services in ensuring that minimum standards are implemented. Further information about the NSF is available from the Department of Health website.[91] The use made by the Healthcare Commission (now the Care Quality Commission) of NSFs in its inspections is discussed in Chapter 17 and on the CQC website.[92] Eventually the NSF standards should become part of the Bolam standard of reasonable care (see Chapter 10). In the same way guidelines published by NICE should become the norm. This does not mean however that the guidelines must be followed whatever the circumstances. If the individual circumstances of a particular patient/client suggest that the guidelines are not appropriate then the health professional must follow his or her professional judgment. Clearly clear documentation would be essential to record the justification for not following the national guidance.

The COT published guidance on the NSF in a briefing note in June 2006.[93] Further information on the NSFs is available from the Department of Health website.[94] The NSF on long term conditions which is discussed in Chapter 24 is also relevant to children and young people and the COT has provided a briefing note on it for those special groups.[95] The DH has also provided specialist advice on young persons suffering from complex needs or disabilities.[96]

Health and safety of the child

Contributory negligence and the child

In Chapter 10 the defence of contributory negligence is discussed. This means that if the client is partly to blame for the harm which has occurred, there may still be liability on the part of the professional but the compensation payable might be reduced in proportion to the client's fault. However, where a child has been harmed, any defence of contributory negligence must take into account the fact that a child is less capable than an adult of taking care of him or herself. The courts have been reluctant to find contributory negligence by a child, where an adult is at fault, as the case of *Gough v Thorne*[97] illustrates.

Occupier's liability and a child

Where a child is allowed on to premises the duty of the occupier to ensure that the visitor is reasonably safe takes into account the fact that children will require a higher standard of care than an adult. Thus the Occupier's Liability Act 1957 states:

The circumstances relevant for the present purpose include the degree of care, or want of care, which would ordinarily be looked for in such a visitor, so that (for example) in proper cases:

a.   an occupier must be prepared for children to be less careful than adults ... (section 2(3))

Practitioners must therefore take into account any reasonably foreseeable harm which could arise if children come into their departments or onto their premises.[98]

Children accompanying patients

A duty of care may also be owed under the Occupier's Liability Act 1957 in respect of children who come onto hospital premises with their parents who are the patients. They would also come under the definition of visitors.

Case: glass door injuries[99]

A 13-year-old pupil was injured when she pushed open the right-hand door of double doors comprising glass panes. Her hand slipped from the push plate on to the adjacent panel of glass. The glass shattered causing severe injuries to her right hand and wrist. The County Council was found liable under the Occupiers' Liability Act 1957 and at common law in failing to fulfil its duty of care. It had failed to comply with the BS standards for glass in doors. There was no finding of contributory negligence.

Precautions therefore have to be taken to prevent children harming themselves in OT departments. Doors should be kept locked to prevent trespassers. Special procedures should be in place if patients are accompanied by children. Other examples of potential dangers include:

- Drugs on the cardiac arrest trolley which needs to be accessible in case of an emergency, but kept in a safe place away from children
- Syringes and needles on trolleys
- Fingers sliced by rise and fall floating top tables
- Potentially dangerous equipment used by OTs
- Substances hazardous to health kept in OT departments.

Equipment, car seats and manual handling

Chapters 11 on health and safety, 15 on equipment and 16 on transport cover the basic principles. However caring for children can present specific problems and the following examples are given of OT concerns:

Review of equipment prescribed

If seating or other equipment for a child is provided, and there are no other ongoing issues, should cases be kept open and reviewed regularly, or could they be discharged, just as OT's working with adults do when the prescription has been made? In Chapter 15 it is suggested that when equipment is issued, a decision should be made as to whether and how frequently a review should be undertaken if at all. OTs have to determine what is the reasonable practice to be expected of their profession and standards will depend upon the type of equipment and the characteristics of the client. The Medicines and Healthcare

Products Regulatory Agency (MHRA) may be able to offer advice and feedback from other prescribers of the equipment should assist in determining standards.

Cot sides

If a hospital bed is provided for a child following multi-level surgery or for another short term period, is there an obligation to include integral cot sides with the bed?

The answer to this depends upon what is seen as reasonable occupational therapy practice and this would probably depend upon the age and capacity of the child and the nature of the surgery or reason for hospital stay. Both the National Patient Safety Agency and the MHRA provide advice on cot-sides and beds. The National Association of Paediatric Occupational Therapists may also provide guidelines, or contribute to the development of standards.

Harnesses and car seats

Parents are currently advised by OTs on car harnesses, trikes, and car seats. However, OTs do not have any specific training in these areas and are not deemed competent. Should they be providing this advice and are they putting themselves at risk as they cannot provide the equipment, or would they be at risk if they did not give their knowledge from a positioning the child perspective? Also, if there is only one harness company and therefore only one company that can be recommended, this does not square with the usual advice not to recommend individual companies.

The OT has a personal and professional responsibility to ensure that she is competent and if she is aware of an area in which she is expected to practise in which she is not competent, then she personally must take steps to secure the necessary training and knowledge to fill this gap. Management has a responsibility under both the common law, contract of employment and health and safety laws to ensure that the employee is competent to perform the activities required and therefore there should be support from management for any occupational therapist wishing to develop her professional competence. Special training in the prescribing of equipment to be used by children is essential for the OT. It cannot be assumed that the knowledge obtained from working with adults is necessarily transferable.

The community equipment advisers discussed in Chapter 15 can advise OTs and whether there are alternative suppliers of harnesses. The OT must ensure that the product meets the requirements of the client and if there is a monopoly supplier, negotiations would be required to ensure the necessary standards are met and the price reasonable.

Moving and handling of children

The area of paediatric moving and handling seems to be a bit of a black hole. Discussions may have been held with risk management regarding the fact that the current mandatory moving and handling training, which is adult-directed, is not helpful for paediatric services and there is no specific paediatric moving and handling available.

The principles set out under the Manual Handling Regulations and considered in Chapter 11 apply to all kinds of manual handling: adults, obese patients and also children. The risk assessment must take account of the characteristics of the client which bring specific risks and where necessary specialist training must be provided. There would be no compliance with the statutory responsibilities if manual handling training for adults was given to those who cared for children, without the specific risks of paediatric handling being considered. Paediatric OTs have a responsibility to ensure that they get the appropriate training for their needs.

There is a struggle to get sling and hoist compatibility. For instance, the community loan store might mainly issues the Huntleigh hoists at home, but the universal paediatric sling for this does not meet most children's needs and so the slings have to be ordered from other companies. This creates a situation where most of the sling companies will give indemnity for their slings to be used with the Huntleigh hoists but not vice versa. Risk management and the moving and handling team might require a risk assessment to be conducted but may not be able to say what should be included in this risk assessment, leaving the door wide open for litigation. In addition, the very nature of a child's life means they move between a number of different areas, e.g. school, respite, home, local leisure services, all of whom have different hoisting equipment. Again, it is impossible to be in all the areas to assess and advise all staff. This situation creates a lot of anxiety. What is the best advice for OTs, and where do they stand?

Advice would be available from the MHRA and/or from the NPSA on carrying out risk assessments on hoist/sling compatibilities. In addition the NHSLA has prepared standards on risk assessments in a variety of settings and may be able to offer further advice. Manufacturers and community equipment stores may also be able to assist the OT.

The responsibility is upon the OT to provide a reasonable standard and to take all reasonable steps to find out what that standard would be. The COT has provided guidance in 2006 on the Manual Handling Regulations,[100] which includes a section on delegation. It may be that where a child is moved from place to place, the OT can instruct others in the safe handling of the child and in the use of equipment.

Research using children

Parents can only give consent to research on their children if there are no (or negligible) risks to the safety of the child. Many organisations have provided advice for research using children. Thus the Royal College of Paediatrics and Childhealth (in its previous identity of the British Paediatric Association) provided a guide to the UN Convention on the Rights of the Child.[101] Subsequently, the Royal College has published guidelines on clinical research involving new born babies and infants[102] and children.[103] A young person of 16 or older could give a valid consent to participating in research on the basis of the common law. The statutory right under section 8 of the Family Law Reform Act 1969 to give consent to treatment (see above) does not cover consent to research. A Gillick competent child under 16 years could also give consent to research, but the capacity of the child must be judged against the nature of the decision to be made and any risks inherent in the research. The research must be approved by a Research Ethics Committee (see Chapter 26).

Conclusions

Care of children can present considerable challenges to the practitioner. Many lessons can be learnt from a clear and consistent monitoring of the service provided and a willingness to learn from weaknesses. There can be no complacency about child protection regimes as the case of Baby P illustrates. The OT working with children faces significant problems in establishing and maintaining high standards of care and in ensuring that the rights of the child are respected. Occupational therapists should be aware of information provided by the COT and its specialist groups, the publications of the Department of Health, the Care Quality Commission and the Office for Standards in Education, Childrens Services and Skills. In 2007 the Government announced a £1 billion plan to improve children's welfare and education with better support for parents and families. This should increase opportunities for the occupational therapist.

Questions and exercises

1 A parent brings to the department a child whom you suspect is subject to abuse. Outline the procedure you would follow.
2 You are involved in the care of a girl with learning disabilities and learn that her mother wishes her to be sterilised. You are of the view that her disability is not severe. What action would you take? (See also Chapter 22.)
3 A child that you are caring for tells you in confidence that she is being abused by her father. She emphasises that she does not want you to take any action. What is the legal situation? Does the age of the child make any difference and if so how?
4 A child on your case list was subsequently the subject of child abuse investigations and a prosecution. You have been asked to attend as a witness at court. How would you prepare for giving evidence? (See also Chapter 13.)

References

1   British Medical Association Consent (2001) *Rights and Choices in Health Care for Children and Young People.* BMJ Books, London.
2   Swee Hong, C. & Howard, L. (eds) (2002) *Occupational Therapy in Childhood.* Whurr Publishers, London.
3   Rodger Sylvia and Ziviani Jenny (2006) *Occupational Therapy with Children; Understanding children's occupations and enabling participation.* Blackwell Publishing.
4   Kucha G and Davidson I (eds) (2008) *Occupational and physical therapy for children with rheumatic disease.* Radcliffe Publishing Oxford.
5   Gibson Caroline, Joanna Grice, Rebecca James and Shona Mulholland (2001) *The Children Act Explained.* Stationery Office, London.
6   HL Paper 117 (incorporating HL paper 98.i and ii of 2003); HC 81 (incorporating HC 1103–1 of 2001–02 and 81–1 of 2002–3). Stationery Office, London.
7   NAPOT/College of Occupational Therapists (1992) *The Children Act 1989 Guidelines for Occupational Therapists.* COT, London.
8   College of Occupational Therapists (2007) Every Child Matters Briefing note 85. COT, London.
9   *In re B(Children)(Care orders: Standard of proof)* The Times Law Report 12 June 2008 HL.
10 *R (on the application of BG) v Medway Council* [2005] EWHC 1932 (Admin); [2005] All ER (D) Sept.
11 *R v Gloucestershire County Council* [1997] 2 All ER 1.
12 *R v E Sussex CC ex p Tandy* (1995) 95 LGR 745.
13 *Holmes-Moorhouse v Richmond upon Thames London Borough Council* [2007] EWCA Civ 970; [2008] LGR 1.
14 Beresford Bryony and Rhodes Dave (2008) Housing and Disabled Children, Joseph Rowntree Foundation, York.
15 *R (on the application of A) v Lambeth London Borough Council; R (on the application of G) v Barnet London Borough Council* and *R (on the application of W) v Lambeth Borough Council* [2003] UKHL 57; [2003] All ER (D) 385 (Oct).

16   *R (on the application of W.) v Lincolnshire County Council* [2006] EWHC Admin 2365.
17   *Associated Provincial Picture Houses Ltd v Wednesbury Corporation* [1948] 1 KB 223. [1947] 2 All ER 680.
18   www.doh.gov.uk/
19   Lougher, L. (ed) (2001) *Occupational Therapy for Child and Adolescent Mental Health*. Churchill Livingstone, Edinburgh.
20   Audit Commission (2007) *Better safe than sorry: preventing unintentional injury to children*. Stationery Office, London.
21   Working Together Under the Children Act 1989: a guide to arrangement for inter-agency co-operation for the protection of children from abuse. Home Office, Department of Health, Department of Education and Science, Welsh Office (1991). HMSO, London.
22   *D v National Society for the Prevention of Cruelty to Children* [1977] 1 All ER 589.
23   *JD v East Berkshire Community NHS Trust, North Staffordshire Hospital NHS Trust and Others*, Lloyd's Rep Med 1 [2003] 9, [2005] UKHL 23, [2005] 2 All ER 443.
24   Mark Macaskill Parents of ill vegan girl may face police The Sunday Times 8 June 2008.
25   Department of Health (2003) *What To Do If You're Worried A Child Is Being Abused*. DH, Home Office and Department for Education and Skills; www.doh.gov.uk/safeguardingchildren/index.htm
26   www.victoria-climbie-inquiry.org.uk/
27   College of Occupational Therapy (2007) Every Child Matters – Change for children Briefing note no 85. COT, London.
28   www.dfes.gov.uk
29   www.everychildmatters.gov.uk
30   HM Government (2006) *Working Together to Safeguard Children*. Stationery Office, London.
31   www.everychildmatters.gov.uk
32   Council for Disabled Children (2006) *Safeguards for Disabled Children – a resource for local safeguarding children boards*. DfES, London; available on www.everychildmatters.gov.uk/
33   HM Government (2008) Safeguarding children in whom illness is fabricated or induced; www.everychild-matters.gov.uk
34   Rosemary Bennett Abused baby might have lived if 30 staff had done their job. The Times 14 February 2008.
35   *R (M) v Hammersmith and Fulham London Borough Council* The Times Law Report 3 March 2008.
36   *R (P) v Nottingham City Council* The Times Law Report 10 June 2008.
37   Lord Laming (2009) *The Protection of Children in England: A Progress Report*. The Stationery Office, London.
38   Rose David Hospitals fail to check children at risk, despite Baby P The Times 19 February 2009.
39   Care Quality Commission (2009) *Review of the involvement and action taken by health bodies in relation to the case of Baby P*. CQC, London.
40   Bennett Rosemary Child services chiefs to be retrained in family risks The Times 12 March 2009.
41   Blom-Cooper, L. et al. (1996) The Case of Jason Mitchell: Report of the Independent Panel of Inquiry. Duckworth, London.
42   *D v NSPCC* [1977] 1 All ER 589.
43   *JD v East Berkshire Community NHS Trust, North Staffordshire Hospital NHS Trust and Others*, Lloyd's Rep Med 1 [2003] 9, [2005] UKHL 23, [2005] 2 All ER 443.
44   *L. v Reading BC* [2006] EWHC 2449 (QB); [2007] BLGR 576.
45   *R.K. and A.K v United Kingdom* The Times Law Report 13 October 2008 Application No. 38000/05.
46   De Bruxelles Simon Damages win for parents falsely suspected of abuse The Times 23 December 2008.
47   www.everychildmatters.gov.uk/socialcare/integratedchildrensystem/
48   Department of Health (1989) An introductory guide to the Children Act for the NHS. HMSO, London.
49   Rosemary Bennett Army of amateurs rides to the rescue of vulnerable families The Times 31 May 2008 page 4.
50   Department of Health (1999) *Working together to safeguard children*. Home Office, Department for Education and Employment, the National Assembly for Wales.

51   LASSL (2001)2 The Children and Family Court Advisory and Support Service (CAFCASS) and complaints about the functioning of child protection conferences.

52   Department of Health (1999) *Working together to safeguard children*. Home Office, Department for Education and Employment, the National Assembly for Wales.

53   Rosemary Bennett Protection Agency staff left children at risk from abuse because of errors. The Times 15 February 2008 page 27.

54   Richard Ford Social Workers' failings put children at risk. The Times 28 May 2008 page 9.

55   Rosemary Bennett Fears for children at risk as care order applications fall by a third The Times 6 May 2008 page 8.

56   *A v The United Kingdom* (100/1997/884/1096) judgment on 23 September 1998.

57   Department of Health (2000) *Protecting Children, Supporting Parents: A consultation document on the physical punishment of children*. DH, London.

58   www.doh.gov.uk/scg/pcspresponse

59   Department of Health Press release 2001/0524, *Protecting Children Supporting Parents No Smacking Ban*. DH, London.

60   Joint Committee on Human Rights. *The UN Convention on the Rights of the Child*, HL Paper 117 (incorporating HL paper 98.i and ii of 2003), HC 81 (incorporating HC 1103-I of 2001–02 and 81-I of 2002–3) Stationery Office, London.

61   Francis Elliott. Parents face total smacking ban as rules are reviewed The Times 16 June 2007 page 11.

62   News item. Total smacking ban is ruled out The Times 26 October 2007.

63   De Bruxelles Simon Boy, 8 is taken into care after mother hit him with hairbrush The Times 10 April 2009.

64   Carers and Disabled Children (Vouchers) (England) Regulations 2003, SI 2003/1216.

65   *R (on the application of J) v Newham LBC* [2001] EWHC Admin 992; (2002) 5 CCL Rep 302.

66   *E and others v United Kingdom* (Application No 33218/96), Times Law Report, 4 December 2002, ECHR.

67   *D.P. and J.C v United Kingdom* (Application No 38719/97), Times Law Report, 23 October 2002, ECHR.

68   *A and another v Essex County Council*, Times Law Report, 24 January 2003.

69   Disability Rights Commission (2002) *Code of Practice for Schools Disability Discrimination Act 1995*. Part 4. Stationery Office, London.

70   *Re W (a minor) (medical treatment)* [1992] 4 All ER 627.

71   *Gillick v W Norfolk & Wisbech Area Health Authority* [1986] 1 AC 112.

72   *R (On the application of Axon) v Secretary of State for Health* [2006] EWCA 37 admin.

73   College of Occupational Therapists (2007) Gillick Competence: The young person's consent to treatment Briefing note no 96. COT, London.

74   *Re M (medical treatment: consent)* [1999] 2 FLR 1097.

75   De Bruxelles Simon Girl wins fight to turn down transplant The Times 11 November 2008.

76   *Re E (a minor) (wardship: medical treatment)* Family Division [1993] 1 FLR 386.

77   British Medical Association Consent (2001) *Rights and Choices in Health Care for Children and Young People*. BMJ Books, London.

78   Britton, C. (1999) A pilot study exploring families' experience of caring for children with chronic arthritis: Views from the inside. *British Journal of Occupational Therapy*, 62(12), 534–42.

79   See further for the rights of the child as applicant in: Wyld, N. (1994) *When Parents Separate*. Children's Legal Centre, London.

80   *Re A (minors) (conjoined twins: surgical separation)*, Times Law Report, 10 October 2000.

81   *Re T (a minor) (wardship: medical treatment)* [1997] 1 All ER 906; Re C (a minor – refusal of parental consent) [1997] 8 Med LR 166.

82   *R v Portsmouth Hospital NHS Trust ex parte Glass* [1999] 2 FLR 905 CA; [1999] Lloyd's Law Reports Med. 367.

83   *Glass v United Kingdom*, Times Law Report, 11 March 2004 ECHR.

84   HC(89)29, para.4.

85   The Data Protection (Subject Access Modification) (Health) Order 2000, SI 2000/413.

86 Stagnitti, K. & Unsworth, C. (2000) The importance of pretend play in child development: An occupational Therapy perspective. *British Journal of Occupational Therapy*, **63**(3), 121–7.

87 Department for Education and Skills and the Department of Health (2003) *Together from the Start*; LASSL (2003)4.

88 LAC (2001)8 Social Care for Deafblind Children and Adults; www.doh.gov.uk/scg/ deafblind

89 Department of Health (2000) *NHS Plan A plan for investment A plan for reform*, Cm 4818–1.

90 Department of Health National Service Framework Children, Young People and Maternity Services October 2004.

91 www.dh.gov.uk/nsf/children

92 www.cqc.org.uk/

93 College of Occupational Therapists (2006) NSF for children, young people and maternity services Briefing note no 60. COT, London.

94 www.doh.gov.uk/nsf/children

95 College of Occupational Therapists (2006) *NSF for long term conditions with relevance to children and young people* Briefing note no 57. COT, London.

96 Department of Health Partnership for children, families and maternity (2008) *Transition: Moving well a good practice guide for health professions and their partners on transition planning for young people with complex health needs or a disability.* DH, London.

97 *Gough v Thorne.* [1966] 3 All ER 398, CA.

98 *Jolley v Sutton London Borough Council*, Times Law Report, 24 May 2000.

99 *J (a minor) v Staffordshire County Council* CLR 1997 Vol 2 3783.

100 College of Occupational Therapists (2006) *Manual Handling*. COT, London.

101 British Paediatric Association (1995) *A Paediatrician's Brief Guide to the UN Convention on the Rights of the Child*. BPA, London.

102 Royal College of Paediatrics and Child Health (1999) *Safeguarding informed parental involvement in clinical research involving newborn babies and infants*. RCPCH, London.

103 Royal College of Paediatrics and Child Health (2000) Guidelines for the ethical conduct of medical research involving children. *Archives of Disease in Childhood*, **82**, 1777–82. RCPCH, London.

24 Older People

It would be a mistake to see older people as a clear client group. From a legal perspective there are no differences between the healthcare rights which apply to those over 75 or 85 or any other age level. However, from a clinical perspective the older that people become, the more likely it is that they have multiple health needs, and that these are likely to be exacerbated by economic and social problems. It is clear that the OT has a major role to play in the care of older patients and they are likely to form an increasing proportion of her case load. Research is necessary to determine the future availability and demands for OTs.

The basic principles of the law relating to patients' rights and to accountability and professional conduct cover adults of all ages. In addition, Article 14 of the European Convention on Human Rights requires that there should be no discrimination in the recognition of the Articles of Human Rights and this would include age (see below). There are, however, specific issues which can arise in the care of older people because a small proportion may lack the competence to make decisions, they may require greater protection from risks and their economic and social situation may cause concerns for the OT. As well as this chapter, reference should be made to the basic principles of law covered in other chapters. (For convenience the discussion on dementia (see below) has been included in this chapter on care of the older person, but dementia can of course affect the young person as well.) Occupational Therapists specialising in care of the elderly may find a book published by Age Concern on the assessment for health and social care of considerable help[1] as well as a book by Gail Mountain.[2] Margaret Richards has written a book on the law and financial planning for Long term care for older people.[3] Age Concern has published the first report from the UK Inquiry into mental health and well being in later life[4] and also a book on public policy and older people.[5] Alan Walker has edited a book on understanding quality of life in old age.[6] See also a book by Derek Wanless on securing good care for older people,[7] a book by A Bradshaw and C Merriman giving a practical guide on caring for the older person[8] and two books by the Open University Press, *Quality of life and older people* by John Bond and Lynne Corner[9] and *Aging well* by Ann Bowling.[10]

The following topics are covered in this chapter:

Legal Aspects of Occupational Therapy, Third Edition By Bridgit Dimond
© 2010 Bridgit Dimond

- Rights of older people: ageism
- Standards of care
- Assessment
- National Service Frameworks for older people
- Autonomy and intermittent incompetence
- Risk taking
- Restraint: the wanderer
- Carers
- Exploitation by relatives
- Abuse of the elderly
- Use of volunteers
- Inter-agency co-operation
- Community care: delayed discharges
- Health and safety manual handling
- Resources

Rights of older people: ageism

There is a tendency for older clients to be treated differently because of their age. Thus it is more likely that relatives will be told the diagnosis and prognosis before the patient, it is more likely that relatives will be asked for their consent for treatments to proceed, and there is a danger that arbitrary age limits will be set, above which certain treatments will not take place. However in law, the basic principles of law of consent and confidentiality and rights to treatment do not change because a person is older. If the client is competent then she alone is able to give consent and should be informed of any diagnosis and should have the right to decide whether or not she wishes this information to be given to the relatives.

Similarly there should be no cut-off points at which certain treatments are not made available. The criteria should be the physical ability of the patient to benefit from the specific treatment being discussed and whether that would be in her best interests, and if she is mentally competent, whether she gives consent.

A private member's bill was introduced into the House of Commons by MP David Winnick on 9 February 1996. If passed it would have made discrimination against the aged in employment unlawful. However, it failed to get Government support and therefore a second reading. Discrimination against the aged would now come under the provision of the Articles of the European Convention on Human Rights (see Appendix 1 and Chapter 6). Article 14 prevents discrimination on any grounds in the implementation of the Articles:

> The enjoyment of the rights and freedoms set forth in this Convention shall be secured without discrimination on any ground such as sex, race, colour, language, religion, political or other opinion, national or social origin, association with a national minority, property, birth or other status.

Whilst age is not specifically mentioned as a ground for discrimination, the list of examples of discrimination is not exhaustive. Consequently if there were evidence that a person was subjected to inhuman or degrading treatment contrary to Article 3 on account of age discrimination, this would be actionable against a public authority. In addition, older people may be able to rely on the Disability Discrimination Act 1995 (see Chapters 19 and 20). However, where they are refused medical treatment, where the duty of confidentiality is broken, or where consent is not obtained, older people have all the rights which the young adult has and which are described in earlier chapters in this book.

It follows therefore that if life-saving treatment or care is withheld from a person purely on the grounds of their age, then that could be a breach of article 14 and article 2. Article 3 and the right not to be subjected to inhuman or degrading treatment or punishment may also apply to older persons. Article 8 and the right to private and family life, home and correspondence may also be breached where the dignity and privacy of an older person is not respected.

The Government launched a national dignity tour on 20 May 2008. It appointed Sir Michael Parkinson as National Dignity Ambassador to ensure that older people using care and health services are treated with dignity and respect at all times. The aim of the tour was to promote the Dignity in Care Campaign which commenced in 2007. The campaign aimed to eliminate tolerance of indignity in health and social care services through raising awareness and inspiring people to take action. In 2008 the campaign was extended from older people to include mental health needs. Information on the campaign, action which is being taken and the extension of the campaign can be obtained from the DH social care website.[11]

The Employment Equality (Age) Regulations which prevent discrimination on grounds of age, only apply to employment. As a consequence the aged now have remedies against employers who discriminate against them. In addition they may be able to rely upon the Disability Discrimination Acts 1995 and 2005. However, a recent Spanish case has held that the Age Discrimination Directive does not apply to those over 65 years where the member country has a retirement age of 65.[12] Subsequently in a case brought by Age Concern which challenged the right of employers to impose retirement at the age of 65 years, the Court of Justice of the European Communities ruled that member states had to justify age discrimination[13] but the burden of proof was on the member state to establish that the discrimination was objectively and reasonably justified (see Chapter 19). Where elderly people are refused medical treatment, where the duty of confidentiality is broken and where consent is not obtained, the elderly have all the rights which the young adult has and which are described in earlier chapters in this book. The Equality Act 2010 widens the protection of the elderly against discrimination (see Chapter 18).

It is important that research on the care of older people is given a high profile, because a significantly larger proportion of the population will be over 65 years and therefore it is important to explore regimes which promote well-being and prevent accidents and deterioration in physical and mental capacity. For example Dawn Skelton and Ann McLaughlin[14] examined the feasibility and acceptability of an exercise class run by healthcare professionals, and whether an eight-week period of moderate intensity exercise could improve the strength, flexibility, balance and selected functional abilities of women aged 74 years and over. They concluded that repeated moderate intensity exercise which involves the practice of functional tasks and mobility can produce substantial increases in strength, balance, flexibility and selected tests of functional ability.

Standards of care

The Bolam test of reasonable professional practice (see Chapter 10) applies to the work of the OT and she must ensure that in caring for older people she follows reasonable professional approved practice. Where policies, guidelines or procedures exist there would be a presumption that these should be followed. However, where there are specific circumstances which make the following of those guidelines inappropriate for a particular patient/client, then the OT should use her professional judgement. It is essential that she should document the reasons why it was not possible to follow the policy. In the NICE[15] guidelines on pressure ulcers, the only level one recommendation (which is the highest level indicating support by research) is that professional judgement should be exercised in following guidelines. NICE published guidance on health – promoting occupational therapy for older people in October 2008.[16] This presents a useful opportunity for occupational therapists to set standards and claim the resources they need to ensure the guidance is implemented. NICE also published in 2008 guidelines on the mental well-being in older people.

Funding of long term care

A Royal Commission was established to consider the funding of long-term care for older people, and reported in 1999.[17] It recommended that Government assistance for nursing and personal care should be provided to older people in nursing and residential homes. A minority report disagreed with this view. As a consequence of the report different parts of the UK have followed different approaches, with Scotland paying all the costs of personal and nursing care, England only paying the nursing costs at three nationally set rates and Wales different levels of payment. The Royal Commission also recommended the establishment of a National Care Commission. (Subsequently the Commission for Social Care Inspection which became absorbed into the Care Quality Commission in April 2009).

NHS responsibilities for arranging care by a registered nurse for people in care homes providing nursing care came into force in October 2001.[18] From April 2003 the funding of the nursing care of around 88 000 residents of care homes providing nursing care, who are receiving care from a registered nurse, transferred from local authorities to the NHS. Guidance for NHS-funded nursing care was provided by the Department of Health.[19] The guidance stresses that primary care trusts should ensure that they have arrangements in place to pay councils for the nursing care of residents.

It is a principle of the NHS that healthcare is provided free at the point of service, unless there are statutory provisions which enable charges to be levied (as there are for prescriptions). In contrast the provision of social services are in general subject to means testing. There are therefore considerable disputes in determining whether the NHS should provide specific services free, or whether they should be provided, on a means tested basis, by social services. In the Grogan case,[20] the court had to determine whether a client was entitled to have services provided by the NHS. The case is considered in Chapter 18.

Following the decision in the Grogan case, the DH announced that new guidelines on determining eligibility for NHS continuing healthcare would be published in October 2007. Assessments for continuing NHS care were to be carried out by a multi-disciplinary team using the concept of 'a primary health need' as the criteria for the receipt of continuing healthcare. The National Framework on NHS Continuing Healthcare and NHS-funded Nursing Care published in October 2007[21] set out the national framework, the legal framework, the primary health need, core values, and principles, eligibility considerations, links to other policies, care planning and provision, review, dispute resolution and governance. It stated that primary health need should be assessed by looking at all of care needs and relating them to four key indicators:

- *nature* – the type of condition or treatment required and its quality and quantity
- *complexity* – symptoms that interact, making them difficult to manage or control
- *intensity* – one or more needs which are so severe that they require regular interventions
- *unpredictability* – unexpected changes in condition that are difficult to manage and present a risk to the patient or to others.

The NHS would make decisions on eligibility for NHS continuing healthcare in collaboration with the local authority through a multi-disciplinary team and with the full and active involvement of the patient and carers. Further information on the National Framework on continuing care is available on the DH website.[22] Answers to frequently asked questions on continuing care are also available.[23]

The annual report for 2006–7 published by CSCI in January 2008[24] summarised the state of social care in England in 2006–7 and painted a picture of a society which was failing to meet the needs of the elderly and disabled. Local authorities under pressure from limited resources were tightening the eligibility criteria for receiving social services and were redefining more narrowly the 'core business' of adult social care and there was now a sharp divide between those people who benefit from the formal system of social care and those who are outside it. There is little consistency both within and between councils as to who is ineligible for care. People, who are lost to the system because they are not eligible for council-arranged services and cannot purchase their care privately, often struggle with fragile informal support arrangements and a poor quality of life. (The House of Lords decided in the Gloucester case[25] that resources could be taken into account when determining the assessment of and the level of social services to be provided by local authorities. This case is considered in Chapter 20.) Those who fund their own care are disadvantaged and lack advice and information about care options. It saw the Government's proposed Green Paper on long-term care funding as an important opportunity to establish a fair and sustainable social care system, where people, whether they pay for their own care or not, as a minimum get good advice, an assessment of their situation , and access to high quality services.

In 2008 the Government initiated a consultation on the future of care and support. It set up a care and support website[26] which can be accessed to take part in the debate. It pointed out that given the longer life expectancy, the cost of disability benefits could increase by 50% in the next 20 years and there could be a £6 billion funding gap for social care. Since the proportion of people of working age in the population would decline, the Government would not be able to raise enough money through tax alone to meet the costs of care and support. A new insurance-based system was seen as a means of funding care for the elderly which was forecast to reach £4 billion in the next 20 years. Feedback is invited in its efforts to find an affordable, fair and sustainable way of delivering and funding a first class care and support system for the 21st century. A letter to the Times[27] from representatives of 12 organisations involved with the care of older and disabled people and their carers pointed out the fact that disabled and older people were being forced to end their support services because they could not afford them. It called for the government to conduct a thorough review of the impact of care charges and for these issues to be addressed in adult care reform.

There is also concern and inconsistency about relatives paying top-up fees.[28] Councils should only ask for top-up fees from relatives if the family has requested a particular care home for their relative than the one chosen by the local authority. Otherwise the LA should pay the fees in full where the assets of the old person are less than £13,500. Where the elderly person has assets of between £13,500 and £22,250 then there is a sliding scale of contribution.

Rationing care

Many local authorities have tightened their criteria for providing social care and are offering help only in critical cases. A legal challenge was brought against Harrow Council by several claimants, who were in receipt of community care services. Harrow had proposed that owing to financial constraints it would limit provision of care services to people with need categorised as critical under the Fair Access to Care Services guidance issued by the Secretary of State. The judge decided that there was a general duty under section 49A of the Disability Discrimination Act 1995 to have due regard to considerations listed therein. Those were important duties which included the need to promote equality of opportunity and to take account of disabilities, even where that involved treating the disabled more favourably than others. There was no evidence that the legal duty and its implications were drawn to the attention of the decision-makers who should have been informed, not just of the disabled as an issue, but of the particular obligations that the law imposed. H's decision-making process had not complied with S 49A of the Act.[29] The implications of this decision are still to be seen.

Green Paper on the funding of long-term care in the future

In July 2009 the long-awaited Green Paper[30] was published. It identified six features that everyone was entitled to expect. These were:

1. The right support to help you stay independent and well for as long as possible and to stop your care and support needs getting worse.
2. Wherever you are in England, you will have the right to have your care and support needs assessed in the same way and you will have a right to have the same proportion of your care and support costs paid for wherever you live.
3. All the services that you need will work together smoothly, particularly when your needs are assessed. ... You will only need to have one assessment of your needs to gain access to a whole range of care and support services.
4. You can understand and find your way through the care and support system easily.
5. The services you use will be based on your personal circumstances and need. Your care and support will be designed and delivered around your individual needs. As part of your care and support plan, you will have much greater choice over how and where you receive support, and the possibility of controlling your own budget wherever appropriate.
6. Your money will be spent wisely and everyone who qualifies for care and support from the state will get some help meeting the cost of care and support needs.

The aim is to build a National Care Service that is fair, simple and affordable. Everyone who qualifies for care and support from the state should get some help with paying for it. Any new system must therefore be:

- fair
- simple and easy to understand
- affordable
- universal, underpinned by national rights and entitlements, and helping everyone who needs care to pay for it
- personalised to individual needs, and flexible enough to support people to live their lives in the ways they want to.

Three funding options are put forward for consultation:

1. *Partnership:* In this system, everyone who qualified for care and support from the state would be entitled to have a set proportion – for example, a quarter or a third – of their basic care and support costs paid for by the state. People who were less well-off would have more care and support paid for – for example, two-thirds – while the least well-off people would continue to get all their care and support for free.
2. *Insurance:* In this system, everyone would be entitled to have a share of their care and support costs met, just as in the Partnership model. But this system would go further to help people cover the additional costs of their care and support through insurance, if they wanted to.
3. *Comprehensive:* In this system, everyone over retirement age who had the resources to do so would be required to pay into a state insurance scheme. Everyone who was able to pay would pay their contribution, and then everyone whose needs meant that they qualified for care and support from the state would get all of their basic care and support for free when they needed it.

The current system with some getting their social care paid for but others receiving no help at all is ruled out as is a tax funded system. In the latter system, people would pay tax throughout their lives, which would be used to pay for all the people who currently need care. When, in turn, people needed care themselves, they would get all their basic care free. This option was ruled out because it places a heavy burden on people of working age. A third system – Pay for Yourself – in which everybody would be responsible for paying for their own basic care and support, when they needed it; they could take out insurance to cover some of these costs, or use their income and savings was also ruled out because it would leave many people without the care and support they need, and is fundamentally unfair because people cannot predict what care and support they will need. The consultation ended on 31 October 2009. In January 2010 the Government's response to the consultation was given in a written statement. An inter-Departmental group on Safeguarding Vulnerable Adults would be established. New legislation would be introduced to put Safeguarding Adult Boards on a statutory basis and new comprehensive multi-agency guidance would be produced. The establishment of the Independent Safeguarding Authority is considered in Chapter 19.

National Service Frameworks for older people

In 2001 the Department of Health published its National Service Framework (NSF) for Older People.[31] Guidance was issued in March 2001.[32] (See Chapter 17 for further details on NSFs.) The NSF for Older People is:

> A strategy to ensure fair, high quality, integrated health and social care services for older people. It is a 10-year programme of action linking services to support independence and promote good health, specialised services for key conditions, and culture change so that all older people and their carers are always treated with respect, dignity and fairness.

The eight standards cover the following areas:

1. rooting out age discrimination
2. person-centred care
3. intermediate care
4. general hospital care
5. stroke
6. falls
7. mental health in older people
8. the promotion of health and active life in older age.

Each standard sets out its aim, defines the standard and identifies its rationale and the key interventions. In addition, a timetable of milestones is set by which specific targets must be achieved. A booklet on medicines and older people is also published to ensure that older people gain maximum benefit from medication and do not suffer unnecessarily from illness caused by excessive, inappropriate or inadequate consumption of medicines. The NSF also identifies how the standards are to be implemented at local level and the national support which will underpin the standards and local action including: finance, workforce, research and development, clinical and practice decision support services and information. The NSF is available on the DH website and the COT has published a review of the NSF and identified the next steps to be taken.[33] NICE (see Chapters 10 and 17) has an important role to play in ensuring that the standards are based on clinically effective research-based practice, and the Care Quality Commission (incorporating from April 2009 the Commission for Health Audit and Inspection (CHAI) and the Commission for Social Care Inspection (CSCI)) ensures through inspections that the standards are implemented across social and health services. In addition, progress overall is overseen by the NHS Modernisation Board and the Older People's Taskforce.

The National Service Framework (NSF) for long-term conditions

More recently the DH has published a strategy for long term conditions setting 5 key outcomes for people with long term conditions.[34] It points out that one in three of the population suffers from a long term condition and the number of people with a long term condition is expected to rise by23% over the next 25 years. A revised edition of the compendium on long term conditions first published in 2004 was published in 2008.[35] The College of Occupational Therapists published a briefing note on supporting people with long term conditions in 2007.[36]

The NSF was published in 2005 sets out 11 quality requirements in health and social case services:

1. a person-centred service
2. early recognition followed by prompt diagnosis and treatment
3. emergency and acute management
4. early and specialist rehabilitation
5. community rehabilitation and support
6. vocational rehabilitation
7. providing equipment and accommodation
8. providing personal care and support
9. palliative care
10. support for family and carers
11. care during admission to hospital.

The COT provided guidance on the NSF for long term conditions in 2005 (briefing note 36).

Stroke services

In 2005 the National Audit Office published a report on stroke services[37] which identified significant deficiencies in stroke services. Subsequently the Government has stated that a dedicated stroke care coordinator should be appointed in every local authority area in England to support survivors and their families. Additional ring fenced funding has been made available to local authorities and to strategic health authorities. A practical manual on stroke care could be a useful source of information for occupational therapists.[38]

Dementia

In January 2008 the Public Accounts Committee of the House of Commons published a report on improving services and support for people with dementia.[39] The report came to the following conclusions:

1. Dementia affects over 560,000 people in England, costs about £14 billion a year but has not been a NHS priority. The National Dementia Strategy now being developed by the DH should have a clear timetable for implementation, and criteria for evaluation and reporting progress. It should also have an effective communication strategy to engage professionals, patient groups, the Royal Colleges, inspectorates and the voluntary sector.
2. Unlike cancer and coronary heart disease, there is no single individual with responsibility or accountability for improving dementia services. The DH should appoint a Senior Responsible Officer.

3.   Between a half and two-thirds of people with dementia never receive a formal diagnosis. Diagnosis should always be made, regardless as to whether interventions are available and could be assisted if: GP practices had greater support from mental health services; if the Royal College of GPs developed a dementia care pathway; and by the Institute of Innovation and Improvement promulgating good diagnostic practice.
4.   There is a poor awareness amongst the public and some professionals of dementia and what can be done to help people with the disease. DH should commission a dementia awareness campaign.
5.   People with dementia require support from multiple health and social care providers but this is often difficult to manage. On diagnosis, people with dementia and their carers should be given a single health or social care professional contact point (e.g. a social worker or CPN) to improve the co-ordination of care.
6.   Carers save the taxpayer £5 billion a year yet between a half and two thirds of all carers do not receive the carer's assessment to which they are entitled. The DH should emphasise to local health organisations and their social care partners that they need to develop an action plan which gives priority to assessing and meeting the needs of carers and develop a commissioning tool kit to demonstrate the cost benefits of the different options for providing support including respite and domiciliary care.
7.   62% of care home residents are currently estimated to have dementia but less than 28% of care home places are registered to provide specialist dementia care. CSCI (now the Care Quality Commission) should assess staff qualifications and training as part of its review of the quality of care for people with dementia and local mental health teams should use the finding when allocating resources to community psychiatric teams.
8.   Hospital care for people with dementia is often not well managed, increasing the risk of longer stays, admission to a care home and deterioration in the patient's health. Hospitals should routinely undertake a mental health assessment. Care records should be shown to paramedics, so that an informed decision on admission to hospital or to care home can be made.

Following the Public Accounts Committee report the DH promised that a national dementia strategy would be developed. As part of an awareness campaign on dementia, the Alzheimer's Society has published in 2008 a booklet (Worried about your Memory) to assist in the identification of Alzheimer's which is available from its website.[40]

The Department of Health published a dementia strategy in February 2009.[41] The key objectives are shown in Figure 24.1. Experts say that dementia will affect at least 1.4 million people and cost the economy £30 billion a year within a generation. The implementation plan published by the DH at the same time as the strategy recognised that all areas would not be able to implement the strategy within 5 years. Therefore seven key priority outcomes were identified that were likely to need focused attention for early delivery:

- early intervention and diagnosis for all;
- improved community personal support services;
- implementing the New Deal for Carers;
- improved quality of care for people with dementia in general hospitals;
- living well with dementia in care homes;
- an informed and effective workforce for people with dementia; and
- a Joint Commissioning strategy for dementia.

£150 million was allocated for dementia care for the first two years of the five year strategy.

Figure 24.1   Key objectives of the National Dementia Strategy from the DH February 2009.

- **Objective 1: Improving public and professional awareness and understanding of dementia.** Public and professional awareness and understanding of dementia to be improved and the stigma associated with it addressed. This should inform individuals of the benefits of timely diagnosis and care, promote the prevention of dementia, and reduce social exclusion and discrimination. It should encourage behaviour change in terms of appropriate help-seeking and help provision.
- **Objective 2: Good-quality early diagnosis and intervention for all.** All people with dementia to have access to a pathway of care that delivers: a rapid and competent specialist assessment; an accurate diagnosis, sensitively communicated to the person with dementia and their carers; and treatment, care and support provided as needed following diagnosis. The system needs to have the capacity to see all new cases of dementia in the area.
- **Objective 3: Good-quality information for those with diagnosed dementia and their carers.** Providing people with dementia and their carers with good-quality information on the illness and on the services available, both at diagnosis and throughout the course of their care.
- **Objective 4: Enabling easy access to care, support and advice following diagnosis.** A dementia adviser to facilitate easy access to appropriate care, support and advice for those diagnosed with dementia and their carers.
- **Objective 5: Development of structured peer support and learning networks.** The establishment and maintenance of such networks will provide direct local peer support for people with dementia and their carers. It will also enable people with dementia and their carers to take an active role in the development and prioritisation of local services.
- **Objective 6: Improved community personal support services.** Provision of an appropriate range of services to support people with dementia living at home and their carers. Access to flexible and reliable services, ranging from early intervention to specialist home care services, which are responsive to the personal needs and preferences of each individual and take account of their broader family circumstances. Accessible to people living alone or with carers, and people who pay for their care privately, through personal budgets or through local authority-arranged services.
- **Objective 7: Implementing the Carers' Strategy.** Family carers are the most important resource available for people with dementia. Active work is needed to ensure that the provisions of the Carers' Strategy are available for carers of people with dementia. Carers have a right to an assessment of their needs and can be supported through an agreed plan to support the important role they play in the care of the person with dementia. This will include good-quality, personalised breaks. Action should also be taken to strengthen support for children who are in caring roles, ensuring that their particular needs as children are protected.
- **Objective 8: Improved quality of care for people with dementia in general hospitals.** Identifying leadership for dementia in general hospitals, defining the care pathway for dementia there and the commissioning of specialist liaison older people's mental health teams to work in general hospitals.
- **Objective 9: Improved intermediate care for people with dementia.** Intermediate care which is accessible to people with dementia and which meets their needs.
- **Objective 10: Considering the potential for housing support, housing-related services and telecare to support people with dementia and their carers.** The needs of people with dementia and their carers should be included in the development of housing options, assistive technology and telecare. As evidence emerges, commissioners should consider the provision of options to prolong independent living and delay reliance on more intensive services.

continued

Figure 24.1 Continued.

- **Objective 11: Living well with dementia in care homes.** Improved quality of care for people with dementia in care homes by the development of explicit leadership for dementia within care homes, defining the care pathway there, the commissioning of specialist in-reach services from community mental health teams, and through inspection regimes.
- **Objective 12: Improved end of life care for people with dementia.** People with dementia and their carers to be involved in planning end of life care which recognises the principles outlined in the Department of Health End of Life Care Strategy. Local work on the End of Life Care Strategy to consider dementia.
- **Objective 13: An informed and effective workforce for people with dementia.** Health and social care staff involved in the care of people who may have dementia to have the necessary skills to provide the best quality of care in the roles and settings where they work. To be achieved by effective basic training and continuous professional and vocational development in dementia.
- **Objective 14: A joint commissioning strategy for dementia.** Local commissioning and planning mechanisms to be established to determine the services needed for people with dementia and their carers, and how best to meet these needs. These commissioning plans should be informed by the World Class Commissioning guidance for dementia developed to support this Strategy and set out in Annex 1.
- **Objective 15: Improved assessment and regulation of health and care services and of how systems are working for people with dementia and their carers.** Inspection regimes for care homes and other services that better assure the quality of dementia care provided.
- **Objective 16: A clear picture of research evidence and needs.** Evidence to be available on the existing research base on dementia in the UK and gaps that need to be filled.
- **Objective 17: Effective national and regional support for implementation of the Strategy.** Appropriate national and regional support to be available to advise and assist local implementation of the Strategy. Good-quality information to be available on the development of dementia services, including information from evaluations and demonstrator sites.

The Alzheimer's Society welcomed the strategy but was surprised that research was not a fundamental component of the strategy and was disappointed that the review of antipsychotic drugs had been delayed.

A report published on 17 March 2009 in a report by a firm of health and social care analysts Laing and Buisson which surveyed 6,000 care homes found that training was "fragmented and ad-hoc" with a third of homes failing to provide staff with specialist instruction. The need for the implementation of the national strategy was obvious. The ethical issues resulting from tagging and tracking those with dementia are considered by Nicola Plastow.[42] She concluded that OTs need to contribute to the multi-disciplinary research that is needed in this area, in order to ensure that if this technology is used, it is for the maintenance or improvement in function of the person with dementia.

Dementia and other legal issues

A person suffering from dementia may involve an OT in many other legal areas and for convenience a guide to the relevant chapters is given below.

- the Mental Capacity Act – see Chapters 7, 21 and 22
- the Mental Health Acts 1983 and 2007 compulsory admission, guardianship, powers of the nearest relative, supervised community treatment order and section 117 – see Chapter 21
- Deprivation of liberty safeguards – see Chapter 22
- Safeguarding adults issues – see Chapter 19
- Financial management and the Court of Protection – see Chapter 22
- Powers of deputy and the Office of Public Guardian – Chapter 22
- Lasting powers of attorney – see below in this chapter
- Advance decisions/Living wills – see Chapter 25

Implications for OTs

Those OTs specialising in this field should ensure that they obtain a copy of the NSF for Older People and use it as a criterion for the minimum level of service provided. If there are shortfalls, these can be identified and the necessary resources and training needs quantified in order to raise standards to the minimum level. Reference could also be made to the article by Claire Ballinger[43] which provides a helpful comment on the relevance of the NSF to the OT. In 2006 the views of OTs on the impact of the NSF for older people on practice were considered.[44] They identified 5 key themes: a raised profile of older people's services, a changing delivery of services, a revisiting of occupational therapy core skills, assessment and resource allocation. The monitoring of services provided also needs to take into account the perceptions of the clients. For example, Darren Awang[45] researched the views of service users on the process of securing adaptations and concluded that older people would welcome a voice in service delivery and some are keen to become more involved in how their services are delivered. Older people's expectations of their stay in an elderly care unit were explored by Karen F Dady and Sue Rugg,[46] who found that the participants in the study had little expectation of any occupational therapy and had little apparent concept of the profession and few expectations about its role in their rehabilitation. They concluded that additional information about OT work and the extent of its services should be targeted at older people in a broad range of institutional and community settings. A useful analysis is provided by Kate Goodacre and others on adapting existing properties to enable older people to stay at home.[47] They concluded that there was a need for OTs to be proactive in relation to housing, that OTs needed to have methods and tools that help identify those factors that increase or decrease the adaptability of a property and OTs, with their knowledge of how disabled people use buildings and space, should use their expertise to influence building design and specific developments such as extra care housing in order to meet the needs of older people.

Whilst patients and carers at present do not have a legal right to sue for breach of statutory duty if the standards are not implemented, they could bring an action for negligence if harm has occurred as a result of a failure to provide a reasonable standard of care, and they could use evidence of failures to comply with the NSF as evidence of the breach of the duty of care. The Health and Social Care (Community Health and Standards) Act 2003 (now incorporated in the Health and Social Care Act 2008) gives powers to the Secretary of State to identify standards and create a statutory duty for health and social services organisations to comply with the set standards (see Chapter 17). The importance of evidence-based practice in the rehabilitation of vulnerable older people is discussed by Gail Mountain in her research paper.[48] The paper sets out the findings from the literature and provides guidance to OTs, with an extensive bibliography. Interestingly she found that:

> the health promotion and preventative role of occupational therapy with vulnerable older people is yet to be realised. However there is indisputable evidence of the value of an established multi-disciplinary team

providing rehabilitation, particularly when team involvement commences early in the treatment process and extends across different agencies.

Assessment

Chapter 2 of the NSF for Older People sets out details of the single assessment process which aims at ensuring that older people receive appropriate, effective and timely responses to their health and social care needs and that professional resources are used effectively. The single assessment process attempts to ensure that the scale and depth of assessment is kept in proportion to older people's needs, that agencies do not duplicate each other's assessment and that professionals contribute to assessments in the most effective way. Further guidance was issued by the Department of Health on the single assessment process for older people.[49] This summarises the key implications for the older people, and health and social care professionals; provides guidance for local implementation; and gives annexes which provide the criteria that localities should use when reviewing and reporting on their progress with implementation. The guidance also suggests that housing needs should be assessed at the same time as health and social care needs so that there can be a co-ordinated response. The standards should be included in the charters which local social services authorities, in conjunction with health and housing departments, are required to prepare and publish.[50]

Autonomy and intermittent incompetence

If the older client is competent, then he or she has the right to give or withhold consent to treatment. The right of a mentally competent adult to refuse treatment was reiterated by the Court of Appeal in a case in 1992.[51] The Court of Appeal stated that it was the duty of the professional to ensure that the refusal was valid, i.e. that the adult had the requisite mental competence, was not under the undue influence of another nor suffering from any disability which impaired his or her capacity to give consent (see Chapter 7). For a person over 16 years there is a presumption of capacity, but this can be rebutted if there is evidence to the contrary.

One of the difficulties facing the OT is the possibility that the client is suffering from intermittent mental incapacity. This may be a feature of Alzheimer's disease. In such situations the OT would be advised to seek the assistance of others who could help to determine the mental capacity of the client.

Situation: refusal to accept residential care

An OT visits a patient at home for treatment following a stroke. She was extremely concerned about the patient's condition. It appeared that she was not able to care for herself properly and no one was helping her. The OT, following an assessment, formed the view that the patient did not have the physical or mental competence to live on her own. What should the OT do?

This is not an unfamiliar situation to many OTs. The OT would have to contact social services and arrange for a community care assessment to be made, with interim assistance being provided until a residential placement could be arranged. Such a plan, of course, depends on persuading the patient to leave home in her best interests. There are statutory powers under the Mental Health Act 1983 to remove the person to a place of safety, but very specific conditions must be shown (see Chapter 21).

Figure 24.2 Section 47 of the National Assistance Act 1948.

This section covers persons:

(a) who are suffering from grave chronic disease or, being aged, infirm or physically incapacitated, are living in insanitary conditions and

(b) are unable to devote to themselves, and are not receiving from other persons, proper care and attention.

They can be removed to a place of safety on an application by the Community Medical specialist (replacing the Medical Officer of Health) who is required to give seven days notice to a magistrate court.

There are also statutory powers under the National Assistance Act 1948 for persons to be removed to a place of safety (see Figure 24.2).

Because of the problems which could arise from this delay in giving notice, an amendment Act was passed in 1951 which enables an order to be made without notice in an emergency.

These provisions have been the subject of review by the Law Commission which, in its consultation paper 130,[52] suggested that section 47 of the National Assistance Act 1948 and the National Assistance (Amendment) Act 1951 should be repealed and replaced by a new scheme giving clearer and more appropriate powers to local social services authorities to intervene to protect incapacitated, mentally disordered or vulnerable people. Draft legislation was included in the final report of the Law Commission.[53] A further consultation paper on mental incapacity was issued by the Lord Chancellor in 1997.[54] This was followed by a White Paper issued by the Lord Chancellor.[55] Subsequently the Department of Health published a draft Mental Incapacity Bill which was reviewed by a committee of the Joint Houses of Parliament (see Chapter 22) and subsequently the Mental Capacity Act 2005 was enacted and brought into force in the main by October 2007.

Where the client refuses to give consent to treatment and care, whatever the reason, the OT cannot usually compel the client to participate in therapy. Many therapies require the intentional involvement of the client. Where this is not so, it would be advisable for the OT to obtain the services of another health professional to determine the competence of the client to give consent. Form 4 of the Department of Health's guidance on implementation of consent[56] to treatment procedures covers the situation where an adult is incapable of giving consent. The form requires the health professional (and it can therefore be used by OTs) to identify the treatment or care to be given, the reasons for the incapacity, and why that treatment is in the best interests of the mentally incapacitated patient. Relatives can sign that they understand that the patient is mentally incapacitated and that the treatment proposed by the clinician is in the best interests of the patient. This is not a consent to treatment by relatives.

Situation: refusal of treatment

An older patient is admitted to hospital with confusion, secondary to an infection. Treatment with antibiotics is implemented. The patient makes a good recovery and the OT is asked to assist in rehabilitation. The patient refuses to attempt to stand. The OT knows the importance of starting rehabilitation as soon as possible. What can the OT do in the face of such opposition?

This common situation requires all the OT's interpersonal skills. A good ploy would be for the OT to be on the ward when the patient is moved from bed to chair or when he or she needs the toilet so that he or she is in a weight bearing situation, and develop mobilisation from that point. If such tactics fail, then taking the patient off the ward to the occupational therapy department to unfamiliar surroundings might assist in persuading the patient to commence rehabilitation. Coercion of a men-tally capacitated person would not be lawful; but where the patient lacks the mental capacity to make her own decisions, then health professionals can act in her best interests in accordance with the provisions of the Mental Capacity Act 2005 (see Chapter 7).

The patient/client who lacks the requisite mental capacity

In the past where the client was incompetent and unable to give consent, the OT could continue to provide care and treatment on the basis of the ruling in the case of *Re F*.[57] In this case the House of Lords established that treatment and care can be given out of necessity to a person who does not have the capacity to give a valid consent. The treatment must be given in the best interests of the person, and the health professional must follow the reasonable standard of care as defined by the Bolam test. The House of Lords confirmed this common law (i.e. judge made law) power to act out of necessity on behalf of a mentally incapacitated adult in the Bournewood case.[58] Subsequently, however, following a long consultation process the Mental Capacity Act 2005 has been enacted and provides a framework for decision-making on behalf of mentally incapacitated adults. In addition deprivation of liberty safeguards have been enacted by amendments to the Mental Capacity Act 2005 and these are discussed in Chapter 22.

Living wills: advance refusals of treatment

If an OT is aware that an older patient wishes to make a living will (advance decision or advance directive) by which the patient is refusing treatments at a future time, when she lacks the requisite mental capacity, she should ensure that the mental competence of the patient to do so is established and that care is taken in recording the patient's wishes. Living wills are considered in detail in Chapter 25 (page 533).

Risk taking

It is recognised that if vulnerable clients are to lead lives with a reasonable quality then certain risks must be faced. Thus it would be less risky keeping clients in an institution rather than taking them out for walks or other activities. The Report[59] on the responses to the Government's Green paper on Independence, Well-being and Choice[60] (see below) points out that "Care cannot and should not strive to be 100% risk free". It recognised that there is a balance to be struck between enabling people to have control over their lives and ensuring that they are free from harm, exploitation and mistreat-ment. The Green paper sought to encourage a more open debate about risk management. The feed-back showed that there was support for the development of a risk management framework to include guidance and training to provide staff with the support they needed to operate in a new culture which favoured greater exposure to risk. The White Paper Our health, our care, our say published in 2006[61] emphasised choice and control as critical components of the future strategy for health and social care. It gave a commitment to developing a national approach to risk management. (The White Paper is considered more fully in Chapter 18). Subsequently the Department of Health issued a guide to independence, choice and risk.[62] The guide can be down loaded from the DH website.[63] The guide provides a risk management framework for use by everyone involved in supporting adults using social care within any setting, including NHS staff working in multi-disciplinary or joint teams. It states that:

> The governing principle is that people have the right to live their lives to the full as long as that doesn't stop others from doing the same. By taking account of the benefits in terms of independence, well-being and choice, it should be possible for a person to have a support plan which enables them to manage risks and to live their lives in ways which best suit them.

The DH has also developed a supported decision tool template which is designed to guide and record the discussion when a person's choices involve an element of risk. This can be adapted to fit into local formats or used as a stand-alone tool.

Counsel and Care has produced advice and guidance to staff who care for older people on risk taking in residential and nursing homes.[64] However, the same principles would apply to the care of an older person in his or her own home or in hospital.

The law would require that reasonable care should be taken to prevent harm arising from reasonably foreseeable risks. This would necessitate a risk assessment, not unlike that required under the health and safety regulations (see Chapter 11).

In the event of harm actually arising to the client or another person, the health professional caring for the client would have to show what risks would have been reasonably foreseeable, what reasonable action was taken to meet those risks and that this was in accordance with the reasonable standards of professional practice.

It follows that it is essential that records are kept of the basis of the decision making and any instructions given to others who are to care for the clients. This is a difficult area for the OT who may feel that she is squeezed between two principles of law: the right of the mentally competent adult to autonomy and the duty of care owed by the health professional to the client.

Falls and risk management

A simple example of risk assessment and management can be seen in the risk of an older person falling. Thus Adele Reece and Janet Simpson[65] discuss the need to teach older people how to cope after a fall. They suggest that older people are slightly more likely to learn successfully how to get up from the floor by the backward chairing method. Those who cannot learn to get up from the floor should be helped by developing alternative strategies for summoning help and for preventing the consequences of the long lie. In a subsequent article, Janet Simpson and others describe guidelines which have been developed for the collaborative rehabilitative management of older people who have fallen.[66] These guidelines are an example of multi-disciplinary planning and working. They set out four aims:

- to improve older people's ability to withstand threats to their balance
- to improve the safety of older people's surroundings
- to prevent older people suffering the consequences of a long lie
- to optimise older people's confidence and, whenever relevant, their carers' confidence, in their ability to move about as safely and independently as possible.

At the heart of the philosophy of such guidelines are the basic principles of risk management: a fall is reasonably foreseeable, therefore simple measures can be introduced to eliminate further risks. The Westmead Home Safety Assessment is described by Lindy Clement and colleagues as an important tool in assessing risk of falling.[67] Sue Kinn and Linda Galloway[68] showed that there is room for improvement in the practice of teaching clients how to rise after a fall. Risk factors and strategies for prevention of falls are considered in a book by Stephen Lord and others.[69]

A home fall and accidents screening tool has been devised as a screening instrument for use in a community preventive care trial for older people.[70] The results showed the complexity of constructing the home safety checklist and the need to test the items included in the checklist in a random controlled trial, so that the magnitude of the risk associated with some hazards can be evaluated.

Helen Buril and colleagues[71] undertook a project to assess whether perceptual dysfunction was a risk factor in falls in older people. They concluded that there was a link, with spatial disorientation posing the greatest risk for falls. OTs and physiotherapists should incorporate adaptive strategies such as visual cues into the strategies for gait, balance and environmental interventions currently being advocated for the prevention of falls in older cognitively impaired people.

Claire Ballinger and Sheila Payne[72] point out the absence of research into the meaning and interpretation of a fall and as a consequence the difficulties in determining effective clinical interventions. A few years later Claire Ballinger and Samuel Nyman reviewed the literature to explore how allied health professionals could improve the update of and adherence to falls preventions interventions.[73] Rhidian Hughes analyses restraint, risk and safety in relation to older people falling out of bed and concluded that it was important to recognise that interventions to stop older people from falling out of bed may also prevent people from leaving their bed voluntarily. A careful balance needs to be struck between respecting people's rights and making decisions about care.[74]

Reference should now be made to the NSF standard six on falls, where key interventions to reduce the number of falls which result in serious injury include:

- public health strategies to reduce the incidence of falls in the population and the identification, assessment and prevention measures for those at most risk of falling
- prevention and treatment of osteoporosis
- new integrated falls services to provide better services for those who have fallen, and provide rehabilitation and long-term support.

NICE has set a clinical practice guideline for the assessment and prevention of falls in older people which includes recommendations for research and audit criteria.[75] As with all NICE guidelines it emphasises that recommendations may not be appropriate for use in all circumstances. A limitation of a guideline is that it simplifies clinical decision-making. A decision to adopt any particular recommendation must be made by the practitioner in the light of:

- available resources
- local services, policies and protocols
- the patient's circumstances and wishes
- available personnel and devices
- clinical experience of the practitioner
- knowledge of more recent research findings

The Department of Health provided a progress report on the prevention of falls in 2007 and suggested that putting in place fully integrated falls prevention services could prevent up to 200 hip fractures annually in each Special Health Authority.[76] An update of the national clinical audit of falls and bone health for older people in 2007 has been provided by Carole MacGregor and Jackie Riglin.[77] An ageline database provides access to a wide range of resources relating to older people[78] as does

Medline Plus.[79] AGILE, ACPC and OCTEP have jointly prepared guidelines for the collaborative rehabilitative management of people who have fallen which is available from the COT website. The College of Occupational Therapists has also published guidance on Falls Management.[80] It assists in the identification of those who are at risk and gives practical guidance on evidence based interventions. It also co-operated with the Chartered Society of Physiotherapy in 2002 in developing a Falls Audit Pack.[81]

Situation: risks in rehabilitation

An OT as part of a treatment plan decides to take an older person to get washed and dressed following a stroke. As she moves him from the chair he lets go his hold on her and falls to the floor, fracturing his pelvis. What is the legal situation of the OT?

The first question which must be asked, is what is the reasonable standard of the OT in this situation? Would any competent OT have acted as she did? Would a simple risk assessment not have suggested that a second person should be at hand to assist? The OT is unlikely to face litigation personally, since her employer would be vicariously liable for her actions (see Chapter 10).

Situation: too risky

A stroke patient, previously active with a full social life, is discharged having made a good recovery. He has been advised that he must contact the DVLA and his insurance company before thinking about driving again. He admits to the OT at the Day Hospital that he has driven but 'only around the village'. What is the OT's legal duty?

The OT should make it clear to the patient that in driving contrary to clinical advice he is breaking the law as well as putting at risk his own safety and that of others. Where she has considerable concerns about his mental and physical capacity to drive safely, there may well be justification in warning the patient that if he fails to notify the DVLA then she may feel obliged as part of her duty of care, to inform them herself. (See Chapter 8 on the exceptions to the duty of confidentiality and Chapter 16 on transport.)

Restraint: the wanderer

Some older people can present special problems because of their disregard for their own health and safety and their inability to make rational decisions. In residential and nursing homes and also hospitals there is a temptation to lock doors or use forms of restraint to prevent the client wandering off into harm. Such forms of restraint are not good practice and ideally there should be sufficient staff to prevent the need for doors to be locked or patients held under restraint. Restraint of those lacking the requisite mental capacity is now covered by the Mental Capacity Act 2005. Sometimes it may be necessary to ensure that the client is protected by the Deprivation of Liberty (Bournewood) safeguards which are discussed in Chapter 22. Guidance is given in the Code of Practice on the Mental Health Act 1983[82] on the care of informal patients who are likely to wander off causing harm to themselves, and the use of a policy and clear documentation on locking doors. Advice is also given by Counsel and Care on minimising the use of restraint in residential and nursing homes for older people.[83] It includes flowcharts to assist in assessing the level of risk and making decisions on the use of restraint. Counsel and Care has also published a discussion document[84] which considers the meaning of restraint, gives examples of why restraint is used and suggests some working principles. Guidance is provided by the RCN on restraint and the care of older people.[85] This guidance is relevant to other health professionals. Anyone using restraint of any sort must ensure that their actions are compatible with Article 3 of the Human Rights Convention which is discussed in Chapter 6 and can be found in Appendix 1. Restraint should not be viewed solely in terms of deliberate locking of doors it could also include harnessing people with severe physical disabilities and/or mental disabilities in special moulded wheelchairs. Consideration must be given to ensuring that they have significant opportunities for freedom of movement. OTs should be concerned with the provision of safe and creative environments with appropriate resources and equipment.

Situation: the wanderer

An OT visits a nursing home where a stroke patient is being cared for. She notes that many of the residents are sitting in seats with tables in front of them or with seats sloping down to the rear so that the resident is effectively trapped in them. She queries this with the home manager who tells her that this is the safest way of preventing them wandering off from the nursing home, because they have been told they cannot lock the doors. The OT wonders if this is lawful.

Restraint can be a form of imprisonment. It may be justified if it is reasonable, of short duration and in the best interests of a mentally incompetent person in accordance with the provisions of the Mental Capacity Act 2005. However, permanent ongoing restraint through clothing or design of furniture is not best practice, and could if brought to court be held unlawful. The OT should discuss alternative systems of keeping the older person safe and the possibility of protecting the patient by using the Deprivation of Liberty Safeguards (Bournewood) which are discussed in Chapter 22. If the managers of the home are not prepared to consider changes, then it may be raised with the registration body, the Care Quality Commission. Where social services have purchased places in the home, they will also be concerned with standards of care and can take issue with the managers if there appears to be a breach in the contract. As a consequence of S.145 of the Health and Social Care Act 2008 private homes providing residential places may now be seen as exercising functions of a public nature and therefore come under the provisions of the Human Rights Act 1998 (see Chapter 6). Residents may therefore be able to bring action against the home on breaches of their human rights.

Carers

The Strategy for carers is considered in Chapter 18. All that has been said in that chapter in relation to the assessment and support of carers would apply to those who look after older people. A useful analysis of carers' perspective on their needs in relation to OT provided within LAs is provided by Lisa Dibsdall and Sue Rugg.[86] They concluded from their small survey that the participants reported poorly integrated community services and little initial awareness of occupational therapy. The authors made recommendations about the information on OT services and other LA services which should be provided to carers and to GPs and the importance of research in underpinning OT practice within local authorities. Similar findings on the need by carers for more information about OT services were reported by Lorraine Birch and Jo Adams.[87] They concluded that more needed to be done to identify and support the needs of carers and there was a lack of professional support from health-care professionals for carers.

Exploitation by relatives and others

The OT may occasionally encounter situations where it is apparent that an older client is being exploited financially. The Court of Protection has since 2007 provided protection for those lacking mental capacity both in relation to personal welfare and also in relation to property and finance. Any concerns that a person lacking the requisite mental capacity is being exploited can be brought before the Court which can appoint a deputy to safeguard that person on a day to day basis in accordance with the instructions of the court. (The appointment of deputies is considered in Chapter 22.) The OT should ensure that the Department of Social Security was notified if the exploitation relates to the use of social security funds. For larger amounts the OT should ensure that there was a referral to the Court of Protection.

Lasting power of attorney

The Mental Capacity Act 2005 enables a person (known as the donor) with the requisite mental capacity to draw up a lasting power of attorney whereby a person (known as the donee) can make decisions on behalf of the donor. The lasting power of attorney can cover decisions relating to personal welfare and also to property and affairs, but the power relating to personal welfare will only come into effect when the donor lacks the requisite mental capacity. In time the lasting power of attorney will replace enduring powers of attorney. Enduring powers of attorney cannot be drawn up after October 2007, whilst those already in place could remain until the donor withdrew them (provided he had the requisite mental capacity) or died. Further information on lasting powers of attorney can be obtained from the author's book[88] and from the website of the Office of Public Guardian.[89] To create a lasting power of attorney a person must be at least 18 years and have the requisite mental capacity. Similarly to be a donee of a power, a person must be at least 18, have the requisite mental capacity and accept the appointment. Sections 9 to14 of the Mental Capacity Act 2005 set down the provisions for the creation and regulation of LPAs. Forms are available from the Office of Public Guardian.

Abuse of older people

Granny bashing and other forms of physical and mental abuse have only recently been recognised as a danger of which all health and social services professionals should be aware. It is estimated by Help the Aged that 500,000 elderly people are believed to be abused at any one time in the UK. Should an OT suspect that her client is the victim of such action, she should take such care as is reasonable in all the circumstances to ensure that the older person is safe. This will probably necessitate referring the client to the community health services and also informing social services. The Social Services Inspectorate has provided a report on confronting abuse of older people. This sets out the ways in which the social services departments respond to and manage cases of 'elder abuse' that arise in domestic settings. It suggests ways in which practice might be improved through clearer policies and guidelines. Claudine McCreadie of the Institute of Gerontology has published an extensive analysis of current research[90] on elder abuse which should be essential reading for every health professional caring for older people. She concludes that the term 'elder abuse' covers diverse situations, that the extent of the problems is still unknown but sufficient to make the case for a service response, that research and training are essential, and she points to the danger that older people who are being abused will fall between existing service provisions and their needs will remain unaddressed, unless action is taken. Information has come to light on the extent of financial abuse and exploitation. Ginny Jenkins, Director of Action on Elder Abuse, stated that it is estimated that one in ten of those granted powers under Enduring Powers of Attorney abuses the trust.[91]

In April 2004 the House of Commons Select Committee of Health published a report on abuse of the elderly. It considered that 500 000 of Britain's elderly are subject to regular abuse by relatives and carers. It has made significant recommendations covering six-monthly assessment of residents in care homes, a national system of data collection on abuse and the creation of guidelines to define where an old person is considered vulnerable. The abused elderly come under the legislation on safeguarding vulnerable adults which is considered in Chapter 19. From 12 October 2009, it will be an offence for any employer to employ someone (paid or unpaid) in regulated activity when he knows the person has been barred by the Independent Safeguarding Authority (ISA). Anyone barred by the ISA commits an offence if they work in regulated activity. Regulated activity will extend to most NHS and social care workers.

Many charities offer guidance in recognising elder abuse and in taking action to prevent its occurrence. Counsel and care published a fact sheet giving advice on abuse and the risk to older people which is available from its website.[92] It covers the types, symptoms, location, of abuse and the likely abusers and abused; the action to be taken if abuse is seen or suspected in a variety of locations and the law which applies. The Domestic Violence Crime and Victims Act (DVCV Act) 2004 requires persons living in a household where there is a child or vulnerable adult to take reasonable steps to prevent the unlawful death of that person. Reasonable steps suggested by Counsel and Care would include:

- reporting suspicions of abuse to the police
- contacting local social services
- making sure that any injuries are treated promptly
- explaining concerns to the GP
- contacting an organisation such as Action on Elder Abuse.

The DVCV Act defines a vulnerable person as:

> any person aged 16 or over whose ability to protect himself from violence, abuse or neglect is significantly impaired through physical or mental disability of illness, through old age or otherwise

In addition under the Mental Capacity Act 2005 it is a criminal offence under section 44(2) to ill-treat or wilfully neglect a person who lacks capacity.

Action on Elder Abuse has a helpline number[93] and website.[94] It has recently launched a Safeguarding Adults Good Practice project together with the Practitioners Alliance for Vulnerable Adults. The project aims to provide practical methods of identifying and disseminating good practice from around the country and the database is available from the Action on Elder Abuse website. Age Concern[95] and Help the Aged[96] also provide information on elder abuse and the action which should be taken. For discussion on the new Independent Safeguarding Authority (ISA) see its website[97] and Chapter 19.

Property and abuse

A consultation document *Safeguarding Adults* was published on 16 October 2008 by four different departments including the Department of Health and the Home Office[98] which aimed at strengthening the *No Secrets* guidance published in 2000[99] to tackle the problem of abuse of the elderly. The consultation ended in January 2009. A study funded by the Department of health and Comic Relief in 2007 found that 342,000 people aged over 66 were being abused in private households at any one time. Figures from Action on Elder Abuse show that in the majority of these cases, abuse is perpetrated by a family member or friend. Safeguarding Adults recommends that banks, building societies an the Financial Services Authority should monitor the accounts of elderly people for unusual cash withdrawals and direct debits and share information with the authorities where theft or fraud is suspected. The problems of exploitation and theft from the elderly are likely to increase as elderly persons opt to receive personal budgets to obtain care in the home. Another recommendation is that social workers should have the power to check up on how older people are being looked after in their own home with the help of their children.[100]

Use of volunteers

One of the principle philosophies of the community care policy is that provision of services for those in need should be based on a partnership between the statutory services, the independent sector, including the voluntary sector, and the family. The OT should be aware of the contribution that voluntary groups and individual volunteers can make towards the care and quality of life of the patient/client, whether at home or in the hospital. She should be alert to the legal implications of delegating tasks to volunteers and should ensure that the principles set out in Chapter 10 on delegation and supervision are observed. An OT who delegated tasks to a volunteer who lacked the knowledge and experience to undertake that activity with reasonable safety, could be liable for any harm which was caused and her employer vicariously liable. Age Concern, which has an extensive programme for volunteers to befriend older persons, provides insurance cover for their volunteers. Many other charities using volunteers also provide cover.

Situation: volunteers

An OT agrees with a volunteer that he can take an older person in the rehabilitation ward on an outing to a restaurant. Unfortunately he had not taken care to make sure that the volunteer had the appropriate insurance cover for his car. The volunteer is involved in an accident and the older person is harmed. Who is liable?

The OT who is responsible for permitting the volunteer to undertake this activity should have ensured that the volunteer had the necessary insurance cover. The volunteer would also be contributorily negligent in not checking up. If the volunteer caused the accident and therefore the injuries to the patient, the patient's compensation would probably be paid by the Motor Insurer's Bureau if the driver himself had no or inadequate insurance cover. If another driver was at fault, then his or her insurance cover should provide compensation. The negligence of the OT may lead to disciplinary proceedings against her by the employer.

Where volunteers are used in health and social care it is important to define who is responsible for giving them clearly defined boundaries within which to work, and ensuring that they have had the necessary training and supervision. If faults can be shown in the delegation to and supervision of the volunteer, then the employer would be vicariously liable for those failures by the delegator. If the volunteer has had appropriate training and instructions and supervision but disobeyed the rules, then although the volunteer is not an employee and so in strict law there is no employer to be vicariously liable, the NHS trust or other employer would probably accept liability, in accordance with Department of Health expectations, since it is directly liable for the patient's safety.

A bill to promote volunteering was debated in Parliament in 2004 but not enacted. It would have provided protection against inherent risks for those organising volunteers.

Inter-agency co-operation

Statutory provisions require health authorities and local authorities to work closely together and with the independent/voluntary sector in the performance of their statutory functions. Other organisations with which the OT may be involved include local authority housing departments, housing associations, care organisations, and many companies and firms which provide services for older people. OTs should be aware of the resources available for the care of older people and from whom further information may be obtained. The Care Quality Commission (which took over the responsibilities of the Commission for Social Care Inspection (CSCI)) publishes the reports of its inspections of care homes which are available on its website.[101] Its website can also be used to find a suitable care home in a particular location check the ratings of any home; and obtain advice and guidance. CSCI ratings are 3 stars excellent; 2 stars good 1 star adequate and 0 star poor. Counsel and Care has also published a fact sheet on *Care Homes: What to look for?* which is available on its website.[102]

The Audit Commission recommended innovative practice and close communication in preventing bed blocking and poor standards of care in its report *The Coming of Age*[103] and in a more recent report it has made strong recommendations on the care of confused older people.[104] In this latter report it emphasises the range of services which those suffering from dementia require, and the need for health and social services to work closely together to make the best use of available resources. The National Audit Office has also reported on the discharge of older patients from NHS acute hospitals.[105] Anita Atwal and others describe occupational therapists' perceptions of pre-discharge occupational therapy home assessments with older adults in acute care and concluded that older adults should be involved in the pre-discharge decision-making process.[106]

Intermediate care

Intermediate care has been described[107] as a

> core element of the Government's programme for improving services for older people. In conjunction with improvements to community equipment services [see Chapter 15], home care support and related services it will enable increased numbers of older people to maintain independent lives at home.

To come within the definition of intermediate care, services must meet *all* the following criteria:

- are targeted at people who would otherwise face unnecessarily prolonged hospital stays or inappropriate admission to acute in-patient care, long-term residential care, or continuing NHS in-patient care
- are provided on the basis of a comprehensive assessment, resulting in a structured individual care plan that involves active therapy, treatment or opportunity for recovery
- have a planned outcome of maximising independence and typically enabling patients/users to resume living at home
- are time-limited, normally no longer than six weeks and frequently as little as 1–2 weeks or less
- involve cross-professional working, with a single assessment framework, single professional records and shared protocols.

Intermediate care is covered in standard three of the NSF for older people.

Various models are envisaged including rapid response, hospital at home, residential rehabilitation, supported discharge and day rehabilitation. The Department of Health has provided guidance on the responsibilities for intermediate care and charging, planning its development, the role of the independent sector, the funding of intermediate care and community equipment services (see Chapter 15), and the evaluation of the service.[108] A work edited by Sian Wade on the intermediate care of older people provides a useful guide to the planning and delivery of intermediate care services for older people.[109] In 2009 the DH published a prevention package for older people designed to ensure that they remained independent for as long as was reasonably practicable. It is available from the DH website and includes a section on intermediate care.

Community care: delayed discharges

Legislation has been passed to prevent discharges from hospital being delayed because of inadequate provision in the community. The Community Care (Delayed Discharges etc.) Act 2003 makes provision for social services authorities to make payments in cases where the discharge of patients is delayed for reasons relating to the provision of community care services or services for carers. Under the Act (whose implementation was delayed by the House of Lords) the responsible NHS organisation can serve notice on a social services authority (in which the patient is ordinarily resident) that a patient is or is expected to become a qualifying hospital patient at a particular hospital and that it is unlikely to be safe to discharge the patient from hospital unless one or more community care services are made available for him. Before issuing a notice the NHS organisation must consult the patient and a carer (if it is aware of the person's identity). Following the notice the responsible authority must carry out an assessment of the patient's needs with a view to identifying any community care services that need to be made available in order for it to be safe to discharge him and, after consulting the NHS body, must decide which of those services, if any, the authority will make available for the patient. The needs of the carer must also be assessed (where the carer has requested such as assessment) in order to identify any services which the authority may provide under section 2 of the Carers and Disabled Children Act 2000 and which need to be made available to the carer in order for it to be safe to discharge the patient, and, after consultation with the responsible NHS body, which services the authority decides to make available to the carer. The NHS body must notify the social services authority of the day it intends to discharge the patient and there must be a period of at least two days between the notice and the day of discharge. (Regulations may stipulate a longer period and provide for the form and content of the notice.) Failure by the social services authority to comply with these statutory duties can lead to the authority being liable to make a payment of the amount prescribed in the regulations for each day of the delayed discharge. Disputes over 'ordinary residence' are to be resolved by the Secretary of State or Welsh Assembly by arrangements to be drawn up by them. Regulations are also to be passed to set up a system for dispute resolution. The Minister is given power to apply these provisions to patients in care homes. In December 2006 the DH in conjunction with the Department of Communities and Local Government issued guidance on hospital admissions and discharges for the homeless or those living in temporary or insecure accommodation.[110]

Regulations[111] came into force on 9 June 2003 which required community equipment (aids and minor adaptations) to be provided free of charge (see Chapter 15) and a period of intermediate care (see earlier section) is to be provided free of charge to any person for a period up to and including 6 weeks.

Health and safety manual handling

The OT who cares for older people should ensure that she follows the principles set out in Chapter 11 in relation to manual handling and other health and safety regulations. Even though she may see some manual handling in the care of her older clients as therapeutic, it still comes under the Manual Handling Regulations and she would be expected to carry out an appropriate risk assessment. She must also ensure that she receives regular updating of her training.

Situation: teaching the carers

An OT watches a husband demonstrate how he gets his wife out of a chair. The patient puts her arm around her husband's neck and pulls, putting him at considerable risk. The OT warns the husband of the dangers, but he says that he has always done it this way and sees no problem with it. Where does the OT stand if he later suffers harm?

It is quite likely in this situation that the husband will ignore the advice of the OT to introduce a different method of lifting his wife. If she arranged for the delivery of a hoist, he may well not use it. However, the OT has a duty to ensure that she gives the appropriate advice in such a way that he can see the serious dangers in his present methods, and that she arranges the supply of any necessary equipment. If having fulfilled her duty of care, the husband ignores her advice and does not use the equipment, then any harm which he suffers is at his own risk and he could not successfully hold the OT liable for it. (For further discussion on manual handling see Chapter 11). Health and safety and equipment issues are considered in Chapters 11 and 15 respectively.

Resources

Older people have not always received the priority in the allocation of resources which their needs require. OTs should be aware of the dangers of using arbitrary age levels to deny services on a blanket basis, rather than assessing patients individually. It may be that a person in her nineties requires treatment which may be contra-indicated in a person much younger, because her physical condition is much better. Because of the mismatch between the demand for services and the resources available, OTs have a duty to ensure that resources are used reasonably. More research comparable to that carried out by Kate Goodacre and others is necessary to obtain clear evidence on the cost of formal care as compared with supplementing care with assistive technology.[112] Pressure on resources may also lead to long waiting times before assessments can be carried out. OTs have a responsibility to ensure that managers are notified of such situations in order to ensure that a reasonable standard of care is provided. Resource issues also arise in relation to asylum seekers and other who visit the UK temporarily as the following situation shows.

Situation: only here for the short term

A Greek woman who had come to the UK for a few months to visit her daughter was found to be suffering from dementia and depression. She had never worked in the UK and she was unable to return to Greece on account of her care needs. Her entitlement to NHS and social services was unclear. What action should the OT take?

The OT has a responsibility to the client to take all action which she requires immediately. She should also contact social services who have a legal department, often well used to advising on entitlements for overseas visitors. Many countries have reciprocal health agreements with the UK and Greece is a member state of the European Community and the Greek visitor would be entitled to NHS care under the EC laws (see Chapter 6). Social care provision may depend upon whether she eventually wishes to return to Greece (she may have other children living there) and that is her home and social services would have the responsibility of liaising with the appropriate Greek organisations. The OT would have the responsibility of drawing up an assessment of her OT needs and accommodation, the situation in the UK and recommendations for the long-term.

Situation: enough is enough

An OT considers that a stroke patient has reached her full potential and would now benefit from feeling 'in charge of her life'. The patient's husband disagrees and wants his wife to continue with regular rehabilitation. Should the OT provide further sessions?

No OT should accept instructions which are contrary to her professional judgment. This applies whoever is giving the instructions: patients, relatives or other professional colleagues, or councillors and MPs. In this situation, it is a matter of professional judgement whether further sessions are clinically justified. If the OT has formed the view that progress will not be made, then she must make this clear to the patient and husband. The patient has no legal right to enforce treatment which is not clinically indicated and this principle was recognised by the Court of Appeal in the Burke case[113] (see Chapter 6). The OT should explain this sensitively since the sessions may be seen by the relative as a necessary (emotional) support and the OT may offer to review the situation after a specified time. She should, of course, ensure that her record keeping is above reproach and should be prepared for the possibility of a complaint arising from the situation. The OT should also explore what other services are available to the client and the carer and give them information about these. The carer may also be eligible for an assessment of his needs as such a request may indicate that he is not ready or able to cope with caring for his wife.

The Community Care (Residential Accommodation) Act 1998 requires local authorities to assist residents in the payment of fees for residential accommodation without undue delay, as soon as their resources fall below a specified level. If the resources fall below a lower specified level the council is obliged to pay all the fees. The Act reinforces the decision of the court in a case brought against Sefton Council by a resident who had had to contribute to the fees even though her resources were well below £10 000. Sefton Council were following a policy of requiring older people to pay their own fees until all they had left was £1500, about the price of a funeral. The court declared Sefton's actions illegal and this decision is incorporated in the 1998 Act (see Chapter 18).

Future initiatives

The government launched an ageing strategy *Building a Society for All Ages* on 13 July 2009. A health prevention package prepared by the Department of Health as part of the ageing strategy which

- brings together information on existing health 'entitlements' including sight tests, flu vaccination and cancer screening;
- promotes best practice around falls prevention and effective fracture management;

- introduces measures to improve access to affordable footcare services;
- updates national intermediate care guidance;
- summarises existing progress on audiology and telecare.

The package can be down loaded from the DH website.

Conclusion

The demographic changes show that those over 65 will increase as a proportion of society and that the numbers of people aged over 80 and 90 are increasing significantly. The figures quoted in the NSF for Older People suggest that between 1995 and 2025 the number of people over the age of 80 is set to increase by almost a half and the number of people over 90 will double. The resource implications for the provision of health and social care as well as pensions and social security are now coming onto the agenda of every political party. It can no longer be assumed that public expenditure can be the main source of assistance. The outcome of the Green Paper on long term funding of health and social care will have significant implications for the occupational therapy services. The care of older people will continue to be one of the principle responsibilities and challenges for the OT.

 Questions and exercises

1   An OT is concerned that an older person living on her own is refusing to accept any assistance and is neglecting herself. What legal powers exist in this situation?
2   An older person visiting a day hospital refuses to have any therapy. What is the legal situation?
3   In a care home, an OT discovers that all the doors are kept locked. When she inquires about this she is told that this is the only way in which the residents can be prevented from going out on to the main road. What action, if any, should she take?
4   An OT is asked by a resident in a home to help her draw up a living will. What action should the OT take? (See also Chapter 25.)

References

1   Heath Hazel and Watson Roger (eds) (2005) *Older People: Assessment for Health and Social Care*. Age Concern, London.
2   Mountain Gail (2004) *Occupational Therapy with Older People*. Whurr Publishing, London.
3   Richards Margaret (2001) *Long-term Care for Older People*. Jordans Bristol.
4   Lee Michelle (2006) *Promoting Mental Health and Well Being in Later Life*. Age Concern, London.
5   Age Concern (2007) *The Age Agenda – Public Policy and Older People*. Age Concern, London.
6   Walker Alan (ed) (2005) *Understanding Quality of Life in Old Age*. Open University Press, Maidenhead.
7   Wanless Derek (2006) *Securing Good Care for Older People – taking a long term view*. Kings Fund, London.
8   Bradshaw A and Merriman C (2007) *Caring for the Older Person- a practical guide in hospital, care home or at home*. Wiley, Chichester.
9   Bond John and Corner Lynne (2004) *Quality of Life for Older People*. Open University Press, Maidenhead.
10 Bowling Ann (2006) *Aging Well: Quality of Life in the 21st Century*. Open University Press, Maidenhead.
11 www.dh.gov.uk/en/SocialCare/Socialcarereform/Dignityincare
12 *Felix Palacios de la Villa v Cortefiel Servicios SA* ECJ [2007] 16 October Case C-411/05; The Times Law Report 23 October 2007.

13   R (Incorporated Trustees of the National Council on Ageing (Age Concern England)) v Secretary of State for Business, Enterprise and Regulatory Reform The Times Law Report 8 March 2009.

14   Skelton, D.A. & McLaughlin, A.W. (1996) Training functional ability in old age. Physiotherapy, 82(3), 159–67.

15   www.nice.org.uk

16   National Council for Health and Clinical Excellence (2008) Occupational therapy interventions and physical activity interventions to promote the mental well-being of older people in primary care and residential care. London, NICE; www.nice.org.uk/nicemedia/pdf

17   Royal Commission (1999) With Respect to Old Age. Stationery Office, London.

18   HSC 2001/17; LAC(2001)26 Guidance on Free Nursing Care; Department of Health. NHS Funded Nursing Care – Practice Guide and Workbook. DH, London.

19   HSC 2003/006; LAC(2003)7 Guidance on NHS-Funded Nursing Care.

20   R (on the application of Grogan) v Bexley NHS Care Trust [2006] EWHC 44 (2006) 9 CCL 188.

21   Department of Health (2007) National Framework for NHS Continuing Healthcare and NHS-funded Nursing Care. DH, London.

22   www.dh.gov.uk/en/Publicationsandstatistics/

23   www.dh.gov.uk/en/SocialCare/Deliveringadultsocialcare/Continuingcare

24   Commission for Social Care Inspection (2008) The State of Social Care in England 2006–7. CSCI, London.

25   R v Gloucestershire County Council [1997] 2 All ER 1.

26   www.careandsupport.direct.gov.uk

27   Adult Care Reform. Letter to the editor The Times 5 June 2008 from Mencap, Age Concern and others.

28   Bennett Rosemary Councils demand care home top-ups from old people. The Times 17 January 2009.

29   R (On the application of Chavda) v Harrow LBC [2007] EWHC 3064 Admin; (2008) 11 C.C.L. Rep 187.

30   Department of Health (2009) Shaping the Future of Care Together. Cm 7673 Stationery Office, London.

31   Department of Health (2001) National Service Framework for Older People. www.doh.gov.uk/NSF/older-peopleexec.htm (for executive summary).

32   HSC 2001/007; LAC(2001)12 National Service Framework for Older People.

33   College of Occupational Therapists (2006) NSF for Older People: Review and next steps. Briefing note no 67. COT, London.

34   www.dh.gov.uk/Healthcare/Longtermconditions/index.htm

35   Department of Health (2008) Raising the Profile of Long Term Conditions Care: A Compendium of Information. DH, London.

36   College of Occupational Therapists (2007) Supporting people with long term conditions. Briefing note 35. COT, London.

37   National Audit Office (2005) Reducing Brain Damage: Faster Access to better stroke care HC 452 Session 2005–6; www.nao.org.uk

38   Harwood Rowan, Huweg Farhad and Good Dawn (2005) Stroke care: A practical manual. Oxford University Press, Oxford.

39   House of Commons Committee of Public Accounts (2008) Improving Services and Support for People with Dementia Sixth Report of Session 2007–8 HC 228 Stationery Office.

40   www.alzheimers.org.uk

41   Department of Health (2009) Living Well with Dementia: A National Dementia Strategy. DH, London.

42   Plastow Nicola Ann (2006) Is Big Brother watching you? Responding to tagging and tracking in dementia care. British Journal of Occupational Therapy, 69(11), 525–7.

43   Ballinger, CB. (2002) Reflections on the National Service Framework for Older People. British Journal of Occupational Therapy, 65(2), 53.

44   Jacob-Lloyd H, Booth J, Ward G, Grant M and Steed A (2006) From paper to practice: the views of occupational therapists on the impact of the NSF for older people on practice. British Journal of Occupational Therapy 69(11), 490–96.

45   Awang, D. (2002) Older people and participation within disabled facilities grant processes. British Journal of Occupational Therapy, 65(6), 261–8.

46 Dady, K.F. & Rugg, S. (2000) An exploration of individual's expectations of their stay on an elderly care unit. *British Journal of Occupational Therapy*, **63**(1), 9–16.
47 Goodacre Kate, McCreadie Claudine, Flanagan Susan and Lansley Peter (2007) Enabling Older People to stay at home: How adaptable are existing properties. *British Journal of Occupational Therapy* **70**(1), 5–15.
48 Mountain, G. (1998) *Rehabilitation of Vulnerable Older People*. COT, London.
49 HSC 2002/001; LAC(2002)1 *Guidance on the Single Assessment process for older people*.
50 HSC 2001/006; LAC(2001)006 *Better Care Higher Standards*.
51 *Re T (adult: refusal of medical treatment)* [1992] 4 All ER 649.
52 Law Commission on Mentally Incapacitated and Other Vulnerable Adults (1993) *Public Law Protection* (the third paper dealing with decision making and the mentally incapacitated adult). HMSO, London.
53 Law Commission (1995) Report No 231 *Mental Incapacity*. HMSO, London.
54 Lord Chancellor (1997) *Who Decides?* Lord Chancellor's Office, London.
55 Lord Chancellor (1999) *Making Decisions*. Lord Chancellor's Office, London.
56 Department of Health (2001) *Good Practice in Consent Implementation Guide*. DH, London.
57 *F v West Berkshire Health Authority and another* [1989] 2 All ER 545.
58 *R v Bournewood Community & Mental Health NHS Trust Ex p1* [1999] 1 AC 458.
59 Department of Health (2005) *Department of Health responses to the Consultation on adult social care in England: analysis of feedback from the Green paper Independence, Well-being and Choice*. DH, London.
60 Department of Health (2005) *Green Paper; Independence, Well-being and Choice*. DH, London.
61 Department of Health (2006) *Our health, our care, our say: A new direction for community services*. DH, London.
62 Department of Health (2007) *Independence, choice and risk: a guide to best practice in supported decision making*. DH, London.
63 www.dh.gov.uk/en/SocialCare/Socialcareform/
64 Residents Taking Risks; Minimising the use of restraint – A guide for care homes. Counsel and Care, Twyman House, 16 Bonny Street, London NW1 9PG; www.counselandcare.org.uk
65 Reece, AC & Simpson, J.M. (1996) Preparing older people to cope after a fall. *Physiotherapy*, **82**(4), 227–35.
66 Simpson, J., Harrington, R. & Marsh, N. (1998) Guidelines for managing falls among elderly people. *Physiotherapy*, **84**(4), 173–7.
67 Clement, L., Fitzgerald, M.H. & Heard, R. (1999) Content validity of an assessment tool to identify home fall hazards: The Westmead Home safety assessment. *British Journal of Occupational Therapy*, **62**(4), 171–9.
68 Kinn, S. & Galloway, L. (2000) Do occupational therapists and physiotherapists teach elderly people how to rise after a fall. *British Journal of Occupational Therapy*, **63**(6), 254–9.
69 Lord Stephen, Sherrington Catherine, Menz Hylton and Close Jacqueline (2007) *Falls in Older People: Risk factors and strategies for prevention*, Cambridge University Press, Cambridge.
70 Mackenzie, M., Byles, J. & Higginbotham, N. (2000) Designing the home falls and accidents screening tool (HOME FAST): Selecting the items. *British Journal of Occupational Therapy*, **63**(6), 260–67.
71 Buril, H., Picton, J. & Dawson, P. (2000) Perceptual dysfunction in elderly people with cognitive impairment: A risk factor for falls. *British Journal of Occupational Therapy*, **63**(6), 248–53.
72 Ballinger, C. & Payne, S. (2000) Falling from grace or into expert hands? Alternative accounts about falling in older people. *British Journal of Occupational Therapy*, **63**(12), 573–9.
73 Nyman Samuel R and Ballinger Claire (2008) A Review to explore how allied health professional can improve uptake of and adherence to falls prevention interventions. *British Journal of Occupational Therapy*, **71**(4), 141–5.
74 Hughes Rhidian (2008) Older people falling out of bed: restraint, risk and safety. *British Journal of Occupational Therapy*, **71**(9), 389–392.
75 National Institute of Health and Clinical Excellence (2004) *Clinical practice guideline for the assessment and prevention of falls in older people*. NICE, London.
76 Ian Philip (2007) *A Recipe for Care – Not a single ingredient*. DH, London.
77 Carole MacGregor and Jackie Riglin (2007) Update on the National Clinical Audit of Falls and Bone Health for Older People. *Agility*, **2**, 20–22.

78   www.aarp.org/research/ageline/about.html
79   www.nlm.nih.gov/medlineplus/seniorshealth.html
80   College of Occupational Therapists (2006) Falls Management. COT, London.
81   College of Occupational Therapists and CSP (2002) Falls Audit Pack. CSP and. COT, London.
82   Department of Health (2008) *Code of Practice on the Mental Health Act 1983*. DH, London.
83   Residents Taking Risks; Minimising the use of restraint – A guide for care homes. Counsel and Care, Twyman House, 16 Bonny Street, London NW1 9PG; www.counselandcare.org.uk
84   Counsel and Care (undated) Showing Restraint: challenging the use of restraint in care homes.
85   Royal College of Nursing (1999) Restraint revisited: rights, risk and responsibility. RCN 000 998.
86   Dibsdall Lisa and Rugg Sue (2008) Carers' perspectives on their needs and Local Authority Ocupational Therapy Practice. *British Journal of Occupational Therapy*, **71**(7), 277–85.
87   Birch Lorraine and Adams Jo (2008) Carers' perceptions of community occupational therapy: Short report. *British Journal of Occupational Therapy*, **71**(5), 205–8.
88   Dimond B. (2008) *Legal Aspects of Mental Capacity*. Blackwell, Oxford.
89   www.guardianship.gov.uk
90   McCreadie, C. (1996) Elder Abuse: Update on Research. Institute of Gerontology.
91   Speaking on Law In Action, BBC Radio 4, 22 October 1998.
92   www.counselandcare.org.uk
93   0808 808 8141.
94   www.elderabuse.org.uk/index.htm
95   www.ageconcern.org.uk
96   www.helptheaged.org.uk
97   www.isa-gov.org.uk
98   Department of Health, Home Office, Criminal Justice System and the Attorney General's Office (2008) Safeguarding Adults *A Consultation on the Review of the 'No Secrets' Guidance*. DH, London.
99   Department of Health and Home Office (2000) *No Secrets: Guidance on developing and implementing multi-agency policies and procedures to protect vulnerable adults from abuse*. DH and Home Office, London.
100 Bennett Rosemary. Elderly to get more protection from thieving relatives The Times 16 October 2008.
101 www.cqc.org.uk
102 www.counselandcare.org.uk
103 Audit Commission (1997) *The Coming of Age: Improving care services for elderly people*. Stationery Office, London.
104 Audit Commission (2000) *'Forget me not': Mental Health services for older people*. Stationery Office, London.
105 National Audit Office. Ensuring the effective discharge of older patients from NHS acute hospitals. HC 392 Parliamentary Session 2002–3; www.nao.gov.uk/publications/vfmsublist/vfm_nhs.htm
106 Atwal Anita, McIntyre Anne, Craik Christine and Hunt Jacki (2008) Occupational therapists' perceptions of predischarge home assessments with older adults in acute care. *British Journal of Occupational Therapy*, **71**(2), 52–7.
107 HSC 2001/01; LAC(2001)1 Intermediate Care.
108 HSC 2001/01; LAC(2001)1 Intermediate Care.
109 Wade San (ed) (2004) *Intermediate Care of Older People*. Whurr Publishers, London.
110 Department of Health and Department of Communities and Local Government.(2006) *Hospital admission and discharge: People who are homeless or living in temporary or insecure accommodation*. DH and CLG, London.
111 The Community Care (Delayed Discharges etc) Act (Qualifying Services) (England) Regulations 2003 SI 2003/1196.
112 Goodacre Kate, McCreadie Claudine, Flanagan Susan and Lansley Peter (2008) Enabling older people to stay at home: the costs of substituting and supplementing care with assistive technology. *British Journal of Occupational Therapy*, **71**(4) 130–40.
113 *R (on the application of Burke) v General Medical Council and Disability Rights Commission and the Official Solicitor to the Supreme Court* [2004] EWHC 1879; [2004] Lloyd's Rep Med 451.

25 Death and the Dying

It is an inevitable fact that occupational therapists across all specialisms will be involved in the care of dying patients. It is important that at such difficult times the occupational therapist has confidence in her knowledge of the law which applies. Very few books for occupational therapists deal directly with this topic, but help can be found in chapters in books dealing with certain conditions. One book of particular relevance is that edited by Jill Cooper on occupational therapy in oncology and palliative care.[1] See also the author's work on this subject.[2] Anna Libby has set up a web site[3] to enable those suffering from breast cancer to access a support group and has written positively on the value of her occupational therapy training to her own survival.[4] This chapter discusses the law relating to the following topics:

- The extent of the duty to maintain life
- Involvement of the court
- Advance decisions/living wills
- Can the court order doctors to provide treatment?
- 'Not for resuscitation' orders

- Parents' refusal to consent to treatment
- Care of the dying patient
- Registration of death and the role of the coroner
- Organ transplants
- Conclusions

The extent of the duty to maintain life

Healthcare professionals can be faced with the problem of whether there is a duty in law to carry out every possible procedure known to science in order to save the life of the patient or whether the law enables a person to be allowed to die. The law draws a distinction between withholding care and taking positive action to end life. The former may or may not be legally permissible depending upon the condition and prognosis of the patient. The latter will always be illegal. It is not therefore

Legal Aspects of Occupational Therapy, Third Edition By Bridgit Dimond
© 2010 Bridgit Dimond

the duty of the health professional to continue to provide high technology care when the patient's prognosis is considered hopeless; and the patient can be allowed to die. Mr Burke, a patient suffering from a chronic debilitating condition, had challenged the GMC guidelines on withholding treatment arguing that he could insist on being treated even when it was contrary to professional judgment. He succeeded in the High Court but the appeal of the GMC was allowed by the Court of Appeal.[5] (The case is discussed in Chapter 6.)

Human Rights and the right to life

Article 2 of the European Convention of Human Rights (see appendix 1) recognises the right to life. However arguments that this right was breached when persons were allowed to die have failed. In a case[6] in 2000, parents lost their attempt to ensure that a severely handicapped baby born prematurely was resuscitated if necessary. The judge ruled that the hospital should provide him with palliative care to ease his suffering, but should not try to revive him as that would cause unnecessary pain. In another case, the President of the Family Division, Dame Elizabeth Butler-Sloss, held that the withdrawal of life-sustaining medical treatment was not contrary to article 2 of the Human Rights Convention and the right to life where the patient was in a persistent vegetative state (PVS). The ruling was made on 25 October 2000 in cases involving Mrs M, a 49-year-old woman, who suffered brain damage during an operation abroad in 1997 and was diagnosed as being in a PVS in October 1998, and in the case of Mrs H, aged 36, who fell ill in America as a result of pancreatitis during Christmas 1999.[7] In the light of these decisions, it would appear that failure to resuscitate a patient, when circumstances justify the decision, would not amount to a breach of article 2 (see also Chapter 6).

In a case to determine whether a hospital was in breach of article 2 following the suicide of a detained mental patient, it was held that the claimant had to show that at the time of the suicide the hospital knew or ought to have known of the existence of a real and immediate risk to her life from self-harm and that it failed to take measures which reasonably might have been expected to avoid that risk.[8] The Court of Appeal did not accept the Trust's argument that the claimant had to establish gross negligence by the defendant. The facts of the case were that the claimant's mother, who had a long history of mental illness had been detained under section 3 of the Mental Health Act 1983. She had made frequent attempts to leave and eventually succeeded and walked to a railway station and jumped in front of a train. The Court of Appeal compared the situation of a detained mentally ill patient to that of a prisoner who were both under the control of a state in a way in which ordinary patients were not. The House of Lords dismissed the appeal.[9] See Chapter 6.

Breach of article 2 has also been alleged in cases where it has been argued that an inadequate inquiry has been held in relation to a death or serious harm in custody. Thus in a case where a young man attempted suicide in Feltham Young Offenders Institution and was left brain damaged, the Court of Appeal held that in such a situation Article 2 rights required that there was a clear obligation on the Secretary of State to ensure that there was an effective inquiry into the near death.[10]

An application for an inquest to be held was granted in the case of *Bicknell v HM Coroner for Birmingham and Solihull* in 2007.[11] The daughter of a man who had died in a care home applied for judicial review of the coroner's decision not to hold an inquest. The father had been suffering from mental health problems and had died soon after admission to the home. Despite the daughter's concern about his treatment, the death was not reported to the coroner and the funeral and cremation took place. The National Care Standards Commission (predecessor to the Commission for Social Care Inspection, now the Care Quality Commission) carried out an inquiry and the owners voluntarily closed the home. The daughter gave to the coroner the report of a medical expert who criticised the medical records in the home and raised concerns about the increased dose of medication and the bucket chair in which he was placed. The coroner held that there was no evidence of unnatural death and refused the request for an inquest. The High Court held that the medical evidence and the daughter's observations gave rise to a reasonable cause to suspect that he had died an unnatural death. In addition the results of the NCSC inquiry revealed concerns about his death.

Murder and manslaughter

To kill a patient may be murder or manslaughter.

> Murder is when a man of sound memory, and of the age of discretion, unlawfully killeth within any country of the realm any reasonable creature *in rerum natura* under the King's peace, with malice aforethought, either expressed by the party or implied by law, so as the party wounded, or hurt, etc. die of the wound or hurt etc. (within a year and a day after the same – these words subsequently deleted). (Coke)

This definition of murder was given in a court case in the 17th century. In 1996 the limitation of time was removed, so that it is not now required that the person dies within a year and a day of the act which caused the death.

Manslaughter is divided into two categories – voluntary and involuntary. Voluntary covers the situation where there is the mental intention to kill or complete indifference to the possibility that death could arise from one's actions (i.e. the mental requirement of a crime (*mens rea*) but there are extenuating factors:

- provocation (abolished by the Coroners and Justice Act 2009; see below)
- death in pursuance of a suicide pact
- diminished responsibility.

The effect of these extenuating factors is that a murder verdict would not be obtained but the defendant could be guilty of voluntary manslaughter.

Involuntary manslaughter exists when the *mens rea* for murder is absent. Such circumstances would include:

- gross negligence
- killing recklessly where the recklessness may be insufficient for it to be murder
- an intention to escape from lawful arrest.

Defences to a charge of murder or manslaughter include:

- killing in the course of preventing crime or arresting offenders
- killing in the defence of one's own person or that of another
- killing in defence of property.

Use of excessive force will negate these defences.

Where the accused is convicted of manslaughter the judge has complete discretion over sentencing, but there may be cases where manslaughter may deserve life imprisonment.[12] In contrast, where there is a murder conviction at present the sentence is a mandatory one of life imprisonment although this has been reviewed by the Law Commission. The Law Commission published a consultation paper in 2006 which set out proposals for a new Homicide Act.[13] It put forward the proposal that the structure of a reformed law of homicide should comprise three general offences plus specific offences: 1st degree murder would have a mandatory life sentence; 2nd degree murder would have a discretionary life sentence, manslaughter would have a fixed term of years maximum imprisonment and specific offences such as assisting suicide and infanticide should have a fixed term of years maximum imprisonment. The Coroners and Justice Act 2009 amended the definition of diminished responsibility which if successfully pleaded can reduce a murder offence to manslaughter. The Act also introduced a new partial defence to murder for loss of control where there is a qualifying trigger. These provisions are shown in Box 25.1. The common law defence of provocation is abolished and the offence of infanticide is amended.

Box 25.1   Sections 52, 54 and 55 of the Coroners and Justice Act 2009.

Section 52

(1)   A person ("D") who kills or is a party to the killing of another is not to be convicted of murder if D was suffering from an abnormality of mental functioning which—
   (a)   arose from a recognised medical condition,
   (b)   substantially impaired D's ability to do one or more of the things mentioned in subsection (1A), and
   (c)   provides an explanation for D's acts and omissions in doing or being a party to the killing.

(1A)   Those things are—
   (a)   to understand the nature of D's conduct;
   (b)   to form a rational judgment;
   (c)   to exercise self-control.

(1B)   For the purposes of subsection (1)(c), an abnormality of mental functioning provides an explanation for D's conduct if it causes, or is a significant contributory factor in causing, D to carry out that conduct.

Section 54 Partial defence to murder: loss of control

(1)   Where a person ("D") kills or is a party to the killing of another ("V"), D is not to be convicted of murder if—
   (a)   D's acts and omissions in doing or being a party to the killing resulted from D's loss of self-control,
   (b)   the loss of self-control had a qualifying trigger, and
   (c)   a person of D's sex and age, with a normal degree of tolerance and self restraint and in the circumstances of D, might have reacted in the same or in a similar way to D.

(2)   For the purposes of subsection (1)(a), it does not matter whether or not the loss of control was sudden.

(3)   In subsection (1)(c) the reference to "the circumstances of D" is a reference to all of D's circumstances other than those whose only relevance to D's conduct is that they bear on D's general capacity for tolerance or self-restraint.

(4)   Subsection (1) does not apply if, in doing or being a party to the killing, D acted in a considered desire for revenge.

(5)   On a charge of murder, if sufficient evidence is adduced to raise an issue with respect to the defence under subsection (1), the jury must assume that the defence is satisfied unless the prosecution proves beyond reasonable doubt that it is not.

(6)   For the purposes of subsection (5), sufficient evidence is adduced to raise an issue with respect to the defence if evidence is adduced on which, in the opinion of the trial judge, a jury, properly directed, could reasonably conclude that the defence might apply.

continued

(7)   A person who, but for this section, would be liable to be convicted of murder is liable instead to be convicted of manslaughter.

(8)   The fact that one party to a killing is by virtue of this section not liable to be convicted of murder does not affect the question whether the killing amounted to murder in the case of any other party to it.

Section 55 Meaning of "qualifying trigger"

(1)   This section applies for the purposes of section 54.

(2)   A loss of self-control had a qualifying trigger if subsection (3), (4) or (5) applies.

(3)   This subsection applies if D's loss of self-control was attributable to D's fear of serious violence from V against D or another identified person.

(4)   This subsection applies if D's loss of self-control was attributable to a thing or things done or said (or both) which—
   (a)   constituted circumstances of an extremely grave character, and
   (b)   caused D to have a justifiable sense of being seriously wronged.

(5)   This subsection applies if D's loss of self-control was attributable to a combination of the matters mentioned in subsections (3) and (4).

(6)   In determining whether a loss of self-control had a qualifying trigger—
   (a)   D's fear of serious violence is to be disregarded to the extent that it was caused by a thing which D incited to be done or said for the purpose of providing an excuse to use violence;
   (b)   a sense of being seriously wronged by a thing done or said is not justifiable if D incited the thing to be done or said for the purpose of providing an excuse to use violence;
   (c)   the fact that a thing done or said constituted sexual infidelity is to be disregarded.

(7)   In this section references to "D" and "V" are to be construed in accordance with section 54.

In February 2008 a husband who had suffocated his sick wife was given a 12-month suspended prison sentence and escaped prison.[14] He had admitted manslaughter on grounds of diminished responsibility and aiding and abetting his wife's suicide. His wife suffered from MS. In another case a woman who tried repeatedly to kill her disabled husband was given 100 hours of community service. The judge was satisfied that her attempts were a cry for help and not a serious attempt to kill her husband.[15] Her husband was crippled by arthritis and she had looked after him every day for 5 years at her home, whilst working full time. The judge accepted that she was unable to cope with the strain of caring for him. In contrast a mother was charged with attempted murder when she gave her daughter who suffered with ME a morphine overdose.[16]

Pain management

It may sometimes occur that in order to control pain, high dosages of medication are required which could reduce life expectancy. It is clear that in law if the intention is to relieve pain and the practitioner is following the reasonable standard of approved practice, no offence is committed.[17] Annie Lindsell, a sufferer from motor neurone disease wanted an assurance that she would be given sufficient pain relief when necessary and that her GP would not be prosecuted for murder if he gave her potentially lethal painkillers. She applied to the court on 28 October 1997. After hearing that a responsible body of medical opinion supported her GP's plan, she withdrew her application. The law draws a clear distinction between administering pain relief with the sole intention of controlling a patient's pain in accordance with responsible medical opinion, and administering painkillers with the intention of ending a patient's life.

Voluntary euthanasia

By this is meant the killing of a person with that person's consent. This is unlawful. It could amount to murder, punishable on conviction by life imprisonment, or it could be seen as manslaughter with the discretion over sentencing. Alternatively, if the act amounts to assistance in a suicide bid, then it is illegal under section 2(1) of the Suicide Act 1961, as amended by the Coroners and Justice Act 2009, shown in Figure 25.1.

Situation: Asking for help

The wife of a patient who was in the terminal stages of a respiratory disease was concerned that the patient found breathing difficult in spite of constant oxygen and no longer wished to carry on living. She asked the occupational therapist if she would provide her with some medicines to help her husband out of his misery. What right of action does the occupational therapist have?

Figure 25.1   The Suicide Act 1961 – section 2(1) (as amended by the Coroners and Justice Act 2009).

(1) A person ("D") commits an offence if—
  (a) D does an act capable of encouraging or assisting the suicide or attempted suicide of another person, and
  (b) D's act was intended to encourage or assist suicide or an attempt at suicide.
(1A) The person referred to in subsection (1)(a) need not be a specific person (or class of persons) known to, or identified by, D.
(1B) D may commit an offence under this section whether or not a suicide, or an attempt at suicide, occurs.
(1C) An offence under this section is triable on indictment and a person convicted of such an offence is liable to imprisonment for a term not exceeding 14 years.
(3) In subsection (2) of that section, for "it" to the end substitute "of a person it is proved that the deceased person committed suicide, and the accused committed an offence under subsection (1) in relation to that suicide, the jury may find the accused guilty of the offence under subsection (1)."
(4) After that section insert—

"2A Acts capable of encouraging or assisting
(1) If D arranges for a person ("D2") to do an act that is capable of encouraging or assisting the suicide or attempted suicide of another person and D2 does that act, D is also to be treated for the purposes of this Act as having done it.
(2) Where the facts are such that an act is not capable of encouraging or assisting suicide or attempted suicide, for the purposes of this Act it is to be treated as so capable if the act would have been so capable had the facts been as D believed them to be at the time of the act or had subsequent events happened in the manner D believed they would happen (or both).
(3) A reference in this Act to a person ("P") doing an act that is capable of encouraging the suicide or attempted suicide of another person includes a reference to P doing so by threatening another person or otherwise putting pressure on another person to commit or attempt suicide.

2B Course of conduct
A reference in this Act to an act includes a reference to a course of conduct, and a reference to doing an act is to be read accordingly.

There is no grey area of law here. Any action on the part of the occupational therapist to assist the wife in ending her husband's misery would constitute a criminal wrong and they could both face murder or manslaughter proceedings or prosecution for an offence under the Suicide Act.

Case of Diane Pretty[18]

In a well publicised case, Diane Pretty, a sufferer of motor neurone disease, appealed to the House of Lords that her husband should be allowed to end her life, and not be prosecuted under the Suicide Act 1961. The House of Lords did not allow her appeal. It held that if there were to be any changes to the Suicide Act to legalise the killing of another person, then these changes should be made by Parliament. As the law stood, the Suicide Act made it a criminal offence to aid and abet the suicide of another person and the husband could not be granted immunity from prosecution were he to assist his wife to die. The House of Lords held that there was no conflict between the human rights of Mrs Pretty as set out in the European Convention on Human Rights. Mrs Pretty then applied to the European Court of Human Rights in Strasbourg, but lost. The Court held that there was no conflict between the Suicide Act 1961 and the European Convention of Human Rights. The Council of Europe issued a press release entitled Chamber judgement in the case of *Pretty v the United Kingdom* published on April 29 2002.[19]

Case of Debbie Purdy

An MS sufferer, Debbie Purdy was allowed to bring an action to the law on assisted suicide. She wished her husband to take her to a Belgian clinic or Switzerland to commit suicide if her condition became unbearably painful and wanted to ensure that he would not be prosecuted for aiding and abetting her suicide.[20] The High Court dismissed her application for further guidance from the Director of Public Prosecutions as to when a prosecution for assisted suicide would be brought. The High Court held that it had great sympathy for Ms Purdy, her husband and others in a similar position to know in advance whether they will face prosecution for doing what many would regard as something that the law should permit, namely to help loved one to go abroad to end their suffering when they are unable to do it on their own. However it said that this would involve a change in the law. The offence of suicide is very widely drawn to cover all manner of different circumstances: only Parliament can change it. The court also held that the Code of Practice for Crown Prosecutors issued by the Director of Public Prosecutions, coupled with the general safeguards of administrative law, satisfied human rights convention standards and met the need for clarity and foreseeability and there was no breach of article 8 of the European Convention on Human Rights and the right to private and family life. She was given leave to appeal but the Court of Appeal dismissed her appeal.[21] It held that she was not entitled to have the specific guidance she was seeking, but that there were broad circumstances in which aiding and abetting suicide would not be prosecuted. Even if there were a prosecution, the court had power to order that the offender should be discharged and might well question publicly the decision to prosecute. It stated that the court was part of the protective system which discouraged and would prevent or extinguish the effect of any arbitrary or unprincipled exercise by the DPP of its responsibilities. The Court of Appeal also said that it was for Parliament to change the law. MS Purdy said afterwards that she felt that she had won her argument, despite having lost the appeal. She did however appeal to the House of Lords which heard the case on 3 June 2009 and gave its judgment on 30 July 2009.[22] The House of Lords unanimously held that the DPP should be required to promulgate a policy identifying the facts and circumstances he would take into account in considering whether to prosecute persons such as the claimant's husband for aiding and abetting an assisted suicide abroad. The lack of clarity on whether there would be a prosecution of relatives who took someone abroad to die was an infringement of Article 8 rights.

Director of Public Prosecution interim policy on assisted suicide prosecutions

The Director of Public Prosecutions has now published its final policy on assisted suicide prosecutions. The interim policy set out the following key facts in relation to the DPP's Interim Policy for Prosecutors in respect of Cases of Assisted Suicide:

- details the public interest factors that CPS prosecutors will consider when deciding whether or not to prosecute someone for assisting suicide*.
- details those public interest factors which carry more weight than others
- supplements the Code for Crown Prosecutors, a publicly available document which gives guidance on the general principles to be applied when making decisions about prosecutions
- will be applied to all current and future cases until a final policy is published in Spring 2010
- applies to all cases where the act(s) of assisting the suicide are carried out in England and Wales, regardless of where the suicide takes place
- applies in cases of attempting to assist a suicide
- does not address euthanasia which remains murder or manslaughter
- does not and cannot provide any individuals with immunity from prosecution
- does not and cannot provide an assurance that individuals will be prosecuted
- does not and cannot decriminalise assisted suicide.

The full document can be obtained from the Crown Prosecution Service website. The final policy was published in the spring of 2010 following the consultation on the interim policy.

The public interest **factors against prosecution** are identified in the interim policy as:

- The victim had a clear, settled and informed wish to commit suicide.
- The victim indicated unequivocally to the suspect that he or she wished to commit suicide.
- The victim asked personally on his or her own initiative for the assistance of the suspect.
- The victim had a terminal illness or a severe and incurable physical disability or a severe degenerative physical condition from which there was no possibility of recovery.
- The suspect was wholly motivated by compassion.
- The suspect was the spouse, partner or a close relative or a close personal friend of the victim, within the context of a long-term and supportive relationship.
- The actions of the suspect, although sufficient to come within the definition of the offence, were of only minor assistance or influence, or the assistance which the suspect provided was as a consequence of their usual lawful employment.

In contrast, the public interest **factors in favour of prosecution** in the interim policy include the following:

- The victim was under 18 years of age,
- The victim's capacity to reach an informed decision was adversely affected by a recognised mental illness or learning difficulty.
- The victim did not have a clear, settled and informed wish to commit suicide; for example, the victim's history suggests that his or her wish to commit suicide was temporary or subject to change,
- The victim did not indicate unequivocally to the suspect that he or she wished to commit suicide.
- The victim did not ask personally on his or her own initiative for the assistance of the suspect.
- The victim did not have a terminal illness; or a severe and incurable physical disability; or a severe degenerative physical condition from which there was no possibility of recovery.

- The suspect was not wholly motivated by compassion; for example, the suspect was motivated by the prospect that they or a person closely connected to them stood to gain in some way from the death of the victim.
- The suspect persuaded, pressured or maliciously encouraged the victim to commit suicide, or exercised improper influence in the victim's decision to do so; and did not take reasonable steps to ensure that any other person did not do so.

The General Medical Council has drafted a consultation document "End of Life Treatment and care" which was published in December 2009 and was considered at its meeting in February 2010. The finalised guidance can be seen on the GMC website.

Even where the parents wish a grossly handicapped baby to die, any professional who intentionally speeds up the process of death could be guilty of causing the death of the child.

Case: *R v Arthur*[23]

A paediatrician was prosecuted for attempting to cause the death of a grossly handicapped baby who was suffering from Down's Syndrome and who had other disabilities when he prescribed dihydrocodeine and nursing care only.

The judge had stated that:

There is no special law in this country that places doctors in a separate category and gives them extra protection over the rest of us...Neither in law is there any special power, facility or license to kill children who are handicapped or seriously disadvantaged in an irreversible way.

Dr Arthur was, however, acquitted by the jury

In contrast, at the other end of life, Dr Nigel Cox[24] was convicted when he prescribed potassium chloride to a terminally ill patient and was sentenced to a year's imprisonment which was suspended for a year. He also had to appear before disciplinary proceedings of the Regional Health Authority, his employers and before the General Medical Council.

The Select Committee of the House of Lords[25] has reported that there should be no change in the law to permit euthanasia. This is also the view put forward by the Law Commission in a report in 1995.[26] Lord Joffe has introduced several Bills into the House of Lords to legalise assisting in a suicide. However none has ever obtained Parliamentary approval and assisting another person to die still remains unlawful.

Letting die

Do these cases mean that it is never lawful to permit patients to die whatever the circumstances of their condition? The answer is that the law does not expect constant medical intervention whatever the prognosis and, in certain circumstances, it is legally permissible to let a patient die. A distinction is drawn between letting die and killing.

Adults

Where an adult wishes to die and refuses treatment, then crucial to the decision making and withholding treatment is their mental capacity to make a decision or the existence of a living will (now known as an advance decision) (see below).

Situation: Coming off a ventilator

A tetraplegic patient attended by the occupational therapist told her that he wished to be allowed to die and come off the ventilator. What is the legal situation?

This is the situation which arose in the Karen Quinlan case in the USA where an extremely long court case resulted in a decision being made that she could come off the ventilator. Once off, ironically, she survived for several years. More recently in the UK a patient who had become paralysed following a haemorrhage was ventilated against her wishes. She applied to court for a declaration that she could lawfully refuse ventilation. The only issue before the judge was whether she had the mental capacity to make such a decision. After hearing evidence of two psychiatrists as to her mental competence the judge had no alternative other than to make the declaration she sought and to find that she had been subjected to a trespass to her person.[27] The case of Ms B is considered in more detail in Chapter 7.

A mentally competent person has the right to refuse treatment. However in this situation the occupational therapist should be careful not to undertake any action which could be interpreted as aiding or abetting a suicide attempt. She should also obtain independent advice on the mental competence of the patient to refuse treatment (see Chapter 7 and the law relating to consent).

Children

The following is an example of the court permitting a child to be allowed to die.

Case: *Re C*[28]

In this case a baby was born suffering from congenital hydrocephalus and had been made a ward of court for reasons unconnected with her medical condition. The local authority sought the court's determination as to the appropriate manner in which she should be treated in the event of her contracting a serious infection or her existing feeding regimes becoming unviable. A specialist paediatrician assessed C's condition as severely and irreversibly brain-damaged, the prognosis of which was hopeless. He recommended that the objective of any treatment should therefore be to ease suffering rather than prolong life. While not specifying the adoption or discontinuance of any particular procedures, he further advised consultation with C's carers as to the appropriate method of achieving that objective. The judge accepted this report and approved the recommendations as being in her best interests. However, he made a very restrictive order to treat the child 'to die'.

The official solicitor who had been appointed *guardian ad litem* (see glossary) of the child, appealed to the Court of Appeal on the ground that the judge had not jurisdiction and was plainly wrong in the exercise of his discretion to make an order that the hospital be at liberty to treat the minor to die.

The Court of Appeal varied the judge's order and the words 'to die' were changed to 'to allow her life to come to an end peacefully and with dignity'. The court emphasised that the decisions on treatment rested with the medical professionals:

The hospital do continue to treat the minor within the parameters of the opinion expressed by [the specialist paediatrician] in his report of 13.4.1989 which report is not to be disclosed to any person other than the health authority.

In *Re J*[29] (1990) the baby was a ward of court and in contrast with the case of *Re C* the baby was not at the point of death.

Case: *Re J* (1990)

J's prognosis was not good and, although he was expected to survive a few years, he was likely to be blind, deaf, unable to speak and have serious spastic quadriplegia. The judge made an order that he should be treated with antibiotics if he developed a chest infection but if he were to stop breathing he should not receive artificial ventilation. The official solicitor on behalf of the child appealed against the order on the grounds that unless the situation was one of terminal illness or it was certain that the child's life would be intolerable, the court was not justified in approving the withholding of life saving treatment.

The Court of Appeal held that the court can never sanction positive steps to terminate the life of a person. However the court could direct that treatment without which death would ensue need not be given to prolong life, even though the child was neither on the point of death nor dying. The court had to undertake a balancing exercise in assessing the course to be adopted in the best interests of the child, looked at from his point of view and giving the fullest possible weight to his desire, if he were in a position to make a sound judgment, to survive, but also taking into account the pain and suffering and quality of life which he would experience if life were prolonged and the pain and suffering involved in the proposed treatment.

The parents do not have the final say, though their wishes must be taken into account in determining the outcome for the child. Ultimately the courts, as is seen in the case of *Re J* (1992) (see page 535), have made it clear that the decision should be in the hands of the health professionals i.e. the doctors. In recent years there have been several contested cases between parents and paediatricians as to whether active treatment should be given to a very severely disabled child. One example is that of the case of Charlotte Wyatt where several applications were made to court for a declaration as to what was in the child's best interests.[30]

The Royal College of Paediatrics and Child Health (RCPCH)[31] has published a framework for practice in determining whether life saving treatment should be withheld or withdrawn. These proposals cover the following situations withholding or withdrawal of treatment could be considered:

- brain dead
- persistent vegetative state
- the 'no chance' situation
- the 'no purpose' situation
- the 'unbearable' situation.

The principles, put forward in the first edition of the RCPCH guidance have been reaffirmed in the second edition, and are set out in Figure 25.2. Figure 25.3 shows the axioms which flow from the fundamental principles set out in The United Nations Convention on the Rights of the Child (1989) as put forward by the Executive Advisory Committee of the RCPCH.

Involvement of the court

When should the consent of the court should be obtained to taking action? There are probably many occasions in practice when a patient is allowed to die without court approval being obtained.

Children and young persons

In the case of a young person under 18 years if there is a dispute with clinicians it is good practice for there to be an application to the court rather than the clinicians ignore the views of the parents

Figure 25.2   Principles set by the Royal College of Paediatrics and Child Health.

(1) To act always in the child's best interests.
(2) It is unrealistic to expect a complete consensus – aim to seek as much ethical common ground as possible.
(3) Seek court intervention if disputes between the healthcare team, the child, the parents and carers cannot be resolved.
(4) Consider each situation on its merits.
(5) There is no ethical difference between the withdrawal and the withholding of treatment.
(6) The duty of care is not absolute.
(7) Redirection of care from life sustaining to palliation is not withdrawal of care.
(8) It is never permissible to withdraw pain relief or contact.
(9) Treatments the primary aim of which is the relief of suffering, but which may incidentally hasten death, may be justified.

as to what is in the best interests of the child. This is the conclusion from the dispute between the mother of Glass and the paediatricians.[32] The case eventually went to the European Court of Human Rights which held that the failure of the NHS trust to seek a declaration from the court before administering diamorphine to her son without her consent and in writing him up for DNR instructions without her knowledge was a breach of her Article 8 rights.

It was reported that a seriously ill baby boy whose parents lost a High Court battle to keep him alive died in hospital after his life support machine was switched off.[33] The nine month old baby was known as OT and the doctors believed that he endured a life of suffering. He suffered from a rare metabolic disease and had brain damage and respiratory failure. The Court of Appeal upheld the Family Court judge's decision that the ventilator should be switched off. The judge held that the father's belief that the baby would get better and come home and go to school was sadly wholly unrealistic.

Mentally competent adults

If an adult (i.e. over 18 years) patient refuses treatment and it is determined that the patient has the capacity to refuse to give consent, then the patient's refusal cannot be overruled (see Chapter 7 and the case of *Re C and Re B.*).

Adults lacking the requisite mental capacity

Where the patient lacks mental competence, if the doctors, the parents and the rest of the multi-disciplinary team are agreed that the prognosis of the patient is extremely poor and that aggressive treatment is inappropriate there is unlikely to be a court hearing. The patient will be allowed to die and 'nature to take its course'. Under the Mental Capacity Act 2005 where the patient lacks the requisite mental capacity to make his or her own decision, in the absence of an advance decision or living will, decisions must be made in his or her best interests. However it is a specific requirement of section 4(5) that "where the determination relates to life-sustaining treatment (the person making

Figure 25.3   Axioms put forward by the Ethics Advisory Committee of the Royal College of Paediatrics and Child Health.

- There is no significant ethical difference between withdrawing (stopping) and withholding treatments, given the same ethical objective.
- Optimal ethical decision-making concerning children requires open and timely communication between members of the Health Care Team and the child and family respecting their values and beliefs and the fundamental principles of ethics and human rights.
- Parents may ethically and legally decide on behalf of children who are unable, for whatever reason, to express preferences, unless they are clearly acting against the child's best interest or are unable, unwilling or persistently unavailable to make decisions on behalf of their child.
- The wishes of a child who has obtained sufficient understanding and experience in the evaluation of treatment options should be given substantial consideration in the decision making process.
- The antecedent wishes and preferences of the child, if known, should also carry considerable weight given that conditions at the time for action match those envisaged in advance.
- In general, resolution of disagreement should be by discussion, consultation and consensus.
- The duty of care is not an absolute duty to preserve life by all means. There is no obligation to provide life sustaining treatment if:
  - ○   its use is inconsistent with the aims and objectives of an appropriate treatment plan
  - ○   the benefits of that treatment no longer outweigh the burden to the patient.
- It is ethical to withdraw life sustaining treatment if refused by a competent child; or from children who are unable to express wishes and preference when the Health Care Team and parent/carers agree that such treatment is not in the child's best interests.
- A redirection of management from life sustaining treatment to palliation represents a change in beneficial aims and objectives and does not constitute a withdrawal of care.
- The range of life sustaining treatments is wide and will vary with the individual circumstances of the patient. It is never permissible to withdraw procedures designed to alleviate pain or promote comfort.
- There is a distinction to be drawn between treatment of the dying patient and euthanasia. When a dying patient is receiving palliative care, the underlying cause of death is the disease process. In euthanasia, the intended action is to cause death.
- It follows that use of medication and other treatments which may incidentally hasten death may be justified if their primary aim is to relieve suffering. The EAC-RCPCH does not support the concept of euthanasia.
- Legal intervention should be considered when disputes between the Health Care Team, the child, parents and carers cannot be resolved by attempts to achieve consensus.

the decision) must not, in considering whether the treatment is in the best interests of the person concerned, be motivated by a desire to bring about his death."

If there are disputes over what is in the best interests of a mentally incapacitated patient, an application could be made to the Court of Protection, which since October 2007 has jurisdiction over issues of the personal welfare as well as the property and affairs of those lacking mental capacity. The following case preceded the establishment of the new Court of Protection but the same principles would apply under the Mental Capacity Act 2005.

The Tony Bland case

Case: *Airedale NHS Trust v Bland*[34]

> The patient was a victim of the football stadium crush at Hillsborough and it was established that, although he could breathe and digest food independently, he could not see, hear, taste, smell or communicate in any way and it appeared that there was no hope of recovery or improvement. Given the importance of the issues involved the matter was referred to the House of Lords which had to decide if it was lawful to permit artificial feeding to be discontinued in the case of a patient in a persistent vegetative state.

The House of Lords held that it would be in the best interests of the patient to discontinue the nasal gastric feed and he was later reported as having died. It specifically recommended that if any similar decisions were required to be made in the future there should be application before the courts and a court in Bristol gave consent in a similar case[35] a few months after the House of Lords decision on Tony Bland.

Court guidance

A practice note was issued by the Official Solicitor[36] following the case and in due course further directions will be issued in the light of the Mental Capacity Act 2005 and hearings before the Court of Protection. Access to the practice directions can be made through HM Courts Service website[37]

Advance decisions or Living wills

A living will (also known as an advance refusal of treatment or advance decision or an advance directive) is a statement, made when a person is mentally competent, over what treatments and care they would wish to refuse at a later time, when they no longer have the mental capacity to make decisions. Statutory provision has been made for advance decisions by the Mental Capacity Act 2005 which came into force in October 2007.

An advance decision is defined in section 24(1) as being a decision made by a person ("P"), after he has reached 18 and when he has capacity to do so, that if:

(a) at a later time and in such circumstances as he may specify, a specified treatment is proposed to be carried out or continued by a person providing healthcare for him, and
(b) at that time he lacks capacity to consent to the carrying out or continuation of the treatment, the specified treatment is not to be carried out or continued.

Whilst the MCA in general covers those over 16 years, 18 years is the minimum age for making a valid advance decision, because of the present power of the court to overrule the refusal of life-saving treatment by a young person under 18 years. (See Chapter 23 and the case of *Re W*[38].)

There is no necessity for the advance decision to be written in a particular format (except for refusal of life-sustaining treatment – see below), since section 24(2) states that a decision may be regarded as specifying a treatment or circumstances even though expressed in layman's terms. However clearly it is essential that the treatment which is being refused is unambiguous and therefore there are considerable advantages if professional help is obtained on its wording.

The Act permits the person who drew up the advance decision to withdraw it or alter it at any time provided that he has the mental capacity to do so. This withdrawal (including a partial withdrawal) need not be in writing. Nor need an alteration be in writing unless as a result of the alteration it now refers to the refusal of life-sustaining treatment, since special statutory provisions apply to life-sustaining treatments.

Life-sustaining treatments

An advance decision is not applicable to life-sustaining treatment unless:

(a)   the decision is verified by a statement by P to the effect that it is to apply to that treatment even if life is at risk, and
(b)   the decision and statement comply with the conditions set down in S.24 (6).

These conditions for an advance decision covering life-sustaining treatments are as follows:

(a)   it is in writing,
(b)   it is signed by P or by another person in P's presence and by P's direction,
(c)   the signature is made or acknowledged by P in the presence of a witness, and
(d)   the witness signs it, or acknowledges his signature, in P's presence.

The effect of an advance decision

An advance decision does not come into effect until the maker has lost the mental capacity to make his own decisions. To be valid it must relate to the treatment in question and to the circumstances envisaged by the maker. If there are reasonable grounds for believing that circumstances exist which the maker of the advance decision (P) did not anticipate at the time of the advance decision and which would have affected his decision had he anticipated them, then the advance decision would not apply.

If the advance decision is valid and the circumstances are as envisaged and the treatment is as specified, then health professionals and others must accept the refusal of the patient, if they have no reason to believe it to be invalid or inapplicable. If a person is satisfied that an advance decision exists which is valid and applicable to the treatment, then he or she could incur liability for carrying out or continuing the treatment contrary to the wishes expressed in the advance decision. On the other hand a person does not incur liability for the consequences of withholding or withdrawing a treatment from P if, at the time, he reasonably believes that an advance decision exists which is valid and applicable to the treatment.

If, however, the maker:

(a)   has withdrawn the decision at a time when he had capacity to do so, or
(b)   has, under a lasting power of attorney created after the advance decision was made, conferred authority on the donee (or, if more than one, any of them) to give or refuse consent to the treatment to which the advance decision relates, or
(c)   has done anything else clearly inconsistent with the advance decision remaining his fixed decision,

then the advance decision will not apply to the situation and is not binding upon those caring for the patient. As an advance statement however it should be taken into account in determining the patient's best interests since this statements is an expression of the patient's view (see Chapter 7 and determination of best interests).

In the event of reasonable doubt about the validity of an advance decision, an application can be made to the Court of Protection for a declaration as to its existence, its validity and its applicability to the treatment in question. In the meantime life-sustaining treatment can be provided or anything which is reasonably believed to be necessary to prevent a serious deterioration in P's condition, while a decision is sought from the court.

Situation: Refusing treatment

A patient, on hearing that he was suffering from Motor Neurone Disease, wrote an advanced refusal of treatment indicating that he would not wish to receive any artificial feeding. He is now finding it more and more difficult to swallow and artificial feeding is seen as the only option. The consultant has stated that this should be commenced and refuses to accept that the living will has any significance to his clinical judgment. What is the law?

Since October 2007 if an advance decision is to cover a refusal of life-sustaining treatment, then the statutory provisions set out above must be satisfied. If these are satisfied, then there is an obligation upon all health professionals to respect the wishes of the patient. If the consultant treats the patient contrary to the wishes expressed in a valid and applicable advance decision, then he is guilty of trespass to the person (see Chapter 7) and those acting on behalf of the patient could instigate an action against him and/or his employer.

Can the court order doctors to provide treatment?

Case: *Re J* (1992)[39]

J was born in January 1991 and suffered an accidental fall when he was a month old with the result that he was profoundly handicapped both mentally and physically. He was severely microcephalic, his brain not having grown sufficiently following the injury. He also had severe cerebral palsy, cortical blindness and severe epilepsy. He was in general fed by a nasal gastric tube.

Medical opinion was unanimous that J was unlikely to develop much beyond his present functioning, that that level might deteriorate and that his expectation of life, although uncertain, would be short. The paediatrician's report stated that, given J's condition, it would not be medically appropriate to intervene with intensive procedures such as artificial ventilation if he were to suffer a life-threatening event.

The baby was in the care of foster parents with whom the local authority shared responsibility. The local authority applied to the court under section 100 of the Children Act 1989 to determine whether ventilation should be given to the child. The mother supported the requirement that the hospital and doctors should be forced to put the baby on a life support machine.

The judge regarded J's best interests as well as the interests of justice in preserving his life as both pointing in favour of the grant of an interim injunction requiring such treatment to take place. The hospital appealed.

In the Court of Appeal Lord Donaldson, Master of the Rolls, stated that he could not at present conceive of any circumstances in which requiring a medical practitioner (or a health authority acting by a medical practitioner) to adopt a course of treatment, which in the *bona fide* clinical judgment of the practitioner was contra-indicated as not being in the patient's best interests, would be other than an abuse of power, as directly or indirectly requiring the practitioner to act contrary to the fundamental duty he owed to his patient.

Lord Donaldson said that the order of the judge, ordering specific treatment to take place, was wholly inconsistent with the law as stated in *Re J*[40] (see above) and in *Re R*[41] and could not be justified on the basis of any known authority. It was also erroneous on two other substantial grounds:

- its lack of certainty as to what was required of the health authority; and
- its failure adequately to take account of the sad fact of life that health authorities might on occasion find that they had too few resources, either human or material or both, to treat all the patients whom they would like to treat in the way they would like to treat them.

It was the health authority's duty to make choices. The court would have no knowledge of competing claims to resources and was in no position to express any view on their deployment of these resources. The Court of Appeal thus held that where a paediatrician caring for a severely handicapped baby considered that mechanical ventilation procedures would not be appropriate the court would not grant an injunction requiring such treatment to take place.

The effect of the Court's decision to set aside the judge's ruling was to leave the health authority and its medical staff free, subject to consent not being withdrawn, to treat J in accordance with their best clinical judgment. That did not mean that in no circumstances should J be subjected to mechanical ventilation.

The reluctance of the court to interfere with the decision making of the doctors in the interests of the patient was seen in a recent case in very different circumstances. In a case[42] where the father of a girl of ten suffering from leukaemia brought an action against the health authority for its refusal to fund a course of chemotherapy followed by a second bone marrow transplant operation, the Court of Appeal took the view that the courts should not intervene in such a decision but that the health authority should follow medical advice as to what was in the best interests of the child. (See Chapter 6 for a fuller discussion of the case.)

In the Burke case the Court of Appeal held that a patient could not insist on being provided with treatment when it was contrary to professional discretion (see Chapter 6).

Under the Mental Capacity Act 2005 decisions relating to extremely serious treatment decisions (for those lacking the requisite mental capacity to make their own decisions) would now go before the Court of Protection. The Code of Practice on the MCA[43] states that. Cases involving any of the following decisions should therefore be brought before a court:

- chemotherapy and surgery for cancer
- electro-convulsive therapy
- therapeutic sterilisation
- major surgery (such as open-heart surgery or brain/neuro-surgery)
- major amputations (for example, loss of an arm or leg)
- treatments which will result in permanent loss of hearing or sight
- withholding or stopping artificial nutrition and hydration, and
- termination of pregnancy.

This list is not exhaustive.

'Not for resuscitation' orders

A joint statement from the British Medical Association, Resuscitation Council (UK) and the Royal College of Nursing[44] provided guidance on decisions relating to cardiopulmonary resuscitation in 1999 (updated in 2001 and 2007). The original guidance was commended to NHS trusts in September 2000 by the NHS Executive[45] in an NHS Circular. Every trust should have in place a policy relating to the use of Not For Resuscitation instructions.

What is the legal significance of such orders?

Competent adults

If patients have the mental competence to understand the situation they are entitled to refuse to give consent to any treatment, even though the treatment is life saving (see Chapter 7 and in particular the case of Re B[46]).

Children and young persons

Whilst a child of 16 or 17 has a statutory right to give consent to treatment, a case in 1992 decided that children cannot refuse treatment which is in their best interests. In the case of *Re W*[47] a girl of 16 years refused to be treated for anorexia nervosa, but her refusal was overruled by the court (see Chapter 23). If, however, the decision made by the minor is considered to be in his or her best interests, then it would be valid for all professional carers of that patient to accept that refusal of care and the instructions that the patient is not to be resuscitated.

Mental incapacity

Where the patient is mentally incapacitated, then the Mental Capacity Act 2005 applies and action must be taken in the best interests of that person, unless the person has, when he or she had the requisite mental capacity, drawn up an advance decision or appointed a lasting power of attorney. If the consultant in charge of the care of the patient decides that it is in the best interests of the patient that he or she should not be resuscitated then this decision would stand. In the event of a dispute over the best interests of the patient, an application could be made to the Court of Protection for a declaration as to what was in the best interests of the mentally incapacitated patient. The steps laid down in section 4 of the MCA should be followed in determining what are the best interests. (See Chapter 7 and Box 7.2).

Relatives and carers

- Could the relatives give 'Not For Resuscitation' or 'Do Not Resuscitate' instructions?

Relatives are able to make day to day decisions on behalf of a mentally incapacitated adult, provided that they make them in the best interests of the patient and follow the statutory principles and steps set down under section 4 of the MCA. Where there is no binding advance decision or lasting power of attorney, the clinical team would normally make serious medical decisions. In the absence of persons who could be consulted, an independent mental capacity advocate should be appointed and would report on the best interests of the patient, according to the statutory provisions. If there are relatives, then the MCA requires full consultation with them in order to satisfy the statutory provisions. If a relative has been appointed under a lasting power of attorney which gives to the donee the power to make decisions about life-sustaining treatment, then that donee would have the right to make a decision as to whether the patient is to be resuscitated. The statutory provisions must however have been complied with. Similarly if the patient had, when competent, drawn up an advance decision which covers resuscitation in the circumstances which now exist, then provided the statutory provisions relating to advance decisions refusing life-sustaining treatment (see above) are complied with, then these NFR instructions must be followed.

Figure 25.4   A matrix for 'Not for Resuscitation'.

Is the patient competent?	No	Yes – and the patient asks for treatment	Yes – but the patient refuses treatment
Good Prognosis	resuscitate	resuscitate	NFR
Bad Prognosis	NFR	The Burke case	NFR

An NFR matrix

Figure 25.4 provides a matrix showing how the factors of mental competence and prognosis impact on each other in NFR decisions.

The Burke case,[48] in the middle box on the bottom line, where the mentally competent patient is asking for treatment when the prognosis is bad, illustrates the general principle that a patient cannot insist on treatment which is clinically contra-indicated. A mentally competent patient does not have an absolute right to insist on treatment when it is contrary to professional judgment. The Burke case is set out in Chapter 6.

Parents' refusal to consent to treatment

An example of where the courts refused to uphold the parents' wish to allow the child to die is seen in the following case.

Case: *Re B*[49]

In *Re B* a child was born suffering from Down's syndrome and an intestinal blockage. She required an operation to relieve the obstruction if she was to live more than a few days. If the operation were performed, the child might die within a few months but it was probable that her life expectancy would be 20 to 30 years. Her parents, having decided that it would be kinder to allow her to die rather than live as a physically and mentally handicapped person, refused to consent to the operation. The local authority made the child a ward of court and, when a surgeon decided that the wishes of the parents should be respected, they sought an order authorising the operation to be performed by other named surgeons.

The judge decided that the parents' wishes should be respected and refused to make the order.
The local authority appealed to the Court of Appeal which allowed the appeal. It stated that:

1. The question for the court was whether it was in the best interests of the child that she should have the operation and not whether the parents' wishes should be respected.
2. Since the effect of the operation might be that the child would have the normal span of life of a Down's syndrome person; and
3. Since it had not been demonstrated that the life of a person with Down's syndrome was of such a nature that the child should be condemned to die;
4. The court would make an order that the operation be performed.

Crucial to the decision in this case was the prognosis of the child. In a contrasting case the parents' refusal was upheld by the courts.

Case: *Re T (a minor)* (wardship: medical treatment[50])

A child was born with a life-threatening liver defect. After unsuccessful treatment, the prognosis was that he would not live beyond two and a half years without a liver transplant. The mother refused to give consent to the operation because she was not willing to permit the child to undergo the pain and distress of invasive surgery. She later moved out of the country. The Local Authority, at the consultants' instigation, applied to the court for permission to carry out the operation and for the child to be returned to the jurisdiction in order that the operation could be carried out. The High Court judge held that the mother's refusal was unreasonable and it was in the child's best interests to undergo the liver transplant. The mother appealed.

The Court of Appeal upheld that appeal. The paramount consideration was the welfare of the child and not the reasonableness of the parent's refusal of consent. However since the welfare of the child depended upon the mother, her views were relevant. The judge had failed to assess the relevance or the weight of the mother's concern as to the benefits to her child of the surgery and post-operative treatment, the dangers of failure both long term as well as short term, the possibility of the need for further transplants, the likely length of life and the effect on her child of all those concerns, together with the strong reservations expressed by one of the consultants about coercing the mother into playing a crucial part in the aftermath of the operation and thereafter.

It must be stressed, however, that *Re T* is an unusual case and there were very special circumstances which led to the court upholding the wishes of the parents over those of the doctors.

The right to insist on treatment

Parents

Parents do not have the right to insist upon care or treatment which the doctors consider is not in the best interests of the child. As has been discussed above, the court would not order the doctors to carry out treatment on a child, which the doctors considered was not in the best interests of the child. (See also the case of Jamie Bowen[51] discussed in Chapter 6.)

Mentally competent adults

Nor do any adults have an absolute right to insist upon treatment. A health professional would be failing in her obligations if she provided treatment, on the patient's insistence, knowing that it was professionally contra-indicated, or even just of no effect. If a patient purported in a living will to direct that treatment be given rather than just refusing treatment in anticipation, this direction is likely to be of little effect if it is not supported by professional judgment as to its appropriateness (see Figure 25.4 above, the Burke case and also Chapter 6).

Care of the dying patient

Children

The Association for Children's Palliative Care (ACT) (formerly the Association for children with life-threatening or terminal conditions and their families) has been active in developing a Charter for their care. Its clauses are set out in Figure 25.5.

Figure 25.5 The ACT charter for children with life-threatening conditions and their families.

- Every child shall be treated with dignity and respect and shall be afforded privacy whatever the child's physical or intellectual ability.
- Parents shall be acknowledged as the primary carers and involved as partners in all care and decisions involving their child.
- Every child shall be given the opportunity to participate in decisions affecting his or her care, according to age and understanding.
- An honest and open approach shall be the basis of all communication.
- Information shall be provided for the parent, the child, the siblings and other relatives, appropriate to age and understanding.
- The family home shall remain the centre of caring whenever possible. Care away from home shall be provided in a child-centred environment by staff trained in the care of children.
- Every child shall have access to a 24-hour multi-disciplinary children's palliative care team for flexible support in the home, and be in the care of a local paediatrician.
- Every child and family shall receive emotional, psychological and spiritual support to meet their needs. This shall begin at diagnosis and continue throughout the child's lifetime, death and in bereavement.
- Every family shall be entitled to a named keyworker who will enable the family to build up and maintain access to an appropriate network of support.
- Every family shall be given the opportunity of a consultation with a paediatric specialist who has particular knowledge of the child's condition.
- Every family shall have access to flexible short term breaks (respite care) both in their own home and away from home, with appropriate children's nursing and medical support.
- Every child shall have access to education and other appropriate childhood activities.
- The needs of adolescents and young people shall be addressed and planned for well in advance.
- Every family shall have timely access to practical support, including clinical equipment, financial grants, suitable housing and domestic help

---

The Department of Health has prepared guidance for health service organisations on caring for the dying patient, which can be accessed on its website.[52] In July 2008 the Government published an end of life strategy for the following 10 years. This stated that patients with terminal conditions should have a care plan setting out how they might be supported with pain relief; that patients should have more choice over where they die and should be encouraged to make their wishes known. "Rapid response" nursing teams should be available to provide care to those who wish to die in the setting they chose. Medical staff should be trained to speak to the patient about his or her prognosis. An extra £286 million was allocated to support the strategy. At the end of the first year, the end of life strategy was reviewed.[53] In the review progress was seen across the three key elements of the strategy (• societal level: actions to raise awareness of, and change attitudes towards, death and dying; • individual level: integrated service delivery based around a care pathway; • infrastructure: workforce development, measurement, research, funding and national support). However in research by the charity Help the Hospices and reported to the Times of 28 primary care trusts sampled only 3 could provide evidence of extra investment in palliative care this year.[54]

General application

The National Council of Palliative Care (NCPC) has published a bulletin on the palliative care needs of older people which would be useful for occupational therapists[55] The Specialist interest section of the COT has also published a research and development strategic vision and action plan[56] Occupational therapists might also find guidance issued for physiotherapists helpful to them as well. The Chartered Society of Physiotherapy has identified the role of the physiotherapist in palliative care in its response to the Health Select Committee's Inquiry into hospice and palliative care.[57] The NSF on long-term conditions published in 2005 contains a section on palliative care which could be used to ensure that the resources are provided to maintain the required standard. The NSF is available on the DH website (see also Chapter 24).

Situation: Am I dying?

> A community occupational therapist was asked by a patient suffering in the terminal stages of MND 'How much longer do I have?' The occupational therapist knew that he was dying but found it difficult to answer since the patient's wife refused to acknowledge to the patient the true nature of his illness.

The answer to the question may require all the occupational therapist's skills and sensitivity. On the one hand she cannot lie to the patient, although in fact she would probably not know the exact answer to the question. Nor should she collude with the spouse in keeping information from the patient. On the other hand she needs to attempt to create some understanding between patient and spouse and should be aware of organisations which could assist in this dilemma.

Registration of death and the role of the coroner

The doctor who attended the patient during the last illness must certify the death and give the cause unless the circumstances are such that the death should be reported to the coroner. These would include the following:[58]

- Where the deceased was not attended in his last illness by a doctor.
- Where the deceased was not seen by a doctor either after death or within the 14 days prior to death.
- Where the cause of death is unknown.
- Where death appears to be due to industrial disease or poisoning.
- Where death may have been unnatural or caused by violence or neglect or abortion or attended by suspicious circumstances.
- Where death has occurred during an operation or before recovery from an anaesthetic.

The following causes of death would therefore be reportable to the coroner:

- deaths following from a criminal offence such as murder, manslaughter or causing death by dangerous driving;
- suicide;
- deaths arising from road traffic accidents, industrial accidents, domestic accidents, etc.;
- death in custody – prison or police custody;
- deaths associated with medical treatment;

- sudden death;
- deaths following abortion, drug dependence or alcoholism;
- infant deaths where no midwife or doctor was present, cot deaths.

Usually individual coroners will make known their requirements in respect of the notification of deaths occurring in hospital. Some, for example, may require reporting of all deaths occurring within 24 hours of emergency admission.[59] The Coroners and Justice Act 2009 now applies.

Once a death has been reported to the coroner, and until the coroner has formally notified the doctor of his decision in relation to the deceased, the body remains under the control of the coroner, i.e. under his jurisdiction. He has the right to request a post mortem and there can be no action taken in respect of the body without his consent.

Situation: Unnatural death

A occupational therapist visits a patient who is terminally ill. When she arrives, she is met by a distraught partner who says that he has just found the patient unconscious in bed with empty bottles of painkillers beside her. He does not know whether the doctor should be called.

It would appear from the few facts given here that the patient has made a suicide attempt. The duty of care owed to the patient would require the occupational therapist to ensure that emergency medical care was summoned. Were the patient to die, the doctor might be unable to certify the cause of death and would need to notify the coroner.

Can relatives view the body?

Once the coroner has jurisdiction over the body, his or her consent must be obtained before the body can be viewed by the relatives.[60]

Post mortem

If the coroner orders a post mortem, the relatives have no right to refuse this. This is so even when the religious views of the deceased would be against a post mortem.[61] On the other hand if the doctor requests a post mortem where the body is not under the jurisdiction of the coroner the person in charge of the body, usually a spouse or relative, could refuse to give consent. The requirements of the Human Tissue Act 2004 must be followed.

Inquest

Where a death has been reported to the coroner he will decide whether or not an inquest will be held. He is obliged by law to hold an inquest:

- where there are reasons to suspect a criminal offence has caused the death
- in cases of industrial accidents and diseases, and
- on deaths in prison or police custody.

The existence of a general discretion to hold an inquest has been doubted.[62] The purpose of the inquest is to ascertain:

1.   who the deceased was; and
2.   how, when and where the deceased came by his death.[63]

Possible verdicts are:

- natural causes
- unlawful killing
- killed lawfully
- suicide
- accidental death
- misadventure
- narrative verdict (e.g. following the deaths of conjoined twins)
- dependence upon a drug
- non-dependent abuse of drugs
- industrial disease
- neglect
- want of attention at birth
- attempted/self-induced abortion.

An open verdict indicates that there is insufficient evidence to determine the nature of the death, i.e. the evidence did not further or fully disclose the means whereby the cause of death arose. A narrative verdict is sometimes given where it is necessary to explain the cause of death. For example where an operation took place which of necessity would lead to the death of one conjoined twin, the coroner gave a narrative verdict.[64] Rule 43 of the Coroner's rules was amended[65] from 17 July 2008 to require a coroner to report circumstances in which further deaths could occur if action is not taken to prevent them. The agency receiving such a report, will be required to give the coroner a written response within 56 days stating what action has been taken. The amendment also allows the coroner to share relevant information with Local Safeguarding Children Boards to enable them to carry out their statutory functions of conducting child death reviews. Copies of the coroners' reports would be sent to other interested parties (including the bereaved families) and to the Lord Chancellor and to be published. This means that reports and responses will be centrally collated for the first time so that any trends can be identified, monitored and lessons learned can be shared widely.

Tom Luce the chair of the Fundamental Review of Coroners and Death Certification in England, Wales and Northern Ireland (2001–3) criticised the use of short-form verdicts such as accidental death, misadventure, unlawful killing in the light of the Coroner's direction to the jury in the De Menezes inquest which ruled out unlawful killing and instructed them to choose between lawful killing and an open verdict.[66] He expressed hope that the Coroners and Justice Bill would get rid of short-form verdicts. Once completed the inquest cannot be resumed but the High Court has the power under section 13(1)(b) of the Coroners Act 1988 to order another inquest to be held. The Coroners and Justice Act 2009 clarified: the coroner's duty to investigate; discontinuance of an investigation the cause of death is revealed by post mortem examination; the matters to be ascertained by an investigation; the duty to hold an inquest, whether a jury is required; assembling a jury and determinations and findings by a jury and the duty or power to suspend or resume investigations; post mortem examinations and the power to remove a body. Schedules to the Act cover the duty or power to suspend or resume investigations; coroner areas; appointment of senior coroners, area coroners and assistant coroners and the powers of coroners.

The occupational therapist and the coroner's court

A occupational therapist might be required to give evidence at an inquest on the events which preceded death. She should be alert to this possibility – for example the occupational therapist may know that a child who has died in an apparent cot death suffered from certain symptoms prior to his death. This information from the occupational therapist may be vital at any inquest.

It is essential that the occupational therapist obtains assistance from a senior manager or lawyer on the preparation of a statement which the coroner's office will require from her. If she is subsequently asked to attend the inquest she should have assistance in preparation for giving evidence. One means of preparation is for the occupational therapist to attend a different inquest so that she can have an understanding of the geography of the court, the procedure which is followed and the level of formality required at a time when she is not personally involved (see Chapter 13 on giving evidence).

She should note that the coroner's court is known as an 'inquisitorial' one. This means that, unlike the magistrates', crown courts and civil courts where an action is brought by one person or organisation against another and the judge controls the proceedings – an 'adversarial' system – the coroner determines the witnesses who will give evidence, the course of the proceedings and he will disallow any question which in his opinion is not relevant or otherwise not a proper one. He can himself examine the witnesses often asking leading questions where information is not disputed to speed up the hearing. Hence the words 'inquisitorial' and 'inquest' (see glossary).

Where the death has been reported to the coroner, no certificate can be issued or registration take place until he has made his decision. If he decides that a post mortem should be carried out, but no inquest is needed, he will issue Form B which is sent or taken to the Registrar. The Registrar will then issue the death certificate and the certificate for disposal which is required by the undertaker before burial can take place. Authorisation for cremation requires an additional medical certificate or the certificate issued by the coroner.

The Registrar General for England and Wales has the right to supply information contained in any register of deaths to a person or body specified in the order for use in the prevention, detection, investigation or prosecution of offences.[67]

Death and miscarriage

Born alive

If a baby is born alive and then dies, there must be a registration of both the birth and the death.

Stillbirth

A stillbirth is defined as:

> Where a child issues forth from its mother after the 24th week of pregnancy, and which did not at any time after being completely expelled from its mother breathe or show any signs of life (Section 41 of the Births and Deaths Registration Act 1953, as amended by section 1 of the Still Birth Act 1992).

The stillbirth has to be registered as such and the informant has to deliver to the Registrar a written certificate that the child was not born alive. This must be signed by the registered medical practitioner or the registered midwife who was in attendance at the birth or who has examined the body. The certificate must state, to the best of the knowledge and belief of the person signing it, the cause of death and the estimated duration of the pregnancy (section 11(1)(a)). Alternatively a declaration in the prescribed form giving the reasons for the absence of a certificate and that the child was not born alive could be made (section 11(1)(b)).

A stillbirth should be disposed of by burial in a burial ground or church yard or by cremation at an authorised crematorium. A health authority should not dispose of a stillbirth without the consent of the parents.

Foetus of less than 24 weeks

If the foetus was delivered without any signs of life, then no registration is necessary. The foetus may be disposed of without formality in any way which does not constitute a nuisance or an affront to public decency. If the foetus, after expulsion, shows signs of life and then dies, it would have to be treated as both a birth and a death.

Health professionals should be sensitive to the fact that parents may suffer the same feelings of bereavement what ever the period of gestation and should therefore arrange for counselling and support as they would if the baby were full term.

Future changes

An Inquiry was set up after the conviction of Harold Shipman for the murder of 15 patients (and possibly another 200) The third report[68] considered the present system for death and cremation certification and for the investigation of deaths by coroners, together with the conduct of those who had operated those systems in the aftermath of the deaths of Shipman's victims. The report noted that the present system of death and cremation certification failed to detect that Shipman had killed any of his 215 victims. The report made significant recommendations for the reform of the coroner's system and the certification of death. Following the 3rd Shipman Report, a position paper was published by the Home Office[69] in March 2004 and constituted the Government's response to the Fundamental Review of Death Certification and Coroner Services[70] and the Shipman Inquiry. In February 2006 the Minister of State for Constitutional Affairs announced the implementation of the first set of reforms: those relating to the Coroners' service.[71] A draft Coroners bill, together with a draft Charter for the bereaved were published in June 2006 to enable pre-legislative scrutiny to be undertaken by the Select Committee for the Department of Constitutional Affairs. The draft Bill was scrutinised by the DCA Select Committee[72] which made strong criticisms about the fact that many of the proposals contained in the Shipman Report and in the position paper were omitted from the Bill, in particular the changes to the death certification system and a national system for the office of coroner. The Select Committee was also concerned that there was inadequate resourcing of the coronial service. The Government responded to these recommendations in November 2006.[73] The Coroners and Justice Act 2009 does not contain all the recommendations of the Shipman Report but more radical changes may follow once it has been brought into force.

Research by Bruce Guthrie at the University of Dundee suggests that even if the reforms were implemented, another Dr Shipman would probably not be identified till after he had killed about 30 patients.[74]

Organ transplants

The donation of organs from a deceased person and from a living person are both regulated by the Human Tissue Act 2004.

Human Tissue Act 2004

This Act covers the use of tissue and organs from the living and the dead.

Transplants from dead donors

If the dying person has been registered as an organ donor with the NHS organ donor register[75] or is carrying a donor card, then that would count as a valid consent for the removal of the organs. Where the deceased person had made it clear that he would wish his organs to be donated, relatives cannot over rule this request unless there is evidence that the deceased changed his mind. In contrast where the deceased has not indicated any views about donation, then consent can be given by any person whom he has nominated to act on his behalf. Where there has been no such nomination, then a person in a qualifying relationship such as a partner or other relative or friend can give consent. The Act sets out the order of precedence of such persons. The Government is at present reviewing the law on organ donation and there are calls for an opt out system to be adopted i.e. unless the deceased person had made a specific request not to be regarded as an organ donor, organs could be taken.

New guidelines were to be published in September 2008 which will allow transplant surgeons to begin removing organs 5 minutes after a donor's heart has stopped in order to tackle the shortage of transplant donors.[76] The new guidelines will give doctors permission to omit a complex set of tests to establish brain stem death which can take 20 minutes. The guidelines have met with concern and considerable debate.

Donation from live donors

Situation: Live donation

> A occupational therapist cares for a renal patient aged 23 years. She has been on dialysis for a number of years but has been advised that a kidney transplant is urgently required. Her mother has offered to be a donor and seeks the advice of the occupational therapist over whether such an offer would be accepted.

This situation would now come under the Human Tissue Act 2004. Donations from living donors can now take place provided strict statutory specifications are followed. These statutory provisions include information being given to the donors and recipients before consent is given. There can be paired donors so that where relatives are not a match, they can be linked with a similar couple or couples who are equally unmatched so that pairings of matched donor/donee can be created. Where the statutory provisions are satisfied, approval to the transplantation from a live donor can be given by the Human Tissue Authority.

Conclusions

In their care of terminally ill patients, occupational therapists need to be confident in their knowledge about the laws which apply. They may, for example, feel great empathy for a tetraplegic patient who no longer has the desire to live. They must be aware, however, that to assist in the death would be to commit a crime under the Suicide Act. Similarly in the care of patients suffering from motor neurone disease they must keep a clear distinction between the right of the mentally capacitated patient to refuse to be treated, including the right of the patient to make an advance decision or appoint a donee under a lasting power of attorney, and the criminal act of killing the patient. Significant changes have been made to the Suicide Act under the Coroner's and Justice Act as discussed above.

 Questions and exercises

1 In what circumstances could a patient facing a terminal illness refuse treatment? (See also Chapter 7.)
2 Draw up the requirements for a valid advance decision which is intended to relate to life-sustaining treatment.
3 Parents of a young person suffering from cystic fibrosis have suggested to you that occupational therapy, physiotherapy and antibiotic treatment should be stopped. What are the legal considerations in this request and what action would you take?
4 Following the death of a patient in hospital who had been receiving occupational therapy you are asked to provide a statement for the coroner. What principles would you bear in mind in preparing the statement? (See also Chapter 13.)

References

1 Cooper Jill (ed) (2006) *Occupational Therapy in Oncology and Palliative Care*. Wiley, Chichester.
2 Dimond, B. (2008) *Legal Aspects of Death*. Quay Publications, Dinton, Wilts.
3 www.liberty-works.co.uk
4 Libby Anna (2007) Staying alive. Letter to the editor. *British Journal of Occupational Therapy*, **70**(9), 400.
5 *R (on the application of Burke) v General Medical Council and Disability Rights Commission and the Official Solicitor to the Supreme Court* [2004] EWHC 1879; [2004] Lloyd's Rep Med 451.
6 *A National Health Service Trust v D* (2000) The Times Law Report 19 July; [2000] Lloyd's Rep Med 411.
7 *NHS Trust A v Mrs M* and *NHS Trust B v Mrs H* Family Division The Times 25 October 2000; [2001] 1 All ER 801; [2001] 2 FLR 367.
8 *Savage v South Essex Partnership NHS Foundation Trust* The Times Law Report 9 January 2008; [2007] EWCA Civ 1375.
9 *Savage v South Essex Partnership NHS Foundation Trust* The Times Law Report 11 December 2008.
10 *R (on the application of JL) v Secretary of State for the Home Department* [2007] EWCA Civ 767.
11 *Bicknell v HM Coroner for Birmingham and Solihull* [2007] EWHC 2547 (Admin) (2008) 99 BMLR 1.
12 *R v Wood (No.2)* The Times Law Report 8 April 2009 CA Crim Div.
13 Law Commission (2006) *A new Homicide Act for England and Wales*. Consultation paper 177.
14 Hannah Fletcher. Husband is spared jail for suffocating sick wife who wanted to die The Times 2 February 2008.

15 Simon de Bruxelles. Freedom for woman who kept trying to kill her husband. The Times 13 May 2008.

16 Bird Steve. Mother on attempted murder charge after daughter with ME dies from morphine overdose The Times 17 April 2009.

17 *R v Bodkin Adams* [1957] Crim LR 365.

18 *R (On the application of Pretty) v DPP* [2001] UKHL 61, [2001] 3 WLR 1598.

19 *Pretty v United Kingdom* ECHR the full judgement is available on www.echr.coe.int/Eng/Press/apr/ Prettyjudepress.htm. (Current law 380 June 2002).

20 *R (On the application of Purdy) v DPP* [2008]) The Times Law Report 17 November 2008.

21 *R (Purdy) v Director of Public Prosecutions* The Times Law Report 24 February 2009.

22 *R (Purdy) v Director of Public Prosecutions* The Times Law Report 31 July 2009 HL.

23 *R v Arthur* reported in The Times 6 November 1981.

24 *R v Cox* [1993] 2 All ER 19.

25 House of Lords: Committee on Medical Ethics, Session 1993–4 (31 January 1994) HMSO, London.

26 Law Commission (1995) Report No. 231 Mental Incapacity. HMSO, London.

27 *Re B (Consent to treatment: capacity)* The Times Law Report, 26 March 2002; [2002] 2 All ER 449.

28 *Re C (a minor) (Wardship; medical treatment)* [1989] 2 All ER 782.

29 *Re J (a minor) (wardship; medical treatment)* [1990] 3 All ER 930.

30 *Wyatt v Portsmouth Hospital NHS Trust* [2004] EWHC Civ 2247; [2005] EWHC 117; [2005] EWHC 693; [2005] EWCA Civ 1181; [2005] EWHC 2293.

31 Royal College of Paediatrics and Child Health (September (2004) Withholding or Withdrawing Life Saving Treatment in Children. A Framework for Practice 2nd edition. RCPCH, London.

32 *R v Portsmouth Hospitals NHS Trust ex p Glass* [1999] 2 FLR 905; [1999] Lloyds RM 367; *Glass v UK*, TLR, 11 March 2004, ECHR.

33 Leppard David. Baby dies after court decision The Sunday Times 22 March 2009.

34 *Airedale NHS Trust v Bland* [1993] 1 All ER 821.

35 *Frenchay Healthcare NHS Trust v S* [1994] 2 All ER 403.

36 Practice Note [1996] 4 All ER 766.

37 www.hmcourts-service.gov.uk

38 *Re W (a minor) (Medical Treatment)* [1992] 4 All ER 627.

39 *Re J* [1992] 4 All ER 614; The Times Law Report, 12 June 1992.

40 *Re J (a minor) (wardship; medical treatment)* [1990] 3 All ER 930.

41 *Re R* [1991] 4 All ER 177.

42 *R v Cambridge and Huntingdon Health Authority ex parte B* The Times Law Report, 15 March 1995. [1995] 2 All ER 129.

43 Ministry of Constitutional Affairs (2007) Code of Practice on Mental Capacity Act 2005 paragraph 10.45; www.justice.gov.uk

44 British Medical Association, Resuscitation Council (UK) and the Royal College of Nursing (1999) *Decisions Relating to Cardiopulmonary Resuscitation.* BMA, London. updated March 2001 and October 2007.

45 NHS Executive, Resuscitation Policy HSC 2000/028, September 2000.

46 *Re B (Consent to treatment: capacity)* The Times Law Report, 26 March 2002; [2002] 2 All ER 449.

47 *Re W (a minor) (medical treatment)* [1992] 4 All ER 627.

48 *R (on the application of Burke) v General Medical Council and Disability Commission and the Official Solicitor to the Supreme Court* [2004] EWHC 1879; [2004] Lloyd's Rep Med 451 [2005] EWCA Civ 1003, 28 July 2005.

49 *Re B (a minor) (wardship; medical treatment)* [1981] 1 WLR 1421.

50 *Re T (a minor) (wardship: medical treatment)* [1997] 1 All ER 906; Re C (sic) (a minor; refusal of parental consent) [1997] 8 Med LR 166.

51 *R v Cambridge and Huntingdon Health Authority, ex parte B* [1995] 2 All ER 129.

52 Department of Health (2005) *When a Patient Dies: Advice on Developing Bereavement Services in the NHS.* DH, London; www.dh.gov.uk/PolicyAnd Guidance/Organisation

53 Department of Health (2009) *End of life care Strategy: First annual report.* DH, London.

54 Rose David. NHS "loses" £286m intended to ease last days of dying patients The Times 15 July 2009.

55   National Council of Palliative Care (2006) The Palliative Care Needs of Older People Briefing bulletin Number 14. NCPC, London.

56   COT SS HIV/AIDS Oncology and Palliative Care (2004) *Research and Development Strategic Vision and Action Plan*. COT, London.

57   Chartered Society of Physiotherapy (2004) Health Select Committee Inquiry into hospice and palliative care – response by the CSP. CSP, London.

58   List taken from The Registration of Births and Deaths Regulations 1987 SI No. 2088; see further Knight, B. (1992) *Legal Aspects of Medical Practice*, 5th edn. Churchill Livingstone, Edinburgh pp 95–102.

59   Knight, B. (1992) *Legal Aspects of Medical Practice*, 5th edn. Churchill Livingstone, Edinburgh, p 96.

60   Dimond, B.C. (1995) Death in the Accident and Emergency Department. *Accident and Emergency Nursing*, 3(1), 38–41 (further details of the coroner's jurisdiction).

61   *R v Westminster City Coroner, ex parte Rainer* (1968) 112 Solicitors Journal 883.

62   *R v Poplar Coroner, ex parte Thomas (CA)* (1993) 2 WLR 547.

63   Coroners and Justice Act 2009 Section 5.

64   *In re A (Minors: conjoined twins: medical treatment)*, The Times Law Report, 10 October 2000.

65   The Coroners (Amendment) Rules 2008 SI No 1652.

66   Luce Tom. Why only radical reform will regain public's confidence. The Times 18 December 2008.

67   Supply of Information (Register of Deaths)(England and Wales) Order 2008 SI 570.

68   Shipman Inquiry Third Report: Death and Cremation Certification, 14 July 2003; www.the-shipman-inquiry.org.uk/reports.asp

69   Home Office. Reforming the Coroner and Death Certification Service. A Position Paper CM 6159 March 2004 Stationery Office.

70   Tom Luce. Chair Fundamental Review of Death Certification and the Coroner Services in England, Wales and Northern Ireland Home Office 2003.

71   Department for Constitutional Affairs (2006) Coroners Service Reform Briefing Note. DCA, London.

72   Department for Constitution Affairs (2006) Select Committee's Report on the Reform of the Coroners' System and Death Certification. DCA, London.

73   Government Response to the Report by the Constitutional Affairs Select Committee (Cm 6943, Session 2005–6) November 2006.

74   Nigel Hawkes. No method in place to stop killing spree by new Shipman The Times 3 May 2008.

75   www.uktransplant.org.uk/ukt/

76   Lois Rogers. Brain-death test dropped to boost organ donation The Sunday Times 29 June 2008.

26

Teaching and Research

Most OTs are in some way involved in the instruction and support of others. Increasingly this role is likely to be formalised and become part of the contract of employment. Even those who are not employed in a teaching capacity might find that their job description includes responsibilities for the education and mentoring of others. Chapter 5 considered the statutory framework for the approval of education programmes leading to the OT's registration. In this chapter we are concerned with the legal issues which can arise in the relationship of lecturer/tutor and student. This chapter also considers the legal aspects of research. Further information on the legal issues arising in the teaching and assessment process can be seen in the author's chapter in *Partners in Learning* (published by Radcliffe Medical, 2002). The College of Occupational Therapists has provided guidance on providing work based learning opportunities for students[1] and also guidance for post-qualifiers.[2]

The following topics are covered in this chapter:

Teaching	Research
• Statutory requirements	• Protection of patients and volunteers
• Duty of care	• International Conventions
• Incompetent or dangerous students	• Professional guidelines on research
• Appeals process	• Consent
• Confidentiality and access to information	• Confidentiality
• Whistle blowing	• Compensation
• Contractual aspects	• Research-based practice
• Health and safety	• Local Research Ethics Committees
• NHS agreements	• Publication
• Writing references	• Intellectual property

Legal Aspects of Occupational Therapy, Third Edition By Bridgit Dimond
© 2010 Bridgit Dimond

Teaching and supervision

Terminology

First, what activities are we considering? Figure 26.1 sets out some of the terminology used in the instruction and support of others.

To make discussion easier, the person who is subject to the instruction, mentorship, etc. at any level (pre or post-registration) will be referred to as the student, even though the person may well be a registered practitioner.

Preceptor

A preceptor is defined by the registration body for nursing, midwifery and health visiting as

a role model and support for about the first four months of practice as a registered practitioner to:

- provide guidance
- be a member of the same team
- judge the appropriate level of responsibility
- agree objectives and outcomes for the period of support
- who may recommend an extension of time to provide support.

A comparable role is clearly of value for support to the newly registered OT and under the Agenda for Change (see Chapter 19) nurses and allied health professionals are required to develop and sustain local programmes of preceptorship. Mary Morley developed (in conjunction with the London group of professional lead OTs) a preceptorship handbook for OTs which was published by the COT in 2006. This handbook provides background information, documentation on the Knowledge and Skills Framework, a Preceptorship toolkit and references and materials together with a CD-ROM. Mary Morely considered the preceptorship process for OTs and its importance in reflective practice.[3] She concluded that preceptorship supported by the NHS Knowledge and Skills Framework provides a robust structure for graduates to maintain good habits of reflecting on practice and recording their learning as part of the ongoing CPD process. The COT has also published a preceptorship training manual.[4] Critical reflection for healthcare professionals is also considered in a work edited by Sylvina Tate and others[5]

Mentor

A mentor is a (usually) older and more experienced person who acts in the nature of a protector for another person for a longer time than would normally be associated with preceptorship, and where

Figure 26.1 Terms used in instructing and supporting others.

- Teacher
- Lecturer
- Clinical instructor
- Preceptor
- Mentor
- Supervisor
- Assessor
- Project manager
- Counsellor

the more experienced person provides guidance, support and a concern for the other's advancement and general progress.

Teacher/instructor/lecturer

This person would usually be based in a college of education and provide education and training for the student. Normally she would also have duties to instruct and assess in the workplace and assess the student's progress.

Supervisor

Clinical supervision, a form of reflective practice, is increasingly recommended for registered health professionals. It was recommended by the UKCC[6] (the predecessor of the NMC) for registered nurses, and is increasingly seen as good practice for OTs. A series of three articles in the *British Journal of Occupational Therapy* by Grace Sweeney and others[7] provides a useful outline of some of the problems which can arise within supervision in OT. A review of the practice of supervision in occupational therapy was conducted by Sue Gaitskell and Mary Morley.[8] They found that there were inconsistencies in the practice and theory of supervision and in the provision of training and recommended that managers in health and social care settings should adopt a theoretical framework for supervision, make their expectations explicit and build an infrastructure, including training and audit, to demonstrate the effectiveness of supervision in improving patient care as well as supporting staff growth. The possibility of using the Knowledge and Skills Framework (KSF) as a useful structure for supervision in order to ensure continual development is considered through a literature review by Helen Kleiser and Diane Cox. They conclude however that the roles of appraiser and supervisor should remain separate.[9]

The COT can provide further information and guidance on the supervisory process.

Situation: An unacceptable supervisor

Supervision has been split between case load supervision carried out by the line manager and clinical supervision to be carried out by mutual agreement between supervisor and supervisees. An OT has been told that her clinical supervisor must be her line manager. Can she refuse? It is essential that clinical supervision (as distinct from management supervision) is to the benefit of the supervisee, who should have respect for the supervisor. To be compelled to accept as a clinical supervisor someone who is not acceptable to the supervisee is unlikely to bode well for the value of the supervision process. It is hoped that an open discussion between those managing the allocation of supervisors and the supervisee could lead to an acceptable solution.

Statutory framework

The HPC has the duty of setting the educational requirements for entry onto the Register for its practitioners (see Chapters 3 and 5 for details of registration and educational requirements). The Rules[10] which came into force on 9 July 2003 require the applicant to provide a reference as to their good character by a person who is not a relative of the applicant and is a person of standing in the community. (A character reference form is provided under Schedule 3 to the Rules.) The applicant must also provide a reference as to their physical and mental health from a person who is not a relative but is the applicant's doctor. (A health reference form is provided under Schedule 4 to the Rules.) (See Chapter 3.)

Duty of care

It is essential to establish the extent of the duty of care owed to the student/trainee. Rarely is the instructor in a line management relationship with the student but there may be a responsibility when it can be seen that harm may occur to the student or to someone else if no action is taken by the instructor. Reference should be made to Chapter 10 on negligence and the basic elements to be established before a successful action can be brought.

The following principles emerge:

- there is no concept of team liability recognised in law
- there is no concept that a superior is vicariously liable for the wrongs of a junior. The superior must be shown to be personally and directly liable
- standards can differ (see the Bolam test and *Maynard* case in Chapter 10)
- liability can exist for negligent advice
- liability can also exist for negligent delegation where the instructor is aware that the student has inadequate experience to undertake a particular activity
- liability can also exist for negligent supervision if the limited experience of the student indicates that a specific level of supervision is required in order to ensure that the client, the student and others are safe.

The HPC has published guidance on conduct and ethics for students which sets the following principles:

1. You should always act in the best interests of your service users.
2. You should respect the confidentiality of your service users.
3. You should keep high standards of personal conduct.
4. You should provide any important information about your conduct, competence or health to your education provider.
5. You should keep your professional knowledge and skills up to date.
6. You should act within the limits of your knowledge and skills.
7. You should maintain proper and effective communications with your service users, practitioners and educators.
8. You should get informed consent to give treatment except in emergencies.
9. You should keep accurate service user records.
10. You should deal fairly and safely with the risks of infection.
11. You should limit your work or stop practising if your performance or judgement is affected by your health.
12. You should behave with integrity and honesty.
13. You should make sure that your behaviour does not damage public confidence in health professionals.

Since students (unless already registered in a different profession) are not registered with the HPC they do not come under its Fitness to Practise procedures for registrants, so it is important that the HPC provides guidance for them.

The extent of the duty of care

One area in which the teacher would be expected to show competence and have a duty of care, would be in ensuring that students were educated in the appropriate areas to obtain registration. The duty is placed upon the lecturer to ensure that the syllabus covered by the student and the standard of teaching, combined with due diligence from the student, are sufficient to enable the student to obtain the necessary qualifications for registration and practice. The lecturer must therefore ensure that she keeps up to date with the statutory requirements for registration.

Delegation to students

Situation – Home visits by unaccompanied students

OT students want to take more and more responsibility on student placement and are encouraged by the OT schools to carry out home visits without a qualified OT accompanying them. The OTs working in the community are concerned about the following issues:

- What happens if a student fails to notice or appropriately address something on the visit resulting in injury to patient?
- What if a complaint is made by patient or relative / carer?
- What if the student encounters abuse whilst on the visit?
- Who is responsible if anything goes wrong?

The same principles which apply to the delegation of activities to healthcare support workers also apply to the delegation of activities to students. The principles are considered in Chapter 10. A student should only be allowed to make an unaccompanied home visit when the supervisor is satisfied from previous accompanied visits that the student has the competence to be able to carry out a home assessment at the reasonable standard of care required of a qualified OT. The student should be aware of the limits of her competence and be prepared to notify the qualified OT of any factors which suggest that her visit should be followed up by that of a qualified OT. If the supervisor has delegated appropriately but the student misses something which a qualified OT would have noticed and acted upon, then the supervisor is not negligent, but the student is and liability would fall upon the college or the NHS trust or PCT depending upon the memorandum of agreement between the college and the organisation. If a complaint is made by a patient or carer that a student visited on her own, this should be investigated and responded to and the complainant reassured that the student from previous supervised visits had the appropriate experience to carry out the home assessment. Any abuse of the student should be dealt with in the same way that abuse of a qualified OT would be dealt with (see Chapter 11 on violence and harassment). Who is responsible if the student causes harm? If it is established that the student should not have been permitted to make the home visit without a supervising qualified OT, then the OT who allocated the visit to the student would be liable. In practice, of course if the OT is employed the employer would be vicariously liable for paying compensation for the harm (see Chapter 10). It is essential that those with the responsibility of supervising a student in the clinical placement do not accept instructions from the college which they consider could lead to harm to patients. Clearly there should be communication between the college lecturers and those supervising the student in the clinical placement over the procedure to be followed in allowing the student to make unaccompanied home visits.

Incompetent or dangerous students

If it is known that the student is likely to refuse or ignore any advice which is offered and if this refusal was likely to endanger clients, then the teacher would have a responsibility to take the appropriate action to prevent harm. In serious situations this might involve reporting a pre-registration student to the head of the education department and recommending that the student be suspended from the course; a post-registration student might be reported to the line manager. In less serious circumstances, and depending on whether the student is registered or not, it might necessitate warning the student that if the advice is ignored then further action will be taken. Should the instructor take the view that it is not her concern and then harm befalls a client, a defence of 'it was not my business' might not prevail in a hearing before the HPC since the instructor would herself be a registered practitioner and therefore subject to a Code of Ethics and Professional Conduct.

A similar situation would arise if the instructor forms the view that the student is too dangerous to practise. In such circumstances the instructor would have a clear professional responsibility to take any action necessary to protect the clients. This would also apply if the instructor feared that the student was mentally disordered. The dangers of such a situation are apparent from the Beverly Allitt[11] case, though there it was not known that the nurse was mentally ill until several children had been killed.

Where the instructor knows that the student is practising outside her sphere of competence, she should ensure that the managers are notified and the necessary training is given to the student to enable her to practise safely.

Sometimes, however, the student might confide in the instructor about confidential matters and disclose information which has been entrusted to her in confidence. For example, she might tell the instructor that she has passed on to the patient information relating to her diagnosis, contrary to the wishes of the consultant who had wanted to keep that information from the patient for the time being. In such a situation the instructor should ensure that the manager of the student is informed and that the patient is receiving all the necessary support. Where the instructor might agree that the student may have been right in her approach, she should be careful not to intervene in a clinical situation for which she is in no way responsible. However, if it appears that the student is in danger of being victimised because she has been a whistle blower, she should ensure that the student obtains the required support (see later section on whistle blowing).

Where the student tells the instructor information about herself in confidence, for example that she is HIV positive or that she has a drink problem or a criminal record, the instructor should make it clear that she cannot keep silent about such facts and should advise the student to notify the line manager, and if she fails to do so, then the instructor would be bound to take the necessary action. Where such information is given to the instructor anonymously the instructor would still have a duty to confront the student and take any necessary action.

Criticisms might also come to the instructor from the ward manager or others about the student's conduct. In such circumstances the instructor would have a duty to give the student advice and counselling and if necessary advise the head of school.

Students may criticise practice to the instructor. For example, a student might inform the instructor that a doctor is incompetent. In such a case, the instructor would have a responsibility to ensure that the student was supported in taking this further, so that appropriate investigations could be carried out by those with managerial responsibility.

Appeals processes

Each education or training institution must ensure that there is a robust, equitable, accessible and just system of appeals. Article 6 of the European Convention on Human Rights (see the Appendix of this book) is of particular importance in the assessment process, since it gives a right to a fair trial and is therefore fundamental to any appeals process where results of the assessment or the actual carrying out of an assessment are challenged. Assessors should ensure that if there is a challenge to their assessment, an independent person reviews the situation and the appropriate appeals machinery is enacted. The principles of natural justice would require that any person involved in hearing an appeal is independent and impartial, hears the evidence from the appellant and ensures that the decision made is in accordance with the evidence received. The decision of an appeals hearing could be challenged in the High Court by way of judicial review if there is an allegation that the principles of natural justice have not been followed or if there is an alleged breach of Article 6. The appeals process should also cover the timing of assessments and examinations. For example, if an assessor fails to carry out an assessment in time to give the student an opportunity for rectifying any shortcomings, and such an opportunity should have been made available to the student, then the student may well have grounds for appeal.

Contractual rights

Pre-registration students may be seen as having a contract with the educational institution and could bring a civil action for breach of contract against the college. Article 6 (see above) would apply to the processing of any such claims. The Court of Appeal held that overseas students could change their course, but if they wanted an extension of stay in the UK, they had to be able to produce evidence of satisfactory progress whether or not on the course named in the application for entry clearance or on another recognised course.[12]

Confidentiality and access to information

Since the instructor will not necessarily be professionally concerned with the care of the patient, what right in law does the instructor have to receive information which the student has received in confidence about the patient? It could be argued that the passing on of such information is in the interests of the patient. However, this is very indirect, and it would have to be shown that unless the instructor had this confidential information harm could arise to the patient. An alternative strategy, and one which would be far more open, is for the patient to be told about the situation relating to the instructor/student role, and the patient's consent obtained to relevant information being passed between them for the education of the student and the protection of the patient.

Where the student is concerned about a hazardous situation on the ward which involves confidential information about a patient, notifying the instructor for advice could be seen as an exception to the duty of confidentiality on the grounds that the disclosure is in the best interests of the patient or in the public interest (see Chapter 8).

Whistle blowing

The student should be guided in relation to the procedure for alerting management of any hazardous situations and the instructor should ensure that she is given the appropriate support. Advice should be given on record keeping and letters which are sent to management, and copies should be kept (see section on whistle blowing in Chapter 19).

Contractual aspects

Occupational therapists employed by trusts

Where an OT, who is employed by an NHS trust, is appointed as an instructor she should ensure that her job description and her terms of service reflect her enlarged duties. Where she is employed by a trust and not by an educational establishment, but is carrying out responsibilities in relation to the latter, she should ensure that her employer is aware of and has agreed to these additional duties and any likely area of conflict is resolved before the agreement is made. If she has any liability towards the educational establishment this should be clarified. She should also have access to the agreement drawn up between the college and the NHS trust in relation to the practical education of OTs and their preceptoring or mentoring, and any provisions relating to liability.

Occupational therapists employed by higher education colleges

OTs employed by colleges of education should ensure that their duties in relation to the clinical placements are spelt out in writing and they should ensure that they have an input into any agreement drawn up between the college and the trust over the clinical training of OTs and continuing education and preceptoring or mentoring. The agreement should clearly establish responsibility for any harm to the OT while she is supervising the student on the clinical placement and which organisation is vicariously liable should the OT cause harm through her negligence. This also applies where the placement is with social services or with another agency. Stipulations about liability for the safety of the OT or any harm caused by the OT should be included in the agreement between the college and the providers of the clinical placement.

Consideration for additional duties

It is unlikely that extra payments would be made for OTs to take on the tasks of being mentors or preceptors or clinical placement supervisors. However, if certain inducements are offered, the OT should ensure that these are put in writing.

Health and safety aspects

Depending on the circumstances of the relationship of instructor to student, the duty of care probably includes duties in relation to health and safety at work. Clearly, where the instructor notes that the student is failing to observe instructions in relation to health and safety, she would have a duty in law to inform the student of the dangers and ensure that those who were supervising the student in the workplace were aware of the situation (Chapter 11).

NHS agreements and agreements with social services authorities and providers of other clinical placements

Agreements for NHS services are increasingly likely to set out the training and educational functions expected of the providers. Those who are involved in the instructing/mentoring of others should ensure that the standards, both in terms of quantity and quality, are detailed in the agreement so that the necessary resources are made available, and that this function is specifically itemised for provision by the NHS trust. Continuing Professional Development responsibilities should be clarified so that continuing education and training is provided.

Continuing professional development

The HPC has set out its principles relating to continuing professional development and registration and these are discussed in Chapter 5. Resourcing for post-registration professional development may not be made centrally available and NHS trusts may differ not only in funding such training but also vary in their provision of paid time off work for study leave. It could be argued, since the employer owes a duty (both under the contract of employment and as part of the duty owed to patients under the law of negligence) to ensure the provision of competent staff, that there is an implied term that the employer will, at its own expense, ensure that the competence of professional staff is maintained and that standards of care are improved.

If such duties are built into the agreements for the provision of OT services, this will strengthen OTs' entitlement to receive regular updating and professional development within their paid hours of work. However, ultimately the duty is on the individual practitioner (see the Code of Ethics and Professional Conduct[13]) to ensure that she keeps up to date and receives the necessary study, whatever the policy of the employer in relation to paid study leave.

References

Liability can arise when an OT is asked to write a reference. If a reference is written negligently then liability can arise both to the recipient of the reference, if in reliance upon that reference he has suffered harm,[14] and also to the person who is the subject of the reference.[15]

Situation: providing a reference

An OT is asked to provide a reference for a student who has had a warning at work for coming into work in a dishevelled state. The OT student asks the OT not to refer to this incident, assuring her that she now takes considerable care over her appearance and cleanliness. What is the position if the OT gives the reference without mentioning this warning, and the student obtains the post, and then the employer blames the OT for an inaccurate reference?

If there is evidence that the student OT is completely reformed then it would probably not be necessary to mention this in the reference, but much depends on the questions which are asked. If inaccurate information is given, the person providing the reference could be liable for negligent advice. The recipient of the reference would have to show that harm had occurred as a result of reliance upon the reference. If a student asks for information to be withheld in a reference, the OT would have to tell the student that she could not give a reference without mentioning specific information. There can also be liability to the person on whose behalf the reference is given, if the reference is written without reasonable care and if harm occurs to the subject of the reference as a result of potential employers relying upon the reference. In one case,[16] Sun Alliance Life Ltd appealed against a decision that it had been negligent in its provision of an unfavourable reference in relation to C, a former employee. The Court of Appeal dismissed the appeal, holding that an employer owed a duty of care in providing a reference in respect of a former employee. Sun Alliance had failed to take reasonable care to be fair or accurate with regard to the reference supplied. The reference had inaccurately implied that C had been suspended for serious matters of dishonesty and that the matters had been thoroughly investigated. However, no charges of dishonesty had ever been put to C, let alone investigated.

Every care should be taken to ensure that a reference is written accurately in the light of the facts available.

If a reference is given with due care but is defamatory of the individual, the writer of the reference should be protected from any successful action of defamation where the comments are correct. If they are incorrect, then provided they were given in a qualified privileged situation without malice by the writer, they are not actionable for defamation.

Conclusion on the law and teachers

More and more pressure is placed upon teaching staff, and also those OTs who, although not teachers, are expected to fulfil the role of preceptor or mentor or undertake a similar activity. Such activities inevitably carry additional legal responsibilities and OTs must ensure that they have an understanding of the legal implications of any such activity they are asked to undertake. As always, clear and comprehensive documentation of how the activity is carried out is essential.

Clarification of the role of the supervisor in contrast to the role of a mentor/preceptor would be beneficial. It is also important to distinguish between a clinical supervisor who is providing a forum for reflective practice and a line manager supervisor who may have direct managerial responsibilities for the OT.

In October 2001 the Department of Health announced the publication of a prospectus for the NHS University.[17] It was the intention that everyone in the NHS (from cleaners to consultants) would begin their career with the NHS University through induction courses and direct training. However after barely 1 year of existence the NHS University was abolished and replaced by the NHS – Institute for Innovation and Improvement. Further information on the activities and strategy of the NHS Institute can be obtained from its website. The statutory provisions for pre and post-registration education are considered in Chapter 5.

Research

This section of the chapter looks at the law relating to research.

Occupational therapists are increasingly likely to be involved in research, either as researchers themselves, or caring for patients who are the subjects of a research project or in using research-based clinically effective practice. Whilst there are clear statutory regulations for the carrying out of research on animals (Animals (Scientific Procedures) Act 1986), for the testing of medicinal products (covered by the Medicines Act 1968), for testing on embryos (covered by the Human Fertilisation and Embryology Act 1990 as amended by the 2008 Act) and more recently European Community law on the conduct of clinical trials,[18] most of the law on research relating to clinical work derives from common law principles, supported by declarations from International Conventions and guidelines from professional registration bodies or associations. These declarations and guidelines, whilst they are frequently incorporated into the standards of professional practice, are not in themselves directly enforceable in the courts in the UK, unless they duplicate an existing common law principle or statute. In contrast the incorporation of the European Convention on Human Rights into the law of this country gives a statutory right to those who consider that they have been treated in an inhuman or degrading way, and this can be applied to participation in research (see Chapter 6 and Appendix 1). As the need for research-based, clinically effective practice increases, there is a greater likelihood that most health professionals will become involved in research, either directly as participants in research projects or indirectly as the provider of services to patients who are research subjects. This section looks at both the protection of patients who are asked to take part in research projects and also the laws which apply to the setting up, carrying out and publication of research work. The College of Occupational Therapy has published research ethics guidelines[19] which provide practical advice for all OTs involved in research, taking them from the start of the project and funding sources to the communications with participants and the laws relating to data protection and consent. It also has a useful explanation of the duty of care in its Appendix C, which could be used in clinical practice generally. Research Ethics are also one of the eleven standards set by the COT in its Professional Standards for Occupational Therapy Practice published in 2007 which sets out the following research ethics standard statements:

1. OT researchers should take steps to prevent or minimise harm to participants, researchers or others through the research.
2. OT researchers should take steps to maximise the potential benefits of research
3. OT researchers should respect everyone involved in research as true partners.
4. OT researchers should create circumstances in which participants are able to act on their own, freely made decisions.
5. OT researchers should act with integrity and honesty
6. OT researchers should act with impartiality and fairness
7. OT researchers should establish and maintain the confidentiality and/or anonymity or participants.

In 2007 the COT established the UK Occupational therapy research foundation (UKOTRF) to build an evidence base for occupational therapy, to increase research capacity within the profession and raise public awareness of the valuable contribution of occupation to people's health and wellbeing. The UKOTRF administers grants to support research in priority areas and to build research capacity. Further information can be obtained from the COT's research and development administrator.

Some of the specialist sections within the COT have also published guidance for research and development. For example the National Association of Paediatric Occupational Therapist have published a research and development strategic vision and action plan.[20] Guidance for research in occupational therapy is also provided in a book edited by Gary Kielhofner.[21] Helpful advice for the OT in evaluating randomised controlled trials is provided by Katherine Ho Deane in two articles[22] and on the use of inferential statistics by Chris Parker and Avril Drummond.[23]

International Conventions

Nuremberg Code

At the end of the second world war, military trials were held in Nuremberg where members of the Nazi party, some of the worst perpetrators of crimes against humanity, were prosecuted. In its

Figure 26.2 Principles for research from Nuremberg Code.

(1) The voluntary consent of the human subject is absolutely essential

(2) The experiment should be such as to yield fruitful results for the good of society, unprocurable by other methods

(3) The experiment should be based on results of animal experiments and a knowledge of the natural history of the disease or other problem so that the anticipated results should justify the performance of the experiment

(4) The experiment should be so conducted as to avoid all unnecessary physical and mental suffering and injury

(5) No experiment should be conducted where there is an a priori reason to believe that death or disabling injury will occur; except, perhaps, in those circumstances where the experimental physicians also serve as subjects

(6) The degree of risk to be taken should never exceed that determined by the humanitarian importance of the problem to be solved by the experiment

(7) Proper preparations should be made and adequate facilities provided to protect the experimental subject against even remote possibilities of injury, disability or death

(8) The experiment should be conducted only by a scientifically qualified person. The highest degree of skill and care should be required through all stages of the experiment by those who conduct or engage in the experiment

(9) During the course of the experiment the human subject should be at liberty to bring the experiment to an end if he had reached the physical or mental state where continuation of the experiment seems to him to be impossible

(10) During the course of the experiment the scientist in charge must be prepared to terminate the experiment at any stage, if he has probable cause to believe, in the exercise of the good faith, superior skill and careful judgment required of him, that a continuation of the experiment is likely to result in injury, disability, or death to the experimental subject

judgment, the court set out ten basic principles which should be observed in order to satisfy moral, ethical and legal concepts. These have become known as the Nuremberg Code.[24] The ten principles are summarised in Figure 26.2.

Declaration of Helsinki

The World Medical Association published a Declaration of Helsinki in 1964 which set out principles for the carrying out of research on human subjects. Amendments were made in 2000 following a conference in Edinburgh.[25]

United Nations Convention on the Rights of the Child

The United Nations Convention on the Rights of the Child was drawn up in 1989[26] and represents clear guidance for the development of rights-based and child-centred healthcare. The UK ratified the Convention in 1991. A biennial report is made on the extent of compliance by the UK with the Convention (see Chapter 23).

Convention on Human Rights and Biomedicine

A Convention for the Protection of Human Rights and Dignity of the Human Being with regard to the application of Biology and Medicine: Convention on Human Rights and Biomedicine[27] also applies to research practice.

Professional guidelines on research

Most health professional organisations have produced guidelines in respect of different aspects of research along the lines of the international conventions. In 1996 the Royal College of Physicians published guidelines on the practice of ethics committees.[28] The COT has also published guidance.[29] (Research using children is considered in Chapter 23.)

Guidance from the General Medical Council

The Standards Committee of the GMC has drafted guidance on medical research: The role and responsibilities of doctors in 2002. This guidance document sets out the core values and principles that it expects doctors to adhere to when they are involved in medical research projects. Subsequently the GMC has undertaken a consultation exercise in order to update its guidance on research practice to take into account its new guidance on consent (2008) and its core guidance "Good Medical Practice" (2006).

The GMC emphasises that the principles set out in its guidance Good Medical Practice, Seeking Patients' Consent: The Ethical Considerations and Confidentiality: Protecting and Providing information must be followed when undertaking research. These principles would apply to research undertaken by the OT or using clients/patients cared for by the OT.

Research governance framework

As part of the clinical governance initiative, the Department of Health published a research governance framework in 2001.[30] This set out the responsibilities of a research sponsor and required that organisations willing to take on these duties be included on a list of recognised sponsors and complete a base line assessment. The framework seeks to establish standards for all those involved in research in health and social care. Standards are set and the appropriate legislation identified, together with other sources of guidance in the areas of:

- ethics
- science
- information
- health, safety and employment
- finance and intellectual property.

The second edition of the research governance framework was published in May 2004.[31] The research governance framework is designed to set standards, define mechanisms to deliver standards, describe the monitoring and assessment arrangements, improve research quality and safeguard the public. It is intended to be used by research participants, those who host research in their organisations, research flinders, research managers and researchers in all environments and levels of health and social care. Regulations were published in April 2004 to implement the EC Directive on clinical trials (see below). The research governance framework for health and social care will incorporate the new regulations.

In 2006 the Department of Health initiated a new programme for research in the NHS called Best Research for Best Health.[32] The strategy and its implementation plans prepared by the new National Institute of Health Research (NIHR) can be downloaded from the DH website.

Consent

The basic principle from all the international declarations and from professional guidance is that the consent of a mentally competent adult is the fundamental requirement in any research. Special procedures must be established for children and mentally incapacitated adults. Failure to obtain consent from a mentally competent patient/volunteer or the Gillick competent child (see Chapter 23) or from parents of children before research is carried out, could lead to an action for trespass to the person (see Chapter 7). It is also essential that all relevant information should be given about any risks of harm from the research. Failure to provide sufficient information could lead to an action for breach of the duty of care to inform. This is on the basis that all researchers have a duty to ensure that a reasonable standard of professional practice is complied with in providing information before the patient gives consent (see Chapter 7). The rights of parents to give consent on behalf of their children to research projects is restricted to situations where there is no undue risk to the child. Further discussion of this difficult area is considered in a BMA publication.[33] Michael Curtin and Jane Murtagh consider the importance of competence, power and representation where children are participating in research.[34] They concluded that more needed to be done to secure the active participation of children and young people in research projects.

A distinction was made in the Helsinki Declaration between therapeutic and non-therapeutic research in the discussion of consent in relation to research. Research which is linked with the treatment of the patient would be described as 'therapeutic', whereas research which has no immediate benefit to that particular patient is described as 'non-therapeutic'. In the discussions which took place between 1998 and 2000 on revisions to the Declaration of Helsinki, it was agreed that the distinction should be dropped from the Declaration. However, in practice there is likely to be a distinction since where the patient/client stands to benefit personally from the research, it could be argued that the research on adults incapable of giving consent could be conducted as part of their treatment plan in their best interests, even though that person lacks the mental capacity to give a valid consent. However, if the individual has no personal benefit from the research and the treatment cannot therefore be given in the best interests of the patient, the research will have to come under the provisions of the Mental Capacity Act 2005 (see below).

The information which is given to the patient/client and the consent form to be signed should be approved by the Local Research Ethics Committee (see below) before the research commences. The importance of involving service users in health and social care research is emphasised in two textbooks, one edited by Lesley Lowes and Ian Hulatt[35] and the other edited by Mike Nolan and others.[36]

Reference should be made to Chapter 23 and the law relating to consent by a child or young person (i.e. a person under 18 years).

Consent to research and the mentally incapacitated adult

The Mental Capacity Act (MCA) 2005 has introduced stringent provisions in relation to research involving those who are over 16 years and who are unable to give consent. The statutory provisions

---

> **Box 26.1   Conditions required for research on those lacking the requisite mental capacity to give consent.**
>
> - that the research is part of a research project
> - which is approved by an appropriate body as defined in section 31
> - complies with the conditions laid down in section 31 (see Box 26.2) and
> - complies with conditions relating to the consulting of carers and additional safeguards. (i.e. sections 32 and 33 see below)

apply to research other than clinical trials. (Clinical trials come under separate EU regulations drawn up as a consequence of the European Directive.[37] (see below))

Under sections 30 to 34 of the MCA the provisions relating to research and the mentally incapacitated adult are set out.

Conditions for intrusive research

The MCA prohibits intrusive research being carried out on, or in relation to a person who lacks the capacity to consent unless certain conditions are met. These conditions are shown in Box 26.1. Intrusive research is defined in section 30(2) as 'research which would be unlawful if carried out on a person capable of giving consent, but without that consent'.

The Code of Practice[38] notes that the Act does not have a specific definition for 'research' and it quotes the definitions used by the Department of Health and National Assembly for Wales publications Research governance framework for health and social care:

> research can be defined as the attempt to derive generalisable new knowledge by addressing clearly defined questions with systematic and rigorous methods.[39]

The Code of Practice points out that research may:

- provide information that can be applied generally to an illness, disorder or condition
- demonstrate how effective and safe a new treatment is
- add to evidence that one form of treatment works better than another
- add to evidence that one form of treatment is safer than another, or
- examine wider issues (for example, the factors that affect someone's capacity to make a decision).

The Code of Practice notes that:[40]

> It is expected that most of the researchers who ask for their research to be approved under the Act will be medical or social care researchers. However, the Act can cover more than just medical and social care research. Intrusive research which does not meet the requirements of the Act cannot be carried out lawfully in relation to people who lack capacity.

Non-intrusive research

Non intrusive research could include research of anonymised records or the use of anonymous tissue or blood left over after it had been collected for use in other procedures Whilst such research is excluded from the provisions of the Mental Capacity Act 2005 it could come under other legislative provisions such as the Data Protection Act 1998 and regulations under the Data Protection Act and the Human Tissue Act 2004.

> **Box 26.2   Conditions for approval of a research project relating to a person lacking the capacity to consent (Section 31).**
>
> (2)   The research is connected with an impairing condition affecting P (the person lacking mental capacity) or its treatment.
>
> (3)   An impairing condition is defined in section 31(3) as a condition which is (or may be) attributable to, or which causes or contributes to, the impairment of, or disturbance in the functioning of, the mind or brain;
>
> (4)   There must be reasonable grounds for believing that the research would not be as effective if carried out only on, or only in relation to, person who have the capacity to consent to taking part in the project
>
> (5(a))   The research must have the potential to benefit P without imposing on P a burden that is disproportionate to the potential benefit to P or
>
> (5(b))   be intended to provide knowledge of the causes or treatment of, or of the care of persons affected by, the same or a similar condition
>
> (6)   If 5(b) applies and not 5(a), there must be reasonable grounds for believing- (a) that the risk to P from taking part in the project is likely to be negligible, and (b) that anything done to, or in relation to, P will not – (i) interfere with P's freedom of action or privacy in a significant way, or (ii) be unduly invasive or restrictive.
>
> (7)   There must be reasonable arrangements in place for ensuring that the requirements of section 32 and 33 are in place (consulting carers and additional safeguards (see below)).

Requirements for approval for intrusive research

The appropriate body (i.e. the person, committee, or other body specified by the Secretary of State in regulations[41]) may not approve a research project relating to a person lacking the capacity to consent unless the conditions shown in Box 26.2 are present.

Consulting of carers

The researcher "R" is required to take reasonable steps to identify a person who is not engaged in a professional capacity nor receiving remuneration but is engaged in caring for P or is interested in P's welfare and is prepared to be consulted by the researcher under section 32.

Subsection (7) makes it clear that the fact that a person is the donee of a lasting power of attorney given by P, or is P's deputy, does not prevent him from being the person consulted under section 32.

If such a person cannot be identified, then R must in accordance with guidance issued by the Secretary of State or the Welsh Assembly nominate a person who is prepared to be consulted by R but has no connection with the project.

R must provide the carer or nominee with information about the project and ask him for advice as to whether P should take part in the project and what, in his opinion, P's wishes and feelings about taking part in the project would be likely to be if P had capacity in relation to the matter. If the person consulted advises R that in his opinion P's wishes and feelings would be likely to lead him to decline to take part in the project (or to wish to withdraw from it), if he had the capacity, then R must ensure that P does not take part, or if he is already taking part, ensure that he is withdrawn from it.

If treatment has commenced it is not necessary to discontinue the treatment if R has reasonable grounds for believing that there would be a significant risk to P's health if it were discontinued.

Urgent research (S.32(8)(9))

Special provisions apply where treatment is to be provided as a matter of urgency and R considers that it is also necessary to take action for the purposes of the research as a matter of urgency, but it is not reasonably practicable to consult under the above provisions of this section.

In these circumstances R must have the agreement of a registered medical practitioner who is not concerned in the organisation or conduct of the research project or where it is not reasonably practicable in the time available to obtain that agreement, he acts in accordance with a procedure approved by the appropriate body at the time when the research project was approved under section 31. When R has reasonable grounds for believing that it is no longer necessary to take the action as a matter of urgency, he cannot continue to act in reliance of these urgent provisions (S32(10)).

Additional safeguards

There are additional safeguards to protect the interests of the person lacking the requisite mental capacity:

- Nothing may be done to, or in relation to a person taking part in the research project who is incapable of giving consent,
- to which he appears to object (whether by showing signs of resistance or otherwise) except where what is being done is intended to protect him from harm or to reduce or prevent pain or discomfort, or
- which would be contrary to an advance decision of his which has effect or any other form of statement made by him and not subsequently withdrawn and R is aware of this.

The MCA expressly states (S33(3)) that the interests of the person must be assumed to outweigh those of science and society.

Loss of capacity during research project

Section 34 applies if P had consented to take part in a research project begun before the commencement of section 30 (1 April 2007) but before the conclusion of the project loses capacity to consent to continue to take part in it. In such a situation regulations may provide that despite his loss of capacity, research of a prescribed kind may be carried out on, or in relation to, P if:

a.   the project satisfies the prescribed requirements
b.   any information or material relating to which is used in the research is of a prescribed description and was obtained before P's loss of capacity and
c.   the person conducting the project takes in relation to P such steps as may be prescribed for the purpose of protecting him.

Regulations[42] covering the situation where an adult who had given consent to participation in research lost the requisite mental capacity during the research project were enacted in 2007. They provide that in such circumstances, despite P's loss of capacity, research for the purposes of the project may be carried out using information or material relating to him if certain specified conditions exist:

(a) the project satisfies the requirements set out in Schedule 1,
(b) all the information or material relating to P which is used in the research was obtained before P's loss of capacity, and

(c) the person conducting the project ("R") takes in relation to P such steps as are set out in Schedule 2.

Schedule 1 is shown in Box 26.3. Schedule 2 of the Regulations is shown in Box 26.4.

Box 26.3   Schedule 1 to the Regulations on loss of capacity during the research project. Requirements which the project must satisfy.

1.   A protocol approved by an appropriate body and having effect in relation to the project makes provision for research to be carried out in relation to a person who has consented to take part in the project but loses capacity to consent to continue to take part in it.
2.   The appropriate body must be satisfied that there are reasonable arrangements in place for ensuring that the requirements of Schedule 2 will be met (see Box 26.4 for Schedule 2).

Box 26.4   Schedule 2 to the Regulations on loss of capacity during the research project. Steps which the person conducting the project must take.

1.   R must take reasonable steps to identify a person who— (a) otherwise than in a professional capacity or for remuneration, is engaged in caring for P or is interested in P's welfare, and (b) is prepared to be consulted by R under this Schedule.
2.   If R is unable to identify such a person he must, in accordance with guidance issued by the Secretary of State, nominate a person who— (a) is prepared to be consulted by R under this Schedule, but (b) has no connection with the project.
3.   R must provide the person identified under paragraph 1, or nominated under paragraph 2, with information about the project and ask him— (a) for advice as to whether research of the kind proposed should be carried out in relation to P, and (b) what, in his opinion, P's wishes and feelings about such research being carried out would be likely to be if P had capacity in relation to the matter.
4.   If, at any time, the person consulted advises R that in his opinion P's wishes and feelings would be likely to lead him to wish to withdraw from the project if he had capacity in relation to the matter, R must ensure that P is withdrawn from it.
5.   The fact that a person is the donee of a lasting power of attorney given by P, or is P's deputy, does not prevent him from being the person consulted under paragraphs 1 to 4.
6.   R must ensure that nothing is done in relation to P in the course of the research which would be contrary to—
(a)   an advance decision of his which has effect, or
(b)   any other form of statement made by him and not subsequently withdrawn, of which R is aware.
7.   The interests of P must be assumed to outweigh those of science and society.
8.   If P indicates (in any way) that he wishes the research in relation to him to be discontinued, it must be discontinued without delay.
9.   The research must be discontinued without delay if at any time R has reasonable grounds for believing that one or more of the requirement set out in Schedule 1 is no longer met or that there are no longer reasonable arrangements in place for ensuring that the requirements of this Schedule are met in relation to P.
10.   R must conduct the research in accordance with the provision made in the protocol referred to in paragraph 1 of Schedule 1 for research to be carried out in relation to a person who has consented to take part in the project but loses capacity to consent to take part in it.

It is hoped that the implementation of these provisions of the MCA are monitored to assess their effectiveness in protecting those incapable of giving consent to participation in a research project and at the same time enabling important research into the underlying conditions of mental incapacity to take place.

Consent and Clinical Trials

Clinical trials which come under the clinical trials regulations,[43] enacted in 2004, are excluded from the statutory provisions of the Mental Capacity Act 2005. Article 5 of the regulations makes provisions for clinical trials on incapacitated adults not able to give informed legal consent.

Confidentiality

Exactly the same principles of confidentiality apply in relation to the personal information obtained from undertaking research. It is probable that the exceptions to the duty to maintain confidentiality recognised by the law in relation to personal information obtained in the course of caring for patients (see Chapter 8) would apply to information obtained through research. For example, if information relating to the health or safety of the patient or of other people were obtained during the research, there may be justification in passing this to the appropriate authorities. In writing case studies it is essential that either the specific consent of the patient to the publication of a case study has been obtained, or the details have either been anonymised or changed to make it impossible for the patient to be identified.

Compensation

At present if a person suffers harm as a result of involvement in a research project, he or she could sue in the tort of negligence and would have to prove that the researcher failed to follow a reasonable standard of care (this could also include the disclosure of information to the patient prior to consent to the research being obtained) and as a consequence the patient has suffered harm.

The Pearson Report[44] in 1978 recommended that both volunteers and patients who take part in medical research and clinical trials and who suffer severe damage as a result, should receive compensation on the basis of strict liability. This recommendation has never been implemented in law, although the Association of British Pharmaceutical Industry has recommended that such persons should obtain compensation without proof of negligence if harm arose as a result of the research project. Research Ethics Committees are required to establish that there has been an agreement to pay compensation before any research on medicinal products takes place.

Research-based practice

In 2001 the COT published a research and development strategic vision and action plan.[45] This reviewed the 1997 strategy[46] and proposed a flexible approach to the next 5 years in collaboration with other health professions, and an approach that was responsive to changes in the policy context and reflected the needs of members, consumers and carers. Objective 6 of this strategy anticipated that all members are expected to promote an evaluative culture to improve practice. The COT was asked to comment on future plans for research policy and funding by the Higher Education Funding Councils of England, Wales, Scotland and Northern Ireland. Their comments, and the implications of the research assessment exercise (RAE) carried out in Higher Education, are considered by Irene Ilott and Elizabeth White.[47] As Rosemary Barnitt[48] has pointed out, there are at present very rarely any occupational therapy submissions to the 5-year RAE carried out by the Higher Education Funding Council and the majority tend to gain a 2 or 3 rating (the maximum is 5). However, she points out the importance of research not just in supporting evidence-based practice but also suggests that 'it is just possible that evidence from research would help us to reduce practice workloads by allowing us to drop activities that have little or no value to the client'.

In the light of the growing expectation that more and more OTs will be personally involved in research, the Association of OTs in Mental Health (AOMH) published an updated list of priorities in mental health research.[49] The revised list reflects the increased awareness of the need to involve users in research, service design and service delivery. The approach could be followed by other special interest groups within OT.

In the COT business plan for 2005–6 there was a commitment to revise the research and development strategic vision and action plan and to develop a UK OT Research Foundation. A research project was commissioned to identify research priorities for OT research. The final report of the POTTER project was published in August 2006.[50] It concluded that, as in 1999, the top research priority for OT research is the effectiveness of OT interventions and the findings of the project were used to develop a strategic overview of research priorities for OT in the UK for use in developing research capacity and commissioning research by COT and other organisations. An overview of the project is provided by Katrina Bannigan et al.[51] In 2007 the COT published its priorities for research based on the work of its R& D group and input from the specialist sections of the COT.[52] The COT has also published a research resources guide for OTs[53] and also guidance on developing a research grant.[54]

The Bolam test, which is discussed in Chapter 10, is the accepted test for defining reasonable, acceptable, professional practice. As discussed, what a reasonable body of responsible practitioners would accept as appropriate practice will change as standards of care improve and develop. The findings from substantiated research will therefore eventually become integrated into accepted practice, and it is essential that the professional keeps abreast of changes in recommended practice. The National Institute for Health and Clinical Excellence should ensure that research-based clinically effective practice is brought to the notice of health professionals and this would become incorporated into the Bolam test of reasonable professional practice. Clare Taylor considers in her book on evidence-based practice for OTs how evidence from clinical trials can be used for practice.[55] The action necessary to change professional practice following research evidence is considered by Anne Roberts and Graeme Barber[56] who show that multifaceted interventions are necessary in order to change practice, including co-ordinated implementation of active methods, such as the combination of continuing education, clinical guidelines, good project management by senior staff and individual ownership. An appeal is made by Karen Whalley Hammell[57] that qualitative research, which is client-centred and not just quantitative research, should be used to support clinical practice.

Local Research Ethics Committees (LREC)

The Department of Health requested each health authority in 1991 to ensure that an LREC[58] was set up to examine research proposals and new guidance was issued in 2001.[59] The new arrangements came into force in April 2002. The Department of Health requires that all research falling within the following categories should be reviewed independently to ensure that it meets the required ethical standards:

(a)   patients and users of the NHS including NHS patients treated under contracts with independent sector institutions
(b)   individuals identified as potential research participants because of their status as relatives or carers of patients and users of the NHS
(c)   access to data, organs or other bodily material of past or present NHS patients
(d)   fetal material and IVF involving NHS patients
(e)   the recently dead in NHS premises
(f)   the use of, or potential access to, NHS premises or facilities.'

The independent review must be obtained from a Research Ethics Committee (REC) recognised for that purpose by the Department of Health. For research in health and social care occurring outside the NHS, it is recommended that an opinion should be obtained from an NHS REC, or from an REC meeting the general standards for NHS RECs laid down in the governance arrangements for NHS RECs. Research may not be started until ethical approval has been obtained. It is the personal responsibility of the person named as principal investigator to apply for approval by the REC and this person retains responsibility for the scientific and ethical conduct of the research.

Section A of the guidance provided by the Department of Health sets out a Statement of General Standards and Principles and covers the following topics:

● role of Research Ethics Committees
● the remit of an NHS REC
● establishment and support of NHS RECs
● membership requirements and process
● composition of an REC
● working procedures
● multi-centre research
● the process of ethical review of a research protocol
● submitting an application
● glossary.

Section B provides more detailed guidance on operating procedures and the requirements for general support for RECs. Section C provides a resource for RECs and collates current advice on ethical issues, and is to be regularly updated.

The governance statement defines the purpose of an REC in reviewing the proposed study as:

to protect the dignity, rights, safety and well-being of all actual or potential research participants. It shares this role and responsibility with others, as described in the *Research Governance Framework for Health and Social Care*.[60]

It is emphasised that the goals of research and researchers, while important should always be secondary to the dignity, rights, safety and well-being of the research participants. Several Local Research Ethic Committees may be set up within each strategic health authority area. Strategic health authorities are accountable for the establishment, support, training and monitoring of all NHS Local Research Ethics Committees within their boundary. The strategic health authority should identify a named officer not otherwise directly involved in REC administration who will have a lead responsibility for the governance of Research Ethics Committees on behalf of the Chief Executive. The

Department of Health is responsible for these functions for Multi-centre Research Ethics Committees. RECs are not accountable to NHS trusts and are separate from trust research and development departments. The appointing authority will take full responsibility for all the actions of a member in the course of their performance as a member of the REC, other than those involving bad faith, wilful default or gross negligence.

Members of RECs are appointed by the strategic health authority according to Nolan standards of public accountability and should include about 18 members providing a sufficiently broad range of experience and expertise so that the scientific, clinical and methodological aspects of a research proposal can be reconciled with the welfare of research participants, and with broader ethical principles. The overall composition should be balanced in age and gender and have a mixture of experts and lay members. Each LREC should provide an annual report to the appointing authority.

Multi-centre research is defined as research carried out within five or more research sites (i.e. the geographical area covered by a single strategic health authority). Where one LREC has approved the proposal, the LRECs in the other areas can accept the opinion without further review by their own LREC, if advised by their own LREC.

Part 9 of Section A covers the process of ethical review and sets down principles relating to the requirements for a favourable opinion, recruitment of research participants, care and protection of research participants, protection of research participants' confidentiality, informed consent process, and community considerations. There is also provision for an expedited review, which is covered in section B of the governance document.

Obtaining the approval of an LREC should ensure that the patient/client is reasonably protected from zealous researchers. However, particular difficulties can arise where the researcher is also the health professional concerned with the treatment of the patient. In such cases, it is not easy to ensure that treatment concerns remain paramount and that the patient is assured that he or she can opt out of the research at any time without suffering any sanction from the health professional.

A Central Office for Research Ethics Committees (COREC) has been established which co-ordinates the development of operational systems for Research Ethics Committees (RECs) in the NHS, manages multi-centre Research Ethics Committees (MRECs) in England, acts as a resource for training for REC members and administrators, and provides advice on policy and operational matters relating to RECs. Occupational therapists interested in taking part in Research Ethic Committee work could contact COREC to obtain further details of the training and the RECs in their area.[61] The College of Occupational Therapists has published a briefing note on applying for ethics approval for research.[62] It gives guidance on why ethics approval is required and how it should be obtained.

Publication

It is extremely wise for researchers to discuss and agree arrangements for possible publication of the research before it is undertaken in order to prevent disputes arising over censorship and control once the outcome is known. Some funding bodies who have sponsored the research may require that they see the findings before they permit publication. This may be seen, however, as an unjustified restraint on the dissemination of the results. Clearly, if major concerns are unearthed during a research investigation and the researcher is an employee of the organisation concerned, the employee would have the protection of the Public Interest Disclosure Act 1998 in bringing to the attention of the appropriate senior management these concerns (see Chapter 19).

Accuracy

If research is published which contains errors of design and interpretation and persons suffer harm as a result of dependence on the conclusions drawn, then there could be liability in negligence. A centre for cancer treatment in women in Bristol suffered financial loss as the result of a research report which suggested that the centre achieved worse results than other treatment centres. It was later learnt that the researchers had failed to take account of the fact that the Bristol centre took patients at a much later stage in their illness compared with other centres and therefore like was not being compared with like. Practitioners who knowingly take part in research which is not sound could face professional conduct proceedings. In addition, there may be liability on the part of LREC members if it has failed to fulfil its functions appropriately and as a consequence someone has suffered harm. The LREC is not itself a statutory body, but the action would lie against the strategic health authority on whose behalf the LREC has acted. Where it is claimed that financial loss has occurred, it would have to be established that there was justifiable and known clear reliance upon statements by the LREC as a consequence of which harm has been caused. Causation would, however, be difficult to establish. The LREC does not necessarily guarantee the scientific validity of research for which it gives its consent. In this case the researchers themselves could be personally liable and if employees, their employers vicariously liable.

Fraud in research

Research misconduct unfortunately takes place and inevitably receives considerable publicity. The BMA has published a book on fraud and misconduct in medical research.[63] A national Committee on Publication Ethics (COPE) has been set up to prevent plagiarism, redundant publication and fraudulent manipulation of data.

Intellectual property and copyright

Sometimes research projects can lead to lucrative rewards, such as for the design of a new piece of equipment or an innovative idea for supporting disabled persons. The right of ownership of any such inventions or innovations depends on the nature of the contract between employer and employee. If the practitioner is undertaking research and development as part of her work as a full-time employee, then the employer would be seen as the owner of the research, though a generous employer may well develop an income sharing scheme with the employee. If on the other hand the research has been developed by the practitioner entirely on her own, with no involvement from the employer or its resources, she would be the owner of the intellectual property. Advice should be taken on patenting the design so that ownership is legally recognised.[64] Guidance is provided in the Department of Health's Research Governance Framework,[65] which was finalised in May 2004.

Ethical issues

Jane Seale and Sue Barnard[66] consider the OTs responsibility to ensure that a research project is ethical, and look at the topics of self respect and dignity, privacy, protection of the research participant, informed consent, information confidentiality, behaving in a professional manner and the role of the ethics committee. Reference should be made to the list of additional reading.

Conclusions on research

Practice must be based on knowledge obtained through research. Evidence-based practice is essential in the twenty-first century and the College of Occupational Therapy is playing its part in encouraging research-based practice and implementing a research and development strategy. Ultimately the Bolam test (see Chapter 10) as to what is the accepted approved practice of the reasonable practitioner should be supported by clinical evidence. The European Convention on Human Rights, as published in Schedule 1 to the Human Rights Act 1998, must be respected in the conduct of research (see Appendix 1). The initiatives set out in the White Paper[67] together with the National Institute for Health and Clinical Excellence, national service framework and the Commission for Health Audit and Inspection should lead to standards being developed across all health specialities and professions. Research should be encouraged, to underpin practice. There is therefore considerable pressure to ensure that the rights of patients and volunteers are protected and that the research complies with the standards set by international declarations and professional guidance.

 Questions and exercises

1   As a lecturer of OTs, you have been told by a student that a fellow student is acting very oddly and appears to be mentally ill. What action would you take?

2   You are employed by an educational institution but have responsibilities within the field of clinical practice. In the event of your being negligent and causing harm to a client, who would be liable: the educational institution or the trust? How would you find out the answer?

3   In litigation, proof of the instruction which has been given is of increasing importance as a defence. Examine your own record keeping in relation to what you teach or mentor.

4   You are wishing to carry out a research project. Draw up a schedule setting out the initial tasks you should undertake before you actually begin the data collection.

5   How do the requirements in relation to consent to participation in a research project apply to mentally competent and mentally incompetent adults and children?

6   Obtain a copy of the local procedure for obtaining the approval of the LREC to a research project and consider the extent to which it protects the interests of patients and volunteers.

References

1   College of Occupational Therapists (2006) *Developing the OT profession – providing new work based learning opportunities for students.* COT, London.

2   College of Occupational Therapists (2006) *Post-qualifying framework- a resource for occupational therapists.* COT, London.

3   Morley Mary (2007) Building reflective practice through preceptorship: the cycles of professional growth. *British Journal of Occupational Therapy,* **70**(1), 40-2.

4   College of Occupational Therapists (2006) *Preceptorship training manual.* COT, London.

5   Tate Sylvina and Gills Margaret (eds) (2004) *The Development of Critical Reflection in the health professions.* Higher Education Academy, London.

6   UKCC (1996) *Position Statement on Clinical Supervision.* UKCC, London.

7   Sweeney, G., Webley, P. & Treacher, A. (2001) Supervision in occupational therapy. *British Journal of Occupational Therapy,* Part 1 the Supervisor's Anxieties, **64**(7), 337–; Part 2 The Supervisee's Dilemma, **64**(8), 380–86; Part 3 Accommodating the Supervisor and Supervisee, **64**(9), 426–31.

8   Gaitskell Sue and Morley Mary (2008) Supervision in Occupational Therapy: How are we doing? *British Journal of Occupational Therapy*, **71**(3), 119–21.

9   Kleiser Helen and Cox Diane L (2008) The Integration of clinical and managerial supervision: a critical literature review. *British Journal of Occupational Therapy*, **71**(1), 2–9.

10 The Health Professions Council (Registration and Fees) Rules Order of Council 2003, SI 2003/1572.

11 The Allitt Inquiry, chaired by Sir Cecil Clothier (1994). HMSO, London.

12 *GO and others v Secretary of State for the Home Department* The Times Law Report 23 July 2008.

13 College of Occupational Therapists (2005) *Code of Ethics and Professional Conduct for Occupational Therapists*. COT, London.

14 *Hedley Byrne v Heller and Partners Ltd* [1963] 2 All ER 575, HL.

15 *Spring v Guardian Assurance plc and others*. Times Law Report, 8 July 1994; [1995] 2 AC 296.

16 *Cox v Sun Alliance Life Ltd* [2001] EWCA Civ 649; [2001] IRLR 448, CA.

17 Department of Health (2001) Press Release 2001/-480, *Introducing the NHS University*.

18 EC Directive 2001/20/EC.

19 College of Occupational Therapists (2003) *Research Ethics Guidelines*. COT, London.

20 National Association of Paediatric Occupational Therapist (2003) *Research and development strategic vision and action plan*. COT, London.

21 Kielhofner Gary (ed) (2006) *Research in Occupational Therapy: Methods of Inquiry for enhancing practice*. FA Davis, Philadelphia.

22 Deane Katherine HO (2006) Randomised Controlled Trials Part 1 Design and Part 2 Reporting. *British Journal of Occupational Therapy*, **69**(5), 217–23 and **69**(6), 248–52.

23 Parker Chris and Drummond Avril ER (2006) From Sample to Population: using and reporting inferential statistics. *British Journal of Occupational Therapy*, **69**(1), 15–21.

24 Kennedy, I. & Grubb, A. (2000) *Medical Law*, 3rd edn. Butterworths, London.

25 European Forum for Good Clinical Practice. *Bulletin of Medical Ethics*, Revising the Declaration of Helsinki: a fresh start, London 3–4 September 1999.

26 United Nations Convention on the Rights of the Child 20, XI.1989; TS 44; CM 1976.

27 Convention for the Protection of Human Rights and Dignity of the Human Being with regard to the application of Biology and Medicine. *Convention on Human Rights and Biomedicine*, 4.iv.1997.

28 Royal College of Physicians (1996) *Guidelines on the Practice of Ethics Committees in Medical Research Involving Human Subjects*, 3rd edn. RCP, London.

29 College of Occupational Therapists (2003) *Research Ethics Guidelines*. COT, London.

30 Department of Health (2001) Research Governance Framework; www.doh.gov.uk/research/rd3/nhsrandd/researchgovernance.htm

31 Department of Health (2004) Research Governance Framework for England, 2nd edn; www.doh.gov.uk/research/rd3/nhsandd/researchgovernance.htm

32 Department of Health (2006) *Best Research for Best Health*. DH, London.

33 British Medical Association (2001) *Consent, Rights and Choices in Health Care for Children and Young People*. BMJ Publications, London.

34 Curtin Michael and Murtagh Jane (2007) Participation of children and young people in research: competence, power and representation. *British Journal of Occupational Therapy*, **70**(2), 67–72.

35 Lowes Lesley and Hulatt Ian (eds) (2005) *Involving Service Users in Health and Social Care Research*. Routledge, London.

36 Nolan Mike, Hanson Elizabeth, Grant Gordon, and Keady John (eds) (2007) *User Participation in Health and Social Care Research: Voices, Values and Evaluation*. Open University Press, Maidenhead.

37 EC Directive 2001/20/EC

38 Code of Practice Mental Capacity Act 2005 Department of Constitutional Affairs February 2007 paragraph 11.2.

39 www.dh.gov.uk/PublicationsAndStatistics/Publications/PublicationsPolicyAndGuidance/PublicationsPolicyAndGuidanceArticle/fs/en?CONTENT_ID=4008777&chk=dMRd/5 and www.word.wales.gov.uk/content/governance/governance-e.htm

40 Code of Practice Mental Capacity Act 2005 Department of Constitutional Affairs February 2007 paragraph 11.5.

41   Mental Capacity Act 2005 (Appropriate Body)(England) Regulations 2006 SI No 2810; Mental Capacity Act 2005 (Appropriate Body)(England)(Amendment) Regulations 2006 SI No 3474.

42   The Mental Capacity Act 2005 (Loss of Capacity during Research Project) (England) Regulations 2007 SI No 679.

43   The Medicines for Human Use (Clinical Trials) Regulations 2004 SI 2004/1031.

44   Royal Commission on Civil Liability and Compensation for Personal Injury, chaired by Lord Pearson. Cmnd 7054 1978 HMSO.

45   College of Occupational Therapists (2001) *Research and Development Strategic Vision and Action Plan*. COT, London.

46   Eakin, P., Ballinger, C., Nicol, M., Walker, M., Alsop, A. & Ilott, I. (1997) College of Occupational Therapists: research and development strategy. *British Journal of Occupational Therapy*, **60**(11), 484–6.

47   Ilott, I. & White, E. (2000) Research and Development Board: the Research Assessment Exercise – Implications for the future of occupational therapy. *British Journal of Occupational Therapy*, **63**(4), 171–6.

48   Barnitt, R. (2002) Research assessment could benefit the client. *British Journal of Occupational Therapy*, **65**(6), 255.

49   Davis, S.F. & Hyde, P. (2002) Priorities in mental health research: an update. *British Journal of Occupational Therapy*, **65**(8), 387–9.

50   Bannigan Katrina, Boniface Gail, Doherty Patrick, Margaret Nicol et al (2006) *Priorities for research in occupational therapy the POTTER Project*. COT, London.

51   Bannigan Katrina, Boniface Gail, Doherty Patrick, Margaret Nicol et al (2008) Priorities for Occupational Therapy research in the UK: Executive summary of the POTTER project. *British Journal of Occupational Therapy*, **71**(1), 13–6

52   College of Occupational Therapy (2007) *Building the evidence for Occupational Therapy – priorities for research*. COT, London.

53   College of Occupational Therapists (2007) Research Resources for Occupational Therapists Briefing note no 75. COT, London.

54   College of Occupational Therapists (2007) Developing a research grant- guidance for specialist sections Briefing note no 79. COT, London.

55   Taylor, M.C. (2000) *Evidence-based Practice for Occupational Therapists*. Blackwell Publishing, Oxford.

56   Roberts, A.E.R. & Barber, G. (2001) Applying research evidence to practice. *British Journal of Occupational Therapy*, **64**(5), 223–7.

57   Whalley Hammell, K. (2001) Using qualitative research to inform the client-centred evidence-based practice of occupational therapy. *British Journal of Occupational Therapy*, **64**(5), 228–34.

58   HSG(91)5

59   Department of Health (2001) *Governance Arrangements for NHS Research Ethics Committees*; replaces HSG(91)5 (the red book) and HSG(97)23 on multi-centre Research Ethics Committees. See www.doh.gov.uk/research/rdl/researchgovernance/corec.htm

60   Department of Health. *Research Governance Framework for England*, 1st edn, 2001; draft 2nd edition, 2003. www.doh.gov.uk/research/rd3/nhsandd/researchgovernance.htm

61   www.corec.org.uk/

62   College of Occupational Therapists (2009) Applying for ethics approval for research Briefing note No. 82 June 2009 COT/BAOT

63   Lock, S.J. & Wells, F. (1999) *Fraud and Misconduct in Medical Research*, 2nd edn. British Medical Association, London.

64   McKeough, J. (1996) Intellectual property and scientific research. *Australian Journal of Physiotherapy*, **42**(3), 235–42.

65   Department of Health. *Research Governance Framework for England*, draft 2nd edn, 2003; www.doh.gov.uk/research/rd3/nhsandd/researchgovernance.htm

66   Seale, J.L. & Barnard, S. (1999) Ethical issues in therapy research. *British Journal of Occupational Therapy*, **62**(8), 371–5.

67   Department of Health (1997) *The New NHS: Modern – Dependable*. Command Paper 3807, HMSO, London.

27 Complementary Medicine

There is no doubt about the interest that now exists in complementary or alternative medicine (CAM). It is estimated that a third of the population have tried the remedies of complementary medicine or visited its practitioners.[1] The Health Education Authority has published an A–Z guide which covers 60 therapies.[2] The Prince of Wales set up a steering group chaired by Dr Manon Williams, his Assistant Private Secretary, to investigate complementary therapies. Four working groups were established which looked at:

- research and development
- education and training
- regulation
- delivery mechanisms.

It reported in 1997 and made extensive recommendations.[3] These included encouraging more research and the dissemination of its results; emphasising the common elements in the core curriculum of all healthcare workers in both orthodox and complementary and alternative medicine; establishing statutory self-regulatory bodies for those professions which could endanger patient safety; and identifying areas of conventional medicine and nursing which are not meeting patients' needs at present. It also recommended the establishment of an Independent Standards Commission for Complementary and Alternative Medicine. The Department of Health, in conjunction with the Centre of Complementary Health Studies at the University of Exeter, also carried out a survey of professional organisations of complementary and alternative medicine in the UK in 1997.[4] An information pack for primary care on complementary medicine has been sponsored by the Department of Health.[5] The pack was initiated after a survey found that one in four adults would use alternative therapies at some point in their lives. The Select Committee on Science and Technology of the House of Lords reported on complementary and alternative therapies in November 2000 and its recommendations are considered below.[6]

Occupational therapists (OTs) are affected by this development in two ways. The OT may be aware that patients are consulting practitioners in complementary medicine therapies and may be taking

Legal Aspects of Occupational Therapy, Third Edition By Bridgit Dimond
© 2010 Bridgit Dimond

medicines, or other treatment, for the same conditions for which the OT herself is giving advice. Conversely, some OTs are themselves undertaking training in a therapy regarded as complementary to conventional medicine. This chapter therefore discusses the definition of complementary therapy and looks at the following topics:

- Definition of complementary therapies
- The client involved in complementary therapy
- Disclosure to the OT
- Ignorance on the part of the OT
- The OT as complementary medicine therapist
- Agreement of employer
- Consent of the patient
- Defining standards
- House of Lords Select Committee
- Department of Health

Definition of complementary therapies

'Complementary is defined as: completing: together making up a whole, ... of medical treatment, therapies, etc ... (l. Complementum – com-, intens. and plere to fill).' (Pamphlet of the British Complementary Medicine Association (BCMA)).[7] Complementary medicine is thus seen to work in parallel with orthodox medicine. The BCMA therefore states that therapy groups which are represented by the BCMA should advise and encourage patients to see their doctor wherever appropriate.

Occupational therapy itself covers a wide range of therapies which on their own might be considered by some as complementary therapies. Thus art and music therapy was seen as an adjunct to traditional medicine and care of the patient. Art and music therapy has now, however, become subject to the registration provisions of the Health Professions Council. Horticultural therapy[8] can be a powerful tool in the work skills assessment, in a psychiatric setting and also useful in a variety of clinical settings.

Client involved in complementary therapy

Disclosure to the OT

When a patient is referred to an OT in the NHS, information relating to that person's care within the NHS would also be given. In addition, where there is a referral within social services, the person referring, whether general practitioner or social worker, would provide the OT with the information required in order to determine priorities and carry out care and treatment. Thus the OT should have basic information about the client in order to determine the care required by the client. In addition, the OT would usually have access to health records kept about the patient, to ensure that her care is compatible with other treatment the patient is receiving.

In contrast, where the patient is receiving treatment from a complementary therapist, there is usually no official way in which this information can be made known to the OT other than through the patient. The OT therefore relies on the openness of the patient in disclosing information which may be relevant to the treatment and care that the OT is offering.

Clearly, the importance of this communication between patient and OT will depend on the relevance of the complementary therapy to the treatment and care that the OT provides. Some therapies may have little effect, while others, such as acupuncture or homeopathy, may have a significant effect on the recommendations the OT may make.

Ignorance on the part of the OT

Does it matter that the OT has no knowledge of the complementary medicine therapy which the patient is undergoing? It may have an important effect and there could be circumstances where, had the OT been aware of certain information about the therapy, she may have advised the patient differently.

Situation

> An OT employed by social services is the key worker for a mentally ill person and is attempting to encourage his regular taking of medication by a programme of positive reinforcement. She is not aware that the client is receiving from outside the NHS a course of hypnotherapy designed to deal with the underlying mental health problems from which he is suffering.

In this situation, it would be of value to the client if the work of the OT (and other members of the multi-disciplinary team) was undertaken in the light of the methods, effects and intentions behind the hypnotherapy course, so that the OT's work complemented this rather than possibly conflicted with it. Unless, however, the OT has a basic understanding of the practice of hypnotherapy, she would be unable to work in parallel.

The OT as complementary medicine therapist

Agreement of employer

It is recognised that many OTs are considering the use of complementary therapies in the treatment of clients. Thus an article in the *British Journal of Occupational Therapy* considers the therapeutic potential of aromatherapy. In a more general article in 1995,[9] Kelly explores the many lessons which OTs can learn from traditional healers and emphasises the value of understanding and the acceptance of patients and their families in a cultural framework. T'ai chi is discussed as a useful skill in mental health.[10] 18 contributions from a variety of health professionals in the USA contribute to a book on the evidence for the efficacy of specific complementary therapies.[11]

If an OT obtains training in a complementary or alternative therapy, she should ensure that she obtains the agreement of the employer before she uses this skill as part of her practice as an OT. If she fails to do this and causes harm to the patient while using her complementary therapy skills, then her employer could argue that she was not acting in the course of employment when she caused the harm. The employer is therefore not vicariously liable and the OT must accept personal liability for the harm which has been caused. The employer would be entitled to check up on her qualifications and competence and the benefits which such treatments could bring to the patient and would have the right to refuse to permit the OT to use these additional skills as part of her practice in that employment. There are advantages if the employer and OT agree a protocol for the use of a specific complementary or alternative therapy comparable to the group patient direction protocol which is the basis for supply of medicines by non-doctors.

Situation

> An OT following training developed skills in acupuncture. One of her NHS patients was suffering from considerable pain and the OT offered to provide acupuncture to relieve the pain. It was arranged that the patient would come to the hospital at the end of the day's clinic. Unfortunately, the OT placed the needle in a nerve and caused permanent damage to the patient. The patient is claiming compensation.

If the NHS trust gave express or implied consent to this work by the OT then her work as an acupuncturist could be seen as being in the course of employment. In this case the NHS trust would be vicariously liable for the harm caused. On the other hand, it could be argued that if the NHS trust were unaware of the work as an acupuncturist then it could not be said that she was acting in the course of her employment and so the OT would have to accept personal liability. Whether or not working without authorisation could be defined in law as being in the course of employment depends upon the application of the House of Lords decision in the case of *Lister and others v Hesley Hall Ltd*[12] which is discussed in Chapter 10. The House of Lords ruled that the owners of a boarding school were vicariously liable for sexual abuse carried out by a warden.

It is also essential for the OT to obtain the consent of the employer if she intends to practise privately during working hours. In the case of case of *Watling v Gloucester County Council* (the full facts are discussed in Chapter 19), an OT was dismissed when he saw private patients for alternative therapy during working hours. His application for unfair dismissal failed.

Consent of the patient

It is also essential that the patient should give explicit consent before the OT is allowed to use any complementary therapies on him. The basic principles of obtaining consent apply (see Chapter 7) but, since a patient would not normally expect an OT to be providing complementary therapies, it is imperative that the OT gives full details of all that is involved and makes it absolutely clear that the patient is fully entitled to continue to receive the conventional treatment usually provided even though he or she refuses the complementary medicine treatment and care. It is preferable to obtain the consent in writing and to put in a leaflet the information which the patient should be told about the treatment. Form 1 or 3 of the forms recommended for use by the Department of Health[13] could be adapted for this purpose.

Westland notes in her articles on massage[14] that:

permission should always be sought before massaging a client and the practitioner should observe for indicators of inconsistency between agreeing verbally to be massaged and non-verbally saying "no" to the touch. These indicators would include breathing more rapidly, breath holding and tensing parts of the body.

Clearly in such a situation, the practitioner should verify that the client is giving a voluntary and real consent.

Defining standards

One of the difficulties of some complementary therapies is that there may not be any clear definition as to what is the expected standard of care. If harm were to occur, to succeed in a claim for compensation the patient would have to establish that the therapist failed to use the reasonable standard of care which the patient was entitled to expect. This may not be easy to prove. A case illustrating the difficulties of determining the standard of care is shown below.

Case: standard of care of a complementary therapist[15]

S, who was suffering from a skin condition, consulted a practitioner of traditional Chinese herbal medicine. After taking nine doses of the herbal remedy, S became ill and later died of acute liver failure, which was attributable to a rare and unpredictable reaction to the remedy. His widow brought proceedings against the practitioner, but failed. The High Court held that on the evidence before it the actions of the defendant had been consistent with the standard of care appropriate to traditional Chinese herbal medicine in accordance with established requirements.

In a recent case in July 2008 there was no agreement on the standard which should have been applied and the claimant won an out of court settlement. Mrs Page, 52 years, won more than £800,000 after she claimed that a radical detox diet left her brain-damaged and epileptic. She said that she had been told to drink four extra pints of water a day and reduce her salt intake to prevent fluid retention and reduce weight.[16] The nutritional therapist and life coach denied any fault and the claim was settled by her insurance company, without any admission of liability. Solicitors for the defendant stated that all allegations of substandard practice were denied and the settlement was less than half the amount claimed.

House of Lords Select Committee

The House of Lords Select Committee on Science and Technology held an inquiry into complementary medicine. It reported[17] in November 2000 and recommended that there should be regulation of complementary and alternative medicines and there should be further research to evaluate their effectiveness. It divided such therapies into three groups:

- Professionally organised therapies, where there is some scientific evidence of their success, though seldom of the highest quality, and there are recognised systems for treatment and training of practitioners. This group includes acupuncture, chiropractic, herbal medicine, homeopathy and osteopathy.
- Complementary medicines, where evidence that they work is generally lacking but which are used as an adjunct rather than a replacement for conventional therapies, so that lack of evidence may not matter so much. Included in this group are the Alexander Technique, aromatherapy, nutritional medicine, hypnotherapy and Bach and other flower remedies.
- Techniques that offer diagnosis as well as treatment, but for which scientific evidence is almost completely lacking. This group cannot be supported and includes naturopathy, crystal therapy, kinesiology, radionics, dowsing and iridology.

The Select Committee of the House of Lords considered that some remedies such as acupuncture and aromatherapy should be available on the NHS, and NHS patients should have wider access to osteopathy and chiropractics. The implementation of these recommendations may lead to fundamental changes in how complementary and alternative therapies are viewed in relation to orthodox medicine and within the NHS.

Department of Health developments

Following the House of Lords report, several working parties were set up by the Department of Health. An acupuncture regulatory working group looked at the necessary developments to secure statutory registration of acupuncturists. Information is available on its meetings and activities.[18] A similar group was set up to progress state registration for herbal medicine practitioners.[19] The Department of Health published a strategy to develop research capacity in complementary and alternative medicine[20] and invited Higher Education Institutions (HEIs) to register their interest in hosting research into this field.[21] The value of complementary and alternative medicine is increasingly likely to feature as a field of inquiry into general research into specific conditions: thus a study was carried out on the use of complementary and alternative therapies among people undergoing cancer treatment,[22] and a report of the working group looking at chronic fatigue syndrome (CFS/ME) considered patients' views on the use of complementary and alternative medicines (CAM) and their value in the management of the illness. Provisions for the registration by the HPC of new health professional groups is considered in Chapter 3.

Following reports by working groups on herbalism and acupuncture in March 2004 the Department of Health put forward proposals for the establishment of a Complementary and Alternative Medicine Council. This would have similar powers to the GMC or NMC and would assess qualifications in herbal medicine and acupuncture; possession of a registration certificate would be required to practise in these fields. There is every likelihood that if research evidence establishes that a complementary therapy is effective, then applications will be made to the new Complementary and Natural Healthcare Council for that therapy to receive recognition by way of state registration.

Complementary and Natural Healthcare Council (CNHC)

The Prince's Foundation for Integrated Health set up a Federal Working Group which spent twelve months considering the formation of a new Council. Its report was published in February 2008.[23] It recommended developing a federal structure for the voluntary self-regulation of complementary healthcare professions ie a single regulatory body rather than a series of regulators for each complementary healthcare profession. The new body is called the Complementary and Natural Healthcare Council and is made up of four elements:

- Federal Regulatory Council
- Profession Specific Boards
- Functional Boards
- Practice Advisory Panel

In May 2009 the CHNC Board agreed to amalgamate the work of the Registration and Education & Standards Committee.

CNHC has four main functions:

- to establish and maintain a voluntary register of complementary healthcare practitioners in the UK who meet our standards of competence and practice
- to make the Register of practitioners available to the general public and to educate them about the CNHC quality mark as a quality standard
- to operate a robust process for handling complaints about registered practitioners
- to work with professional bodies in the complementary healthcare field to further develop and improve standards of professional practice

The CNHC describes itself as the national voluntary regulator for complementary healthcare practitioners. The Members of the Council and the functional boards are lay people, appointed independently; each Profession Specific Board (one for each profession) has a lay Chair and four registrants from the appropriate profession. Each Profession Specific Board select one of its practitioner members to sit on the Practice Advisory Panel which provides a pool of expertise to support the Council. The report recommended robust procedures for handling complaints and fitness to practise issues, along with a code of conduct and ethics based on the code used by the Health Professions Council. The complementary healthcare professions that are, or have been, part of the Foundation for Integrated Health's regulation programme have developed, or are developing, the competencies necessary for entry to the Register. Full public and professional liability insurance will be mandatory, as will continuing professional development. The Federal Working Group has suggested that an independent, external organisation be invited to review the work of the Complementary and Natural Healthcare Council from time to time, to ensure that it remains fit for purpose and that it meets the needs of all who have an interest in its work. The Department of Health has provided start-up funding but the aim is for the Complementary and Natural Healthcare Council to be financed solely by registration fees. The Department of Health will also ensure that the principles underpinning professional regulation as set out in its White Paper Trust, Assurance and Safety[24] are implemented (see Chapter 3). The Council's register was in place in January 2009 with massage therapy and nutritional therapy, Aromatherapy was added in May 2009 and over the next year further therapies including Alexander technique; Bowen technique; Cranial therapy; Homeopathy; Naturopathy; Reflexology; Reiki; Shiatsu; and Yoga therapy will be included on the register.

To be eligible for registration, a practitioner must have undertaken a programme of education and training which meets, as a minimum, the National Occupational Standards for that profession/discipline or achieved competency to the same level by means of relevant experience and assessment. The Register can be checked on the CNHC's website.[25]

The overall intention is that the Council will provide enhanced consumer confidence and safety through a credible, robust and professional voluntary regulatory structure for the practice of complementary healthcare in the UK.

The CNHC's key objectives in its first year were:

- to register at least 10,000 complementary healthcare practitioners around the UK
- to achieve recognition of the the CNHC quality mark by healthcare practitioners and commissioners as the quality benchmark for NHS referrals
- to achieve recognition of the CNHC quality mark by private healthcare companies as the quality benchmark for re-imbursement purposes
- to have the CNHC quality mark recognised as a gateway to wider advertising of practitioners' services in national listings such as Yellow Pages and Thomsons
- to build awareness amongst the general public of the CNHC quality mark as a symbol of quality service

The CNHC describes its key function as follows:

> Our key function is to enhance **public protection**, by setting standards for registration with CNHC. We anticipate that obtaining the CNHC "quality mark" will swiftly be recognised as the hallmark of quality for the sector. Over time, the general public and those who commission the services of complementary healthcare practitioners will be able to choose with confidence, by looking for the CNHC quality mark.

Registrants are able to make use of the CNHC logo next to their own logo on headed paper or business cards. They will also be able to put on display a certificate, incorporating the CNHC quality mark which provides an independent indications of quality to those wishing to use complementary and natural health services. The quality mark can also be used on websites, promotional literature and elsewhere as confirmation to the public that the CNHC registrant meets the standards set by the CNHC.

> By using the CNHC quality mark you are demonstrating to members of the general public and other healthcare providers that you conform to national standards of practice in your work.

The NHS spends £50 million a year on therapies which will come under the Council. It was reported that NHS homoeopathy, which will come under the Council, is in sharp decline with only 37% of Trusts offering homoeopathic treatment.[26]

A petition to the Government criticised the fact that CNHC registrants would use the certificate provided by the CNHC to imply efficacy and safety, yet the CNHC's approval of the therapy did not involve any actual evidence of efficacy and safety. The Government responsed to this petition by stating that

> The CNHC does not promote the efficacy of disciplines practised by its registrants. The aim of the CNHC is protection of the public. Registration means that the practitioner has met certain entry standards (in terms of having an accredited qualification or relevant experience) and that they subscribe to a set of professional standards. The public will have the reassurance that the practitioner they choose meets these standards and will be subject to fitness to practise procedures should they behave inappropriately.
>
> Regulation, whether statutory or voluntary, is about protecting the public. For this reason, the Government fully supports the work of the CNHC. If patients choose to use complementary or alternative therapy, the Government's advice is to choose a practitioner registered with a reputable voluntary registration body such as the CNHC.

A consultation on the Report to Ministers from the DH Steering Group on the Statutory Regulation of Practitioners of Acupuncture, Herbal Medicine, Traditional Chinese Medicine and Other Traditional Medicine Systems Practised in the UK ended on 2 November 2009.

Conclusions

There is every likelihood that the interest and demand for CAM will continue to grow and will be accompanied by a requirement that therapies should be provided within the NHS. This is already occurring as GPs and primary care trusts make agreements to buy such therapies for their patients. More and more OTs are likely to acquire double qualifications and to be caring for clients who are recipients of alternative therapies. The greater the use by and training of OTs in additional therapies, the more likely they are to become concerned at the content and meaning of occupational therapy in itself (see discussion in Chapter 1). More detailed information on law and complementary medicine can be found in the author's book.[27] A turning point for many complementary and alternative therapies has now arrived with the establishment of the Complementary and Natural Healthcare Council and the emphasis on research-based effective treatments. Those therapists whose treatments which are not proven to be effective on the basis of research evidence will not be registered by Council nor will they obtain funding from the NHS. Further information on complementary therapies can be obtained from the website of the Complementary Healthcare Information Service[28] and from the CNHC.[29]

   Questions and exercises

1   You have decided that you would like to undertake a training in aromatherapy and eventually use it as part of your practice as an OT. What actions would you take to ensure that your plans are compatible with your role as an OT?

2   You are visiting a patient in the community and become concerned that she appears to be paying a lot of money to a psychotherapist and her condition does not seem to be improving – in fact you consider that it is deteriorating. What action, if any, would you take?

3   Do you consider that all complementary therapies that so wished, should be permitted to have registered status under the Health Professions Council or the Complementary and Natural Healthcare Council ? (Refer also to Chapter 3.) If not, what criteria would you lay down for a profession to receive registered status?

References

1   Laurance, J. (1996) 'Alternative health: An honest alternative or just magic?' *The Times*, 5 February, p. 11.
2   Health Education Authority (2006) *A-Z guide on complementary therapies* available on the website: www.internethealthlibrary.com.
3   *Integrated Healthcare: A Way Forward for the Next Five Years*. Foundation for Integrated Medicine, 1997.
4   www.doh.gov.uk/public/altmed.htm
5   Complementary Medicine, Information Pack for Primary Care. www.doh.gov.uk
6   House of Lords Select Committee on Science and Technology, 6th Report, *Complementary and Alternative Medicine*, 21 November 2000, Session 1999–2000.
7   Further information can be obtained from the BCMA, Exmoor Street, London W10 6DZ.
8   Goodban, A. & Goodban, D. (1990) Horticultural therapy: A growing concern, Parts 1 and 2. *British Journal of Occupational Therapy*, **53**(10), 425–9, (11), 468–70.
9   Kelly, L. (1995) What occupational therapists can learn from traditional healers. *British Journal of Occupational Therapy*, **58**(3), 111–14.
10 Amhed Odusanya (2003) T'ai chi for mental health. *Occupational Therapy News*, **11**(5), 30.
11 Davis Carol M ed.(2004) Complementary Therapies in rehabilitation: Evidence for efficacy in therapy, prevention and wellness Slack Incorporated.
12 *Lister and others v Hesley Hall Ltd* Times Law Reports, 10 May 2001, HL; [2001] 2 WLR 1311.
13 Department of Health (2001) *Good Practice in Consent Implementation Guide*. DoH, London.
14 Westland, G. (1993) Massage as a therapeutic tool. *British Journal of Occupational Therapy*, **56**(4), 129–34, (5), 177–80.
15 *Shakoor (Administratix of the Estate of Shakoor (Deceased)) v Situ* (T/A Eternal Health Co), The Independent, 25 May 2000.
16 Alexi Mostrous £800,000 for brain injury 'caused by high-fluid diet' The Times 23 July 2008 page 16.
17 House of Lords Select Committee on Science and Technology, 6th Report, *Complementary and Alternative Medicine*, 21 November 2000, Session 1999–2000.
18 www.doh.gov.uk/acupuncturerwg/index.htm
19 www.doh.gov.uk/herbalmedicinerwg/tor.htm
20 Pighills, A. & Bailey, C. (2002) Developing Research Capacity in Complementary and Alternative Medicine: A strategy for Action. DoH, London.
21 www.doh.gov.uk/research/rdl/cam.htm
22 www.doh.gov.uk/research/rd3/nhsandd/cam/28_02.htm
23 The Prince's Foundation for Integrated Health A Federal Approach to Professionally-Led Voluntary Regulation for Complementary Healthcare: A plan for Action 2008.
24 Department of Health (2007) White Paper 'Trust, Assurance and Safety: the Regulation of Health Professionals in the 21st Century Cmnd 7013.
25 www.cnhc.org.uk
26 David Rose NHS homoeopathy in sharp decline The Times 30 January 2008.
27 Dimond, B. (1998) *Legal Aspects of Complementary Therapy Practice*. Churchill Livingstone, London.
28 www.chisuk.org.uk
29 www.cnhc.org.uk

28 Independent Practice

An increasing number of occupational therapists (OTs) are deciding to work as self-employed independent contractors and there is every likelihood that this number will grow as NHS trusts, primary care trusts, other health service bodies, social services authorities and groups such as charitable organisations and independent healthcare providers have the capacity to contract with self-employed individuals for services.

The following topics are covered in this chapter:

- Variety of contracts and work
- Running a business
- Accountability and the independent practitioner
- Documentation
- Essential contract law
- Contract law and the tort of negligence contrasted
- The independent practitioner and health and safety

- Professional issues
- Independent practice and alternative statutory provision
- Compensation claims – expert witness and witness of fact
- Complaints and unprofessional conduct by others
- Part-time independent practice

Variety of contracts and work

Figure 28.1 shows some of the different contracting partners for the OT who works as an independent contractor. In 1989 the College of Occupational Therapists (COT) established a Private Practice Directory[1] and published standards and policies and proceedings for OTs in private practice.[2] These standards were revised in November 1994[3] and a further guidance has been provided by the OTs

Figure 28.1 Contracts and the independent practitioner.

- with private patients
- with NHS trusts and primary care trusts
- with health authorities
- with general practitioners
- with private hospitals
- with agencies
- with local authorities
- with charities
- with solicitors
- with residential and nursing homes

in Independent Practice Specialist Group. It published a Code of Practice for OTs in Independent Practice in 2005 which was revised in 2008. This covers the setting up in business and maintaining an ethical business practice.[4] Other publications by the COT include research and development strategic vision and action plan for OTs in Independent Practice in 2004 which identified six objectives to be achieved in the following years, based on the COT's own research and development strategic vision and action plan published in 2001. The COT has published a briefing note on managing a budget[5] which may be helpful to those in private practice.

Andreas Diamantis explored the assessment methods used by OTs working with children in Independent Practice in the UK in a MSc thesis.[6]

The COT identified six settings where an OT may undertake private practice:

- setting up a practice (sole trader, partnership or company)
- becoming an employee or partner in an established practice
- being employed as a consultant
- working under contract (negotiated for work limited by type or time)
- undertaking litigation work
- working in private residential homes, nursing homes, hospitals, hospices, etc.

Legal issues for the self-employed

There are significant legal implications in becoming a self-employed practitioner. The most obvious one is that self-employed professionals do not have an employer who will be vicariously liable for their actions and therefore pay out compensation arising from their negligence. Instead, as self-employed, independent practitioners who offer a contract for services with others, they are personally responsible for their own negligence and also vicariously liable for any harm resulting from the negligence or other wrongful acts of their employees (if any) which are committed in the course of employment. Some of the differences are shown in Figure 28.2.

The relationship between the independent contractor and the contracting party is not a contract of employment but a contract for services. All the benefits which the employment legislation gives to employees (see Chapter 19), such as time off work for specific purposes, protection against unfair dismissal and redundancy and guaranteed payments, are not there for the self-employed.

Since self-employed persons have to pay personally any compensation arising out of their negligence, they have to have insurance cover in respect of public liability and for all the benefits that they would receive if they had employee status, such as cover for sickness. In addition, they cannot look to an employer for protection in relation to health and safety and should take out their own personal accident cover. As employers themselves they must ensure that they recognise the employment rights of their employees, have relevant insurance cover, and also provide all reasonable care to protect their employees' health and safety.

Figure 28.2   Legal issues and the self-employed practitioner.

*Contract for Services **not** Contract of Employment*

- No vicarious liability (except as regards their own employees)
- No employee rights (except for those they employ)
- No indemnity *by* another
- Personal liability for health and safety of self and others
- Liability for breach of contract

Running a business

The COT has published standards for OTs in independent practice.[7] These cover standards for Good Business Practice, Marketing and Advertising, Office Procedures and Administration and Accounts. In addition, Occupational Therapists in Private Practice has published a business start-up pack.[8] OTs in Independent Practice should also refer to the Code of Business Practice published by the COT in 2005. The Code covers the following topics:

- The Practitioner and her professional requirements
- Giving your business an identity
- Ensuring a robust business and protecting against risk
- Providing a quality service
- Promoting your business honestly

   OTs in private practice are also subject to the professional standards set by the COT for all OTs. The COT has published a briefing note on writing a business case which OTs in private practice should find of assistance.[9]

   In running a business OTs should seek professional help on the areas shown in Figure 28.3.

   It is essential that the practitioner takes legal advice before deciding on the type of arrangement she should have if working with another person or persons. For example, it may seem preferable to set up a partnership so that the profits and overheads can be shared. However, each partner would be responsible for the debts of the partnership even if she has not personally incurred them.

Accountability and the independent practitioner

Figure 28.4 illustrates the arenas of accountability for independent practitioners. For the most part these are similar to those of the professional who works as an employee. However, instead of being accountable to an employer, the independent practitioner has a contract of services with a purchaser (see Figures 28.1 and 28.2). If there is a breach of contract, the referral is not to the employment tribunal but to the civil courts.

Documentation

It should be obvious from the great potential for different conflicts which can arise in independent practice that the documentation which the independent practitioner keeps is extremely important

Figure 28.3   The independent practitioner and business law.

- HM Revenue and Customs/VAT
- National Insurance
  - self
  - others
- Insurance and indemnity
  - Personal accident cover
- Health and Safety regulations
- Contracts for supplies/services
- Training and development
- Employment law
- Data Protection
- Pensions and sickness
- Formation of business
  - Type of business
    sole trader
    partnership
    limited company
    co-operative

- Name
- Protection
  patents
  registered designs
- Premises
  planning permission
  building regulations
  the lease
  special trades
- Trading laws
  Sale of goods and services
  Trade Descriptions Act
  Unfair Contract Terms Act
- Taxation and starting up
  capital allowances
  deciding on tax year

Figure 28.4   Accountability and the independent practitioner.

To the public: criminal law
To the patient: civil law of negligence and contract law
To the purchaser: civil law: contract for services
To the profession: conduct and competence committee of the Health Professions Council

– not only in establishing the care that is given to the patient and the terms on which it is to be given in the event of any referral or dispute, but also in relation to the management of a small business. She needs to ensure that she is able to respond to the many statutory requests for information about her practice from the HM Revenue and Customs as well as respond to any queries from statutory health and social services providers. The COT guidelines, on page 5, emphasise the importance of keeping concise factual records and reports (see also Chapter 12). The self-employed practitioner also needs to ensure that she is registered with the Information Commissioner in respect of holding confidential personal information under the Data Protection Act 1998 (see Chapter 8).

Essential contract law

The independent practitioner must have a good understanding of the law of contract. The essential features of contract law are shown in Figure 28.5 and some are also touched on in Chapter 19.

Figure 28.5   Elements of contract law.

Formation: invitation to treat
offer and acceptance

Contents: fundamental terms
implied and express terms

Performance

Breach: remedies for breach
right of election

Termination: by performance
by breach
by agreement
by notice
by frustration

Formation of contract

There may often be a lengthy period of negotiation before a contract is formed. There may for example be an opening 'invitation to treat' by the one party that is on quite different terms to those eventually arrived at. The contract is reached when one party can be said to have made an offer (either in response to the invitation to treat or as a 'counter offer') and the other party accepts that offer. If an offer is made and the other party responds by offering alternative conditions, this is a counter offer which, if accepted by the other party, constitutes the agreement and therefore the contract. The contract may not be entirely in writing. It may be partly in writing and partly by word of mouth. If, following a dispute, one party argues that additional terms discussed during negotiations became part of the contract and are therefore binding, it is a question of interpretation as to what was said and any other evidence to establish what were the agreed terms of the contract.

The three essential elements to make a contract binding are:

1. An agreement
2. Consideration
3. An intention to create legal relations.

Consideration need not necessarily be payment of money in return for the performance of the agreement by the other side. It could be a benefit in kind or it could be an agreement releasing the other from something which they had a duty to do. It need not necessarily equate with what the other is prepared to do. For example, an OT who has an independent practice may agree that, because a client is extremely short of funds but runs an aromatherapy clinic, she will forego any payment on the understanding that she will be given two sessions of aromatherapy. On that basis the agreement is made and she provides the occupational therapy. If the aromatherapist client then goes back on that agreement, she is in breach of contract. The OT has the right to seek damages for breach of contract in the civil courts. In practice she may prefer not to attract the publicity which such an action would bring.

It is essential that the OT in private practice agrees a fee and the likely number of sessions before the course of treatment commences. It is also extremely important for this agreement to be recorded in writing and that the client is aware of the services which could be obtained for free from the NHS.

In commercial contracts the intention to create legal relations would normally be presumed. In domestic matters, there is a presumption that there is no such intention. Where a practitioner is carrying out independent work it is essential for her to make it absolutely clear that it is the intention to create a binding agreement, in order to be able to enforce the contract through the courts.

Where possible the independent practitioner should ensure that all the terms of the contract are put in writing to protect herself in the event of a dispute.

Breach of contract

If it is claimed that one party is in fundamental breach of the contract, then the innocent party has the right of election. She can either elect to treat the contract as at an end and seek damages, i.e. compensation for breach of contract, or she can elect to see the contract as continuing but seek compensation for the loss to her (financial or otherwise) of it being less than she had bargained for. It is important that the innocent party makes it clear which she chooses; if she delays and carries on regarding the contract as subsisting, it could be said that by her conduct she has treated the contract as continuing and has therefore lost the right of election.

Termination of contract

It is advisable to consider at the beginning of the contract how it should end. Is it for a specific number of treatments? Is it for a certain length of time? Is it for a specified number of weeks after hospital discharge? Can it be ended on notice by one party to the other? How long should that notice be?

In the absence of notice provisions in an employment contract, the courts will imply a reasonable notice provision into the contract and there are statutory minimum periods. However, these statutory minimum periods do not exist for contracts for services and it would be more difficult to determine what is reasonable notice.

Frustration

Frustration of the contract arises when an event takes place which was outside the contemplation of the parties when the contract was made.

Situation

An OT agreed to provide occupational therapy services to a client in the community. Her main task was to carry out an assessment of the equipment and support that the client would need to live on her own. She had almost completely carried out this task and compiled a suggested list of equipment and suppliers when the client informed her that her niece was coming to live with her and she would not therefore require any aids and help from the OT. The OT claimed the money due to her for the work she had already done. The client refused to pay on the grounds that she no longer required help.

In this case the client or OT could argue that the contract had been frustrated by the unforeseen event of the niece's arrival. However, the OT should be able to obtain reimbursement for the work she had already undertaken. As a result of the Law Reform (Frustrated Contracts) Act 1943, generally all sums paid before the contract was frustrated are repayable and any money due to be paid but not paid before frustration ceases to be payable. However, the court will look to the justice of the situation and work done will be paid for. This Act does not apply where the contract itself makes provision for any frustrating event and it would therefore be possible for the independent practitioner to include in the agreement a provision defining what rights would exist were a specified frustrating event to occur.

If the client refuses to pay

Payment is the passing of consideration from the one party to the contract to the other in return for the provision of some service. Time of payment is not normally a fundamental term unless the contract clearly makes it so. It is therefore advisable for the professional to include in the contract a term in relation to when the fee should be paid – in advance, in instalments at each session, after each session, monthly, etc. When she is negotiating with a health service body or NHS trust there might not be much choice for her, but it is essential that she should establish this, so it is clear when there has been a breach of contract and when she is entitled to commence action for recovery.

The guidelines issued by the COT on private practice emphasise that fees should be discussed prior to the delivery of any form of occupational therapy and, whenever possible, an estimate of the planned number of sessions and costs should be given. The guidelines identify a wide range of fees including fees for:

- consultation/assessment
- treatment
- continuing care
- domiciliary or clinic-based sessions
- sessional rates as a consultant
- a specific commission
- litigation work.

The guidelines also highlight the need to identify any VAT payable, and the costs incurred for professional development, travelling and out of pocket expenses. Taxation must also be provided for.

Situation

An OT contracted with an NHS trust for occupational therapy services to be provided for four sessions a week on the basis that payment would be made every month in arrears on completion and submission of a return certified by the unit manager. The OT duly performed the services and submitted the return but several months later was still without payment. Should she cease to work?

Failure to pay could be regarded as breach of a fundamental clause of the contract and looking back at the section on breach of contract, it will be recalled that the innocent party therefore has the right of election, i.e. to decide whether to recognise the contract as continuing or see it ended by the breach of contract. The occupational therapist could therefore see the contract as at an end and sue for the outstanding payment and damages for the breach of contract. Alternatively, if there is every likelihood that she would eventually be paid, she might well prefer to elect to see the contract as continuing and continue to perform her sessions, meanwhile chasing for the outstanding payments.

Should she eventually be forced into taking legal action she could, depending on the amount outstanding, take the case to the small claims court (up to £5000), to the County Court (up to £50 000) or to the High Court (over £50 000). The new procedures for civil cases are considered in Chapter 13. With the contract in writing and evidence of the sessions she has carried out, the OT should quickly and easily obtain judgment for her payments with no valid defence being available against her. However, if she were suing a private individual rather than an organisation, the practicalities of getting the money from someone who may have no assets and no job is another matter.

Contract law and the tort of negligence contrasted

It may be bewildering to non-lawyers that there are two overlapping duties: the duty owed to a client under the law of negligence and the duty owed to a client under the law of contract. However, this is the legal situation and an aggrieved client who had suffered harm as a result of the activities of the independent practitioner could sue for both breach of contract and breach of the duty of care at common law. The duties are not identical, since the former derives from the contract which has been agreed between client and practitioner, including the implied terms, and the latter is set by common law. It has been stated by the Court of Appeal that, where a duty of care in tort arose between the parties to a contract, wider obligations could be imposed by that duty than those arising as implied terms under the contract.[10]

The independent practitioner and health and safety

While there is no employer responsible for the self-employed practitioner, she may be an employer herself and therefore have responsibilities to her employees. The duty to take reasonable care of the health and safety of the employee exists whether the employee is full or part-time. The self-employed practitioner also has a duty under the health and safety legislation to take care of the safety of others who may be affected by her work, and if she operates from premises which clients attend she could be liable as 'occupier' if harm befalls them as a result of a foreseeable hazard (see Chapter 11). The Management of Health and Safety at Work Regulations 1999 refer specifically to the self-employed in Regulation 3(2), as shown in Figure 28.6.

Health and safety violence and self-defence

Situation

A private practitioner who has her own premises which clients attend, was carrying out a session when a client became extremely violent and threatening. The professional was working on her own and there was no-one who could come to her aid.

In such a situation she is entitled to use reasonable force in self-defence. What is reasonable depends on the circumstances, the danger she is in and the amount of violence she faces, the nature of the

Figure 28.6   Regulation 3(2) and (3) – the self-employed.

(2)   Every self-employed person shall make a suitable and sufficient assessment of—
    (a)   the risks to his own health and safety to which he is exposed whilst he is at work; and
    (b)   the risks to the health and safety of persons not in his employment arising out of or in connection with the conduct by him of his undertaking,

for the purpose of identifying the measures he needs to take to comply with the requirements and prohibitions imposed upon him by or under the relevant statutory provisions.

(3)   Any assessment such as is referred to in paragraph (1) [employers] or (2) shall be reviewed by the employer or the self-employed person who made it if—
    (a)   there is reason to suspect that it is no longer valid; or
    (b)   there has been a significant change in the matters to which it relates;

and where as a result of any such review changes to an assessment are required, the employer or self-employed person concerned shall make them.

training she has received, her own size and that of her assailant, and the type of weapons to hand. Where grievous bodily harm is feared, more force might be justified. Her actions should, however, always be defensive not aggressive.

Professional issues

Matters of health and safety for clients or for the professional herself can also be bound up with acting in a duly professional manner.

Situation

An OT works as a self-employed practitioner and has a caseload of clients for whom she provides services. One client is extremely demanding and is very anxious to obtain a chair-lift from the social services. The OT forms the view that a lift is neither appropriate nor practicable and in fact, given the client's particular circumstances, could be dangerous. The OT is told by the client that unless she is prepared to support her claim their contract for services will be ended. What should the OT do?

The answer should be clear: she must abide by her professional standards and not be demand-led by the client into recommending equipment which is entirely unsuitable. The difference between the employee status and the self-employed status is, however, apparent. If employees refuse to agree with clients on professional grounds, their employment should not be endangered. If it is the employer who is putting pressure on them to act unprofessionally, then provided they have the continuous service requirement, they could claim constructive dismissal before the employment tribunal. However, self-employed professionals have no such protection. If they keep to their professional standards they might lose that client and suffer economically. However, there is no alternative if they wish to remain as registered professionals.

Independent practice and alternative statutory provision

It is essential (and this is identified in the COT guidelines) that, when discussing the costs of treatment and equipment, the independent practitioner should make it clear what is available on the NHS so that clients do not assume that they have no option other than to pay privately for the care and equipment. Page 7 of the COT guidelines, paragraph 2, on statutory services states that:

> Where the service being offered by a private practitioner is subject to statutory provision, consumers should be informed of their rights under statute, so that the option to pay for services is taken with full knowledge of the fact that these services may be available free of charge through the NHS or local authority. This is particularly relevant in the provision of daily living equipment. It also applies to recommendations for adaptations where local authorities have budgets or grants available for these services.

Compensation claims – expert witness and witness of fact

An increasing part of the practitioner's work is the provision of expert reports for those who have been involved in litigation and are seeking compensation. The practitioner might be asked by the plaintiff's solicitor or the defendant's solicitor for an expert report on the situation and the prognosis in order to assess the amount of compensation (known as quantum). This, and the need to give the accurate picture even if this does not 'help' the client's case, are considered in Chapter 13 on giving evidence in court. The independent practitioner specialist section of the COT has prepared standards for practice for expert witnesses[11] which is also useful for employed OTs and is discussed in Chapter 13.

Complaints and unprofessional conduct by others

Because the independent practitioner often works on her own, she is more vulnerable in pointing out low standards of care provided by other professionals. She lacks a management hierarchy and does not belong to a large organisation (other than her own professional association) to be able to take action effectively without herself becoming a scapegoat or losing out financially.

Situation

> An OT provides services at a residential care home. She is horrified to discover that the residents have a very low standard of care. There appear to be only two sessions a week when they receive any occupational activities and for the most part they sit around the walls of the room with very little to do despite the fact that many of them have active minds and are capable of undertaking a variety of activities. She tried to point this out discreetly to the manager, but unfortunately the manager reacts badly at the implied criticism, suggests she is merely touting for more sessions and says the funds do not exist for more activities to be undertaken and the staff are too busy as it is.

It may be possible for the OT to suggest to the manager ways in which the OT herself could teach the care assistants simple activities that they could carry out with the residents to make use of their physical and mental capabilities. If she were able to do this within the hours she is already working, this would not necessarily lead to any additional expenditure. However, if the manager is adamant that no action will be taken, the OT may consider it necessary to take things further in order to improve the quality of life of the residents.

There are several options open to the OT but all are likely to end her association with the home:

- She could report the situation to the owners or senior management.
- If a registered health professional were at fault this could be reported to the registration body (e.g. NMC, HPC or GMC).
- She could complain to the Care Quality Commission (which replaced the Commission for Social Care Inspection (CSCI) and the Commission for Healthcare Audit and Inspection (CHAI) in April 2009).
- She could also report the situation to the contract department of the LA which funded places in the home for clients (or of the primary care trust if the place was funded by the NHS).
- In extremely serious cases where it would appear that criminal activities are taking place, she could report the situation to the police.

Unfortunately, none of these courses of action are likely to ensure that her work with the home will continue.

What if the unsound or unsafe practice she witnesses, is the conduct of another professional?

Situation

An OT visits an older person who lives alone and is always profusely grateful for the help and attention she receives. She notices that on the dresser the client keeps a few notes of money. She questions her about the advisability of keeping money in the house and on the dresser. The client explains that she always gives the ambulance driver £5 after each visit to the day hospital. The OT fears that the ambulance man might be exploiting the old lady. What action, if any, should she take?

The OT would first have to verify the facts: is there in fact an ambulance service provided free for the clients? If this were so, then one course would be to explain to the client that the service provided by the ambulance is free and no payment need be made. If the client says that the ambulance men expect it, what does the OT do then? One possibility is for her to take up the complaint with the director of the ambulance service. This would be preferable to writing an anonymous letter or complaining indirectly. However, she may find that she becomes ostracised as a result.

It is essential, however, that she takes appropriate action and does not ignore the dangers to the client. She has a duty of care to the client and if harm were eventually to befall the client and it were ascertained that a professional had been aware of the situation but had taken no action, she could face professional misconduct proceedings.

Part-time independent practice

Some OTs might try to develop an independent practice as well as being employed part-time. Some OTs, for example, may develop skills in complementary therapies and undertake these on an independent basis (see Chapter 27). In such a situation they must ensure that they do not exploit their employed situation to increase their independent practice, by taking clients away from their employer. This would be regarded as a breach of the implied term of loyalty to their employer in their contract of employment (see Chapter 19). Similarly, they should keep their independent practice entirely separate from their employment and not attempt to see private clients in working hours without the express consent of their employer, nor should they use any of the employer's facilities for their private work (e.g. telephones, equipment, secretarial services or stationery). In the case of *Watling v*

Gloucestershire County Council (see Chapter 19 for the full facts) Mr Watling, an OT employed by the County Council, was dismissed since he continued to see private clients during his working hours, and the dismissal was held to be fair.

College of Occupational Therapy and Private Practice

The College of OT provides considerable support and information for those working in private practice, whether full or part time. The COT specialist section for independent practice (COTSS-IP) provides guidance for members in private practice including briefing notes on copyright (101), VAT (89), Professional indemnity insurance (66), writing a business case (73) OTs as facilitators of telecare (83) and briefings on medico-legal issues from its medical-legal forum. COTSS-IP has set up a free telephone enquiry line for those seeking to contact independent practitioners. The service has been evaluated to assess who uses it, why and how.[12]

Conclusion

Not everyone is content with healthcare developments outside the NHS. There may, for example, be some general practitioners and primary care trusts who refuse to contract with independent practitioners. What action can the independent practitioners take? The primary care trusts have the statutory freedom to obtain services from those providers that they consider would be best for their patients. They cannot be forced to go outside the NHS nor can they be forced to stay within it. If a GP practice refuses to use the services of the independent sector there is no action which can be taken other than to hope that, in terms of quality and price, the independent service will eventually be seen to offer services of equal or superior standing to those within the NHS. As with employed OTs, it is vital that research should take place in relation to independent practice. For example a large research project investigating the assessment practices of paediatric occupational therapists in independent practice in the UK is showing valuable results.[13] There is likely to be an increase in the numbers self-employed OTs offering their services in the community and to primary care and hospital trusts. To move outside employed status is often a courageous step and the OT who is considering such a step should seek professional advice and take note of the topics briefly discussed in this chapter. Reference should be made to general law books (see the further reading list) and to the publications recommended by the COT.

   Questions and exercises

1   Identify the differences in law between the situation of the OT in independent practice and the employed occupational therapist.
2   A colleague has suggested that there may be considerable advantages in the OTs withdrawing from employed status within the NHS and setting up a consortium of independent practitioners to sell their services to the NHS trusts and primary care trusts. Draw up a list of benefits and weaknesses of this suggestion.
3   An OT in independent practice has two sessions at a independent nursing home. She is concerned at the low standards of patient care. What action could she take?

References

1 College of Occupational Therapists (1989) *Private Practice Directory*. COT, London.
2 College of Occupational Therapists (1989) *Guidelines for Occupational Therapists in Private Practice*, SPP 100. COT, London.
3 College of Occupational Therapists (1994) *Statement on Occupational Therapy in Private Practice*, SPP 100A. COT, London.
4 College of Occupational Therapists (2008) Specialist section – Independent practitioners (2008) *Code of Business Practice*. COT, London.
5 College of Occupational Therapists (2007) Management Briefing: Managing a budget briefing note no 91. COT, London.
6 Andreas Diamantis. Assessment methods used by OTs working with children in Independent Practice in the UK. Coventry University, MSc Thesis 2004.
7 College of Occupational Therapists (2003) *Professional Standards for Occupational Therapy Practice*. COT, London.
8 Occupational Therapists in Private Practice (2001) Business start-up information pack for new members. Contact via COT, London.
9 College of Occupational Therapists (2006) Management Briefing: Writing a business case Briefing note no 73. COT, London
10 *Holt and another v Payne Skillington (a firm) and another*, The Times, 22 December 1995.
11 College of Occupational Therapist (2009) Medical Legal Forum Standards for practice for expert witnesses. COT, London
12 Bristow Anna, Rugg Sue and Drew Julie (2008) The Occupational Therapists in Independent Practice National Telephone Enquiry Line: Who uses it, why and how? *British Journal of Occupational Therapy*, **71**(6), 234–40.
13 Diamantis Andreas D (2008) Use of Assesment methods in Paediatrics: The Practice of Private Occupational therapists. *British Journal of Occupational Therapy*, **71**(12), 524–30.

29 The Future

In July 2008, to link in with the 60th anniversary of the establishment of the NHS on 5 July 1948, the final report of Professor Lord Darzi, *High Quality of Care for All* on the future of the NHS was published.[1] It had been preceded by an interim report in October 2007 which set out the vision of an NHS which was fair, personalised, effective and safe and which outlined the immediate steps to be taken before the final report, which included the PCTs ensuring greater access to GP services at weekends and out of hours. The interim report was followed on 9 May 2008 by a review *Leading Local Change* in which 74 local clinical working groups had developed models of care for their regions. This document set out 5 pledges for the changes to the NHS:

- changes will always be to the benefit of patients
- change will be clinically driven
- all change will be locally-led
- patients, carers, the public and other key partners will be involved
- existing services will not be withdrawn until new and better services are available to patients so they can see the difference.

The final report was the culmination of extensive consultation and review with over 60,000 people participating including 2,000 clinicians, and other health and social care professionals from every NHS region in England. Its aim was to create an NHS that is focussed on helping people to stay healthy. The publication of the final report was preceded by an announcement that 150 large health centres, known as polyclinics were to be established which would be run by nurses. Nurses would be encouraged to set up not-for-profit firms to run the practises by being allowed to opt out of the NHS without losing pension rights.

The review saw the immediate steps as being:

Legal Aspects of Occupational Therapy, Third Edition By Bridgit Dimond
© 2010 Bridgit Dimond

a. Every primary care trust will commission comprehensive wellbeing and prevention services, in partnership with local authorities, with the services offered personalised to meet the specific needs of their local populations
b. A Coalition for Better Health, with a set of new voluntary agreements between the Government, private and third sector organisations on actions to improve health outcomes.
c. Raised awareness of vascular risk assessment through a new 'Reduce Your Risk' campaign
d. Support for people to stay healthy at work
e. Support for GPs to help individuals and their families stay healthy.

Patients were to be given more rights and control over their own health by:

- Extending choice of GP practice
- Introducing a new right to choice in a NHS Constitution
- Ensuring everyone with a long-term condition has a personalised care plan
- Piloting personal health budgets
- Guaranteeing patients access to the most clinically and cost-effective drugs and treatments

High quality care was to be at the centre of the NHS and to secure this the following measures will be taken:

- New enforcement powers for the Care Quality Commission
- Independent quality standards and clinical priority setting
- Systematic publications on quality of care including reports from patients and quality accounts to be provided by law by all registered healthcare providers
- Funding to reflect quality of care that patients receive
- Strengthen clinical excellence awards scheme for doctors
- Easy access for NHS staff to information about high quality care
- Measures to ensure continuous improvement in the quality of primary and community care
- New best practice tariffs focused on areas for improvement

Other measures were to be taken to strengthen the involvement of clinicians in decision making in the NHS including the appointment of medical directors and quality boards at regional and national level.

A new Quality Observatory was to be established in every region of the NHS to inform local quality improvement efforts. Innovation and advances in the NHS are to be encouraged: SHAs would have a new legal duty to promote innovation; with new funds and prizes being made available; clinically and cost-effective innovation in medicines and medical technologies was to be encouraged with new partnerships between the NHS, universities and industry.

Frontline staff were to be empowered with re-invigorated practice based commissioning, encouragement of social enterprise organisations and easy transfer of NHS staff with protected pension rights; improvements in the quality of NHS education and training; a three-fold increase in investment in nurse and midwife preceptorships and doubling investment in apprenticeships for healthcare support staff.

The NHS constitution

The Darzi report included, in a draft format, an NHS constitution[2] which can be seen in Appendix 2 of this book in its finalised format. The constitution sets out the 7 key principles which guide the NHS; the rights and responsibilities of patients, the rights and responsibilities of staff and the values underpinning the NHS. It thus attempts to consolidate all the existing legal rights of patients, staff and public in one document and to set down some pledges such as:

> The NHS will strive to provide all staff with personal development, access to appropriate training for their jobs, and line management support to succeed. (pledge)

The NHS Constitution is to be accompanied by a statement of accountability. All organisations providing NHS services will be obliged by law to take account of the Constitution and its principles and values in their decisions and actions.

One danger resulting from a constitution is the possibility of increasing litigation within the NHS. Most of the rights of the patients are to be found in statute or common law (as this book shows). The rights of staff are also embodied in health and safety legislation and are terms of the contract of employment. However many of the pledges such as staff development set out above are not implied terms of the contract nor explicit statutory rights. Does a pledge mean that it is actionable in a court of law? Is there a danger that it could become smooth talk with no substance? The extent to which more laws can provide the answer to problems within the NHS is highly questionable.

Other criticisms of the report were that the new powers given to the Care Quality Commission and the amalgamation of the existing inspectorates in the new body were unnecessary and would not decrease costs nor lead to greater efficiency. It remains to be seen from the way in which the CQC functions whether this criticism is well founded.

It is inevitable that any major proposals for change within the NHS will lead to controversy and debate and the DH website published the reaction of the media. One major criticism from the chief executive of King's Fund health think tank who welcomed a new era where patients will be able to check on the quality of the services was that there were no estimates of how much all this would cost. The absence of financial costings was serious in view of the proposal that all patients would have access to the drugs approved by NICE. Nor was there any indication of just how the different the government expects the quality of health services to be in 5 or 10 years' time.

Nor was there any indication of the timescale within which the proposals will be implemented. The report proposed that quality service would be rewarded both to individual trusts and to individual staff, but there was no discussion of how low quality providers would be treated.

However the Darzi review does set out a strategy which can be used by health professionals to develop their own services according to established values and clear standards. For example it is planned that about 15 million clients with long-term conditions will have individual care plans. Occupational therapists should already have individual care plans for each of their clients and can ensure that they are developed on a multi-disciplinary basis including social services.

The implementation of the final Darzi proposals will constitute a significant development in the future.

The Health Act 2009 provides the statutory enactment of the Darzi proposals and the NHS review. The contents of the Act are set out in Figure 29.1 and the sections relating to the NHS Constitution are set out in Appendix 3 to this book.

Direct payments for healthcare

Included in the Health Act 2009 was provision for direct payments of healthcare to the patient or a person nominated by the patient with the patient's consent (new S12A of the NHS Act 2006 as added by section 11 of the Health Act 2009).

Figure 29.1   Health Act 2009.

PART 1
QUALITY AND DELIVERY OF NHS SERVICES IN ENGLAND

CHAPTER 1
NHS CONSTITUTION
  1   NHS Constitution
  2   Duty to have regard to NHS Constitution
  3   Availability and review of NHS Constitution
  4   Other revisions of NHS Constitution
  5   Availability, review and revision of Handbook
  6   Report on effect of NHS Constitution
  7   Regulations under section 3 or 4

CHAPTER 2
QUALITY ACCOUNTS
  8   Duty of providers to publish information
  9   Supplementary provision about the duty
10   Regulations under section 8

CHAPTER 3
DIRECT PAYMENTS
11   Direct payments for health care
12   Jurisdiction of Health Service Commissioner
13   Direct payments: minor and consequential amendments

CHAPTER 4
INNOVATION
14   Innovation prizes

PART 2
POWERS IN RELATION TO HEALTH BODIES

CHAPTER 1
POWERS IN RELATION TO FAILING NHS BODIES IN ENGLAND
De-authorisation of NHS foundation trusts
15   De-authorisation of NHS foundation trusts

Trust special administrators
16   Trust special administrators: NHS trusts and NHS foundation trusts
17   Trust special administrators: Primary Care Trusts

Consequential amendments
18   Trust special administrators: consequential amendments

CHAPTER 2
SUSPENSION
19   NHS and other health appointments: suspension

PART 3
MISCELLANEOUS
Tobacco
20   Prohibition of advertising: exclusion for specialist tobacconists
21   Prohibition of tobacco displays etc
22   Power to prohibit sales from vending machines
23   Power to prohibit sales from vending machines: Northern Ireland
24   Tobacco: minor and consequential amendments

continued

Figure 29.1   Continued.

Pharmaceutical services in England
25   Pharmaceutical needs assessments
26   New arrangements for entry to pharmaceutical list
27   Pharmaceutical lists: minor amendment
28   Breach of terms of arrangements: notices and penalties
29   LPS schemes: powers of Primary Care Trusts and Strategic Health Authorities

Pharmaceutical services in Wales
30   Pharmaceutical lists: minor amendment
31   Breach of terms of arrangements: notices and penalties
32   LPS schemes: powers of Local Health Boards

Private patient income
33   Private patient income of mental health foundation trusts

Optical appliances
34   Payments in respect of costs of optical appliances

Adult social care
35   Investigation of complaints about privately arranged or funded adult social care

Disclosure of information
36   Disclosure of information by Her Majesty's Revenue and Customs

PART 4
GENERAL
37   Power to make transitional and consequential provision etc
38   Repeals and revocations
39   Extent
40   Commencement
41   Short title
Schedule 1—Direct payments: minor and consequential amendments
Schedule 2—De-authorised NHS foundation trusts
Schedule 3—NHS and other health appointments: suspension
Part 1—Amendments of enactments
Part 2—Supplementary
Schedule 4—Tobacco: minor and consequential amendments
Schedule 5—Investigation of complaints about privately arranged or funded adult social care
Part 1—New Part 3A for the Local Government Act 1974
Part 2—Minor and consequential amendments
Schedule 6—Repeals and revocations

Personal budgets have been used in social care since the mid 1990's and include cash payments with which an individual can buy social care. Direct payments for healthcare will be tested in 2009 with a view to implementation across England in 2012. The statutory provisions are shown in Appendix 3.

Implications for OTs

It cannot be said with any certainty what will be the impact for the occupational therapist of the Darzi reforms and in particular the NHS Constitution and direct payments for healthcare. There may be the possibility that patients will be aware of their rights and confront the OT with impossible demands. Alternatively the patient may prefer to spend sums allocated for occupational therapy on alternative services and OTs might find the demand for their services diminishing. Whatever the changes, there is no doubt that the OT faces a challenging time. It is thus essential that the OT is aware of the law which applies to her practice, the rights of the patient and the point at which she needs to seek legal advice.

It is hoped that this third edition will continue to assist occupational therapists in developing their awareness of the legal context within which they practice and in meeting the many challenges to come.

References

1   Department of Health (2008) *High Quality of Care for All Cm 7432*. DH, London.
2   Available on the DH website with supporting documents; dh.gov.uk

Appendix 1
Articles of the European Convention on Human Rights

Section 1(3)

Human Rights Act 1998
SCHEDULE 1
The Articles

Part I
The Convention – Rights and Freedoms

Article 2
Right to life

1. Everyone's right to life shall be protected by law. No one shall be deprived of his life intentionally save in the execution of a sentence of a court following his conviction of a crime for which this penalty is provided by law.
2. Deprivation of life shall not be regarded as inflicted in contravention of this Article when it results from the use of force which is no more than absolutely necessary:
    (a)   in defence of any person from unlawful violence;
    (b)   in order to effect a lawful arrest or to prevent the escape of a person lawfully detained;
    (c)   in action lawfully taken for the purpose of quelling a riot or insurrection.

Article 3
Prohibition of torture

No one shall be subjected to torture or to inhuman or degrading treatment or punishment.

Article 4
Prohibition of slavery and forced labour

1. No one shall be held in slavery or servitude.
2. No one shall be required to perform forced or compulsory labour.
3. For the purpose of this Article the term 'forced or compulsory labour' shall not include:
   (a) any work required to be done in the ordinary course of detention imposed according to the provisions of Article 5 of this Convention or during conditional release from such detention;
   (b) any service of a military character or, in case of conscientious objectors in countries where they are recognised, service exacted instead of compulsory military service;
   (c) any service exacted in case of an emergency or calamity threatening the life or well-being of the community;
   (d) any work or service which forms part of normal civic obligations.

Article 5
Right to liberty and security

1. Everyone has the right to liberty and security of person. No one shall be deprived of his liberty save in the following cases and in accordance with a procedure prescribed by law:
   (a) the lawful detention of a person after conviction by a competent court;
   (b) the lawful arrest or detention of a person for non-compliance with the lawful order of a court or in order to secure the fulfilment of any obligation prescribed by law;
   (c) the lawful arrest or detention of a person effected for the purpose of bringing him before the competent legal authority on reasonable suspicion of having committed an offence or when it is reasonably considered necessary to prevent his committing an offence or fleeing after having done so;
   (d) the detention of a minor by lawful order for the purpose of educational supervision or his lawful detention for the purpose of bringing him before the competent legal authority;
   (e) the lawful detention of persons for the prevention of the spreading of infectious diseases, of persons of unsound mind alcoholics or drug addicts or vagrants;
   (f) the lawful arrest or detention of a person to prevent his effecting an unauthorised entry into the country or of a person against whom action is being taken with a view to deportation or extradition.
2. Everyone who is arrested shall be informed promptly, in a language which he understands, of the reasons for his arrest and of any charge against him.
3. Everyone arrested or detained in accordance with the provisions of paragraph 1(c) of this Article shall be brought promptly before a judge or other officer authorised by law to exercise judicial power and shall be entitled to trial within a reasonable time or to release pending trial. Release may be conditioned by guarantees to appear for trial.
4. Everyone who is deprived of his liberty by arrest or detention shall be entitled to take proceedings by which the lawfulness of his detention shall be decided speedily by a court and his release ordered if the detention is not lawful.
5. Everyone who has been the victim of arrest or detention in contravention of the provisions of this Article shall have an enforceable right to compensation.

Article 6
Right to a fair trial

1. In the determination of his civil rights and obligations or of any criminal charge against him, everyone is entitled to a fair and public hearing within a reasonable time by an independent and impartial tribunal established by law. Judgment shall be pronounced publicly but the press and public may be excluded from all or part of the trial in the interest of morals, public order or national security in a democratic society, where the interests of juveniles or the protection of the private life of the parties so require, or to the extent strictly necessary in the opinion of the court in special circumstances where publicity would prejudice the interests of justice.
2. Everyone charged with a criminal offence shall be presumed innocent until proved guilty according to law.
3. Everyone charged with a criminal offence has the following minimum rights:
    (a) to be informed promptly, in a language which he understands and in detail, of the nature and cause of the accusation against him;
    (b) to have adequate time and facilities for the preparation of his defence;
    (c) to defend himself in person or through legal assistance of his own choosing or, if he has not sufficient means to pay for legal assistance, to be given it free when the interests of justice so require;
    (d) to examine or have examined witnesses against him and to obtain the attendance and examination of witnesses on his behalf under the same conditions as witnesses against him;
    (e) to have the free assistance of an interpreter if he cannot understand or speak the language used in court.

Article 7
No punishment without law

1. No one shall be held guilty of any criminal offence on account of any act or omission which did not constitute a criminal offence under national or international law at the time when it was committed. Nor shall a heavier penalty be imposed than the one that was applicable at the time the criminal offence was committed.
2. This Article shall not prejudice the trial and punishment of any person for any act or omission which, at the time when it was committed, was criminal according to the general principles of law recognised by civilised nations.

Article 8
Right to respect for private and family life

1. Everyone has the right to respect for his private and family life, his home and his correspondence.
2. There shall be no interference by a public authority with the exercise of this right except such as is in accordance with the law and is necessary in a democratic society in the interests of national security, public safety or the economic wellbeing of the country, for the prevention of disorder or crime, for the protection of health or morals, or for the protection of the rights and freedoms of others.

Article 9
Freedom of thought, conscience and religion

1. Everyone has the right to freedom of thought, conscience and religion; this right includes freedom to change his religion or belief and freedom, either alone or in community with others and in public or private, to manifest his religion or belief, in worship, teaching, practice and observance.
2. Freedom to manifest one's religion or beliefs shall be subject only to such limitations as are prescribed by law and are necessary in a democratic society in the interests of public safety, for the protection of public order, health or morals, or for the protection of the rights and freedoms of others.

Article 10
Freedom of expression

1. Everyone has the right to freedom of expression. This right shall include freedom to hold opinions and to receive and impart information and ideas without interference by public authority and regardless of frontiers. This Article shall not prevent States from requiring the licensing of broadcasting, television or cinema enterprises.
2. The exercise of these freedoms, since it carries with it duties and responsibilities, may be subject to such formalities, conditions, restrictions or penalties as are prescribed by law and are necessary in a democratic society, in the interests of national security, territorial integrity or public safety, for the prevention of disorder or crime, for the protection of health or morals, for the protection of the reputation or rights of others, for preventing the disclosure of information received in confidence, or for maintaining the authority and impartiality of the judiciary.

Article 11
Freedom of assembly and association

1. Everyone has the right to freedom of peaceful assembly and to freedom of association with others, including the right to form and to join trade unions for the protection of his interests.
2. No restrictions shall be placed on the exercise of these rights other than such as are prescribed by law and are necessary in a democratic society in the interests of national security or public safety, for the prevention of disorder or crime, for the protection of health or morals or for the protection of the rights and freedoms of others. This Article shall not prevent the imposition of lawful restrictions on the exercise of these rights by members of the armed forces, of the police or of the administration of the State.

Article 12
Right to marry

Men and women of marriageable age have the right to marry and to found a family, according to the national laws governing the exercise of this right.

Article 14
Prohibition of discrimination

The enjoyment of the rights and freedoms set forth in this Convention shall be secured without discrimination on any ground such as sex, race, colour, language, religion, political or other opinion, national or social origin, association with a national minority, property, birth or other status.

Article 16
Restrictions on political activity of aliens

Nothing in Articles 10, 11 and 14 shall be regarded as preventing the High Contracting Parties from imposing restrictions on the political activity of aliens.

Article 17
Prohibition of abuse of rights

Nothing in this Convention may be interpreted as implying for any State, group or person any right to engage in any activity or perform any act aimed at the destruction of any of the rights and freedoms set forth herein or at their limitation to a greater extent than is provided for in the Convention.

Article 18
Limitation on use of restrictions on rights

The restrictions permitted under this Convention to the said rights and freedoms shall not be applied for any purpose other than those for which they have been prescribed.

Part II
The First Protocol

Article 1
Protection of property

Every natural or legal person is entitled to the peaceful enjoyment of his possessions. No one shall be deprived of his possessions except in the public interest and subject to the conditions provided for by law and by the general principles of international law.

The preceding provisions shall not, however, in any way impair the right of a State to enforce such laws as it deems necessary to control the use of property in accordance with the general interest or to secure the payment of taxes or other contributions or penalties.

Article 2
Right to education

No person shall be denied the right to education. In the exercise of any functions which it assumes in relation to education and to teaching, the State shall respect the right of parents to ensure such education and teaching in conformity with their own religious and philosophical convictions.

Article 3
Right to free elections

The High Contracting Parties undertake to hold free elections at reasonable intervals by secret ballot, under conditions which will ensure the free expression of the opinion of the people in the choice of the legislature.

Part III
The Sixth Protocol

Article 1
Abolition of the death penalty

The death penalty shall be abolished. No one shall be condemned to such penalty or executed.

Article 2
Death penalty in time of war

A State may make provision in its law for the death penalty in respect of acts committed in time of war or of imminent threat of war; such penalty shall be applied only in the instances laid down in the law and in accordance with its provisions. The State shall communicate to the Secretary General of the Council of Europe the relevant provisions of that law.

Appendix 2
NHS Constitution

The NHS belongs to the people.

It is there to improve our health and well-being, supporting us to keep mentally and physically well, to get better when we are ill and, when we cannot fully recover, to stay as well as we can to the end of our lives. It works at the limits of science – bringing the highest levels of human knowledge and skill to save lives and improve health. It touches our lives at times of basic human need, when care and compassion are what matter most.

The NHS is founded on a common set of principles and values that bind together the communities and people it serves – patients and public – and the staff who work for it.

This Constitution establishes the **principles** and **values** of the NHS in England. It sets out **rights** to which patients, public and staff are entitled, and **pledges** which the NHS is committed to achieve, together with **responsibilities** which the public, patients and staff owe to one another to ensure that the NHS operates fairly and effectively. All NHS bodies and private and third sector providers supplying NHS services will be required by law to take account of this Constitution in their decisions and actions.

The Constitution will be renewed every 10 years, with the involvement of the public, patients and staff. It will be accompanied by the Handbook to the NHS Constitution, to be renewed at least every three years, setting out current guidance on the rights, pledges, duties and responsibilities established by the Constitution. These requirements for renewal will be made legally binding. They will guarantee that the principles and values which underpin the NHS are subject to regular review and recommitment; and that any government which seeks to alter the principles or values of the NHS, or the rights, pledges, duties and responsibilities set out in this Constitution, will have to engage in a full and transparent debate with the public, patients and staff.

1. Principles that guide the NHS

Seven key principles guide the NHS in all it does. They are underpinned by core NHS values which have been derived from extensive discussions with staff, patients and the public. These values are set out at the back of this document.

1. **The NHS provides a comprehensive service, available to all** irrespective of gender, race, disability, age, sexual orientation, religion or belief. It has a duty to each and every individual that it serves and must respect their human rights. At the same time, it has a wider social duty to promote equality through the services it provides and to pay particular attention to groups or sections of society where improvements in health and life expectancy are not keeping pace with the rest of the population.

2. **Access to NHS services is based on clinical need, not an individual's ability to pay.** NHS services are free of charge, except in limited circumstances sanctioned by Parliament.

3. **The NHS aspires to the highest standards of excellence and professionalism** – in the provision of high-quality care that is safe, effective and focused on patient experience; in the planning and delivery of the clinical and other services it provides; in the people it employs and the education, training and development they receive; in the leadership and management of its organisations; and through its commitment to innovation and to the promotion and conduct of research to improve the current and future health and care of the population.

4. **NHS services must reflect the needs and preferences of patients, their families and their carers.** Patients, with their families and carers, where appropriate, will be involved in and consulted on all decisions about their care and treatment.

5. **The NHS works across organisational boundaries and in partnership with other organisations in the interest of patients, local communities and the wider population.** The NHS is an integrated system of organisations and services bound together by the principles and values now reflected in the Constitution. The NHS is committed to working jointly with local authorities and a wide range of other private, public and third sector organisations at national and local level to provide and deliver improvements in health and well-being.

6. **The NHS is committed to providing best value for taxpayers' money and the most effective, fair and sustainable use of finite resources.** Public funds for healthcare will be devoted solely to the benefit of the people that the NHS serves.

7. **The NHS is accountable to the public, communities and patients that it serves.** The NHS is a national service funded through national taxation, and it is the Government which sets the framework for the NHS and which is accountable to Parliament for its operation. However, most decisions in the NHS, especially those about the treatment of individuals and the detailed organisation of services, are rightly taken by the local NHS and by patients with their clinicians. The system of responsibility and accountability for taking decisions in the NHS should be transparent and clear to the public, patients and staff. The Government will ensure that there is always a clear and up-to-date statement of NHS accountability for this purpose.

2a.   Patients and the public – your rights and NHS pledges to you

Everyone who uses the NHS should understand what legal rights they have. For this reason, important legal rights are summarised in this Constitution and explained in more detail in the Handbook to the NHS Constitution, which also explains what you can do if you think you have not received what is rightfully yours. This summary does not alter the content of your legal rights.

The Constitution also contains pledges that the NHS is committed to achieve. Pledges go above and beyond legal rights. This means that pledges are not legally binding but represent a commitment by the NHS to provide high quality services.

Access to health services:

You have the right to receive NHS services free of charge, apart from certain limited exceptions sanctioned by Parliament.

You have the right to access NHS services. You will not be refused access on unreasonable grounds.

You have the right to expect your local NHS to assess the health requirements of the local community and to commission and put in place the services to meet those needs as considered necessary.

You have the right, in certain circumstances, to go to other European Economic Area countries or Switzerland for treatment which would be available to you through your NHS commissioner.

You have the right not to be unlawfully discriminated against in the provision of NHS services including on grounds of gender, race, religion or belief, sexual orientation, disability (including learning disability or mental illness) or age.[1]

The NHS also commits:

- to provide convenient, easy access to services within the waiting times set out in the Handbook to the NHS Constitution (pledge);
- to make decisions in a clear and transparent way, so that patients and the public can understand how services are planned and delivered (pledge); and
- to make the transition as smooth as possible when you are referred between services, and to include you in relevant discussions (pledge).

Quality of care and environment:

You have the right to be treated with a professional standard of care, by appropriately qualified and experienced staff, in a properly approved or registered organisation that meets required levels of safety and quality.[2]

You have the right to expect NHS organisations to monitor, and make efforts to improve, the quality of healthcare they commission or provide.

The NHS also commits:

- to ensure that services are provided in a clean and safe environment that is fit for purpose, based on national best practice (pledge); and
- to continuous improvement in the quality of services you receive, identifying and sharing best practice in quality of care and treatments (pledge).

Nationally approved treatments, drugs and programmes:

You have the right to drugs and treatments that have been recommended by NICE[3] for use in the NHS, if your doctor says they are clinically appropriate for you.

You have the right to expect local decisions on funding of other drugs and treatments to be made rationally following a proper consideration of the evidence. If the local NHS decides not to fund a drug or treatment you and your doctor feel would be right for you, they will explain that decision to you.

You have the right to receive the vaccinations that the Joint Committee on Vaccination and Immunisation recommends that you should receive under an NHS-provided national immunisation programme.

The NHS also commits:

- to provide screening programmes as recommended by the UK National Screening Committee (pledge).

Respect, consent and confidentiality:

You have the right to be treated with dignity and respect, in accordance with your human rights.

You have the right to accept or refuse treatment that is offered to you, and not to be given any physical examination or treatment unless you have given valid consent. If you do not have the capacity to do so, consent must be obtained from a person legally able to act on your behalf, or the treatment must be in your best interests.[4]

You have the right to be given information about your proposed treatment in advance, including any significant risks and any alternative treatments which may be available, and the risks involved in doing nothing.

You have the right to privacy and confidentiality and to expect the NHS to keep your confidential information safe and secure.

You have the right of access to your own health records. These will always be used to manage your treatment in your best interests.

The NHS also commits:

● to share with you any letters sent between clinicians about your care (pledge).

Informed choice:

You have the right to choose your GP practice, and to be accepted by that practice unless there are reasonable grounds to refuse, in which case you will be informed of those reasons.

You have the right to express a preference for using a particular doctor within your GP practice, and for the practice to try to comply.

You have the right to make choices about your NHS care and to information to support these choices. The options available to you will develop over time and depend on your individual needs. Details are set out in the Handbook to the NHS Constitution.

The NHS also commits:

● to inform you about the healthcare services available to you, locally and nationally (pledge); and

● to offer you easily accessible, reliable and relevant information to enable you to participate fully in your own healthcare decisions and to support you in making choices. This will include information on the quality of clinical services where there is robust and accurate information available (pledge).

Involvement in your healthcare and in the NHS:

You have the right to be involved in discussions and decisions about your healthcare, and to be given information to enable you to do this.

You have the right to be involved, directly or through representatives, in the planning of healthcare services, the development and consideration of proposals for changes in the way those services are provided, and in decisions to be made affecting the operation of those services.

The NHS also commits:

● to provide you with the information you need to influence and scrutinise the planning and delivery of NHS services (pledge); and

● to work in partnership with you, your family, carers and representatives (pledge).

Complaint and redress:

You have the right to have any complaint you make about NHS services dealt with efficiently and to have it properly investigated.

You have the right to know the outcome of any investigation into your complaint.

You have the right to take your complaint to the independent Health Service Ombudsman, if you are not satisfied with the way your complaint has been dealt with by the NHS.

You have the right to make a claim for judicial review if you think you have been directly affected by an unlawful act or decision of an NHS body.

You have the right to compensation where you have been harmed by negligent treatment.

The NHS also commits:

- to ensure you are treated with courtesy and you receive appropriate support throughout the handling of a complaint; and the fact that you have complained will not adversely affect your future treatment (pledge);
- when mistakes happen, to acknowledge them, apologise, explain what went wrong and put things right quickly and effectively (pledge); and
- to ensure that the organisation learns lessons from complaints and claims and uses these to improve NHS services (pledge).

2b.   Patients and the public – your responsibilities

The NHS belongs to all of us. There are things that we can all do for ourselves and for one another to help it work effectively, and to ensure resources are used responsibly:

You should recognise that you can make a significant contribution to your own, and your family's, good health and well-being, and take some personal responsibility for it.

You should register with a GP practice – the main point of access to NHS care.

You should treat NHS staff and other patients with respect and recognise that causing a nuisance or disturbance on NHS premises could result in prosecution.

You should provide accurate information about your health, condition and status.

You should keep appointments, or cancel within reasonable time. Receiving treatment within the maximum waiting times may be compromised unless you do.

You should follow the course of treatment which you have agreed, and talk to your clinician if you find this difficult.

You should participate in important public health programmes such as vaccination.

You should ensure that those closest to you are aware of your wishes about organ donation.

You should give feedback – both positive and negative – about the treatment and care you have received, including any adverse reactions you may have had.

3a.   Staff – your rights and NHS pledges to you

It is the commitment, professionalism and dedication of staff working for the benefit of the people the NHS serves which really make the difference. High quality care requires high quality workplaces, with commissioners and providers aiming to be employers of choice.

All staff should have rewarding and worthwhile jobs, with the freedom and confidence to act in the interest of patients. To do this, they need to be trusted and actively listened to. They must be treated with respect at work, have the tools, training and support to deliver care, and opportunities to develop and progress.

The Constitution applies to all staff, doing clinical or non-clinical NHS work, and their employers. It covers staff wherever they are working, whether in public, private or third sector organisations.

Staff have extensive **legal rights**, embodied in general employment and discrimination law. These are summarised in the Handbook to the NHS Constitution. In addition, individual contracts of employment contain terms and conditions giving staff further rights.

The rights are there to help ensure that staff:

- have a good working environment with flexible working opportunities, consistent with the needs of patients and with the way that people live their lives;
- have a fair pay and contract framework;
- can be involved and represented in the workplace;
- have healthy and safe working conditions and an environment free from harassment, bullying or violence;
- are treated fairly, equally and free from discrimination; and
- can raise an internal grievance and if necessary seek redress, where it is felt that a right has not been upheld.

In addition to these legal rights, there are a number of **pledges**, which the NHS is committed to achieve. Pledges go above and beyond your legal rights. This means that they are not legally binding but represent a commitment by the NHS to provide high-quality working environments for staff.

The NHS commits:

- to provide all staff with clear roles and responsibilities and rewarding jobs for teams and individuals that make a difference to patients, their families and carers and communities (pledge);
- to provide all staff with personal development, access to appropriate training for their jobs and line management support to succeed (pledge);
- to provide support and opportunities for staff to maintain their health, well-being and safety (pledge); and
- to engage staff in decisions that affect them and the services they provide, individually, through representative organisations and through local partnership working arrangements. All staff will be empowered to put forward ways to deliver better and safer services for patients and their families (pledge).

3b.   Staff – your responsibilities

All staff have responsibilities to the public, their patients and colleagues.

Important legal duties are summarised below.

You have a duty to accept professional accountability and maintain the standards of professional practice as set by the appropriate regulatory body applicable to your profession or role.

You have a duty to take reasonable care of health and safety at work for you, your team and others, and to co-operate with employers to ensure compliance with health and safety requirements.

You have a duty to act in accordance with the express and implied terms of your contract of employment.

You have a duty not to discriminate against patients or staff and to adhere to equal opportunities and equality and human rights legislation.

You have a duty to protect the confidentiality of personal information that you hold unless to do so would put anyone at risk of significant harm.

You have a duty to be honest and truthful in applying for a job and in carrying out that job.

The Constitution also includes **expectations** that reflect how staff should play their part in ensuring the success of the NHS and delivering high-quality care.

You should aim:

- to maintain the highest standards of care and service, taking responsibility not only for the care you personally provide, but also for your wider contribution to the aims of your team and the NHS as a whole;
- to take up training and development opportunities provided over and above those legally required of your post;
- to play your part in sustainably improving services by working in partnership with patients, the public and communities;
- to be open with patients, their families, carers or representatives, including if anything goes wrong; welcoming and listening to feedback and addressing concerns promptly and in a spirit of co-operation. You should contribute to a climate where the truth can be heard and the reporting of, and learning from, errors is encouraged; and
- to view the services you provide from the standpoint of a patient, and involve patients, their families and carers in the services you provide, working with them, their communities and other organisations, and making it clear who is responsible for their care.

NHS values

Patients, public and staff have helped develop this expression of values that inspire passion in the NHS and should guide it in the 21st century. Individual organisations will develop and refresh their own values, tailored to their local needs. The NHS values provide common ground for co operation to achieve shared aspirations.

Respect and dignity. We value each person as an individual, respect their aspirations and commitments in life, and seek to understand their priorities, needs, abilities and limits. We take what others have to say seriously. We are honest about our point of view and what we can and cannot do.

Commitment to quality of care. We earn the trust placed in us by insisting on quality and striving to get the basics right every time: safety, confidentiality, professional and managerial integrity, accountability, dependable service and good communication. We welcome feedback, learn from our mistakes and build on our successes.

Compassion. We respond with humanity and kindness to each person's pain, distress, anxiety or need. We search for the things we can do, however small, to give comfort and relieve suffering. We find time for those we serve and work alongside. We do not wait to be asked, because we care.

Improving lives. We strive to improve health and well-being and people's experiences of the NHS. We value excellence and professionalism wherever we find it – in the everyday things that make people's lives better as much as in clinical practice, service improvements and innovation.

Working together for patients. We put patients first in everything we do, by reaching out to staff, patients, carers, families, communities, and professionals outside the NHS. We put the needs of patients and communities before organisational boundaries.

Everyone counts. We use our resources for the benefit of the whole community, and make sure nobody is excluded or left behind. We accept that some people need more help, that difficult decisions have to be taken – and that when we waste resources we waste others' opportunities. We recognise that we all have a part to play in making ourselves and our communities healthier.

References

1   The Government intends to use the Equality Bill to make unjustifiable age discrimination against adults unlawful in the provision of services and exercise of public functions. Subject to Parliamentary approval, this right not to be discriminated against will extend to age when the relevant provisions are brought into force for the health sector.

2   The registration system will apply to some NHS providers in respect of infection control from 2009, and more broadly from 2010. Further detail is set out in the Handbook to the NHS Constitution.

3   NICE (the National Institute for Health and Clinical Excellence) is an independent NHS organisation producing guidance on drugs and treatments. 'Recommended' means recommended by a NICE technology appraisal. Primary care trusts are normally obliged to fund NICE technology appraisals from a date no later than three months from the publication of the appraisal.

4   If you are detained in hospital or on supervised community treatment under the Mental Health Act 1983 different rules may apply to treatment for your mental disorder. These rules will be explained to you at the time. They may mean that you can be given treatment for your mental disorder even though you do not consent.

(Produced by the Department of Health. © Crown Copyright 2009.)

Appendix 3
Sections 1–6 of the Health Act 2009 and section 11 introducing provisions for Direct Payments for health care into the NHS Act 2006

1 NHS Constitution

(1) In this Chapter the "NHS Constitution" means—
    (a) the document entitled "The NHS Constitution" published by the Secretary of State on 21 January 2009, or
    (b) any revised version of that document published under section 4.
(2) In this Chapter the "Handbook" means—
    (a) the document entitled "The Handbook to the NHS Constitution" published by the Secretary of State on 21 January 2009, or
    (b) any revised version of that document published under section 5.

2 Duty to have regard to NHS Constitution

(1) Each of the bodies listed in subsection (2) must, in performing its NHS functions, have regard to the NHS Constitution.
(2) The bodies are—
    (a) Strategic Health Authorities;
    (b) Primary Care Trusts;
    (c) National Health Service trusts;
    (d) Special Health Authorities;
    (e) NHS foundation trusts;
    (f) the Independent Regulator of NHS Foundation Trusts;
    (g) the Care Quality Commission.
(3) In subsection (1) an "NHS function" means any function under an enactment which is a function concerned with, or connected to, the provision, commissioning or regulation of NHS services.
(4) Each person who—

(a)   provides NHS services under a contract, agreement or arrangements made under or by virtue of an enactment listed in subsection (6), or

(b)   provides or assists in providing NHS services under arrangements under section 12(1) of the National Health Service Act 2006 (c. 41), must, in doing so, have regard to the NHS Constitution.

(5)   Each person who—

(a)   in pursuance of a contract, agreement or arrangements as mentioned in subsection (4)(a) or (b), makes arrangements ("sub-contracting arrangements") for another person to provide or assist in providing NHS services, or

(b)   provides or assists in providing NHS services under sub-contracting arrangements, must, in doing so, have regard to the NHS Constitution.

(6)   The enactments referred to in subsection (4)(a) are the following provisions of the National Health Service Act 2006—

(a)   section 83(2)(b) (arrangements made by PCTs for provision of primary medical services);

(b)   section 84(1) (general medical services contracts);

(c)   section 92 (other arrangements for the provision of primary medical services);

(d)   section 100(1) (general dental services contracts);

(e)   section 107(1) (other arrangements for the provision of primary dental services);

(f)   section 117(1) (general ophthalmic services contracts);

(g)   section 126(1) (pharmaceutical services);

(h)   section 127(1) (additional pharmaceutical services);

(i)   Schedule 12 (local pharmaceutical services schemes).

(7)   In this Chapter "NHS services" means health services provided in England for the purposes of the health service continued under section 1(1) of the National Health Service Act 2006 (c. 41).

(8)   References in this section to the provision of services include references to the provision of services jointly with another person.

3   Availability and review of NHS Constitution

(1)   The Secretary of State must ensure that the NHS Constitution continues to be available to patients, staff and members of the public.

(2)   At least once in any period of 10 years the Secretary of State must carry out a review of the NHS Constitution (a "10 year review").

(3)   The following must be consulted about the NHS Constitution on a 10 year review—

(a)   patients and bodies or other persons representing patients,

(b)   staff and bodies or other persons representing staff,

(c)   carers,

(d)   local authorities,

(e)   members of the public,

(f)   the bodies and persons listed in section 2(2), (4) and (5), and

(g)   such other persons as the Secretary of State considers appropriate.

(4)   The first 10 year review must be completed not later than 5 July 2018.

(5)   The guiding principles may not be revised as a result of a 10 year review, except in accordance with regulations made by the Secretary of State setting out the revision to be made.

(6)   The Secretary of State must publish the NHS Constitution after any revision made as a result of a 10 year review.

(7)   In this Chapter—
"carers" means persons who, as relatives or friends, care for other persons to whom NHS services are being provided;
"the guiding principles" means—
(a)   the 7 principles described in the NHS Constitution published on 21 January 2009 as "the principles that guide the NHS", or
(b)   any revised version of those principles set out in the NHS Constitution published under this section or section 4;
"patients" means persons to whom NHS services are being provided;
"staff" means—
(a)   persons employed by a body listed in section 2(2) or otherwise working for such a body (whether as or on behalf of a contractor, as a volunteer or otherwise) in, or in connection with, the provision, commissioning or regulation of NHS services;
(b)   persons employed by a person listed in subsection (4) or (5) of section 2 or otherwise working for such a person (whether as or on behalf of a contractor, as a volunteer or otherwise) in, or in connection with, the provision of NHS services or assistance or the making of arrangements as mentioned in the subsection in question.
(8)   For the purposes of subsection (3), each of the following is a local authority—
(a)   a county council in England;
(b)   a district council in England, other than a council for a district in a county for which there is a county council;
(c)   a London borough council;
(d)   the Common Council of the City of London;
(e)   the Council of the Isles of Scilly.

4   Other revisions of NHS Constitution

(1)   This section applies to any revision of the NHS Constitution made other than as a result of a 10 year review (including any such revision which revises the guiding principles).
(2)   Before any revision the Secretary of State must undertake appropriate consultation about the proposed revision.
(3)   The persons consulted must include such patients, staff, members of the public and other persons as appear to the Secretary of State to be affected by the proposed revision.
(4)   The guiding principles may not be revised, except in accordance with regulations made by the Secretary of State setting out the revision to be made.
(5)   The Secretary of State must publish the NHS Constitution after any revision.

5   Availability, review and revision of Handbook

(1)   The Secretary of State must ensure that the Handbook continues to be available to patients, staff and members of the public.
(2)   At least once in any period of 3 years the Secretary of State must carry out a review of the Handbook.
(3)   The first review must be completed not later than 5 July 2012.
(4)   The Secretary of State must publish the Handbook after any revision.

6   Report on effect of NHS Constitution

(1)   The Secretary of State must publish a report every 3 years on how the NHS Constitution has affected patients, staff, carers and members of the public, since the last report was produced under this subsection.

(2)   The first report must be published not later than 5 July 2012.

(3)   The Secretary of State must lay before Parliament a copy of each report under subsection (1).

11   Direct payments for health care

In Part 1 of the National Health Service Act 2006 (c. 41), after section 12 insert—

"Direct payments for health care

12A   Direct payments for health care

(1)   The Secretary of State may, for the purpose of securing the provision to a patient of anything to which this subsection applies, make payments, with the patient's consent, to the patient or to a person nominated by the patient.

(2)   Subsection (1) applies to—

    (a)   anything that the Secretary of State may or must provide under section 2(1) or 3(1);

    (b)   anything for which the Secretary of State must arrange under paragraph 8 of Schedule 1;

    (c)   vehicles that the Secretary of State may provide under paragraph 9 of that Schedule.

(3)   Subsection (1) is subject to any provision made by regulations under section 12B.

(4)   If regulations so provide, a Primary Care Trust may, for the purpose of securing the provision for a patient of services that the trust must provide under section 117 of the Mental Health Act 1983 (after-care), make payments, with the patient's consent, to the patient or to a person nominated by the patient.

(5)   A payment under subsection (1) or under regulations under subsection (4) is referred to in this Part as a "direct payment".

(6)   A direct payment may be made only in accordance with a pilot scheme under regulations made by virtue of section 12C.

12B   Regulations about direct payments

(1)   The Secretary of State may make regulations about direct payments.

(2)   The regulations may in particular make provision—

    (a)   as to circumstances in which, and descriptions of persons and services in respect of which, direct payments may or must be made;

    (b)   as to circumstances in which direct payments may or must be made to a person nominated by the patient;

    (c)   as to the making of direct payments (and, in particular, as to persons to whom payments may or must be made) where the patient lacks capacity to consent to the making of the payments;

(d)   as to conditions that the Secretary of State or the Primary Care Trust must comply with before, after or at the time of making a direct payment;

(e)   as to conditions that the patient or (if different) the payee may or must be required to comply with before, after, or at the time when a direct payment is made;

(f)   as to the amount of any direct payment or how it is to be calculated;

(g)   as to circumstances in which the Secretary of State or the Primary Care Trust may or must stop making direct payments;

(h)   as to circumstances in which the Secretary of State or the Primary Care Trust may or must require all or part of a direct payment to be repaid, by the payee or otherwise;

(i)   as to monitoring of the making of direct payments, of their use by the payee, or of services which they are used to secure.

(j)   as to arrangements to be made by the Secretary of State or the Primary Care Trust for providing patients, payees or their representatives with information, advice or other support in connection with direct payments;

(k)   for such support to be treated to any prescribed extent as a service in respect of which direct payments may be made.

(3)   If the regulations make provision in the case of a person who lacks capacity to consent to direct payments being made, they may apply that provision, or make corresponding provision, with or without modifications, in the case of a person who has lacked that capacity but no longer does so (whether because of fluctuating capacity, or regaining or gaining capacity).

(4)   The regulations may provide for a sum which must be repaid to the Secretary of State or the Primary Care Trust by virtue of a condition or other requirement imposed by or under the regulations to be recoverable as a debt due to the Secretary of State or the Primary Care Trust.

(5)   The regulations may make provision—

(a)   for a service in respect of which a direct payment has been made under section 12A(1) to be regarded, only to such extent and subject to such conditions as may be prescribed, as provided or arranged for by the Secretary of State under an enactment mentioned in section 12A(2);

(b)   displacing functions or obligations of a Primary Care Trust with respect to the provision of after-care services under section 117 of the Mental Health Act 1983, only to such extent and subject to such conditions as may be prescribed.

(6)   In this section—

(a)   "service" includes anything in respect of which direct payments may be made;

(b)   references to a person lacking capacity are references to a person lacking capacity within the meaning of the Mental Capacity Act 2005.

12C   Direct payments pilot schemes

(1)   Regulations under section 12B may provide for the Secretary of State to have power—

(a)   to make pilot schemes in accordance with which direct payments may be made;

(b)   to include in a pilot scheme, as respects payments to which the scheme applies, any provision within section 12B(2), subject to any provision made by the regulations.

(2)   The regulations may in particular make provision, or provide for the pilot scheme to make provision, as to—

(a)   the geographical area in which a pilot scheme operates;

(b)   the revocation or amendment of a pilot scheme.

(3)   A pilot scheme must, in accordance with the regulations, specify the period for which it has effect, subject to the extension of that period by the Secretary of State in accordance with the regulations.

(4)   The regulations must make provision as to the review of a pilot scheme, or require the pilot scheme to include such provision.

(5)   Provision as to the review of a pilot scheme may in particular include provision—
    (a)   for a review to be carried out by an independent person;
    (b)   for publication of the findings of a review;
    (c)   as to matters to be considered on a review.

(6)   Those matters may in particular include any of the following—
    (a)   the administration of the scheme;
    (b)   the effect of direct payments on the cost or quality of care received by patients;
    (c)   the effect of direct payments on the behaviour of patients, carers or persons providing services in respect of which direct payments are made.

(7)   After any review of one or more pilot schemes, the Secretary of State may make an order under subsection (8) or (10).

(8)   An order under this subsection is an order making provision for either or both of the following—
    (a)   repealing section 12A(6) and subsections (1) to (4) of this section;
    (b)   amending, repealing, or otherwise modifying any other provision of this Act.

(9)   An order may make provision within subsection (6)(b) only if it appears to the Secretary of State to be necessary or expedient for the purpose of facilitating the exercise of the powers conferred by section 12A(1) or by regulations under section 12A(4).

(10)   An order under this subsection is an order repealing sections 12A, 12B, 12D and this section.

12D   Arrangements with other bodies relating to direct payments

(1)   The Secretary of State may arrange with any person or body to give assistance in connection with direct payments.

(2)   Arrangements may be made under subsection (1) with voluntary organisations.

(3)   Powers under this section may be exercised on such terms as may be agreed, including terms as to the making of payments by the Secretary of State."

Glossary

acceptance an agreement to the terms of an offer which leads to a binding legal obligation, i.e. a *contract*.

accusatorial a system of court proceedings where the two sides contest the issue (contrast with *inquisitorial*)

Act of Parliament, *statute*

action legal proceedings

actionable per se A court action where the claimant does not have to show loss, *damage* or harm to obtain compensation, e.g. an action for *trespass to the person*.

actus reus the essential element of a crime which must be proved to secure a conviction, as opposed to the mental state of the accused (*mens rea*)

adversarial the approach adopted in an accusatorial system

advocate a person who pleads for another: could be paid and professional, such as a *barrister or solicitor*, or could be a lay advocate either paid or unpaid; a witness is not an advocate

affidavit a statement given under oath

alternative dispute resolution methods to resolve a dispute without going to court, such as mediation

approved social worker a social worker qualified for the purposes of the Mental Health Act

arrestable offence an offence defined in section 24 of the Police and Criminal Evidence Act 1984 which gives to the citizen the power of arrest in certain circumstances without a warrant

assault a threat of unlawful contact (see *trespass to the person*)

balance of probabilities the standard of proof in *civil* proceedings

barrister a lawyer qualified to take a case in court

battery an unlawful touching (see *trespass to the person*)

bench the *magistrates*, Justice of the Peace

Bolam test The test laid down by Judge McNair in the case of *Bolam v. Friern HMC* on the standard of care expected of a professional in cases of alleged *negligence*

burden of proof the duty of a party to litigation to establish the facts, or in criminal proceedings the duty of the prosecution to establish both the *actus reus* and the *mens rea* of the alleged offence

cause of action   the facts that entitle a person to sue

certiorari   an action taken to challenge an administrative or judicial decision (literally: to make more certain)

civil action   proceedings brought in the civil courts

civil wrong   an act or omission which can be pursued in the civil courts by the person who has suffered the wrong (see *torts*)

claimant   the person bringing a civil action (originally *plaintiff*)

committal proceedings   hearings before the magistrates to decide if a person should be sent for *trial* in the crown court

common law   law derived from the decisions of judges, case law, judge made law.

conditional fee system   a system whereby client and lawyer can agree that payment of fees is dependent upon the outcome of the court action; also known as 'no win, no fee'

conditions   terms of a *contract* (see *warranties*)

constructive dismissal   when an employer is in fundamental breach of the contract of employment, the employee can elect to see this as ending the contract and therefore a constructive dismissal situation, and claim for unfair dismissal. Alternatively, the employee can elect to see the contract as continuing and seek compensation

constructive knowledge   knowledge which can be obtained from the circumstances

continuous service   the length of service which an employee must have served to be entitled to receive certain statutory or contractual rights

contract   an agreement enforceable in law

contract for services   an agreement, enforceable in law, whereby one party provides services, not being employment, in return for payment or other consideration from the other party

contract of service   a contract for employment

contributory negligence   when a claimant makes an allegation of negligence, the defendant can allege that the complainant was (partly) to blame for the harm which the complainant has suffered. If this allegation is accepted, the judge can reduce the amount payable in compensation to the claimant according to the extent of the claimant's fault

coroner   a person appointed to hold an inquiry (inquest) into a death in unexpected or unusual circumstances

counter-offer   a response to an offer which suggests different terms and is therefore counted as an offer not an acceptance

cross-examination   questions asked of a witness by the lawyer for the opposing side; leading questions can be asked

criminal wrong   an act or omission which can be pursued in the criminal courts

damages   a sum of money awarded by a court as compensation for a tort or breach of contract

declaration   a ruling by the court, setting out the legal situation

disclosure   documents made available to the other party

dissenting judgment   A judge who disagrees with the decision of the majority of judges

distinguished (of cases)   the rules of precedent require judges to follow decisions of judges in previous cases, where these are binding upon them. However, in some circumstances it is possible to come to a different decision because the facts of the earlier case are not comparable to the case now being heard, and therefore the earlier decision can be 'distinguished'

examination in chief   The witness is asked questions in court by the lawyer of the party who has asked the witness to attend; leading questions cannot be asked

ex gratia   as a matter of favour, e.g. without admission of *liability*, of payment offered to a claimant

expert witness   evidence given by a person whose general opinion based on training or experience is relevant to some of the issues in dispute (contrast with *witness of fact*)

ex turpi causa non oritur actio   no right of action derives from a base cause

frustration (of contracts)   the ending of a contract by operation of law, because of the existence of an event not contemplated by the parties when they made the contract, e.g. imprisonment, death, blindness

Re F **ruling**   a professional who acts in the best interests of an incompetent person who is incapable of giving consent, does not act unlawfully if he follows the accepted standard of care according to the *Bolam test.*

guardian *ad litem*   a person with a social work and child care background who is appointed to ensure that the court is fully informed of the relevant facts which relate to a child and that the wishes and feelings of the child are clearly established. The appointment is made from a panel set up by the local authority

guilty   a finding in a criminal court of responsibility for a criminal offence

hearsay   evidence which has been learnt from another person

hierarchy   the recognised status of courts which results in lower courts following the decisions of higher courts (see *precedent*). Thus decisions of the House of Lords must be followed by all lower courts unless they can be *distinguished*

indictment   a written accusation against a person, charging him with a serious crime, triable by jury

informal   of a patient who has entered hospital without any statutory requirements

injunction   an order of the court restraining a person

inquisitorial   a system of justice whereby the truth is revealed by an inquiry into the facts conducted by the judge, e.g. coroner's court

invitation to treat   the early stages in negotiating a contract, e.g. an advertisement, or letter expressing interest. An invitation to treat will often precede an offer which, when accepted, leads to the formation of an agreement which, if there is consideration and an intention to create legal relations, will be binding

judicial review   an application to the High Court for a judicial or administrative decision to be reviewed and an appropriate order made, e.g. declaration

Justice of the Peace (JP)   a lay *magistrate*, i.e. not legally qualified, who hears summary (minor) offences and sometimes indictable (serious) offences in the magistrates court in a group of three (*bench*)

liable/liability   responsible for the wrong doing or harm in civil proceedings

litigation   civil proceedings

magistrate   a person (see *JP* and *stipendiary*) who hears summary (minor) offences or indictable offences which can be heard in the magistrates court

mens rea   the mental element in a crime (contrasted with *actus reus*)

negligence   a civil action for compensation, also a failure to follow a reasonable standard of care

next friend   a person who brings a court action on behalf of a minor

offer   a proposal made by a party which if accepted can lead to a contract. It often follows an *invitation to treat*

ombudsman   a commissioner (e.g. health, Local Government) appointed by the Government to hear complaints

payment into court   an offer to settle a dispute at a particular sum, which is paid into court. The claimant's failure to accept the offer means that the claimant is liable to pay costs, if the final award is the same or less than the payment made

pedagogic   of the science of teaching

plaintiff   term formerly used to describe one who brings an action in the civil courts. Now the term *claimant* is used

plea in mitigation   a formal statement to the court aimed at reducing the sentence to be pronounced by the judge

practice direction   guidance issued by the head of the court to which it relates, on the procedure to be followed

pre-action protocol   Rules of the Supreme Court provide guidance on action to be taken before legal proceedings commence

precedent   a decision which may have to be followed in a subsequent court hearing (see *hierarchy*)

prima facie   at first sight, or sufficient evidence brought by one party to require the other party to provide a defence

privilege   in relation to evidence, being able to refuse to disclose it to the court

privity   the relationship which exists between parties as the result of a legal agreement

professional misconduct   conduct of a registered health practitioner which could lead to conduct and competence proceedings by the registration body

proof   evidence which secures the establishment of a claimant's or prosecution's or defendant's case

prosecution   the pursuing of criminal offences in court

quantum   the amount of compensation, or the monetary value of a claim

Queen's Counsel (QC)   a senior barrister, also known as a 'silk'

reasonable doubt   to secure a conviction in criminal proceedings the prosecution must establish 'beyond reasonable doubt' the guilt of the accused

rescission   where a contract is ended by the order of a court, or by the cancellation of the contract by one party entitled in law to do so

solicitor   a lawyer who is qualified on the register held by the Law Society

statute law (statutory)   law made by Acts of Parliament

stipendiary magistrate   a legally qualified magistrate who is paid (i.e. has a stipend)

strict liability   liability for a criminal act where the mental element does not have to be proved; in civil proceedings liability without establishing *negligence*

subpoena   an order of the court requiring a person to appear as a witness (*subpoena ad testificandum*) or to bring records/documents (*subpoena duces tecum*)

summary offence   a lesser offence which can only be heard by *magistrates*

summary judgment   a procedure whereby the claimant can obtain judgment without the defendant being permitted to defend the action

tort   a civil wrong excluding breach of contract. It includes: *negligence, trespass* (*to the person*, goods or land), nuisance, breach of statutory duty and defamation

trespass to the person   a wrongful direct interference with another person. Harm does not have to be proved

trial   a court hearing before a judge

ultra vires   outside the powers given by law (e.g. of a statutory body or company)

vicarious liability   the liability of an employer for the wrongful acts of an employee committed while in the course of employment

volenti non fit injuria   to the willing there is no wrong; the voluntary assumption of risk.

ward of court   a minor placed under the protection of the High Court, which assumes responsibility for him or her, and all decisions relating to his or her care must be made in accordance with the directions of the court

warranties   terms of a contract which are considered to be less important than the terms described as conditions: breach of a condition entitles the innocent party to see the contract as ended, i.e. repudiated by the other party (breach of warranties entitles the innocent party to claim damages)

Wednesbury principle   the court will intervene to prevent or remedy abuses of power by public authorities if there is evidence of unreasonableness or perversity. Principle laid down by the Court of Appeal in the case of *Associated Provincial Picture House Ltd* v. *Wednesbury Corporation*

without prejudice   without detracting from or without disadvantage to. The use of the phrase prevents the other party using the information to the prejudice of the one providing it

witness of fact   a person who gives evidence of what they saw, heard, did or failed to do (contrast with *expert witness*)

writ   a form of written command, e.g. the document which used to commence civil proceedings. Now a claim form is served

Further Reading

Appelbe, G.E. & Wingfield, J. (eds) (2001) *Dale and Appelbe's Pharmacy: Law and Ethics*, 7th edn, The Pharmaceutical Press, London.

Andrew, A. & Hunter, C. (2003) *Manual of Housing Law*, 7th edn. Sweet and Maxwell, London.

Beauchamp, T.L. & Childres, J.F. (1989) *Principles of Biomedical Ethics*, 3rd edn. Oxford University Press, Oxford.

Benn Piers (1998 reprinted 2005) *Ethics*. Routledge, Oxford.

Blom-Cooper, L. et al. (1996) *The Case of Jason Mitchell: Report of the Independent Panel of Inquiry*. Duckworth, London.

Blom-Cooper, L., Hally, H. & Murphy, E. (1996) *The Falling Shadow – One patient's mental health care 1978–1993* (Report of an Inquiry into the death of an occupational therapist at Edith Morgan Unit, Torbay 1993). Duckworth, London.

Brazier, M. (1992) *Medicine, Patients and the Law*. Penguin, London.

Brazier, M. & Murphy, J. (ed.) (1999) *Street on Torts*. Butterworth, London.

British Medical Association (1998) *Medical Ethics Today*. BMJ Publishing, London.

Campbell, A.V. (1984) *Moral Dilemmas in Medicine*. Churchill Livingstone, Edinburgh.

Card, R. (1998) *Cross and Jones' Criminal Law*, 14th edn. Butterworth, London.

Carey Peter (2004) *Data Protection: a Practical Guide to UK and EU Law*, 2nd edn. Oxford University Press, Oxford.

Carson David and Bain Andy (2008) *Professional Risk and Working with People: Decision making in health, social care and criminal justice*. Jessica Kingsley Publishers, London.

Clements, L. (2000) *Community Care and the Law*, 2nd edn. Legal Action Group, London.

Committee of Experts Advisory Group on AIDS (1994) *Guidance for health care worker's protection against infection with HIV and Hepatitis*. HMSO, London.

Cooper, J. & Vernon, S. (1996) *Disability and the Law*. Jessica Kingsley Publishers, London.

Cooper, J. (ed.) (2000) *Law, Rights and Disability*. Jessica Kingsley Publishers, London.

Creek, J. & Loughes, L. (eds) (2008) *Occupational Therapy and Mental Health*, 4th edn. Churchill Livingstone, Edinburgh.

Department of Education and Employment (2001) *Towards Inclusion – Civil rights for disabled people*. DfEE.

Department of Health (1993) *AIDS/HIV Infected Health Care Workers*.

Denis, I.H. (1999) *The Law of Evidence*. Sweet and Maxwell, London.

Dimond, B.C. (1999) *Patients' Rights, Responsibilities and the Nurse*, 2nd edn. Central Health Studies, Quay Publishing, Dinton, Salisbury.

Dimond, B.C. (2003) *Legal Aspects of Consent*. Quay Publications, Mark Allen Press, Dinton, Salisbury.

Dimond, B.C. (2010) *Legal Aspects of Patient Confidentiality*, 2nd edn. Quay Publications, Mark Allen Press, Dinton, Salisbury.

Dimond, B.C. (2010) *Legal Aspects of Pain Management*, 2nd edn. Quay Publications, Mark Allen Press, Dinton, Salisbury.

Dimond, B.C. (1996) *Legal Aspects of Child Health Care*. Mosby, London.

Dimond, B.C. (2005) *Legal Aspects of Midwifery*, 3rd edn. Books for Midwives Press, Cheshire.

Dimond, B.C. & Barker, F. (1996) *Mental Health Law for Nurses*. Blackwell Science, Oxford.

Dimond, B.C. (1997) *Legal Aspects of Care in the Community*. Macmillans Press, London.

Dimond, B.C. (1998) *Legal Aspects of Complementary Therapy Practice*. Churchill Livingstone, Edinburgh.

Dimond, B.C. (2009) *Legal Aspects of Physiotherapy*, 2nd edn. Blackwell Science, Oxford.

Dimond, B.C. (2010) *Legal Aspects of Nursing*, 6th edn. Pearson Education, London.

Dimond, B.C. (1997) *Mental Health (Patients in the Community) Act 1995: An introductory text*. Mark Allen Publications, London.

Doyle, B.J. (1996) *Disability Discrimination: the New Law*. Jordans, Bristol.

Ellis, N. (1994) *Employing Staff*, 5th edn. British Medical Journal, London.

Faulder, C. (1985) *Whose Body Is It?* Virago, London.

Finch, J. (ed.) (1994) *Speller's Law Relating to Hospitals*, 7th edn. Chapman and Hall Medical, London.

Fletcher, N. & Holt, J. (1995) *Ethics law and nursing*. Manchester University Press, Manchester.

Gann, R. (1993) *The NHS A to Z*, 2nd edn. The help for Health Trust, Winchester.

Gibson Caroline, Joanna Grice Rebecca James and Shona Mulholland (2001) *The Children Act Explained*. The Stationery Office London.

Glover, J. (1984) *Causing Death and Saving Lives*, Penguin, London.

Glover, J. (1984) *What Sort of People Should There Be?* Penguin, London.

Grainger, I. & Fealy, M. with Spencer M. (2000) *Civil Procedure Rules in Action*, 2nd edn. Cavendish Publishers, London.

Ham, C. (1991) *The New National Health Service*. NAHAT.

Harris, P. (1997) *An Introduction to Law*, 5th edn. Butterworths, London.

Health and Safety Commission (1999) *Management of Health and Safety at work Regulations Approved code of practice*. HMSO, London.

Health and Safety Commission (1992) *Manual Handling Regulations and approved code of practice*. HMSO, London.

Health and Safety Commission (1992) *Guidelines on Manual Handling in the Health Services*. HMSO, London.

Hepple, B.A. & Matthews, M.H. (1991) *Tort Cases and Materials*, 4th edn. Butterworths, London.

Heywood, F. (2001) *Money well spent: the effectiveness and value of housing adaptations*. The Policy Press, Bristol, for Joseph Rowntree Foundation.

Hoggett, B. (2002) *Mental Health Law*, 4th edn. Sweet and Maxwell, London.

Howells, G. & Weatherill, S. (1995) *Consumer Protection Law*. Dartmouth Publishing, Aldershot.

Hunt, G. & Wainright, P. (eds), *Expanding the Role of the Nurse*. Blackwell Publishing, Oxford.

Hurwitz, B. (1998) *Clinical Guidelines and the Law*. Radcliffe Medical Press, Oxford.

Ingman, T. (1996) *The English Legal Process*, 6th edn. Blackstone Publishing, London.

Jay, R. & Hamilton, A. (1999) *Data Protection Law and Practice*. Sweet and Maxwell, London.

Jones, M. (2003) *Medical Negligence*, 3rd edn. Sweet and Maxwell, London.

Jones, R. (2003) *Mental Health Act Manual*, 8th edn. Sweet and Maxwell, London.

Keenan, D. (1992) *Smith and Keenan's English Law*, 10th edn. Pitman Publishing, London.

Kennedy, I. & Grubb, A. (2000) *Medical Law*, 3rd edn. Butterworth, London.

Kennedy, T. (1998) *Learning European Law*. Sweet and Maxwell, London.

Kidner, R. (1993) *Blackstone's Statutes on Employment Law*, 3rd edn. Blackstone Press, London.

Kloss, D. (2000) *Occupational Health Law*, 3rd edn. Blackwell Publishing, Oxford.

Knight, B. (1992) *Legal Aspects of Medical Practice*, 5th edn. Churchill Livingstone, Edinburgh.

Leathard Audrey and McLaren Susan eds. (2007) *Ethics: Contemporary Challenges in Health and Social Care*. The Policy Press Bristol.

Lee, R.G. & Morgan, D. (2001) *Human Fertilisation and Embryology Act 1990*. Blackstone Press, London.

Leigh-Pollit Piers and Mullock James (2001) *The Data Protection Act explained*, 3rd edn. The Stationery Office, London.

Mandelstam, M. (1998) *An A-Z of Community Care Law*. Jessican Kingsley Publishers, London.

Mandelstam, M. (2009) *Community Care Practice and the Law*, 4th edn. Jessica Kingsley, London.

Mandelstam, M. (1997) *Equipment for Older or Disabled People and the Law*. Jessica Kingsley, London.

Markesinis, B.S. & Deakin, S.F. (1999) *Tort Law*, 4th edn. Clarendon Press, Oxford.

Mason, D. & Edwards, P. (1993) *Litigation: A Risk Management Guide for Midwives*. Royal College of Midwives, London.

Mason, J.K. & McCall-Smith, A. (1999) *Law and Medical Ethics*, 5th edn. Butterworths, London.

McHale, J. & Fox, M. with Murphy, J. (1997) *Health Care Law*. Sweet and Maxwell, London.

McHale, J. & Tingle, J. (2001) *Law and Nursing*. Butterworth Heineman, London.

Metzer, A. & Weinberg J. (1998) *Criminal Litigation*. Legal Action Group, London.

Miers, D. & Page, A. (1990) *Legislation*, 2nd edn. Sweet and Maxwell, London.

Montgomery, J. (2003) *Health Care Law*, 2nd edn. Oxford University Press, Oxford.

National Association of Theatre Nurses (1993) *The Role of the Nurse as First Assistant in the Operating Department*. NATN, Harrogate.

Oliver Paul (2003) *The Student's Guide to Research Ethics*. Open University Press Maidenhead.

Pearse, P. et al. (1988) *Personal Data Protection in Health and Social Services*. Croom Helm, London.

Pitt, G. (2000) *Employment Law*, 4th edn. Sweet and Maxwell, London.

Pyne, R.H. (1991) *Professional Discipline in Nursing, Midwifery and Health Visiting*, 2nd edn. Blackwell Publishing, Oxford.

Read Janet and Clements Luke (2002) *Disabled Children and the Law*. Jessica Kingsley, London.

Richards, P. (1999) *Law on Contract*. Financial Times and Pitman Publishing, London.

Royal College of Nursing (1992) *Focus on Restraint*, 2nd edn. RCN, London.

Rowson, R. (1990) *An Introduction to Ethics for Nurses*. Scutari Press, London.

Rumbold, G. (1993) *Ethics in Nursing Practice*, 2nd edn. Baillière Tindall, London.

Salvage, J. (1988) *Nurses at Risk: Guide to Health and Safety at Work*. Heinemann, London.

Salvage, J. & Rogers, R. (1988) *Health and Safety and the Nurse*. Heinemann, London.

Saunders, P. (1989) *The A-Z of Disability Directory of Information, Services, Organisations, Equipment and Manufacturers*. The Crowood Press, Ramsay, Marlborough.

Seedhouse David (2003) *Ethics: The Heart of Health Care*. Wiley, Chichester.

Sellars, C. (2002) *Risk Assessment with People with Learning Disabilities*. Blackwell Publishing, Oxford.

Selwyn, N. (2000) *Selwyn's Law of Employment*, 11th edn. Butterworth, London.

Selwyn, N. (1982) *Selwyn's Law of Safety at Work*, Butterworth, London.

Slapper, G. & Kelly, D. (2001) *The English Legal System*. Cavendish Publishing, London.

Sims, S. (2000) *Practical Approach to Civil Procedure*, 4th edn. Blackstone Press, London.

Skegg, P.D.G. (1998) *Law, Ethics and Medicine*, 2nd edn. Oxford University Press, Oxford.

Smith, K. & Keenan, D. (1992) *English Law*, 10th edn. Pitman, London.

Sim Julian (1997) *Ethical Decision Making in Therapy Practice*. Butterworth Heinemann, Oxford.

Social Security Inspectorate, Department of Health (1993) *No Longer Afraid: Safeguard of Older People in Domestic Settings*. HMSO, London.

Finch, J. (ed.) (1994) *Speller's Law Relating to Hospitals*, 7th edn. Chapman and Hall Medical, London.

Stauch, M., Wheat, K. & Tingle, J. (2002) *Source Book on Medical Law*, 2nd edn. Cavendish Publishing, London.

Steiner, J. (1992) *Textbook on EC Law*, 3rd edn. Blackstone Press, London.

Stone, J. & Matthews, J. (1996) *Complementary Medicine and the Law*. Oxford University Press, Oxford.

Taylor, M.C. (2000) *Evidence-based practice for Occupational Therapists*. Blackwell Publishing, Oxford.

Thompson, R. & Thompson, B. (1993) *Dismissal: A basic introduction to your legal rights*. Robin Thompson and Partners and Brian Thompson and Partners, London.

Thompson, R. & Thompson, B. (1993) *Equal Pay*. Robin Thompson and Partners and Brian Thompson and Partners, London.

Thompson, R. & Thompson, B. (1993) *Health and Safety at Work*. Robin Thompson and Partners and Brian Thompson and Partners, London.

Thompson, R. & Thompson, B. (1993) *Injuries at Work and Work-related Illnesses*. Robin Thompson and Partners and Brian Thompson and Partners, London.

Thompson, R. & Thompson, B. (1993) *Women at Work*. Robin Thompson and Partners and Brian Thompson and Partners, London.

Tingle, J. & Cribb, A. (eds.) (1995) *Nursing Law and Ethics*. Blackwell Publishing, Oxford.

Tolley's Health and Safety at Work Handbook, 15th edn, (2003) Tolley, Croydon.

Tschudin, V. & Marks-Maran, D. (1993) *Ethics: A Primer for Nurses*. Baillière Tindall, London.

Turner, A., Foster, M. & Johnson, S.E. (eds.) (2002) *Occupational Therapy and Physical Dysfunction*, 5th edn. Churchill Livingstone, Edinburgh.

Vincent, C. *et al.* (1993) *Medical Accidents*. Oxford University Press, Oxford.

Vincent, C. (ed.) (1995) *Clinical Risk Management*. BMJ, London.

Warnock Mary (2002) *An Intelligent Person's Guide to Ethics*. Duckworths, London.

Watt Helen (2000) *Life and Death in Healthcare Ethics – a short introduction*. Routledge, London.

Wheeler, J. (2002) *The English Legal System*. Pearson Education, Harlow.

White, R., Carr, P. & Lowe, N. (2002) *A Guide to the Children Act 1989*, 3rd edn. Butterworth, London.

Wilkinson, R. & Caulfield, H. (2000) *The Human Rights Act: a Practical Guide for Nurses*. Whurr Publishers, London.

Young, A.P. (1989) *Legal Problems in Nursing Practice*. Harper & Row, London.

Young, A.P. (1994) *Law and Professional Conduct in Nursing*, 2nd edn. Scutari Press, London.

Zander, M. (1995) *Police and Criminal Evidence Act*, 3rd ed. Sweet and Maxwell, London.

Useful Websites

Action for advocacy	www.actionforadvocacy.org
Action on Elder Abuse	www.elderabuse.org.uk
Advisory Conciliation and Arbitration Service	www.acas.org.uk
Age Concern	www.ageconcern.org.uk
Alert	www.donoharm.org.uk
Alzheimer's Research	www.Alzheimers-research.org.uk
Alzheimer's Society	www.alzheimers.org.uk
ASA Advice	www.advice.org.uk
Association of Contentious Trust and Probate Solicitors	www.actaps.com
Audit Commission	www.audit-commission.gov.uk
Bailii (case law resource)	www.bailii.org/ew/cases
CARERS UK	www.carersonline.org.uk
	www.carersuk.org
Care Quality Commission	www.cqc.org.uk
Care Services Improvement Partnership	www.csip.org.uk
Citizens Advice Bureaux	www.citizensadvice.org.uk
Citizen Advocacy Information and Training	www.citizenadvocacy.rg.uk
Civil Procedure Rules	www.open.gov.uk/lcd/civil/procrules_fin/crules.htm
Clinical Negligence Scheme for Trusts	www.nhsla.com/Claims/Schemes/CNST/
Equality and Human Rights Commission	www.equalityhumanrights.com
Commission for Racial Equality	www.cre.gov.uk/
Commission for Social Care and Inspection	www.csci.gov.uk
Community Legal Service Direct	www.clsdirect.org.uk
Complementary Healthcare Information Service	www.chisuk.org.uk
Contact the Elderly	www.contact-the-elderly.org

Convention on the International Protection of Adults	www.hcch.net/index_en.php
Council for Healthcare Regulatory Excellence	www.chre.org.uk
Commission for Patient and Public Involvement in Health	www.cppih.org/
Counsel and Care	www.counselandcare.org.uk
Court Funds Office	www.hmcourts-service.gov.uk/infoabout/cfo/index.htm
Court of Protection	via the Office of Public Guardian or HM Courts Services
Central Office for Research Ethics Committees	www.corec.org.uk
Dementia Care Trust	www.dct.org.uk
Department for Business Enterprise and Regulatory Reform	www.berr.gov.uk/employment
Department for Education and Skills	www.dfes.gov.uk
Department for Work and Pensions	www.dwp.gov.uk/
Department of Health	www.dh.gov.uk
Department of Trade and Industry	www.dti.gov.uk/
Disability Law Service	www.dls.org.uk/
Domestic Violence	www.domesticviolence.gov.uk
Down's Syndrome Association	ww.downs-syndrome.org.uk www.dsa-uk.com
Equality and Human Rights Commission	www.equalityhumanrights.com
Family Carer Support Service	www.familycarers.org.uk
Family Mediation Helpline	www.familymediationhelpline.co.uk
Foundation for People with Learning Disabilities	www.learningdisabilities.org.uk
General Medical Council	www.gmc-uk.org
Headway – brain injury Association	www.headway.org.uk
Health and Safety Commission	www.hsc.gov.uk
Health and Safety Executive	www.hse.gov.uk
Help the Aged	www.helptheagedorg.uk
Help the Hospices	www.hospiceinformation.info
Healthcare Commission	www.healthcarecommission.org.uk/
Health Professions Council	www.hpc-uk.org
HM Courts Service	www.hmcourts-service.gov.uk
Home Farm Trust	www.hft.org.uk
Human Fertilisation and Embryology Authority	www.hfea.gov.uk/
Human Genetics Commission	www.hgc.gov.uk
Human Rights	www.humanrights.gov.uk
Independent Mental Capacity Advocate	www.dh.gov.uk.imca
Information Commissioner's Office	www.ico.gov.uk
Independent Safeguarding Authority	www.isa-gov.org.uk
Law Centres Federation	www.lawcentres.org.uk
Law Society	www.lawsociety.org.uk/
Legal cases (England and Wales)	www.bailli.org/ew/cases
Legislation	www.opsi.gov.uk/legislation or
Linacre Centre for Healthcare Ethics	www.linacre.org

Making Decisions Alliance	www.makingdecisions.org.uk
Manic Depression Fellowship	www.mdf.org.uk
MedicAlert Foundation	www.medicalert.org.uk
Medicines and Healthcare Products Regulatory Agency	www.mhra.gov.uk
MENCAP	www.mencap.org.uk
Mental Capacity Implementation Programme	www.dca.go.uk/legal-policy/mental-capacity/index.htm
Mental Health Act Commission	www.mhac.org.uk/
Mental Health Foundation	www.mentalhealth.org.uk
Mental Health Lawyers Assoc	www.mhla.co.uk
Mental Health Matters	www.mentalhealthmatters.com/
Mind	www.mind.org.uk
Ministry of Justice	www.justice.gov.uk
Motor Neurone Disease Association	www.mndassociation.org.uk
National Audit Office	www.nao.gov.uk
National Autistic Society	www.nas.org.uk;www.autism.org.uk
National Care Association	www.nca.gb.com
National Family Carer Network	www.familycarers.org.uk
National Health Service Litigation Authority	www.nhsla.com
National Information and Governance Board for Health and Social Care	www.nigb.nhs.uk
National Mediation Helpline,	www.nationalmediationhelpline.com
National Patient Safety Agency	www.npsa.gov.uk
National Perinatal Epidemiology Unit	www.npeu.ox.ac.uk/
National Treatment Agency	www.nta.nhs.uk/
NHS website	www.nhs.uk
NHS Direct	www.nhsdirect.nhs.uk
NHS Institute for Innovation and Improvement	www.institute.nhs.uk/
NHS Professionals	www.nhsprofessionals.nhs.uk
NICE	www.nice.org.uk
Nursing and Midwifery Council	www.nmc-uk.org/
Office of Public Guardian	www.guardianship.gov.uk
Office of Public Sector Information	www.opsi.gov.uk
Official Solicitor	www.officialsolicitor.gov.uk
Open Government	www.open.gov.uk
Pain website	www.pain-talk.co.uk
Patient's Association	www.patients-association.org.uk
Patient Concern	www.patientconcern.org.uk
People First	www.peoplefirst.org.uk
Prevention of Professional Abuse Network	www.popan.org.uk
Princess Royal Trust for Carers	www.carers.org/
Relatives and Residents Association	www.releres.org/
RESCARE (The National Society for mentally disabled people in residential care)	www.rescare.org.uk
Respond	www.respond.org.uk

Rethink (formerly the National Schizophrenia Fellowship)	www.rethink.org
Royal College of Nursing	www.rcn.org.uk
Royal College of Psychiatrists	www.rcpsych.ac.uk
SANE	www.sane.org.uk
Scope	www.scope.org.uk
Sense	www.sense.org.uk
Solicitors for the Elderly	www.solicitorsfortheelderly.com
Speaking Up	www.speakingup.org/
Speakability	www.speakability.org.uk
Shipman Inquiry	www.the-shipman-inquiry.org.uk/reports.asp
Solicitors for the Elderly	www.solicitorsfortheelderly.com
Stroke Association	www.stroke.org.uk
Together: Working for Wellbeing	www.together-uk.org
Turning Point	www.turning-point.co.uk
UK Homecare Association	www.ukhca.co.uk
UK Parliament	www.parliament.uk
United Response	www.unitedresponse.org.uk
Values into Action	www.viauk.org
Veterans Agency	www.veteransagency.org.uk
VOICE UK	www.voiceuk.clara.net
Voluntary Euthanasia Society	www.ves.org.uk
Welsh Assembly Government	www.wales.gov.uk
World Medical Association	www.wma.net/e/policy/b3.htm

Table of Cases

Table of Statutes

Index

Keep up with critical fields

Would you like to receive up-to-date information on our books, journals and databases in the areas that interest you, direct to your mailbox?

Join the **Wiley e-mail service** - a convenient way to receive updates and exclusive discount offers on products from us.

Simply visit **www.wiley.com/email** and register online

We won't bombard you with emails and we'll only email you with information that's relevant to you. We will ALWAYS respect your e-mail privacy and NEVER sell, rent, or exchange your e-mail address to any outside company. Full details on our privacy policy can be found online.

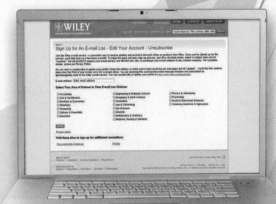

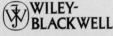